D0918988

ASPERGER SYNDROME

Also from James C. McPartland, Ami Klin, and Fred R. Volkmar

FOR PROFESSIONALS

**Autism Spectrum Disorders in Infants and Toddlers:
Diagnosis, Assessment, and Treatment**
*Edited by Katarzyna Chawarska,
Ami Klin, and Fred R. Volkmar*

FOR GENERAL READERS

**A Parent's Guide to High-Functioning Autism Spectrum Disorder, Second Edition:
How to Meet the Challenges and Help Your Child Thrive**
*Sally Ozonoff, Geraldine Dawson,
and James C. McPartland*

ASPERGER SYNDROME

Assessing and Treating
High-Functioning Autism Spectrum Disorders

SECOND EDITION

Edited by
James C. McPartland
Ami Klin
Fred R. Volkmar

Foreword by Maria Asperger Felder

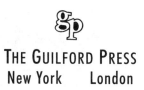

THE GUILFORD PRESS
New York   London

© 2014 The Guilford Press
A Division of Guilford Publications, Inc.
72 Spring Street, New York, NY 10012
www.guilford.com

Printed in the United States of America

This book is printed on acid-free paper.

Last digit is print number: 9 8 7 6 5 4 3 2 1

The authors have checked with sources believed to be reliable in their
efforts to provide information that is complete and generally in accord with
the standards of practice that are accepted at the time of publication. However, in view of the possibility of human error or changes in behavioral,
mental health, or medical sciences, neither the authors, nor the editors and
publisher, nor any other party who has been involved in the preparation or
publication of this work warrants that the information contained herein is
in every respect accurate or complete, and they are not responsible for any
errors or omissions or the results obtained from the use of such information. Readers are encouraged to confirm the information contained in this
book with other sources.

Library of Congress Cataloging-in-Publication Data

Asperger syndrome : assessing and treating high-functioning autism
    spectrum disorders / edited by James C. McPartland, Ami Klin,
    Fred R. Volkmar ; foreword by Maria Asperger Felder. — Second edition.
        pages cm.
    Includes bibliographical references and index.
    ISBN 978-1-4625-1414-4 (hardback : acid-free paper)
    1. Asperger's syndrome. I. McPartland, James C., editor of
compilation. II. Klin, Ami, editor of compilation. III. Volkmar,
Fred R, editor of compilation.
RC553.A88A788 2014
616.85′883200835—dc23
                                                            2008021106

To the memory of our colleague
Dr. Sara S. Sparrow—teacher, mentor, and friend

About the Editors

James C. McPartland, PhD, is Assistant Professor, Director of the Developmental Disabilities Clinic, and Associate Director of the Developmental Electrophysiology Laboratory at the Yale Child Study Center, Yale University School of Medicine. Dr. McPartland's research focuses on the clinical neuroscience of autism spectrum disorders from infancy through adulthood. He is a recipient of honors including the Behavioral Science Track Award for Rapid Transition and a Patient-Oriented Research Career Development Award from the National Institute of Mental Health, the NARSAD Atherton Young Investigator Award, the Young Investigator Award from the International Society for Autism Research, and the Klerman Prize for Exceptional Achievement in Clinical Research from the Brain and Behavior Research Foundation.

Ami Klin, PhD, is Director of the Marcus Autism Center at Children's Healthcare of Atlanta and Professor and Chief of the Division of Autism and Related Disabilities at Emory University School of Medicine. He is also a Georgia Research Alliance Eminent Scholar and a faculty member at Emory's Center for Translational Social Neuroscience. He formerly was Professor at the Yale Child Study Center, where he directed the Autism Program. Dr. Klin's research focuses on the social development and well-being of individuals with autism spectrum disorders from infancy through adulthood. He directs the National Institutes of Health Autism Center of Excellence at the Marcus Autism Center and Emory University, which includes genetic, social, and behavioral neuroscience studies in human infants and in model systems.

Fred R. Volkmar, MD, is Irving B. Harris Professor of Child Psychiatry, Pediatrics, and Psychology and Director of the Yale Child Study Center at the Yale University School of Medicine. He is also Chief of Child Psychiatry at Yale–New Haven Hospital. Dr. Volkmar was the primary author of the American Psychiatric Association's DSM-IV autism and pervasive developmental disorders section. He is the author of several hundred scientific papers and chapters as well as a number of books, and serves as Editor of the *Journal of Autism and Developmental Disorders*.

Contributors

Tony Attwood, PhD, Minds and Hearts, West End, Queensland, Australia

Jane Thierfeld Brown, EdD, University of Connecticut School of Law, Hartford, Connecticut

Jonathan M. Campbell, PhD, Department of Educational, School, and Counseling Psychology, University of Kentucky, Lexington, Kentucky

Yu-Chi Chou, PhD, Special Education Department, University of Kansas, Lawrence, Kansas

Susan E. Folstein, MD, Department of Psychiatry, Miller School of Medicine, University of Miami, Miami, Florida

Caitlin M. Hudac, PhD, Developmental Brain Laboratory, University of Nebraska–Lincoln, Lincoln, Nebraska

Carrah L. James, PhD, private practice, Spokane, Washington

Ami Klin, PhD, Marcus Autism Center, Children's Healthcare of Atlanta, and Emory University School of Medicine, Atlanta, Georgia

Dana Kober, MD, Department of Pediatric Medicine, Texas Children's Hospital, Baylor College of Medicine, Houston, Texas

Rebecca Landa, PhD, Kennedy Krieger Institute, Baltimore, Maryland

Hyo Jung Lee, PhD, Department of Education, Dongguk University, Seoul, South Korea

James W. Loomis, PhD, Yale Child Study Center, Yale University School of Medicine, New Haven, Connecticut; and The Center for Children with Special Needs, Glastonbury, Connecticut

James C. McPartland, PhD, Yale Child Study Center, Yale University School of Medicine, New Haven, Connecticut

Brenda Smith Myles, PhD, Ziggurat Group, Columbus, Ohio

Rhea Paul, PhD, Department of Speech–Language Pathology, College of Health Professions, Sacred Heart University, Fairfield, Connecticut

Kevin A. Pelphrey, PhD, Yale Child Study Center, Yale University School of Medicine, New Haven, Connecticut

Michael D. Powers, PsyD, Yale Child Study Center, Yale University School of Medicine, New Haven, Connecticut; and The Center for Children with Special Needs, Glastonbury, Connecticut

Emily Rubin, MS, Marcus Autism Center, Atlanta, Georgia

Sarah Shultz, PhD, Marcus Autism Center, Atlanta, Georgia

Elizabeth Simmons, MS, Yale Autism Program, Yale University, New Haven, Connecticut

Sheila M. Smith, PhD, Ohio Center for Autism and Low Incidence, Columbus, Ohio

Kai-Chien Tien, PhD, Department of Special Education, National Changhua University of Education, Changhua, Taiwan

Katherine D. Tsatsanis, PhD, Yale Child Study Center, Yale University School of Medicine, New Haven, Connecticut

Brent C. Vander Wyk, PhD, Yale Child Study Center, Yale University School of Medicine, New Haven, Connecticut

Sarah F. Vess, PhD, Department of Special Education, High Point University, High Point, North Carolina

Fred R. Volkmar, MD, Yale Child Study Center, Yale University School of Medicine, New Haven Connecticut

Avery Voos, BA, The Gevirtz School, University of California at Santa Barbara, Santa Barbara, California

Alexander Westphal, MD, Yale Child Study Center, Yale University School of Medicine, New Haven, Connecticut

Marc Woodbury-Smith, MD, PhD, Department of Psychiatry and Behavioral Neurosciences, McMaster University, Hamilton, Ontario, Canada

Lorraine Wolf, PhD, Department of Psychiatry, Boston University School of Medicine, Boston, Massachusetts

Foreword

Hans Asperger used to love telling the story of his life; thus all I have to do is retell it. He was born in Vienna in 1906. His grandfather's family had been farmers east of the capital of the Austro-Hungarian Monarchy for many generations. As a high school student, he became acquainted with the "German Youth Movement." It was in this movement that this achievement-oriented and intellectual young man was to find all those things he valued most throughout his lifetime. There he discovered friendship, mountaineering, nature, art as a source of strength and repose, and literature—the medium in which he moved and lived.

In 1931 he graduated from medical school and started working for the Children's Hospital of the University of Vienna, the institution to which he devoted most of his working years. He remained a pediatrician at heart until the end of his life. However, his first publication (Siegl & Asperger, 1934) already showed that his primary interest was not in symptoms and treatment methods only but, rather, in the child who was suffering, his or her environment, and the interplay between constitutional and environmental factors. This approach to medicine and his work as the director of the Unit for Special Education ("Heilpädagogik") at the Children's Hospital led him to coin the term "autistic psychopathy," which he first used in the article "Das psychisch abnorme Kind" (Asperger, 1938). Despite the fact that notions of genetic hygiene or racial determinism severely undermined human values at the time, Hans Asperger favored unpredictability and the idea that development resulted from the interplay between genetic and environmental factors ("predisposition is not fate but rather a possible fate").

In 1944, Hans Asperger published his postgraduate thesis, "Die 'Autistischen Psychopathen' im Kindesalter" ("'Autistic Psychopathy' in

Childhood"), an excellent and comprehensive description of the children who deeply interested him. By describing the ways they expressed themselves, he tried to gain insight into their being, consciously refusing to impose any underlying system of explanation:

> The path [to understanding] necessarily begins with the individual himself . . . [it] looks for parallels between an outer region and an inner one, between physical constitution and emotional factors, motor activity, facial expression and gestures, between autonomic effects (that reflect emotions), between speech modulation and manner of speaking and character traits. (Asperger, 1944, p. 44)

Hans Asperger (1944) believed that this disorder was determined by genetic factors:

> In light of the homogeneity and the distinctiveness of this type of mentally disturbed children, the question of genetic determination necessarily must emerge. The question as to whether abnormal conditions are determined by constitution and are thus heritable has long been resolved. . . . Over the past 10 years, we have studied over 200 children who evidence a more or less severe autistic disorder. In the process we also got to know their parents and other relatives of theirs and found abnormal traits in their relatives.

During the war, Hans Asperger served as a medical officer in Croatia (1944–1945). After the war he returned to Vienna. In 1957 he became the director of the Children's Hospital of the University of Innsbruck and in 1963 he was named the director of the Children's Hospital of the University of Vienna. Although he kept abreast of the treatment of physical illnesses and the rapid developments in the field of medicine, children themselves and their emotions were his main interest. He tried to adopt an intuitive approach to understanding them rather than an intellectual one:

> A doctor . . . needs more than mere book knowledge; he needs not to have lost the ability to "look," which is a very holistic function of recognition and in which intuitive, instinctive, pre-intellectual skills play an important role. They lead us to the innermost regions of the child to be assessed because whatever a child expresses comes out of the innermost parts of him or herself. (Asperger, 1975, p. 8)

This is what he referred to as "medical art," a skill he considered to be important not only for physicians but also for all those working in the field of education, particularly special education. Thus, although the medical approach seemed to be particularly useful in diagnosing and understanding a child's personality and disorders, pedagogical methods were the first and foremost methods of treating them:

We believe that an exclusively medical approach to the treatment of mentally disturbed children, even psychiatric therapy, can only be effective to
a limited extent. Only pedagogical methods in the broadest sense of the
word can really change people to the better, or put more precisely, can
pinpoint the best of the developmental alternatives that are at a child's
disposal and make it possible for him or her to develop along these lines.
(Asperger, 1950, p. 105)

From 1949 onward, Hans Asperger published several articles comparing the disorder he had been describing with the one that Leo Kanner had
called "early infantile autism." He pointed out not only the characteristics
that both disorders had in common (impairment in social responsiveness
or interest in others, and serious communicative impairment) but also the
differences in personality structure and cognitive skills. Yet, despite their
common interests, Kanner and Hans Asperger were never to meet.

Hans Asperger was never to lose his lifelong interest in and his curiosity about all living creatures (*naturae curiosus*), which explained why
he was elected to the Academy of Nature Researchers in Halle. However,
what interested him was not conducting large studies as a method of gain-
ing insight into the meaning of things but, rather, the act of watching as
a means to gain insight into the underlying laws that govern life. That is
why the words spoken by Lynkeus, the tower watchman in Goethe's *Faust*,
meant a great deal to him and guided him:

> Born to see
> Called for to watch
> Pledged to the tower
> I like the world.

Hans Asperger died in Vienna in 1980, after a short illness. He was an
active, interested, and committed person until the very end.

MARIA ASPERGER FELDER, MD
Child and Adolescent Psychiatrist/Psychotherapist
Zurich, Switzerland

REFERENCES

Asperger, H. (1938). Das psychisch abnorme Kinde. *Wiener Klinische Wochenschrift, 51,*
    1314–1317.
Asperger, H. (1944). Die "Autistischen Psychopathen" im Kindesalter. *Archiv für Psychiatrie
    und Nervenkrankheiten, 117,* 76–136.
Asperger, H. (1950). Die medizinischen Grundlagen der Heilpädagogik. *Monatsschrift für
    Kinderheilkunde, 99*(3), 105–115.
Asperger, H. (1975). Erlebte Heilpädagogik. In H. Asperger (Ed.), *Heilpädagogik Gegen-
    wart und Zukunft.* Berlin: Springer.
Siegl, J., & Asperger, H. (1934). Zur Behandlung der Enuresis. *Archiv für Kinderheilkunde,
    102,* 88–102.

Contents

CHAPTER 1

Asperger Syndrome

An Overview

Fred R. Volkmar
Ami Klin
James C. McPartland

Asperger syndrome (AS) is a serious and chronic neurodevelopmental disorder characterized by significant and severe social deficits along with restricted interests, as in autism, but, in contrast to autism, relatively and selectively preserved language and cognitive abilities. As presented in Table 1.1, formal diagnostic criteria for AS in the text revision of the fourth edition of the *Diagnostic and Statistical Manual of Mental Disorders* (DSM-IV-TR; American Psychiatric Association, 2000) and the 10th edition of the *International Classification of Diseases* (ICD-10; World Health Organization, 1993; see Table 1.1) ruled out individuals who meet criteria for autistic disorder. The fifth and most recent edition of the DSM (DSM-5; American Psychiatric Association, 2013) eliminated AS as an official diagnosis, collapsing it into a presumably broader category of autism spectrum disorder (ASD). In the following chapters, discussion of AS refers to the disorder as defined by the most recent DSM-IV-TR and ICD-10 criteria. Clearly, the absence of an official diagnostic category does not render the information contained herein less relevant to the many individuals who have carried a diagnosis of AS, as well as to the many families, support groups, and advocacy organizations associated with AS.

TABLE 1.1. ICD-10 Research Diagnostic Guidelines for Asperger Syndrome

1. There is no clinically significant general delay in spoken or receptive language or cognitive development. Diagnosis requires that single words should have developed by 2 years of age or earlier and that communicative phrases be used by 3 years of age or earlier. Self-help skills, adaptive behavior, and curiosity about the environment during the first 3 years should be at a level consistent with normal intellectual development. However, motor milestones may be somewhat delayed and motor clumsiness is usual (although not a necessary diagnostic feature). Isolated special skills, often related to abnormal preoccupations, are common but are not required for the diagnosis.

2. There are qualitative abnormalities in reciprocal social interaction (criteria for autism).

3. The individual exhibits an unusual intense, circumscribed interest or restricted, repetitive, and stereotyped patterns of behavior interests and activities (criteria for autism; however, it would be less usual for these to include either motor mannerisms or preoccupations with part-objects or nonfunctional elements of play materials).

4. The disorder is not attributable to other varieties of pervasive developmental disorder; simple schizophrenia, schizotypal disorder, obsessive–compulsive disorder, anakastic personality disorder, reactive and disinhibited attachment disorders of childhood.

Note. From World Health Organization (1993, pp. 153–154). Copyright 1993 by the World Health Organization. Reprinted by permission.

Narrative text in both the DSM-IV-TR (American Psychiatric Association, 2000) and ICD-10 (World Health Organization, 1993) noted that motor awkwardness and/or clumsiness are common and that, in contrast to autism, the restricted interests observed often take the form of unusual, intense, and highly circumscribed interest(s). Although not explicitly discussed, implication of diagnostic criteria was that generally the onset of AS (or at least its recognition) was usually after age 3. Before that, age problems in social interaction, communication, and responses to the environment must not be of the type seen in autism or must not be accompanied by the characteristic behavioral features of autism (see Kamp-Becker et al., 2010, for a recent study suggesting several areas of differences in the onset of the conditions).

Although described the year after autism (Kanner, 1943), the body of research on AS is much less extensive than that for autism; nevertheless, research has advanced markedly since official recognition (about 75 papers between 1944 and 1994, but over 1,800 papers from 1994 to 2010). During the 1970s and 1980s considerable progress occurred in the attempt to provide better definitions of autism, and it was on this body of work that DSM-IV-TR criteria rested. The official definition of autism was revised twice in the 14 years separating DSM-III (American Psychiatric Association, 1980) from DSM-IV (American Psychiatric Association, 1994), and even when it appeared in DSM-III for the first time, a considerable body of work on diagnosis and definition of autism had accumulated. Its subsequent revision illustrates the importance of a deliberate, data-based approach to the problem. In this chapter we review the history of the diagnostic concept of AS; the rationale for, and limitations of, the extant diagnostic approaches; the validity of the concept; current controversies in diagnosis; with a final summary and recommendations for the future.

EVOLUTION OF THE CONCEPT: 1944–1994

The most recent definitions of AS evolved Asperger's original (1944) description of the condition he termed *autistic psychopathy* or *autistic personality disorder*.[1] This evolution has not been straightforward. As with autism, modifications in Asperger's description were proposed, initially by Wing (1981) and subsequently by many others (Klin & Volkmar, 2003; Klin, Pauls, Schultz, & Volkmar, 2005). Some of these changes moved the concept away from the one originally envisioned by Asperger, who regarded the condition as quite separate from autism and one that was, in many ways, more a personality than a developmental disorder (Asperger, 1979). Partly because of its ambiguous diagnostic status, markedly divergent views of the condition developed. Sometimes these alternative views are of only minimal interest from the perspective of nomenclature, but in other cases they are more critical. For example, the convention of viewing AS a synonymous term for adults with autism is of little interest, in that such a convention simply reifies an existing diagnostic concept around an important but nonessential characteristic (in this case, age). Similarly, the convention of equating AS with either pervasive developmental disorder not otherwise specified (PDD-NOS) or higher-functioning autism (HFA) has little importance from the point of view of nomenclature, since it simply substitutes one term for another (Volkmar & Tsatsanis, 2005). The much more critical question is whether AS differs in some important way or ways from autism, PDD-NOS, and other conditions in terms of its natural history, course and outcome, family history or genetic involvement, neuropsychological profiles, and important associated features, relative to implications for treatment and intervention, and so forth. These differences must be truly "external" ones, avoiding circularity of reasoning or of research strategy in that differences, if found, must reflect factors independent of original diagnostic assignment (Volkmar, Chawarska, Carter, & Lord, 2007; Rutter, 2011). Put another way, the issues are (1) whether AS can be separated from autism and other conditions in a reliable and empirical fashion, and, if so, (2) whether this discrimination has meaningful importance (e.g., for research or clinical work). Practical issues involved in diagnostic practice

---

[1]Note that, as is true of autism, it is likely that cases with what now would be viewed as AS were seen even before Asperger's 1944 work; see Wolff (1996, 2004).

associated with AS have not yet fully benefited from recent improvements in diagnostic instrumentation seen in autism (see Campbell, James, & Vess, Chapter 2, this volume) although more rating scales are now available.

Finally, another set of complicating issues has arisen because several alternative concepts have been proposed that share at least some fundamental similarity with AS; semantic–pragmatic disorder, right-hemisphere learning disability, nonverbal learning disability, and schizoid disorder are some of these alternative concepts (Klin, McPartland, & Volkmar, 2005). All involve some degree of impairment in complex social skills. These concepts have their own histories of development and emerge from diverse disciplines. Before considering the uses and limitations of current official diagnostic approaches to AS, we therefore consider the various alternatives to definition of the condition that have arisen over the years, as well as the potential overlap between AS and these alternative diagnostic concepts. Given the centrality of Asperger's report, it is appropriate to begin with a discussion of his views of the concept before moving to alternative views and the centrally important role of Wing's (1981) paper in the evolution of the diagnostic concstruct.

ASPERGER'S REPORT: 1944

In 1944, Hans Asperger, a medical student, reported four cases (all boys) with marked difficulties in social interaction despite apparently adequate to excellent cognitive and verbal skills. In addition, these boys exhibited motor difficulties and unusual and intense circumscribed interests, and their fathers often exhibited similar problems. Asperger made the important point that these interests were so intense as to interfere with learning (i.e., were a source of impairment) and that family life often also centered around them.

At the time of Asperger's original (1944) work there was, of course, not the considerable interest in operational definitions that has characterized psychiatry so much since the 1970s (Klin, McPartland, et al., 2005; Spitzer, Endicott, & Robbins, 1978). As with Kanner (1943), Asperger provided a clinical account of what appeared to him to be a new syndrome. His description of this condition was inspired by his work with these boys, ages 6–11, who had marked problems in social interaction despite having what appeared to be good language and cognitive skills (see Frith, 1991, for an English translation). These four boys, however, were said to be representative of a much larger sample of children presenting with the profile described. In addition to the *problems in social interaction*, which Asperger emphasized by the use of the word *autism* in his original name for the condition (*Autistischen Psychopathen im Kindesalter*, or autistic personality disorders in childhood). He also noted other features that were commonly present. These included *egocentric preoccupations* with unusual and circumscribed interests that were the focus of much of the child's life and which interfered with acquisition of skills in other areas; for example, the child might be fascinated with train schedules but be unable to plan or anticipate his own daily routine. Affectively, Asperger noted that these children had *difficulties in dealing with their feelings*, often tending to intellectualize them, and had poor empathy and difficulties in understanding social cues. In addition, Asperger mentioned that they had *motor vulnerabilities* and typically were awkward and clumsy, with odd posture and gait and generally poor awareness of the movement of the body in space; graphomotor skills were also poor and the ability to participate in group sports activities was compromised. In terms of language and communication skills, Asperger described these boys as like "little professors" who talked (often at great length) about the topic of their interest but who had *difficulties with nonverbal and pragmatic aspects of communication*, for example, in use of facial expressions and gestures, in modulation of their voice, and in responding appropriately to the nonverbal cues of their conversational partners. Behavioral difficulties included *noncompliance and negativism* often leading to aggression and other conduct problems. These difficulties stemmed from the marked egocentrism and highly circumscribed interests as well as from the poor social understanding and peer relations these children exhibited at school. Asperger's original paper also *emphasized familial factors*; that is, similar traits were seen in relatives, particularly fathers.

In terming this condition *autistic personality disorder*, Asperger (1944), like Kanner the year before (1943), used Bleuler's much earlier (1911) term *autism* in describing the marked social vulnerability. Bleuler's earlier term was created to capture "a loss of contact, a retirement into self and a disregard of the outside world" observed in schizophrenia (Asperger, 1979, p. 46). In his use of the term, Asperger was careful to contrast the condition he described from schizophrenia. Because of World War II, Asperger was unaware of Kanner's similar use of the term the year previously. Asperger's observation of similar traits in family members may also have led him to be more optimistic about ultimate outcome

ASPERGER'S DISORDER: 1944–1981

Originally published in German, Asperger's paper was the focus of relatively little interest in the English-speaking literature until Wing's seminal (1981) review a year following Asperger's death. The rather small body of work on AS prior to 1981 included discussion of AS as a personality, rather than as a developmental, disorder (van Krevelan, 1971, 1973; van Krevelen & Kuipers, 1962) and what are probably some of the first case reports of the condition in the English language literature, albeit by individuals unaware of Asperger's work (Robinson & Vitale, 1954).

In 1962, van Krevelen and Kuipers attempted to distinguish AS from Kanner's autism, suggesting that the latter was present from the first months of life, that language was absent or delayed, that there was a lack of interest in others, and that prognosis was poor. They contrasted this profile with the later onset/recognition of AS as well as the often precocious language development ("the child talked before he walked"); the one-sided, eccentric social style, which caused problems in social interaction despite social interest; and the apparently better prognosis. These views were elaborated by van Krevelen again in 1971 in an article in the first issue of the *Journal of Autism and Childhood Schizophrenia,* where he attempted to draw clear distinctions between autism and AS. Similar attempts had been made in the German literature, some of which were translated into English at around the same time (see Bolte & Bosch, 2004).

Despite van Krevelan's attempt to distinguish between the two conditions, considerable confusion arose about AS. This confusion stemmed from several sources. Firstly, it took several decades before investigators and clinicians were sure of the validity of autism, for example, apart from childhood schizophrenia, and indeed it was not until 1980 that autism was first officially recognized as a diagnosis. This naturally delayed evaluation of other, similar diagnostic concepts. Secondly, as research on autism was conducted in the 1950s and 1960s, it became clear that Kanner's original concept had to be modified; Kanner originally thought, for example, that autism was probably associated with normal intellectual levels, but it became apparent that many individuals with autism functioned in the intellectually disabled range.

Another source of confusion stemmed from the use of the same word, *autism,* by both Asperger and Kanner. This term reflected the core disability present in the children described in their accounts. In addition, both groups of patients had difficulties in the areas of affective reaction, nature and range of interests, and social use of language. The main differences in the two conditions appeared to be that in AS, early speech and formal language skills were acquired on time if not precociously, motor deficits were more common, and in contrast to autism, the apparent onset of the condition was after the first several years of life. In addition, all of the original cases described by Asperger had been boys, whereas Kanner had noted some girls with autism in his original report.

Other areas of divergence in the accounts included differences in speech and language skills, motor mannerisms, circumscribed interests, and ultimate outcome. Some of the differences in the original syndrome descriptions may relate to the nature of differences in the groups being reported; that is, whereas Kanner was describing more impaired and younger children, Asperger was describing older and apparently less severely impaired individuals. These differences contributed to the subsequent tendency to equate Kanner's syndrome with the "classically" lower-functioning autistic child and Asperger's description with the nonretarded and verbal child with autism. It is important to note that Asperger himself emphasized the differences from autism once he became aware of the latter concept (Asperger, 1979), and indeed information on cases subsequently seen by him is consistent with this view (Hippler & Klicpera, 2003, 2005).

WING'S REVIEW: 1981

Wing's highly influential 1981 review brought Asperger's concept to the attention of a much larger audience. It provided a summary of Asperger's account, suggested some ways his description might be modified, emphasized the possible connection to autism, and provided a series of case reports. She suggested the term *Asperger's syndrome* for the condition. Her publication generated considerable interest and an expanding literature on the condition related both to a possible connection to autism, on the one hand (based on family history), and the possibility that AS was a possible transitional disorder with schizophrenia (see Klin, Volkmar, & Sparrow, 2000; Klin, McPartland, et al., 2005; Volkmar & Tsatsanis, 2005).

Wing's (1981) report of over 30 cases was important in that she was able to identify a group of individuals whose histories and clinical presentations were very similar to Asperger's account, as well as another group of cases in which the current clinical presentation was consistent but early history was not. In addition to summarizing Asperger's original work, Wing proposed some modifications of the concept based on her case series; these modifications were primarily related to the issue of early development and early clinical presentation. She suggested that difficulties might be apparent early in life (i.e., in the first 2 years) and might take the form of lack of interest in others, early language deficits, and imaginative play; also, her cases suggested that Asperger's speculation that these children talked before they walked was not always correct. Finally, she noted that sometimes the condition was apparently associated with mild mental retardation and could be seen in both males and females. Her use of the eponymous label *Asperger syndrome* avoided potential confusion in English regarding the use of the word *psychopathy* adopted by Asperger (who intended the term to suggest a personality).

Wing's (1981) description increased interest in this condition and prefigured much of the subsequent debate about boundaries, or lack thereof, with autism. She emphasized that despite her interest in Asperger's work, she fundamentally viewed the disorder as part of the autistic spectrum and was more concerned with broadening, rather than narrowing, Asperger's original concept. Not surprisingly, the modifications she proposed thus tended to blur the distinctions between AS and autism originally suggested by van Krevelen (1971). The latter had been reemphasized by Asperger himself just the year before (1979) when he noted areas of difference from autism (see also Hippler & Klicpera, 2003, for a review of cases seen by

Asperger over the years). These differences include the preserved language abilities as well as motor problems and the apparently later recognition of AS as well as differences in other clinical features (e.g., circumscribed interests).

ASPERGER SYNDROME: 1981–1994

Although not providing truly operational categorical diagnostic criteria, Wing's (1981) paper served as the basis for much subsequent work as authors attempted (with somewhat different areas of emphasis) to adapt her description into an operationalized definition. As a result of a series of approaches, all in some ways derivative of Wing (1981) but in other ways rather divergent, arose. Clearly for purposes of official systems such as DSM-IV and ICD-10, it clearly was important that AS differ from autism in some relevant and meaningful way or ways. Unfortunately, the lack of consistency in diagnostic approach complicated this discussion but did set the stage for possible inclusion of the concept in DSM-IV and ICD-10— that is, whether any substantive data on differences in clinical presentation course or treatment could be used to justify its inclusion (Szatmari, Bartolucci, & Bremner, 1989; Szatmari, Bremner, & Nagy, 1989; Tantam, 1988a, 1988b).

The DSM-IV field trial (Volkmar et al., 1994) primarily focused on autism, but as part of this work almost 50 cases of AS (based on clinician diagnosis) were submitted from sites around the world over the course of a year. This large sample of cases had some advantages in that comparisons could readily be made with relevant IQ-matched groups for which clinicians had diagnosed autism or PDD-NOS. Interesting significant differences were, in fact, observed both relative to HFA and PDD-NOS (different patterns of verbal–performance IQ in AS and greater frequency of circumscribed interests as well as greater social symptom severity than in PDD-NOS). And as result a tentative decision was made to include the condition in DSM as well as in ICD-10 (World Health Organization, 1993; Volkmar et al., 1994).

Unfortunately, the ambivalence over including this category was reflected in several last-minute changes in diagnostic approach, so that, in practice, the ICD-10 and DSM-IV definitions use age of onset as a primary differentiating feature and also give autism precedence (the "precedence rule"). As a result, many individuals who appear to have relatively prototypical forms of the condition are given an autism diagnosis instead (Volkmar, Klin, Schultz, Rubin, & Bronen, 2000; Volkmar & Klin, 2000). This approach reflects a concern that autism not be "overshadowed" by AS (the former being the much more well-known concept), an awareness that earlier diagnosis was more likely now than in the past (given greater parental and professional sophistication), and some degree of skepticism about the validity of AS as a distinctive concept.

Very quickly the DSM-IV and ICD-10 approach was criticized widely, and even with the major changes in the text description that occurred in DSM-IV-TR (American Psychiatric Association, 2000) the approach continued to be criticized as overly narrow (Eisenmajer et al., 1996; Szatmari et al., 1995; Mayes, Calhoun, & Crites, 2001; Miller & Ozonoff, 1997). Table 1.2 summarizes key points of similarity and difference in these various diagnostic approaches.

ASPERGER SYNDROME POST-DSM-IV/ICD-10

Official recognition of AS clearly has stimulated a considerable body of research but, as noted previously, has not resolved some of the continued (and continuing) controversies to diagnosis. Clearly, comparisons across approaches are complex; Ghaziuddin, Ghaziuddin, and Tsai (1992) summarized some of these issues even before DSM-IV appeared. As a result of these issues and a lack of a generally agreed-upon diagnostic approach, several rather disparate approaches to diagnosis remain in common use and complicate interpretation of research findings.

The *spectrum approach* views AS as one manifestation of the broader spectrum of autism (e.g., Baron-Cohen, 2000a, 2000b; Constantino & Todd, 2003). The *speech-by-age-2 approach* focuses on the presence/ absence of language delay in the first years of life; that is, in the absence of language and cognitive delay, AS becomes the default diagnosis (Gilchrist et al., 2001; Szatmari, Bartolucci, & Bremner, 1989). The *DSM-IV approach* represents a variation of the language delay approach (with the additional complexity of specifying the precedence of autism as a concept and specification of relatively normal early development). The *strict diagnostic approach*, likely more consistent with Asperger's original one, attempts to emphasize unique features of clinical presentation as well as history: for example, motor difficulties, circumscribed interests, and nature of early developmental processes (see Volkmar & Klin, 2000). This last approach emphasizes features more unique to AS, and in one study comparing these approaches, it was this last approach that was more likely to produce significant differences in IQ profiles, comorbidity of the proband, and family history of psychiatric symptom (Klin, Pauls, et al., 2005).

A growing body of literature on issues relevant to diagnosis/differential diagnosis of AS and HFA, although still relatively small, has now developed. In the following sections we summarize the limited available literature that directly assesses the impact of diagnostic approach as well as some of the relevant literature in specific areas: neuropsychology, psychiatric comorbidity, and family genetics. As will become apparent, the

TABLE 1.2. Comparison of Six Sets of Clinical Criteria Defining Asperger Syndrome

Clinical feature	Asperger (1944, 1979)	Wing (1981)	Gillberg & Gillberg (1989)	Tantam (1988a)	Szatmari, Brammers, et al. (1989)	DSM-IV (American Psychiatric Association, 1994)
Social impairment						
Poor nonverbal communication	Yes	Yes	Yes	Yes	Yes	Yes
Poor empathy	Yes	Yes	Yes	Yes	Yes	Yes
Failure to develop friendships	Yes	Yes	Yes	Yes	(implied)	Yes
Language/communication						
Poor prosody and pragmatics	Yes	Yes	Yes	Yes	Yes	Not stated
Idiosyncratic language	Yes	Yes	Not stated	Not stated	Yes	Not stated
Impoverished imaginative play	Yes	Yes	Not stated	Not stated	Not stated	Not stated
All-absorbing interest	Yes	Yes	Yes	Yes	Not stated	Of ten
Motor clumsiness	Yes	Yes	Yes	Yes	Not stated	Of ten
Onset (0–3 years)						
Speech delays/ deviance	No	May be present	May be present	Not stated	Not stated	No
Cognitive delays	No	May be present	Not stated	Not stated	Not stated	No
Motor delays	Yes	Sometimes	Not stated	Not stated	Not stated	May be present
Exclusion of autism	Yes (1979)	No	No	No	Yes	Yes
Mental retardation	No	May be present	Not stated	Not stated	Not stated	No

Note. From Klin, McPartland, and Volkmar (2005, p. 94). Copyright 2005 by John Wiley & Sons, Inc. Reprinted by permission.

available data vary quite dramatically across these three areas, and it is always important in interpreting this literature to be aware that fundamental differences in approaches to diagnosis may, of course, significantly impact the results obtained.

Direct Comparison of Diagnostic Approaches

Klin, Pauls, Schultz, and Volkmar (2005) directly compared three different approaches to the diagnosis of AS in 65 individuals with good cognitive skills but with severe social disability. In this study comparisons were made relative to IQ profiles, comorbid symptoms, and familial aggregation of social and other psychiatric symptoms. The three approaches compared were the DSM-IV criteria, the "absence-of-speech-delay" approach (presence of communicative speech by age 3; Szatmari et al., 2000), and a method more consistent with Asperger's (1944) approach (the "prototypic" approach). They noted the issues with DSM-IV but also emphasized the potential limitations of the speech-delay approach, in that it tended to minimize other features that might well contribute in important ways to the presentation of AS with what they suggested was considerable potential for increasing type II errors (i.e., of not finding differences that otherwise would be observed with a more specific approach). The prototypic approach was consistent with Asperger's report (see also Hippler & Klicpera, 2003; Volkmar & Klin, 2000). In this approach the features more unique to AS were emphasized (e.g., social interest but social insensitivity; language not just present but precocious, with the inclusion of one-sided verbosity as a necessary communication criterion; and factual, circumscribed interests that interfere with both general learning and with reciprocal social conversation). For the prototypic or strict diagnosis approach the DSM-IV precedence rule (autism being given precedence over AS) was reversed.

The Autism Diagnostic Interview—Revised (ADI-R) and the Autism Diagnostic Observation Schedule (ADOS) were administered in all cases and used to operationalize the three diagnostic approaches (see Klin, Pauls, et al., 2005, for additional information). The 65 cases (61 male and 4 female) were evaluated using a standard set of assessments, including the ADI-R, ADOS, Wechsler IQ test, and structured psychiatric interviews. The mean IQ of the sample (primarily adolescents and young adults) was 98, but all had severe delays in social skills development; for example, standard scores on the socialization domain of the Vineland Adaptive Behavior Scales—Expanded Edition (Sparrow, Balla, & Cicchetti, 1984) were more than two SDs below the mean. In terms of psychological and psychiatric assessments, special care was taken to avoid bias by having evaluators blind to history and diagnosis. Best-estimate psychiatric diagnoses (for comorbidity and family psychiatric disorders) were completed by two senior clinicians not otherwise familiar with the cases.

In this study four individuals were excluded for having failed to meet a threshold for PDD. Of the remaining individuals there were major shifts in case assignment depending on which diagnostic system was used. Using the DSM-IV system, over 50% of cases had a diagnosis for autistic disorder and only 24% AS (with the remainder receiving a PDD-NOS diagnosis); with the speech-present approach the situation was essentially reversed, with 50% of cases receiving an AS diagnosis and only 14% a diagnosis of autistic disorder. With the presumably more prototypic approach, 38% of individuals met criteria for AS and 28% for autistic disorder. Over half of the sample (56%) was noted to have at least two different diagnoses using the three approaches. In the IQ data there were no overall differences for Full Scale, Verbal, or Performance IQ over the three systems, but the verbal–performance IQ difference that had previously been noted for AS was noted in individuals with this diagnosis in either the prototypic or DSM-IV approach. Differences in proband comorbidity were most robust with the prototypic approach. As expected, rates of anxiety and mood disorders were increased with some suggestion of differences across the various systems and categories. Interestingly, the prototypic approach to the diagnosis of AS was associated with higher rates of the broader autism phenotype in relatives of probands with a diagnosis of AS in that system.

Similarly, Ghaziuddin (2005) examined family psychiatric history in nearly 60 subjects (diagnosed using DSM-IV). They noted that all subjects (mean age, 13 years) had normal IQ, significant social deficits, special interests, and pedantic speech, but no previous diagnosis of autism. Of the siblings of these individuals, four had AS (no cases of autism) and rates of AS were increased in other first-degree relatives. Both schizophrenia and depression were also more frequent than in the comparison group with HFA. Thus it appears that, perhaps not surprisingly, the stringency of diagnostic approach has major implications for research findings and that lack of consistency in diagnostic approach remains a major complication for interpretation of available research (Susan, Libby, Wing, Gould, & Gillberg, 2000).

NEUROPSYCHOLOGY

The area of neuropsychology has, without doubt, been one of the most productive in the literature on AS and its similarities and differences from autism and PDD-NOS. This issue is discussed in greater detail by Tsatsanis (Chapter 3, this volume). Differences in patterns of neuropsychological functioning are of considerable theoretical and practical interest. From the research side such differences can suggest potential differences in pathogenesis, mechanisms, or even relative to end phenotypes. Many of the topics that continue to be the focus of research were raised by Asperger in his original (1944) paper—for example, relatively preserved or advanced verbal abilities, motor difficulties, clumsiness, and so forth. From the clinical side these issues may have particular importance for differences in intervention strategies. As has been discussed previously, the diversity in diagnostic practice and approach is a considerable complication in the comparison of research studies, as are other methodological issues (e.g., small sample size and lack of statistical power or diversity in ages of subjects studied). Accordingly, when relevant, the possible limitations of studies are noted.

Asperger's original report (1944) suggested some areas of variability in cognitive profile. In subsequent reviews of Asperger's cases (Hippler & Klickpera, 2003, 2005), differences in cognitive profiles were noted, with Verbal IQ preserved relative to performance or nonverbal abilities. A series of studies using more stringent diagnostic approaches has also demonstrated significant scatter in IQ test profiles—but a pattern of scatter rather different from that usually seen in autistic disorder, in which verbal, rather than nonverbal/perceptual, skills are preserved (e.g., Ehlers et al., 1997; Ghaziuddin, Mohammad, & Mountain-Kimchi, 2004; Koyama, Tomonori, Tachimori, Hisateru, Osada, et al., 2007; Lincoln, Courchesne, Allen, Hanson, & Ene, 1998; Ozonoff, South, & Miller, 2000). In addition, the specific pattern of assets and deficits has also been noted to be highly consistent with a nonverbal learning disability (NLD; Rourke, 1989), has been proposed to be characteristic of individuals with AS, and potentially could serve as a source of external validity for the syndrome (Klin et al., 1995; Klin & Volkmar, 1997).

The NLD subtype, which emerged from research on children with learning disabilities, represents a distinct profile of neuropsychological functioning characterized by better developed verbal skills, relative to visual, tactile, and complex motor skills, in addition to deficits in novel problem solving and concept formation. In Rourke's (1989) model, it is proposed that this pattern of neuropsychological assets and deficits eventuates in a specific pattern of strengths and weaknesses in academic (e.g., well-developed single-word reading and spelling relative to mechanical arithmetic) and social (e.g., overreliance on language to learn about themselves and the world and to navigate social situations, with less efficient use of nonverbal information) functioning. Individuals with NLD are increased at risk for internalizing disorders such as depression and anxiety. Clearly descriptive accounts of individuals with AS show considerable overlap with the clinical manifestations of the NLD syndrome.

In addition, an extensive investigation comparing the neuropsychological profiles of well-characterized individuals with AS or HFA offered strong support for a relationship between AS and NLD (Klin, Sparrow, et al., 1995). The sample in this study consisted of 19 individuals with HFA and 21 individuals with AS, diagnosed using stringent criteria modified from ICD-10 (World Health Organization, 1993). The neuropsychological records showed that a highly significant association between AS and NLD was obtained (n = 18) but not for autism (n = 1). Areas of deficit associated with AS include problems with fine motor skills, visual–motor integration, visual–spatial perception, nonverbal concept formation, gross motor skills, and visual memory. Similarly the IQ profiles revealed a significant verbal–nonverbal split, with higher verbal than nonverbal skills; this pattern was not seen in the HFA group. Subsequent studies have both supported the association with NLD (Gunter, Ghaziuddin, & Ellis, 2002) and questioned it (Ambery, Russell, Perry, Morris, & Murphy, 2006), with other work focused more broadly on patterns of neuropsychological strength/weakness in ASD in general (see Tsatsanis, Chapter 3, this volume; Tager-Flusberg & Joseph, 2003; Noterdaeme, Wriedt, & Hohne, 2010). Differences in verbal fluency between the two conditions have been reported (Spek, Schatorjé, Scholte, & van Berckelaer-Onnes, 2009), although differences in diagnostic approach must be considered in evaluating these studies. Clearly, the study of distinctive cognitive profiles in AS, in particular, and in the broader autism spectrum group remains of much interest.

A smaller body of work on memory issues in AS suggests some differences relative to specific functions. For example, fact recall and semantic memory may be a strength, but aspects of spatial working memory (Morris et al., 1999) and visual memory (Ambery et al., 2006) may be impaired and impact on social processes. Similarly, difficulties may be observed in the range of abilities subsumed within the concept of *executive functions*: problem solving, forward planning, self-monitoring, set shifting, inhibition, organization, flexibility, and working memory (Bennetto, Pennington, & Rogers, 1996; Goldstein, Johnson, & Minshew, 2001; Minshew, Meyer, & Goldstein, 2002; Ozonoff, Strayer, McMahon, & Filloux, 1994; Verté, Geurts, Roeyers, Oosterlaan, & Sergeant, 2006; Joseph, McGrath, & Tager-Flusberg, 2005). As with memory problems, these difficulties also can adversely impact social judgment and social decision making. Clearly, executive functioning difficulties are also seen in autism, although some suggestion of difference has been reported (e.g., Kleinhans, Akshoomoff, & Delis, 2005).

Motor and sensory issues have been the focus of some research resources. A range of problems, including in motor integration and broader relationships to sensory issues, have been noted as well (see Tsatsanis, Chapter 3, this volume). Consistent with Asperger's original report, persistent motor difficulties in AS samples (e.g., Ghaziuddin, Butler, Tsai, & Ghaziuddin, 1994; Manjiviona & Prior, 1995; Miyahara et al., 1997; Green et al., 2002) have been reported. Although suffering from various shortcomings, the earliest work in this area suggested significant impairment in motor skills in patients with AS, as compared to those with autism (e.g., Tantam, 1988a; Gillberg, 1989; Szatmari, Bartolucci, et al., 1989). Subsequent work has been better controlled and more equivocal in its findings, although again it suffers from the issues of diagnostic consistency (Ghaziuddin et al., 1994; Manjiviona & Prior, 1999; Ghaziuddin & Butler, 1998). A major issue in the interpretation of this literature has been a general lack of attention to important changes in the nature of motor tasks; for example, over time social or imitation elements may be more central. An important and unresolved issue is the degree to which difficulties with organization and executive function impact motor difficulties (e.g., Rinehart et al., 2006). The severity of motor skills deficits has been noted to correlate with overall severity of AS (Hilton, Wente, LaVesser, Ito, Reed, et al., 2007).

Motor difficulties have both clinical and research implications. Difficulties in these areas present obstacles for information processing and pose challenges for learning, particularly when combined with strengths in other areas (e.g., verbal). The child may learn, over time, to develop compensatory abilities even when core difficulties remain. A further complication in interpreting results obtained.

Compared to autism, work in this area for AS is less extensive. Dunne and colleagues (Dunn, Myles, & Orr, 2002) reported difficulties relative to both under- and overresponsiveness on the Sensory Profile (Dunn, 1999). Other studies note differences in tactile sensitivity (Blakemore et al., 2006; Cascio et al., 2008). Similarly, studies of visual perception have noted differences relative to perceptual organization (Tsatsanis et al., in press). In individuals with AS, difficulties with organization and with seeing the "whole" image both impact on recall.

Issues of auditory processing suggest similar areas of difficulty in both children (Lepistö et al., 2006; Kujala et al., 2007) and fathers as well (Korpilahti et al., 2007). These difficulties may contribute to communication problems more generally.

Despite the limitations, the bulk of available evidence provides reasonably strong support for the notion that motor impairment is frequent in AS (and more frequent than in autism, although the evidence here is less strong). A major complication is the degree to which motor and sensory issues are (usually) intertwined with other developmental processes and the potentially very significant impact that social dysfunction may have on motor processes.

PSYCHIATRIC COMORBIDITIES

Issues of psychiatric comorbidity are complex (see Volkmar & Woolston, 1997; Rutter, 1997; Westphal, Kober, Voos, & Volkmar, Chapter 9, this volume). Comorbidities also appear to vary significantly over the course of development, with higher presenting complaints of attention and impulse problems in children but greater rates of mood difficulties and disorders in adolescents and adults. One reason, of course, for the greater interest in this topic is the substantially greater verbal abilities of individuals with AS, as compared with individuals who exhibit more classic cases of autism, wherein language problems limit the usefulness of many instruments.

Attentional problems have historically been one of the most frequent clinical complaints for children with AS, often as an initial presenting complaint, and have been the focus of some research (e.g., Hanson, 2003; Rinehart, Bradshaw, Brereton, & Tonge, 2001; Rinehart, Bradshaw, Moss, Brereton, & Tonge, 2001; Semrud-Clikeman, Walkowiak, Wilkinson, & Minne, 2010; Tani et al., 2006). These deficits can be expressed as isolated attentional problems, in the form of impulsivity, or as a combination of the two. In contrast to the typical child with attention-deficit/hyperactivity disorder (ADHD), individuals with AS may demonstrate excellent attention in some areas (e.g., in a focus on a topic of interest), but social and organizational difficulties contribute to difficulties with attention in other situations—a pattern rather different than seen in autism (see Rinehart et al., 2001). Paradoxically the "hyperfocus" on a topic of special interest can coexist with other types of attentional problems. The complex processes involved in attention to more complex tasks have been reviewed elsewhere (e.g., Townsend, Harris, & Courchesne, 1996; Wainwright-Sharp & Bryson, 1996; Hanson, 2003; Joshi et al., 2010), although the literature specific to AS is rather limited (see Pelphry et al., Chapter 13, this volume). The data are of interest in that they seem to suggest difficulties rather the opposite of those more typical in classical autism; that is, difficulties with sustained attention but not on shifting attention. The caveat is that the studies are few and constructs across studies not necessarily measured the same way; but this area is worthy of further and more systematic study. The ASD criteria published in DSM-5 permit concurrent diagnoses of ASD and ADHD, a change that will hopefully foster deeper understanding of the overlap between social and attentional difficulties in individuals with AS. As discussed by Westphal et al. (Chapter 9, this volume), attention difficulties are a frequent cause for pharmacological intervention.

In adolescents and adults, anxiety and depression are very frequent (Hanson, 2003; Humphrey, 2008; Kim, Szatmari, Bryson, Streiner, & Wilson, 2000). Anxiety may come from an appropriate awareness of the difficulties with social information processing, feelings of being overwhelmed by demands of typical peer interactions, and an awareness of the lack of understanding of the nuances of the social world. Depression may be viewed as a result of repeated failure experiences, over time, coupled with an awareness of social isolation and lack of interpersonal supports. Estimates of the rates of comorbid anxiety and/or depression in individuals with AS are high, with over 50% exhibiting one or more of these problems (Ellis, Ellis, Fraser, & Deb, 1994; Fujikawa, Kobayashi, Koga, & Murata, 1987; Ghaziuddin & Butler, 1998; Ghaziuddin, 2002; Ghaziuddin & Greden, 1998; Green, Gilchrist, Burton, & Cox, 2000; Howlin & Goode, 1998). On the other hand, individuals with HFA may also be at risk for these problems, and some reports find no differences between groups (e.g., Szatmari et al., 2000), although this may reflect the particular diagnostic approach used and the age of the sample. It has been our experience that more able individuals with autism suffer less from depression and anxiety partly because of their lack of social interest and motivation, but this topic continues to merit study. In one report from our center, rates of these conditions in both probands and family members were higher in individuals with AS (Klin, Pauls, et al., 2005).

Other conditions have been described in association with AS (see Folstein, Chapter 14, this volume), although often this literature is based on case reports, which are then difficult to place in a broader context. Conditions observed have included Tourette syndrome (Kerbeshian & Burd, 1986; Littlejohns, Clarke, & Corbett, 1990; Marriage, Miles, Stokes, & Davey, 1993), obsessive–compulsive disorder (Fontenelle et al., 2004; Gallucci, Hackerman, & Schmidt, 2005; Kraemer, Delsignore, Gundelfinger, Schnyder, & Hepp, 2005; Ruta, Mugno, d'Arrigo, Vitiello, & Mazzone, 2010; Wendland et al., 2008) and gender identity disorder (Gallucci et al., 2005; Kraemer et al., 2005). Reported associations with psychotic conditions have included both major depression and bipolar disorder as well as schizophrenia (Stewart et al., 2006; Fontenelle et al., 2004; Duggal, 2003; Bejerot & Duvner, 1995; Gillberg, 1985; Wolff, 1998). Difficulties with diagnosis arise because of the social isolation of individuals with AS and their tendency to verbalize many of their thoughts (Ryan, 1992). One small study suggested differences in indices of thought disorder in AS versus in HFA (Ghaziuddin, Leininger, & Tsai, 1995). Some attention has focused on the association of schizophrenia with AS and suggested that AS might, in some sense, be a "bridging condition" (Wolff & McGuire, 1995). Some support for this possibility is noted in the literature (e.g., Nagy & Szatmari, 1986), although other studies fail to support it (Ghaziuddin et al., 1995). Family studies, although limited, do not seem to suggest higher rates of schizophrenia in family members; rather, mood and social problems appear more frequently (and are discussed subsequently).

Another line of work, again mostly limited to case reports, has noted conduct problems and violent behavior (e.g., Mawson, Grounds, & Tantam, 1985; Baron-Cohen, 1988; Hall & Bernal, 1995; Everall & LeCouteur, 1990; Scragg & Shah, 1994). In their review of the topic Ghaziuddin, Tsai, and Ghaziuddin (1991) found little support for this notion. Similar findings are noted by Hippler, Viding, Klicpera, and Happé (2010). In our experience it is much more likely that individuals with AS are victims and not victimizers; they are often teased and bullied (e.g., Sofronoff, Dark, & Stone, 2011), and their oddity and isolation make them frequent targets for others; this issue is addressed in greater detail by Woodbury-Smith, Chapter 12, this volume). Somewhat paradoxically, it is their tendency to rely rigidly on rules that may pose challenges for them (i.e., via failures to make appropriate exceptions and accommodations), and this can, at times, bring these individuals into conflict with school and legal authorities. With the onset of adolescence and increased sexual interest, lack of sophistication may lead them to make highly one-sided and inappropriate overtures (e.g., verbal sexual requests). At times, an all-absorbing interest may even lead to legal difficulties.

The specificity of difficulties associated with AS, rather than with HFA, remains debated, but strong suggestion of differential patterns has emerged, and certainly better verbal skills would suggest important implications for treatments (see Volkmar, Klin, & McPartland, Chapter 5, this volume). Clearly, more systematic and comprehensive study is needed to understand both clinical service implications and, more broadly, potential implications for research conceptualizations.

SOCIAL FUNCTIONING

Over the past two decades research has increasingly focused on understanding the social difficulties associated with autism and AS. One major line of work has focused on difficulties in the ability to understand the mental life of others and their own subjectivity—what is usually termed *theory-of-mind* abilities (ToM; Baron-Cohen, 1989). The initial assumption was that a fundamental deficit in this area accounted for a major portion, if not all, of the individual's social disability. Although several lines of work have now questioned this view as overly simplistic, studies differentiating the performance of individuals with AS or HFA have been conducted and are of interest in clarifying the nature of the social disturbance seen in these conditions. For example, Ozonoff et al. (Ozonoff, Pennington, & Rogers, 1991; Ozonoff, Rogers, & Pennington, 1991) noted differences, with individuals with autism exhibiting significant impairment in relation to both AS and an age- and IQ-matched control groups. Similar results were noted by Bowler (1992) and Ziatas, Durkin, and Pratt (2003). Consistent with Asperger's (1944) original impression regarding the later ages of parental concern reported in AS, various studies have suggested that the social issues (e.g., problems in joint attention and play) are frequent early signs of autism in very young children (Baird et al., 2000), whereas parental concern arises later for individuals with AS (Klin, McPartland, et al., 2005).

Other work has suggested differences in the expression of ToM skills in the two conditions (Kaland et al., 2002). A difference was also observed in one positron emission tomography (PET) study using ToM tasks (Happé et al., 1996). No differences have also been reported, although issues of diagnostic assignment complicate interpretation of all these results (e.g., Dahlgren & Trillingsgaard, 1996). On balance, Frith (2004) concluded that the available data to that point suggested a milder degree of social impairment (at least, as expressed in ToM tasks) for individuals with AS, also noting that this finding might simply reflect higher verbal abilities.

Careful review of Asperger's original report emphasized the nature of adaptive ("real life") social difficulties. Van Krevelen (1971) emphasized this point in his description of the lack of empathy and intuitive understanding and the difficulties in dealing with face-based social interaction. The tendency of individuals with AS to use words, logic, and thinking to negotiate the social world is encompassed in this view and offers an additional area of relevance both to differentiation from HFA and for purposes of intervention (see also Klin, Jones, Schultz, & Volkmar, 2003, who emphasize the importance of ecological context on results obtained). Tager-Flusberg, Joseph, and Folstein (2001) differentiated social perception for social reasoning and suggested that whereas in autism both are adversely impacted, in AS it is social perception, rather than cognition, that is primarily involved. As discussed below and elsewhere in this volume, this observation has important implications for intervention.

ONSET PATTERNS

In contrast to Kanner (who speculated that the condition he described was congenital), Asperger suggested that parents typically were not concerned for some years, although they had frequently reported an atypical pattern of early development characterized by precocious language skills and delayed motor abilities. This pattern was consistent with his description of parents frequently reporting that children with AS "talk before they walk," that words become an early and enduring "lifeline" for social connectedness, and of his eventual impression that the condition he described was, in some respects, more a personality trait than a developmental disorder. The observations of relatively more preserved patterns of verbal (as compared to nonverbal or performance) abilities are consistent with this description. On the other hand, it is possible that the delay in parental concern might reflect other factors: for example, the higher the cognitive potential, as a group, of the children with AS, the better the verbal skills (a frequently used proxy of overall ability that can mask areas of disability). Similarly, it might be that, to some extent, social interest is more preserved in AS and/or that it takes a different form than in autism.

Careful and meticulous history taking often does reveal some slightly unusual aspects of early development; for example, the child's speech may be precocious, but the "little professor" quality noted by Asperger may predominate with odd (for age) language use, pedantic speech quality, and so forth. Interestingly, parents do *not* typically report obvious signs of social disability (although these become much more obvious when children are required to interact with typical peers); attachment to family members seems unremarkable, and the level of social disability (at least at this age) appears to be more subtle usually than that typically seen in autism. Interactions with other children (peers or family members) may be more a source of early concern, in contrast to interactions with parents and older individuals who "scaffold" the child's social overtures and typically assume a less demanding social interactional pattern than peers. Accordingly, as

Asperger first suggested, it remains typical for parental concern to arise only as the child is routinely exposed to typical peers (e.g., in nursery and preschool settings) (see Klin, McPartland, et al., 2005).

The issue of onset in AS was considered in a recent study by Kamp-Becker and colleagues (2010), which considered early presentation of AS and ADHD (the latter condition also diagnosed later than autism and one frequently confused with AS in younger children). Parents of large groups of children with AS or ADHD were interviewed, and the authors reported that 10 features distinguished the groups, including problems in social development and communication, repetitive behaviors, and interests.

Clearly much more work in this area is needed, given our necessary reliance on parent report; that is, identification of younger children with AS would contribute significantly to formation of a research literature. The strong potential for children (of all types) to develop specific compensatory mechanisms and learn, at least eventually, to rely on areas of strength to cope with social disability also underscores the value of identifying the condition in younger children.

SPECIAL INTERESTS

In autism the issue of special interests has, in fact, tended to center in important ways on unusual *abilities*: on either peak skills (e.g., block design in IQ tests) or, in a small percentage of cases, on some isolated or "savant" ability (Hermelin, 2001). In Asperger's (1944) original description, he was careful to point out that the children he described had very significant and circumscribed *interests* that both interfered with their learning (e.g., of other skills) and also intruded on the family's life. From Asperger's description the interests of the children he described tended to center on amassing facts about some isolated area of interest, whereas the cases described by Kanner (1943) were more likely to have special abilities involving memory (e.g., for birthdays) or in terms of visual nonverbal abilities. As noted previously, Robinson and Vitale (1954) provided vivid descriptions of three children with unusual and all-encompassing interests that were very suggestive of Asperger's earlier work (of which Robinson and Vitale were unaware). In their report one child was focused on aspects of chemistry, another on astronomy, and a third on a transportation system. Kanner (1954) was the discussant of the paper and noted similarities and differences from the children he had described with autism (e.g., the interference of the behavior as was true of resistance to change behaviors in autism and significant social-communication problems, but also the context of more preserved social skills use of special interests to try to connect with others).

Given the early interest and Asperger's clear "demarcation" of this as an area of possible differentiation from autism, focused work on the topic has been remarkably limited. Baron-Cohen (1989) provided results of a survey of a large group of children with ASD whose focus was obsessions (in some ways, different from special interests). They noted a high proportion of interest in fact-based knowledge in science and taxonomy. South, Ozonoff, and McMahon (2005) studied 40 higher-functioning individuals (with autism or AS) and reported interests in a range of topics that included science (space and physics), animals, video games, dinosaurs, and so forth. Interests were rather similar in both clinical samples. Klin, Danovitch, Merz, and Volkmar (2007) studied nearly 100 individuals with IQs in the normal range and a mix of diagnoses, using a special interest survey. The parent-completed ratings included descriptions of topic and degree of interference. Topics were grouped into eight overarching categories (facts and verbal memory, facts and visual memory, sensory behaviors, math, classification, dates/time, hoarding, and letters/numbers). Over 250 specific topics of interest were coded for the 96 individuals. Reliability of coding was high, using a chance-corrected statistic. Some developmental trends were noted, with shifts in interest over age (from preschool to school age). Interestingly, the degree of interference of these skills, as reported by parents, .correlated significantly in a negative direction with Vineland socialization scores for preschoolers and similarly in a negative direction with communication abilities in the school-age children. About two-thirds of the preschoolers and three-fourths of the school-age children had interests that centered around amassing facts, and it was noted that particularly when children were left to their own devices, they tended to gravitate to their special area of interest.

Other investigators have described the longitudinal course of special interests in AS. For example, Atwood (2003) noted that both the number and focus of the special interest shifts over time (with a shift sometimes being triggered by a specific event). Atwood also emphasized (as did Asperger) the degree to which the family may be forced to accommodate the child's special interest. This important point is very much in keeping with Asperger's original emphasis on how these interests potentially interfered with the child's learning and development as well as with family life. Accordingly, some intervention strategies focus on reducing or minimizing, to the extent possible, the degree to which these interests serve as a barrier to social interaction. On the other hand, sometimes these interests can be used productively, particularly if they have some potential social or ultimate vocational utility. Interests that are less highly unusual and idiosyncratic may also be easier topics of conversation and social interaction.

NEUROBIOLOGY AND GENETICS

Various lines of work have focused on neurobiological factors as possibly differentiating AS from HFA. As in other areas, the lack of consistency in diagnostic approach and small samples (particularly with neuroimaging studies) pose major obstacles for interpretation. As with autism, early work (particularly case reports) suggested potential associations of AS with birth complications and various medical conditions (Miles & Capelle, 1987; Tantam, Evered, & Hersov, 1990; Ghaziuddin, Shakal, et al., 1995; Haglund & Kallen, 2011).

Given possible differences in neuropsychological profiles, neuroimaging studies are of great interest—particularly given the apparent similarity of AS to the concept of "right-hemisphere syndrome" or "developmental disabilities of the right hemisphere" (Ellis et al., 1994; Gold & Faust, 2010; Gunter et al., 2002; Sandson, Manoach, Rentz, & Weintraub, 1994; Semrud-Clikeman & Hynd, 1990; Shields, 1991; Weintraub, Mesulam, & Kramer, 1981). In essence, this model suggests relative preservation of the left cerebral cortex (reflected in the many aspects of language preserved in AS but not in HFA), whereas right-hemisphere deficits would be reflected in social (pragmatic) and semantic problems and perhaps the NLD profile).

The available literature does suggest some areas of possible difference relative to cortical organization (Berthier, Starkstein, & Leiguarda, 1990), gray tissue abnormalities (McAlonan et al., 2008), limbic areas (McAlonan et al., 2002), and abnormalities in the temporal lobe (Jones & Kerwin, 1990). One recent meta-analysis (Yu, Cheung, Chua, & McAlonan, 2011) found significant differences, with reduced gray matter volume in the amygdala, hippocampal gyros, and prefrontal lobe. Semrud-Clikeman and Fine (2011) noted abnormalities in the occipital region, although others, such as, Via, Radua, Cardoner, Happé, and Mataix-Cols (2011), reported minimal differences. In contrast, Semrud-Clikeman and Fine (2011) noted that individuals with NLD and AS were more likely to exhibit specific abnormalities. Case reports from our center have included a father and son with AS (Volkmar et al., 1996) who exhibited right-hemisphere abnormalities and individual also with right-hemisphere abnormalities (Volkmar, et al., 2000; Korpilahti et al., 2007) and problems suggestive of NLD. Differences have also been found using proton magnetic resonance spectroscopy (see Murphy et al., 2002, 2006; Lotspeich et al., 2004; Berthier, Bayes, & Tolosa, 1993). White matter differences relative to normal controls and those with autism have been observed (Bloemen et al., 2010; McAlonan et al., 2008; McAlonan, Cheung, et al., 2009). Prefrontal cortex problems have also been noted in AS (Iwanami et al., 2011). One recent study suggested differences in cortical folding in the higher lobe as well as individuals with autism, but not AS, having higher folding levels (Jou, Minshew, Keshavan, & Hardan, 2010), although others (Williams, Goldstein, Kojkowski, & Minshew, 2008) did not notice this pattern (see also Hardan et al., 2008, on possible differences in other areas).

Given Asperger's (1944) initial observation of high rates of social disability in the fathers of the children in his cases, the issue of genetic mechanisms is of great interest, particularly since the recognition of the "broader autism phenotype" in family members of children with autism only became apparent many years after Kanner's first description of autism. There have been reports of families with multiple children with AS or with a positive family history for the condition (Cederlund & Gillberg, 2004; Ghaziuddin et al., 1993; Gillberg, 1991). On the other hand, and starting with Wing's (1981) report, other investigators have suggested strong links between AS and autism (Folstein & Santangelo, 2000; see also Folstein, Chapter 14, this volume). Complexities around diagnosis complicate the interpretation of the limited work available. For example, DeLong and Dwyer (1988) reported high rates of AS in relatives of individuals with HFA as well as higher rates of bipolar disorder in family members of individuals with AS. Many case reports have emphasized the increased rate of social disabilities in first-degree relatives (Bowman, 1988; DeLong & Dwyer, 1988; Gillberg, Gillberg, & Steffenburg, 1992; Volkmar et al., 1996). In one study Klin, Pauls, and colleagues (2005) noted that about half of first-degree relatives of AS probands exhibited high rates of social vulnerability if a strict diagnostic approach to AS was used (further underscoring the importance of use and reporting of the diagnostic approach).

The observation that autism and AS might co-occur in the same family has been suggested to indicate that the two conditions are related. The complexity of autism genetics (Rutter, 2005) offers the possibility that with multiple genes involved in autism, some subset of genes might also be involved in AS (one of many possibilities), but this, of, does not necessarily imply that the two disorders are "the same" in a fundamental sense. The literature on the genetics of AS, per se, remains small (e.g., Anneren, Dahl, Uddenfeldt, & Janols, 1995; Saliba & Griffiths, 1990; Bartolucci & Szatmari, 1987; Tentler, Johannesson, Johansson, Rastam, Gillberg, et al., 2003) and the issue remains important, with recent work suggesting areas of similarity and difference (Sciutto & Cantwell, 2005).

COURSE AND OUTCOME

The relatively recent recognition of AS complicates, to some degree, interpretation of data on outcome. Howlin (2005) noted that early differences from HFA tend to diminish over time (interestingly, the same is true for autism, more broadly defined, and for severe language disorder). In some ways there is a general tendency toward improvement over time, although adolescence may provide special risks for teenagers with AS, given increased social and academic demands and looming challenges of work or college (Volkmar & Wiesner, 2009). There does appear to be increased risk for comorbid problems, particularly anxiety and depression. Neuromata vulnerabilities and organizational problems often appear to persist (see Murphy et al., 2006; Brown & Wolf, Chapter 11, this volume) also appear to persist.

For adults AS can present with sometimes subtle difficulties, especially in communication, social relationships and interests (see Powers & Loomis, Chapter 10, this volume), underscoring Asperger's original impression that the condition he described was more a personality style/pattern. It is frequently noted that either with help or on his or her own, the individual with AS may learn to use a host of compensatory strategies. For example, in one case seen in our clinic a child managed to markedly increase his nonverbal IQ by learning (on his own) to turn nonverbal problems into verbal ones (making Block Design on the IQ into a verbal problem of matrix algebra; Volkmar et al., 1996).

Studies of AS frequently suggest that, for many individuals, improvement over time is sufficiently great that, as adults, they no longer qualify for or need this diagnosis (i.e., they move past the boundary of disorder into the broader category of eccentricity in the normal population). This transition may happen in as many as 20%, or so, of individuals (Woodbury-Smith & Volkmar, 2009). As noted previously, there does appear to be increased risk for anxiety and depression, which can impact functional outcome (Woodbury-Smith & Volkmar, 2009; McPartland & Klin, 2006).

Although comparison to autism is complex, if one considers the entire range of autism, the outcome in AS is much better (Larsen & Mouridsen, 1997; Cederlund, Hagberg, Billstedt, Gillberg, & Gillberg, 2008; Szatmari, 1991). The more complex and interesting question is the issue of outcome in AS as compared to the most cognitively able persons with autism.

Very long-term follow-up studies as well as cross-sectional studies of various age groups (with careful report of diagnostic approach used) would help to clarify these issues. Positive factors in AS include better preserved verbal abilities along with a strong desire for social contact. These factors are reflected in our observation that whereas we have rather rarely met a person with autism who is married, it is not uncommon to find individuals with AS who have done so (and, in fact, support books and resources for spouses are now available; Renty & Roeyers, 2007).

As a practical matter many adults with AS face various challenges in securing and maintaining employment. These challenges include persistent vulnerabilities in social abilities, pragmatic communication, and organization (Mawhood & Howlin, 1999). These challenges can take the form of poor adaptive skills, comorbid psychiatric conditions, and vocational issues and challenges—all of which require appropriate support. Supportive placements that maximize strengths and minimize social and neuropsychological challenges are important. Thus jobs involving less intensive social demands, less time pressure, and fewer organizational/executive skills and decisions are often better (Mawhood & Howlin, 1999; Muller, Schuler, Burton, & Yates, 2003). Computer-related occupations (with minimal direct interpersonal demands) may often be highly appropriate.

TREATMENT IMPLICATIONS

The issue of treatment implications of AS is discussed more extensively in the remainder of this volume. For purposes of this chapter our focus is specifically on the issues related to AS as a diagnostic concept apart from other disorders (see Volkmar et al., Chapter 5, this volume). As we have discussed elsewhere (Klin, Pauls, et al., 2005; Klin, McPartland, et al., 2005), treatment is essentially supportive and symptomatic, with some degree of overlap in treatment approaches relative to more able persons with autism but also with some important potential differences. The similarities include supporting social skill acquisition. Differences involve (1) different neuropsychological profiles (typically with much more preserved verbal skills in individuals with AS as compared to HFA) and (2) usually higher levels of social motivation in individuals with AS. Over the last several years the body of work in this area has increased dramatically with several hundred papers focusing on treatment issues. We emphasize that, in considering treatment options, it is also important to maintain an awareness of any comorbid conditions present and the possibility that these may be addressed through psychotherapy or medication (see Westphal et al., Chapter 9, this volume).

Pharmacological treatments can be used to address inattention, anxiety, or depression, although, to date, the core social disability has not been directly targeted (see Westphal et al., Chapter 9, this volume; Tsai, 2007, for reviews). Unfortunately, much of this literature has consisted of case reports or open clinical trails; double-blind studies focusing solely on the AS population are limited.

Psychological and educational interventions have been much more extensively discussed in the literature, with several books on the topic highlighting specific strategies (e.g., Ozonoff, Dawson, & McPartland, 2002; Atwood, 2003; Howlin, 1999; Myles, 2005; Chapters 5–8, this volume). As might be expected, interventions have typically focused on facilitating better verbal skills and particular areas of strength in AS, with an emphasis on developing and implementing compensatory strategies for weaknesses and providing environmental supports to maximize effective learning and functioning, with the important provision that all such supports be designed in the context of a comprehensive assessment (Klin et al., 2005). Typical supports include those involved in teaching basic social and communication skills, adaptive functioning, and (depending on what is developmentally appropriate) academic or vocational skills; as with autism, issues of generalization across settings are important (Lee & Park, 2007).

We have emphasized the importance of explicit teaching and rote learning, using a parts-to-whole verbal instruction approach (Klin, McPartland, et al., 2005). Motor (including graphomotor and visuomotor) deficits also require support via physical and occupational therapies and, where available, the use assistive technologies (e.g., using a laptop to type assignments rather than writing, using electronic organizers). Occupational therapy that emphasizes the integration of activities with the learning of visual–spatial concepts and orientation, as well as body awareness, has been advocated. Similarly, an explicit focus on adaptive skills and generalization has been repeatedly emphasized as critical (Lee & Park, 2007). Unfortunately, the tendency of individuals with AS toward a rigid focus on familiarity and routine can pose challenges for generalization; on the other hand, these same tendencies can be used to encourage positive coping strategies.

Behavioral and emotional issues are frequently challenges to effective intervention and arise because social disability is associated with problems in regulation and self-awareness. The use of explicit problem-solving strategies such as rules/scripts/"self-talk" can be helpful. An increased body of work has focused on strategies derived from cognitive-behavioral therapy (CBT; e.g., Wood, Drahota, Sze, Har, Chiu, et al., 2009; Cardaciotto & Herbert, 2004; Weiss & Lunsky, 2010; Farrugia & Hudson, 2006). Speech pathologists can also be helpful (both through direct intervention and consultation) in focusing on development of pragmatic skills. In general, the focus should be on explicit teaching/modeling/feedback of relevant tasks such as self-monitoring, topic management, turn taking, conversational rules, volume of speech, prosody, and so forth (Paul, Orlovski, Marcinko, & Volkmar, 2009; Shriberg et al., 2001; Weintraub et al., 1981; Paul, Landa, & Schoen, Chapter 4, and Rubin, Chapter 6, this volume).

Unfortunately, the social skills gap begins to increase more dramatically as individuals enter adolescence, often further exacerbating social isolation and leading to the potential for anxiety as well as the likelihood of bullying (Shtayermman, 2007; Carter, 2009; Dubin, 2007; McManus, 2008; Myles et al., Chapter 7, this volume). The latter problem increases dramatically in adolescence for many individuals, given their apparent good language skills, which can mislead both teachers and peers. Lack of appreciation of social nuance and difficulties in understanding humor and figurative language lead to further isolation, since the teenager with AS is frequently laughed at (for behaviors that others understandably see as humorous but are not usually meant to be); conversely, not being able to successfully use humor with peers (making what are meant to be jokes either about arcane topics of special interest or topics that usually would be considered too sensitive for discussion; see McCormick, 2001; Samson & Hegenloh, 2010) is equally stigmatizing.

Although evidence-based research is relatively limited, it does appear that a range of procedures can be used to teach social skills. These include direct work with a therapist, social skills groups, and peer modeling (see Paul, 2003). As with other areas (and in some ways even more so), the complexity of social interaction requires explicit teaching of rules (what can and can't be discussed and with whom), conversational and interactional strategies, and so forth (Kaland, Mortensen, & Smith, 2011; Rubin & Lennon, 2004; Saulnier & Klin, 2007). The individual's often strong motivation to establish friendships and peer connections and the often strong verbal and rote-memory skills are important strengths than be used effectively in this process. The range of social skills teaching methods has also dramatically increased over the past decade and can be used for individuals of various ages (see Beaumont & Sofronoff, 2008; Macintosh & Dissanayake, 2006; Muller, 2010; Patrick, 2008). These groups may or may not involve typically developing peers and sometimes make excellent use of siblings as part of the group process. Psychotherapy (particularly if more conceptualized around a longer-term "life coaching" model) can be productive for this population as well (Munro, 2010; Mero, 2002; Volkmar, et al., 2011).

ASPERGER SYNDROME AND DSM-5

DSM-5, published in May 2013 (American Psychiatric Association, 2013), removed AS as a formal diagnosis. The decision to "drop" AS as a formal diagnosis has been the source of much controversy (see Volkmar & Reichow, in press). The broad conceptual focuses of DSM-5 likely impacted this decision by eliminating "subthreshold" categories, subtypes of PDDs used inconsistently by clinicians, alongside an emphasis on standardized diagnostic instruments for criteria. These problems were particularly relevant for AS, given the continued discussions of how best to "draw the line" separating the condition from HFA, the perception by many of AS as a specific personality style (as Asperger himself originally suggested; see also Rutter, 2011), and the relative dearth (not surprisingly, given the other controversies) of extensively developed diagnostic instruments demonstrating specificity for AS versus other forms of ASD (Taheri & Perry, 2012).

SUMMARY AND DIRECTIONS FOR THE FUTURE

The official recognition of AS as a diagnostic concept in 1994 markedly increased both scientific and public awareness of this condition (Wing, 2005). This increased awareness has resulted in a substantial and growing body of research and a similarly growing body of work focused on intervention strategies. This body of work also is a testament to an important clinical need.

In reviewing this work, it is clear that major differences in diagnostic approach have remained, reflecting both the DSM/ICD ambivalence about the category, but also, to some extent, the debate on validity of the concept apart from autism and the variability in its usage by clinicians (Lord et al., 2012). Both of these challenge have existed since Wing's (1981) seminal report. The decision to drop (rather than refine) the concept in DSM-5 will complicate research and clinical activities that could further clarify the validity and clinical utility of AS as an official diagnosis. The current state of research on the "validity" of AS as a distinct disorder might best be summarized as "inconclusive," leaving the door open to further research (Volkmar, 2010; see also Ghaziuddin, 2010, 2011; Rutter, 2011). The loss of the diagnostic term may, particularly in the United States, result in a loss of services for individuals residing in states that recognize AS as a handicapping condition. There will be a need to foster awareness of the DSM-5 stipulation that, for individuals previously meeting criteria for one of the PDDs as defined in DSM-IV, eligibility for services should continue even if they are now found not to meet the new set of DSM-5 criteria for ASD (American Psychiatric Association, 2013).

Given what increasingly appears to be the complexity of autism as a condition and the neural basis of social behavior, it seems likely that there may be many underlying paths of pathophysiology that result in it and in autistic-like conditions, so that perhaps the use of the term *autisms,* rather than ASD, might be more appropriate. Within the overarching category it seems likely that the identification of specific and more homogeneous subtypes could enhance both clinical work and research. There is some suggestion, from the data reviewed in this chapter, that a concept closer to that originally proposed by Hans Asperger may be most productive in this regard, but the issue remains an open one.

REFERENCES

Ambery, F. Z., Russell, A. J., Perry, K., Morris, R., & Murphy, D. G. (2006). Neuropsychological functioning in adults with Asperger syndrome. *Autism, 10*(6), 551–564.

American Psychiatric Association. (1980). *Diagnostic and statistical manual of mental disorders* (3rd ed.). Washington, DC: Author.

American Psychiatric Association. (1987). *Diagnostic and statistical manual of mental disorders* (3rd ed., rev.). Washington, DC: Author.

American Psychiatric Association. (1994). *Diagnostic and statistical manual of mental disorders* (4th ed.). Washington, DC: Author.

American Psychiatric Association. (2000). *Diagnostic and statistical manual of mental disorders* (4th ed., text rev.). Washington, DC: Author.

American Psychiatric Association. (2013). *Diagnostic and statistical manual of mental disorders* (5th ed.). Arlington, VA: Author.

Anneren, G., Dahl, N., Uddenfeldt, U., & Janols, L. O. (1995). Asperger syndrome in a boy with a balanced de novo translocation. *American Journal of Medical Genetics, 56*(3), 330–331.

Asperger, H. (1944). Die "autistichen Psychopathen" im Kindersalter. *Archiv für Psychiatrie und Nervenkrankheiten, 117,* 76–136.

Asperger, H. (1979). Problems of infantile autism. *Communication, 13,* 45–52.

Atwood, T. (2003). Frameworks for behavioral intervention. *Child and Adolescent Psychiatric Clinics of North America, 12,* 65–86.

Baird, G., Charman, T., Baron-Cohen, S., Cox, A., Swettenham, J., Wheelwright, S., et al. (2000). A screening instrument for autism at 18 months of age: A 6-year follow-up study. *Journal of the American Academy of Child and Adolescent Psychiatry, 39*(6), 694–702.

Baron-Cohen, S. (1988). An assessment of violence in a young man with Asperger's syndrome. *Journal of Child Psychology and Psychiatry, 29*(3), 351–360.

Baron-Cohen, S. (1989). Do autistic children have obsessions and compulsions? *British Journal of Clinical Psychology, 28*(Pt. 3), 193–200.

Baron-Cohen, S. (2000a). Autism: Deficits in folk psychology exist alongside superiority in folk physics. In S. Baron-Cohen, H. Tager-Flusberg, & D. J. Cohen (Eds.), *Understanding other minds: Perspectives from developmental cognitive neuroscience* (2nd ed., pp. 73–82). New York: Oxford University Press.

Baron-Cohen, S. (2000b). Is Asperger syndrome/high-functioning autism necessarily a disability? *Development and Psychopathology, 12*(3), 489–500.

Bartolucci, G., & Szatmari, P. (1987). Possible similarities between the fragile X and Asperger's syndromes. *American Journal of Diseases of Children, 141*(6), 601–602.

Beaumont, R., & Sofronoff, K. (2008). A multi-component social skills intervention for children with Asperger syndrome: The Junior Detective Training Program: Errata. *Journal of Child Psychology and Psychiatry, 49*(8), 895.

Bejerot, S., & Duvner, T. (1995). Asperger's syndrome of schizophrenia? *Nordic Journal of Psychiatry, 49*(2), 145.

Bennetto, L., Pennington, B. F., & Rogers, S. J. (1996). Intact and impaired memory functions in autism. *Child Development, 67*(4), 1816–1835.

Berthier, M. L., Bayes, A., & Tolosa, E. S. (1993). Magnetic resonance imaging in patients with concurrent Tourette's disorder and Asperger's syndrome. *Journal of the American Academy of Child and Adolescent Psychiatry, 32*(3), 633–639.

Berthier, M. L., Starkstein, S. E., & Leiguarda, R. (1990). Developmental cortical anomalies in Asperger's syndrome: Neuroradiological findings in two patients. *Journal of Neuropsychiatry and Clinical Neurosciences, 2*(2), 197–201.

Blakemore, S.-J., Tavassoli, T. C., Susana, T. R., & Haggard, P. (2006). Tactile sensitivity in Asperger syndrome. *Brain and Cognition, 61*(1), 5–13.

Bleuler, E. (1911). *Dementia praecox oder Gruppe der Schizophrenien* (J. Zinkin, Trans.). New York: International Universities Press.

Bloemen, O. J., Deeley, Q., Sundram, F., Daly, E. M., Barker, G. J., Jones, D. K., et al. (2010). White matter integrity in Asperger syndrome: A preliminary diffusion tensor magnetic resonance imaging study in adults. *Autism Research, 3*(5), 203–213.

Bolte, S., & Bosch, G. (2004). Bosch's cases: A 40 year follow-up of patients with infantile autism and Asperger syndrome. *German Journal of Psychiatry, 7*(1), 10–13.

Bowler, D. M. (1992). "Theory of mind" in Asperger's syndrome. *Journal of Child Psychology and Psychiatry, 33*(5), 877–893.

Bowman, E. P. (1988). Asperger's syndrome and autism: The case for a connection. *British Journal of Psychiatry, 152*, 377–382.

Cardaciotto, L., & Herbert, J. D. (2004). Cognitive behavior therapy for social anxiety disorder in the context of Asperger's syndrome: A single-subject report. *Cognitive and Behavioral Practice, 11*(1), 75–81.

Carter, S. (2009). Bullying of students with Asperger syndrome. *Issues in Comprehensive Pediatric Nursing, 32*(3), 145–154.

Cascio, C., McGlone, F., Folger, S., Tannan, V., Baranek, G., Pelphrey, K. A., et al. (2008). Tactile perception in adults with autism: A multidimensional psychophysical study. *Journal of Autism and Developmental Disorders, 38*(1), 127–137.

Cederlund, M., & Gillberg, C. (2004). One hundred males with Asperger syndrome: A clinical study of background and associated factors. *Developmental Medicine and Child Neurology, 46*(10), 652–660.

Cederlund, M., Hagberg, B., Billstedt, E., Gillberg, I., & Gillberg, C. (2008). Asperger syndrome and autism: A comparative longitudinal follow-up study more than 5 years after original diagnosis. *Journal of Autism and Developmental Disorders, 38*(1), 72–85.

Constantino, J. N., & Todd, R. D. (2003). Autistic traits in the general population: A twin study. *Archives of General Psychiatry, 60*(5), 524–530.

Dahlgren, S. O., & Trillingsgaard, A. (1996). Theory of mind in non-retarded children with autism and Asperger's syndrome: A research note. *Journal of Child Psychology and Psychiatry, 37*(6), 759–763.

DeLong, G. R., & Dwyer, J. T. (1988). Correlation of family history with specific autistic subgroups: Asperger's syndrome and bipolar affective disease. *Journal of Autism and Developmental Disorders, 18*(4), 593–600.

Dubin, N. (2007). *Asperger syndrome and bullying: Strategies and solutions.* London, UK: Jessica Kingsley.

Duggal, H. (2003). Bipolar disorder with Asperger's disorder [Comment/reply]. *American Journal of Psychiatry, 160*(1), 184–185.

Dunn, W. (1999). *The Sensory Profile: Users manual.* San Antonio, TX: Psychlogical Corporation.

Dunn, W., Myles, B. S., & Orr, S. (2002). Sensory processing issues associated with Asperger syndrome: A preliminary investigation. *American Journal of Occupational Therapy, 56*(1), 97–102.

Ehlers, S., Nyden, A., Gillberg, C., Dahlgren Sandberg, A., Dahlgren, S., & et al. (1997). Asperger syndrome, autism, and attention disorders: A comparative study of the cognitive profiles of 120 children. *Journal of Child Psychology and Psychiatry and Allied Disciplines, 38*(2), 207–217.

Eisenmajer, R., Prior, M., Leekam, S., Wing, L., Gould, J., et al. (1996). Comparison of clinical symptoms in autism and Asperger's disorder. *Journal of the American Academy of Child and Adolesecent Psychiatry, 35*(11), 1523–1531.

Ellis, H. D., Ellis, D. M., Fraser, W., & Deb, S. (1994). A preliminary study of right hemisphere cognitive deficits and impaired social judgments among young people with Asperger syndrome. *European Child and Adolesecent Psychiatry, 3*(4), 255–266.

Everall, I. P., & LeCouteur, A. (1990). Firesetting in an adolescent boy with Asperger's syndrome. *British Journal of Psychiatry, 157,* 284–287.

Farrugia, S., & Hudson, J. (2006). Anxiety in adolescents with Asperger syndrome: Negative thoughts, behavioral problems, and life interference. *Focus on Autism and Other Developmental Disorders, 21*(1), 25–35.

Folstein, S. E., & Santangelo, S. L. (2000). Does Asperger syndrome aggregate in families? In A. Klin & F. R. Volkmar (Eds.), *Asperger syndrome* (pp. 159–171). New York: Guilford Press.

Fontenelle, L. F., Mendlowicz, M. V., Bezerra de Menezes, G., dos Santos Martins, R. R., & Versiani, M. (2004). Asperger syndrome, obsessive–compulsive disorder, and major depression in a patient with 45,X/46,XY mosaicism. *Psychopathology, 37*(3), 105–109.

Frith, U. (Ed.). (1991). *Autism and Asperger syndrome.* New York: Cambridge University Press.

Frith, U. (2004). Emanuel Miller lecture: Confusions and controversies about Asperger syndrome. *Journal of Child Psychology and Psychiatry, 45*(4), 672–686.

Fujikawa, H., Kobayashi, R., Koga, Y., & Murata, T. (1987). A case of Asperger's syndrome in a nineteen-year-old who showed psychotic breakdown with depressive state and attempted suicide after entering university. *Japanese Journal of Child and Adolesecent Psychiatry, 28*(4), 217–225.

Gallucci, G., Hackerman, F., & Schmidt, C. W. (2005). Gender identity disorder in an adult male with Asperger's syndrome. *Sexuality and Disability, 23*(1), 35–40.

Ghaziuddin, M. (2002). Asperger syndrome: Associated psychiatric and medical conditions. *Focus on Autism and Other Developmental Disabilities, 17*(3), 138–144.

Ghaziuddin, M. (2005). A family history study of Asperger syndrome. *Journal of Autism and Developmental Disorders, 35*(2), 177–182.

Ghaziuddin, M. (2010). Brief report: Should the DSM-V drop Asperger syndrome? *Journal of Autism and Developmental Disorders, 40*(9), 1146–1148.

Ghaziuddin, M. (2011). Asperger disorder in the DSM-V: Sacrificing utility for validity. *Journal of the American Academy of Child and Adolesecent Psychiatry, 50*(2), 192–193.

Ghaziuddin, M., & Butler, E. (1998). Clumsiness in autism and Asperger syndrome: A further report. *Journal of Intellectual Disability Research, 42*(Pt. 1), 43–48.

Ghaziuddin, M., Butler, E., Tsai, L., & Ghaziuddin, N. (1994). Is clumsiness a marker for Asperger syndrome? *Journal of Intellectual Disability Research, 38*(Pt. 5), 519–527.

Ghaziuddin, M., Ghaziuddin, N., & Tsai, L. (1992). Comorbidity of autistic disorder in children and adolescents. *European Child and Adolesecent Psychiatry, 1*(4), 209–213.

Ghaziuddin, M., & Greden, J. (1998). Depression in children with autism/pervasive developmental disorders: A case–control family history study. *Journal of Autism and Developmental Disorders, 28*(2), 111–115.

Ghaziuddin, M., Leininger, L., & Tsai, L. (1995). Thought disorder in Asperger syndrome: Comparison with high-functioning autism. *Journal of Autism and Developmental Disorders, 25*(3), 311–317.

Ghaziuddin, M., & Mountain-Kimchi, K. (2004). Defining the intellectual profile of Asperger syndrome: Comparison with high-functioning autism. *Journal of Autism and Developmental Disorders, 34*(3), 279–284.

Ghaziuddin, M., Shakal, J., & Tsai, L. (1995). Obstetric factors in Asperger syndrome: comparison with high-functioning autism. *Journal of Intellectual Disability Research, 39*(Pt. 6), 538–543.

Ghaziuddin, M., Tsai, L., & Ghaziuddin, N. (1991). Brief report: Violence in Asperger syndrome—a critique. *Journal of Autism and Developmental Disorders, 21*(3), 349–354.

Ghaziuddin, N., Metler, L., Ghaziuddin, M., Tsai, L., et al. (1993). Three siblings with Asperger syndrome: A family case study. *European Child and Adolescent Psychiatry, 2*(1), 44–49.

Gilchrist, A., Green, J., Cox, A., Burton, D., Rutter, M., & Le Couteur, A. (2001). Development and current functioning in adolescents with Asperger syndrome: A comparative study. *Journal of Child Psychology and Psychiatry and Allied Disciplines, 42*(2), 227–240.

Gillberg, C. (1985). Asperger's syndrome and recurrent psychosis: A case study. *Journal of Autism and Developmental Disorders, 15*(4), 389–397.

Gillberg, C. (1991). Clinical and neurobiological aspects of Asperger syndrome in six family studies. In U. Frith (Ed.), *Autism and Asperger syndrome* (pp. 122–146). Cambridge University Press.

Gillberg, C., Gillberg, I., & Steffenburg, S. (1992). Siblings and parents of children with autism: A controlled population-based study. *Developmental Medicine and Child Neurology, 34*(5), 389–398.

Gillberg, I. C., & Gillberg, C. (1989). Asperger syndrome—some epidemiological considerations: A research note. *Journal of Child Psychology and Psychiatry and Allied Disciplines, 30*(4), 631–638.

Gold, R., & Faust, M. (2010). Right hemisphere dysfunction and metaphor comprehension in young adults with Asperger Syndrome. *Journal of Autism and Developmental Disorders, 40*, 800–811.

Goldstein, G., Johnson, C. R., & Minshew, N. J. (2001). Attentional processes in autism. *Journal of Autism and Developmental Disorders, 31*(4), 433–440.

Green, D., Baird, G., Barnett, A. L., Henderson, L., Huber, J., & Henderson, S. E. (2002). The severity and nature of motor impairment in Asperger's syndrome: A comparison with specific developmental disorder of motor function. *Journal of Child Psychology and Psychiatry and Allied Disciplines, 43*(5), 655–668.

Green, J., Gilchrist, A., Burton, D., & Cox, A. (2000). Social and psychiatric functioning in adolescents with Asperger syndrome compared with conduct disorder. *Journal of Autism and Developmental Disorders, 30*(4), 279–293.

Gunter, H. L., Ghaziuddin, M., & Ellis, H. D. (2002). Asperger syndrome: Tests of right hemisphere functioning and interhemispheric communication. *Journal of Autism and Developmental Disorders, 32*(4), 263–281.

Haglund, N. G., & Kallen, K. B. (2011). Risk factors for autism and Asperger syndrome: Perinatal factors and migration. *Autism, 15*(2), 163–183.

Hall, I., & Bernal, J. (1995). Asperger's syndrome and violence [Comment/reply]. *British Journal of Psychiatry, 166*(2), 262.

Hanson, E. M. (2003). A comparison of individuals with Asperger syndrome and autism on neuropsychological measures sensitive to the ability to shift attention. *Dissertation Abstracts International Section B: Sciences and Engineering, 64*(1-B), 420.

Happé, F., Ehlers, S., Fletcher, P., Frith, U., Johansson, M., Gillberg, C., et al. (1996). "Theory of mind" in the brain: Evidence from a PET scan study of Asperger syndrome. *NeuroReport, 8*(1), 197–201.

Hardan, A. Y., Girgis, R. R., Adams, J., Gilbert, A. R., Melhem, N. M., Keshavan, M. S., et al. (2008). Abnormal association between the thalamus and brain size in Asperger's disorder. *Journal of Autism and Developmental Disorders, 38*(2), 390–394.

Hermelin, B. (2001). *Bright splinters of the mind: A personal story of research with autistic savants*. London: Jessica Kingsley.

Hilton, C., Wente, L., LaVesser, P., Ito, M., Reed, C., & Herzberg, G. (2007). Relationship between motor skill impairment and severity in children with Asperger syndrome. *Research in Autism Spectrum Disorders, 1*(4), 339–349.

Hippler, K., & Klicpera, C. (2003). A retrospective analysis of the clinical case records of "autistic psychopaths" diagnosed by Hans Asperger and his team at the University Children's Hospital, Vienna. *Philosophical Transactions of the Royal Society of London Series B: Biological Sciences, 358*(1430), 291–301.

Hippler, K., & Klicpera, C. (2005). Hans Asperger and his patients: A retrospective examination of the spectrum of autistic disorders. *Zeitschrift für Kinder- und Jugendpsychiatrie und Psychotherapie, 33*(1), 35–47.

Hippler, K., Viding, E., Klicpera, C., & Happé, F. (2010). No increase in criminal convictions in Hans Asperger's original cohort. *Journal of Autism and Developmental Disorders, 40*(6), 774–780.

Howlin, P. (2005). Outcomes in autism spectrum disorders. In F. R. Volkmar, A. Klin, R. Paul, & D. J. Cohen (Eds.), *Handbook of autism and pervasive developmental disorders* (3rd ed., Vol. 1, pp. 201–222). Hoboken, NJ: Wiley.

Howlin, P., & Asgharian, A. (1999). The diagnosis of autism and Asperger syndrome: Findings from a survey of 770 families. *Developmental Medicine and Child Neurology, 41*(12), 834–839.

Howlin, P., & Goode, S. (1998). Outcome in adult life for people with autism and Asperger's syndrome. In F. R. Volkmar (Ed.), *Autism and pervasive developmental disorders: Cambridge monographs in child and adolescent psychiatry* (pp. 209–241). New York: Cambridge University Press.

Humphrey, A. (2008). Anxiety and Asperger's disorder. In P. Appleton (Ed.), *Children's anxiety: A contextual approach* (pp. 121–128). New York: Routledge/Taylor & Francis Group.

Iwanami, A., Okajima, Y., Ota, H., Tani, M., Yamada, T., Hashimoro, R., et al. (2011). Task dependent prefrontal dysfunction in persons with Asperger's disorder investigated with multi-channel near-infrared spectroscopy. *Research in Autism Spectrum Disorders, 5*(3), 1187–1193.

Jones, P. B., & Kerwin, R. W. (1990). Left temporal lobe damage in Asperger's syndrome. *British Journal of Psychiatry, 156*, 570–572.

Joseph, R. M., McGrath, L. M., & Tager-Flusberg, H. (2005). Executive dysfunction and its relation to language ability in verbal school-age children with autism. *Developmental Neuropsychology, 27*(3), 361–378.

Joshi, G., Petty, C., Wozniak, J., Henin, A., Fried, R., Galdo, M., et al. (2010). The heavy burden of psychiatric comorbidity in youth with autism spectrum disorders: A large comparative study of a psychiatrically referred population. *Journal of Autism and Developmental Disorders, 40*(11), 1361–1370.

Jou, R. J., Minshew, N. J., Keshavan, M. S., & Hardan, A. Y. (2010). Cortical gyrification in autistic and asperger disorders: A preliminary magnetic resonance imaging study. *Journal of Child Neurology, 25*, 1462–1467.

Kaland, N., Moller-Nielsen, A., Callesen, K., Mortensen, E. L., Gottlieb, D., & Smith, L. (2002). A new "advanced" test of theory of mind: Evidence from children and adolescents with Asperger syndrome. *Journal of Child Psychology and Psychiatry and Allied Disciplines, 43*(4), 517–528.

Kaland, N., Mortensen, E. L., & Smith, L. (2011). Social communication

impairments in children and adolescents with Asperger syndrome: Slow
response time and the impact of prompting. *Research in Autism Spectrum
Disorders, 5*(3), 1129–1137.

Kamp-Becker, I., Wulf, C., Bachmann, C. J., Ghahreman, M., Heinzel-Gutenbrun-
ner, M., Gerber, G., et al. (2010). Early symptoms of Asperger syndrome in
childhood: A retrospective study. *Kindheit und Entwicklung, 19*(3), 168–176.

Kanner, L. (1943). Autistic disturbances of affective contact. *Nervous Child, 2,*
217–250.

Kanner, L. (1954). Discussion of Robinson and Vitale's paper on childen with circumscribed interests. *American Journal of Orthopsychiatry 24*, 764–766.

Kerbeshian, J., & Burd, L. (1986). Asperger's syndrome and Tourette syndrome:
The case of the pinball wizard. *British Journal of Psychiatry, 148*, 731–736.

Kim, J. A., Szatmari, P., Bryson, S. E., Streiner, D. L., & Wilson, F. J. (2000). The
prevalence of anxiety and mood problems among children with autism and
Asperger syndrome. *Autism, 4*(2), 117–132.

Kleinhans, N., Akshoomoff, N., & Delis, D. C. (2005). Executive functions in
autism and Asperger's disorder: Flexibility, fluency, and inhibition. *Developmental Neuropsychology, 27*(3), 379–401.

Klin, A., Danovitch, J. H., Merz, A. B., & Volkmar, F. R. (2007). Circumscribed
interests in higher functioning individuals with autism spectrum disorder: An
exploratory study. *Research and Practice for Persons with Severe Disabilities,
32*(2), 890–899.

Klin, A., Jones, W., Schultz, R., & Volkmar, F. R. (2003). The enactive mind, or
from actions to cognition: Lessons from autism. *Philosophical Transactions
of the Royal Society of London—Series B: Biological Sciences, 358*(1430),
345—360.

Klin, A., McPartland, J., & Volkmar, F. R. (2005). Asperger syndrome. In F. R.
Volkmar, A. Klin, R. Paul, & D. J. Cohen (Eds.), *Handbook of autism and
pervasive developmental disorders* (3rd ed., pp. 88–125). Hoboken, NJ:
Wiley.

Klin, A., Pauls, D., Schultz, R., & Volkmar, F. R. (2005). Three diagnostic
approaches to Asperger syndrome: Implications for research. *Journal of
Autism and Developmental Disorders, 35*(2), 221–234.

Klin, A., Sparrow, S. S., Volkmar, F. R., Cicchetti, D. V., & Rourke, B. P. (1995).
Asperger syndrome. In B. P. Rourke (Ed.), *Syndrome of nonverbal learning
disabilities: Neurodevelopmental manifestations* (pp. 93–118). New York:
Guilford Press.

Klin, A., & Volkmar, F. R. (1997). Asperger syndrome. In D. J. Cohen & F. R.
Volkmar (Eds.), *Handbook of autism andpervasive developmental disorders*
(2nd ed., pp. 94–122). New York: Wiley.

Klin, A., & Volkmar, F. R. (2003). Asperger syndrome: Diagnosis and external validity. *Child and Adolescent Psychiatric Clinics of North America, 12*(1), 1–13.

Klin, A., Volkmar, F. R., & Sparrow, S. S. (Eds.). (2000). *Asperger syndrome.* New
York: Guilford Press.

Korpilahti, P., Jansson-Verkasalo, E., Mattila, M.-L., Kuusikko, S., Suominen, K.,
Rytky, S., et al. (2007). Processing of affective speech prosody is impaired in
Asperger syndrome. *Journal of Autism and Developmental Disorders, 37*(8),
1539–1549.

Koyama, T., Tachimori, H., Osada, H., Takeda, T., & Kurita, H. (2007). Cognitive and symptom profiles in Asperger's syndrome and high-functioning autism. *Psychiatry and Clinical Neurosciences, 61*(1), 99–104.

Kraemer, B., Delsignore, A., Gundelfinger, R., Schnyder, U., & Hepp, U. (2005). Comorbidity of Asperger syndrome and gender identity disorder. *European Child and Adolesecent Psychiatry, 14*(5), 292–296.

Kujala, T., Aho, E., Lepistö, T., Jansson-Verkasato, E., & Viemen-von Wendt, T. (2007). Atypical pattern of discriminating sound features in adults with Asperger syndrome as reflected by the mismatch negativity. *Biological Psychology, 75*(1), 109–114.

Larsen, F., & Mouridsen, S. (1997). The outcome of children with childhood autism and Asperger syndrome originally diagnosed as psychotic: A 30-year follow-up study of subjects hospitalized as children. *European Child and Adolescent Psychiatry, 6*(4), 181–190.

Lee, H. J., & Park, H. R. (2007). An integrated literature review on the adaptive behavior of individuals with Asperger syndrome. *Remedial and Special Education, 28*(3), 132–139.

Lepistö, T., Silokallio, S., Nieminen-von Wendt, T., Alku, P., Naatanen, R., & Kujala, T. (2006). Auditory perception and attention as reflected by the brain event-related potentials in children with Asperger syndrome. *Clinical Neurophysiology, 117*(10), 2161–2171.

Lincoln, A., Courchesne, E., Allen, M., Hanson, E., & Ene, M. (1998). Neurobiology of Asperger syndrome: Seven case studies and quantitative magnetic resonance imaging findings. In E. Schopler, G. B. Mesibov, & L. J. Kunc (Eds.), *Asperger syndrome or high functioning autism?* (pp. 145–166). New York: Plenum Press.

Littlejohns, C. S., Clarke, D. J., & Corbett, J. A. (1990). Tourette-like disorder in Asperger's syndrome. *British Journal of Psychiatry, 156*, 430–433.

Lord, C., Petkova, E., Hus, V., Gan, W., Lu, F., et al. (2012). A multisite study of the clinical diagnosis of different autism spectrum disorders. *Archives of General Psychiatry, 69*(3), 306–313.

Lotspeich, L., Kwon, H., Schumann, C. M., Fryer, S. L., Goodlin-Jones, B. L., Buonocore, M. H., et al. (2004). Investigation of neuroanatomical differences between autism and Asperger syndrome. *Archives of General Psychiatry, 61*(3), 291–298.

Macintosh, K., & Dissanayake, C. (2006). Social skills and problem behaviours in school-aged children with high-functioning autism and Asperger's disorder. *Journal of Autism and Developmental Disorders, 36*(8), 1065–1076.

Manjiviona, J., & Prior, M. (1995). Comparison of Asperger syndrome and high-functioning autistic children on a test of motor impairment. *Journal of Autism and Developmental Disorders, 25*(1), 23–39.

Manjiviona, J., & Prior, M. (1999). Neuropsychological profiles of children with Asperger syndrome and autism. *Autism, 3*(4), 327–356.

Marriage, K., Miles, T., Stokes, D., & Davey, M. (1993). Clinical and research implications of the co-occurrence of Asperger's and Tourette syndromes. *Australian and New Zealand Journal of Psychiatry, 27*(4), 666–672.

Mattila, M.-L., Kielinen, M., Linna, S. L., Jussila, K., Ebeling, H., et al. (2011). Autism spectrum disorders according to DSM-IV-TR and comparison with DSM-5 draft criteria: An epidemiological study. *Journal of the American Academy of Child and Adolesecent Psychiatry, 50*(6), 583–592.

Mawhood, L., & Howlin, P. (1999). The outcome of a supported employment scheme for high-functioning adults with autism or Asperger syndrome. *Autism, 3*(3), 229–254.

Mawson, D. C., Grounds, A., & Tantam, D. (1985). Violence and Asperger's syndrome: A case study. *British Journal of Psychiatry, 147,* 566–569.

Mayes, S. D., Calhoun, S. L., & Crites, D. L. (2001). Does DSM-IV Asperger's disorder exist? *Journal of Abnormal Child Psychology, 29*(3), 263–271.

Mazefsky, C. A., McPartland, J. C., Gastgeb, H. Z., & Minshew, N. J. (2013). Comparability of DSM-IV and DSM-5 ASD research samples. *Journal of Autism and Developmental Disorders, 43*(5), 1236–1242.

McAlonan, G., Cheung, C., Cheung, V., Wong, N., Suckling, J., & Chua, S. (2009). Differential effects on white-matter systems in high-functioning autism and Asperger syndrome. *Psychological Medicine: A Journal of Research in Psychiatry and the Allied Sciences, 39*(11), 1885–1893.

McAlonan, G. M., Daly, E., Kumari, V., Critchley, H. D., van Amelsvoort, T., Suckling, J., et al. (2002). Brain anatomy and sensorimotor gating in Asperger's syndrome. *Brain, 125*(Pt. 7), 1594–1606.

McAlonan, G. M., Einne, M., Suckling, J., Wong, N., Cheung, V., & Chua, S. E. (2008). Distinct patterns of grey matter abnormality in high-functioning autism and Asperger's syndrome. *Journal of Child Psychology and Psychiatry and Allied Disciplines, 49*(12), 1287–1295.

McCormick, J. B. (2001). The effect of Asperger's syndrome on the humor perception and production of teenage boys. *Dissertation Abstracts International Section B: Sciences and Engineering, 62*(4-B), 2068.

McManus, M. (2008). Review of Asperer syndrome and bullying: Strategies and solutions. *Support for Learning, 23*(1), 50.

McPartland, J., Reichow, B., & Volkmar, F. R. (2011). Sensitivity and specificity of proposed DSM-5 diagnostic criteria for autism spectrum disorder. *Journal of the American Academy of Child and Adolescent Psychiatry, 51*(4), 368–383.

Mero, M.-M. (2002). Asperger syndrome with comorbid emotional disorder—treatment with psychoanalytic psychotherapy. *International Journal of Circumpolar Health, 61*(Suppl. 2), 80–89.

Miles, S. W., & Capelle, P. (1987). Asperger's syndrome and aminoaciduria: A case example. *British Journal of Psychiatry, 150,* 397–400.

Miller, J. N., & Ozonoff, S. (1997). Did Asperger's cases have Asperger's disorder?: A research note. *Journal of Child Psychology and Psychiatry, 38*(2), 247–251.

Minshew, N. J., Meyer, J., & Goldstein, G. (2002). Abstract reasoning in autism: A dissociation between concept formation and concept identification. *Neuropsychology, 16*(3), 327–334.

Minshew, N. J., & Williams, D. L. (2007). The new neurobiology of autism: Cortex, connectivity, and neuronal organization. [Erratum appears in *Archives of Neurology,* 2007, *64*(10), 1464.] *Archives of Neurology, 64*(7), 945–950.

Miyahara, M., Tsujii, M., Hori, M., Nakanishi, K., Kageyama, H., & Sugiyama, T. (1997). Motor incoordination in children with Asperger syndrome and learning disabilities. *Journal of Autism and Developmental Disorders, 27*(5), 595–603.

Morris, R. G., Rowe, A., Fox, N., Feigenbaum, J., Miotto, E., & Howlin, P. (1999). Spatial working memory in Asperger's syndrome and in patients with focal frontal and temporal lobe lesions. *Brain and Cognition, 41*(1), 9–26.

Muller, E., Schuler, A., Burton, B. A., & Yates, G. B. (2003). Meeting the vocational support needs of individuals with Asperger syndrome and other autism spectrum disabilities. *Journal of Vocational Rehabilitation, 18*(3), 163–175.

Muller, R., (2010). Will you play with me?: Improving social skills for children with Asperger syndrome. *International Journal of Disability, Development and Education, 57*(3), 331–334.

Munro, J. (2010). An integrated model of psychotherapy for teens and adults with Asperger syndrome. *Journal of Systemic Therapies, 29*(3), 82–96.

Murphy, D. G., Critchley, H. D., Schmitz, N., McAlonan, G., Van Amelsvoort, T., Robertson, D., et al. (2002). Asperger syndrome: A proton magnetic resonance spectroscopy study of brain. *Archives of General Psychiatry, 59*(10), 885–891.

Murphy, D. G., Daly, E., Schmitz, N., Toal, F., Murphy, K., Curran, S., et al. (2006). Cortical serotonin 5-HT2A receptor binding and social communication in adults with Asperger's syndrome: An *in vivo* SPECT study. *American Journal of Psychiatry, 163*(5), 934–936.

Myles, B. S. (2005). *Children and youth with Asperger syndrome: Strategies for success in inclusive settings.* Thousand Oaks, CA: Corwin Press.

Nagy, J., & Szatmari, P. (1986). A chart review of schizotypal personality disorders in children. *Journal of Autism and Developmental Disorders, 16*(3), 351–367.

Noterdaeme, M., Wriedt, E., & Hohne, C. (2010). Asperger's syndrome and high-functioning autism: Language, motor and cognitive profiles. *European Child and Adolesecent Psychiatry, 19*(6), 475–481.

Ozonoff, S., Dawson, G., & McPartland, J. (2002). *A parent's guide to Asperger syndrome and high-functioning autism: How to meet the challenges and help your child thrive.* New York: Guilford Press.

Ozonoff, S., Pennington, B. F., & Rogers, S. J. (1991). Executive function deficits in high-functioning autistic individuals: Relationship to theory of mind. *Journal of Child Psychology and Psychiatry, 32*(7), 1081–1105.

Ozonoff, S., Rogers, S. J., & Pennington, B. F. (1991). Asperger's syndrome: Evidence of an empirical distinction from high-functioning autism. *Journal of Child Psychology and Psychiatry, 32*(7), 1107–1122.

Ozonoff, S., South, M., & Miller, J. N. (2000). DSM-IV-defined Asperger syndrome: Cognitive, behavioral and early history differentiation from high-functioning autism. *Autism, 4*(1), 29–46.

Ozonoff, S., Strayer, D. L., McMahon, W. M., & Filloux, F. (1994). Executive function abilities in autism and Tourette syndrome: An information processing approach. *Journal of Child Psychology and Psychiatry, 35*(6), 1015–1032.

Patrick, N. J. (2008). *Social skills for teenagers and adults with Asperger syndrome: A practical guide to day-to-day life.* London: Jessica Kingsley.

Paul, R. (2003). Promoting social communication in high-functioning individuals with autistic spectrum disorders. *Child and Adolescent Psychiatric Clinics of North America, 12*(1), 87–106.

Paul, R., Orlovski, S. M., Marcinko, H. C., & Volkmar, F. R. (2009). Conversational behaviors in youth with high-functioning ASD and Asperger syndrome. *Journal of Autism and Developmental Disorders, 39*(1), 115–125.

Renty, J., & Roeyers, H. (2007). Individual and marital adaptation in men with autism spectrum disorder and their spouses: The role of social support and coping strategies. *Journal of Autism and Developmental Disorders, 37*(7), 1247–1255.

Rinehart, N. J., Bradshaw, J. L., Brereton, A. V., & Tonge, B. J. (2001). Movement preparation in high-functioning autism and Asperger disorder: A serial choice reaction time task involving motor reprogramming. *Journal of Autism and Developmental Disorders, 31*(1), 79–88.

Rinehart, N. J., Bradshaw, J. L., Moss, S. A., Brereton, A. V., & Tonge, B. J. (2001). A deficit in shifting attention present in high-functioning autism but not Asperger's disorder. *Autism, 5*(1), 67–80.

Rinehart, N. J., Tonge, B. J., Bradshaw, J. L., Iansek, R., Enticott, P. G., & McGinley, J. (2006). Gait function in high-functioning autism and Asperger's disorder: Evidence for basal-ganglia and cerebellar involvement? *European Child and Adolesecent Psychiatry, 15*(5), 256–264.

Robinson, J., F., & Vitale, L. J. (1954). Children with circumscribed interest patterns. *American Journal of Orthopsychiatry, 24,* 755–767.

Rourke, B. P. (1989). *Nonverbal learning disabilities: The syndrome and the model.* New York: Guilford Press.

Rubin, E., & Lennon, L. (2004). Challenges in social communication in Asperger syndrome and high-functioning autism. *Topics in Language Disorders, 24*(4), 271–285.

Ruta, L., Mugno, D., D'Arrigo, V. G., Vitiello, B., & Mazzone, L. (2010). Obsessive–compulsive traits in children and adolescents with Asperger syndrome. *European Child and Adolesecent Psychiatry, 19*(1), 17–24.

Rutter, M. (1997). Comorbidity: Concepts, claims and choices. *Criminal Behaviour and Mental Health, 7*(4), 265–285.

Rutter, M. (2005). Genetic influences and autism. In F. R. Volkmar, A. Klin, R. Paul, & D. J. Cohen (Eds.), *Handbook of autism and pervasive developmental disorders* (3rd ed., Vol. 1, pp. 425–452). Hoboken, NJ: Wiley.

Rutter, M. (2011). Research review: Child psychiatric diagnosis and classification: Concepts, findings, challenges and potential. *Journal of Child Psychology and Psychiatry and Allied Disciplines, 52*(6), 647–660.

Ryan, R. M. (1992). Treatment-resistant chronic mental illness: Is it Asperger's syndrome? *Hospital and Community Psychiatry, 43*(8), 807–811.

Saliba, J. R., & Griffiths, M. (1990). Brief report: Autism of the Asperger type associated with an autosomal fragile site. *Journal of Autism and Developmental Disorders, 20*(4), 569–575.

Samson, A. C., & Hegenloh, M. (2010). Stimulus characteristics affect humor processing in individuals with Asperger syndrome. *Journal of Autism and Developmental Disorders, 40*(4), 438–447.

Sandson, T. A., Manoach, D., Price, B, P., Rentz, D., & Weintraub, S. (1994). Right hemisphere learning disability associates with left hemisphere dysfunction anomalous dominance and development. *Journal of Neurology, Neurosurgery, and Psychiatry, 57,* 1129–1132.

Saulnier, C. A., & Klin, A. (2007). Brief report: Social and communication abilities and disabilities in higher functioning individuals with autism and Asperger syndrome. *Journal of Autism and Developmental Disorders, 37*(4), 788–793.

Sciutto, M. J., & Cantwell, C. (2005). Factors influencing the differential diagnosis of Asperger's disorder and high-functioning autism. *Journal of Developmental and Physical Disabilities, 17*(4), 345–359.

Scragg, P., & Shah, A. (1994). Prevalence of Asperger's syndrome in a secure hospital. *British Journal of Psychiatry, 165*(5), 679–682.

Semrud-Clikeman, M., & Fine, J. (2011). Presence of cysts on magnetic resonance images (MRIs) in children with Asperger disorder and nonverbal learning disabilities. *Journal of Child Neurology, 11*, 1–5.

Semrud-Clikeman, M., & Hynd, G. W. (1990). Right hemisphere dysfunction in nonverbal learning disabilities: Social, academic, and adaptive functioning in adults and children. *Psychological Bulletin, 107*, 196–209.

Semrud-Clikeman, M., Walkowiak, J., Wilkinson, A., & Minne, E. P. (2010). Direct and indirect measures of social perception, behavior, and emotional functioning in children with Asperger's disorder, nonverbal learning disability, or ADHD. *Journal of Abnormal Child Psychology, 38*(4), 509–519.

Shields, J. (1991). Semantic–pragmatic disorder: A right hemisphere syndrome? *British Journal of Disorders of Communication, 26*(3), 383–392.

Shriberg, L. D., Paul, R., McSweeny, J. L., Klin, A. M., Cohen, D. J., & Volkmar, F. R. (2001). Speech and prosody characteristics of adolescents and adults with high-functioning autism and Asperger syndrome. *Journal of Speech, Language, and Hearing Research, 44*(5), 1097–1115.

Shtayermman, O. (2007). Peer victimization in adolescents and young adults diagnosed with Asperger's syndrome: A link to depressive symptomatology, anxiety symptomatology and suicidal ideation. *Issues in Comprehensive Pediatric Nursing, 30*(3), 87–107.

Sofronoff, K., Dark, E., & Stone, V. (2011). Social vulnerability and bullying in children with Asperger syndrome. *Autism, 15*(3), 355–372.

South, M., Ozonoff, S., & McMahon, W. M. (2005). Repetitive behavior profiles in Asperger syndrome and high-functioning autism. *Journal of Autism and Developmental Disorders, 35*(2), 145–158.

Sparrow, S. S., Balla, D., & Cicchetti, D. V. (1984). *Vineland Adaptive Behavior Scales (Survey Form).* Circle Pines, MN: American Guidance Service.

Spek, A., Schatorjé, T., Scholte, E., & van Berckalaer-Onnes, I. (2009). Verbal fluency in adults with high-functioning autism or Asperger syndrome. *Neuropsychologia, 47*(3), 652–656.

Spitzer, R. L., Endicott, J. E., & Robbins, E. (1978). Resarch diagnostic criteria. *Archives of General Psychiatry, 35*, 773–782.

Stewart, M. E., Barnard, L., Pearson, J., Hasan, R., & O'Brien, G. (2006). Presentation of depression in autism and Asperger syndrome: A review. *Autism, 10*(1), 103–116.

Susan, L., Libby, S., Wing, L., Gould, J., & Gillberg, C. (2000). Comparison of ICD-10 and Gillberg's criteria for Asperger syndrome. *Autism, 4*(1), 11–28.

Szatmari, P. (1991). Asperger's syndrome: Diagnosis, treatment, and outcome. *Psychiatric Clinics of North America, 14*(1), 81–93.

Szatmari, P., Archer, L., Fisman, S., Streiner, D. L., et al. (1995). Asperger's syndrome and autism: Differences in behavior, cognition, and adaptive functioning. *Journal of the American Academy of Child and Adolesecent Psychiatry, 34*(12), 1662–1671.

Szatmari, P., Bartolucci, G., & Bremner, R. (1989). Asperger's syndrome and autism: Comparison of early history and outcome. *Developmental Medicine and Child Neurology, 31*(6), 709–720.

Szatmari, P., Bremner, R., & Nagy, J. (1989). Asperger's syndrome: A review of clinical features. *Canadian Journal of Psychiatry, 34*(6), 554–560.

Szatmari, P., Bryson, S. E., Streiner, D. L., Wilson, F., Archer, L., & Ryerse, C. (2000). Two-year outcome of preschool children with autism or Asperger's syndrome. *American Journal of Psychiatry, 157*(12), 1980–1987.

Tager-Flusberg, H., Joseph, R. M., & Folstein, S. (2001). Current directions in research on autism. *Mental Retardation and Developmental Disabilities Research Reviews, 7*(1), 21–29.

Tager-Flusberg, H., & Joseph, R. M. (2003). Identifying neurocognitive phenotypes in autism. *Philosophical Transactions of the Royal Society of London Series B: Biological Sciences., 358*(1430), 303–314.

Taheri, A., & Perry, A. (2012). Exploring the proposed DSM-5 criteria in a clinical sample. *Journal of Autism and Developmental Disorders, 42*(9), 1810–1817.

Tani, P., Tuisku, K., Lindberg, N., Virkkala, J., Nieminen-von Wendt, T., von Wendt, L., et al. (2006). Is Asperger syndrome associated with abnormal nocturnal motor phenomena? *Psychiatry and Clinical Neurosciences, 60*(4), 527–528.

Tantam, D. (1988a). Asperger's syndrome. *Journal of Child Psychology and Psychiatry, 29*(3), 245–255.

Tantam, D. (1988b). Lifelong eccentricity and social isolation: II. Asperger's syndrome or schizoid personality disorder? *British Journal of Psychiatry, 153*, 783–791.

Tantam, D., Evered, C., & Hersov, L. (1990). Asperger's syndrome and ligamentous laxity. *Journal of the American Academy of Child and Adolescent Psychiatry, 29*(6), 892–896.

Tentler, D., Johannesson, T., Johansson, M., Rastam, M., Gillberg, C., Orsmark, C., et al. (2003). A candidate region for Asperger syndrome defined by two 17p breakpoints. *European Journal of Human Genetics, 11*(2), 189–195.

Townsend, J., Harris, N. S., & Courchesne, E. (1996). Visual attention abnormalities in autism: Delayed orienting to location. *Journal of the International Neuropsychology Society, 2*(6), 541–550.

Tsai, L. Y. (2007). Asperger syndrome and medication treatment. *Focus on Autism and Other Developmental Disabilities, 22*(3), 138–148.

van Krevelen, D. A. (1971). Early infantile autism and autistic psychopathy. *Journal of Autism and Childhood Schizophrenia, 1*(1), 82–86.

van Krevelen, D. A. (1973). Problems of differential diagnosis between mental retardation and autismus infantum. *Acta Paedopsychiatrica, 39*(8), 199–203.

van Krevelen, D. A., & Kuipers, C. (1962). The psychopathology of autistic psychopathy. *Acta Paedopsychiatrica, 29*(1), 22–31.

Verté, S., Geurts, H. M., Roeyers, H., Oosterlaan, J., & Sergeant, J. A. (2006). Executive functioning in children with an autism spectrum disorder: Can we differentiate within the spectrum? *Journal of Autism and Developmental Disorders, 36*(3), 351–372.

Via, E., Radua, J., Cardoner, N., Happé, F., & Mataix-Cols, D. (2011). Meta-analysis of gray matter abnormalities in autism spectrum disorder: Should Asperger disorder be subsumed under a broader umbrella of autistic spectrum disorder? *Archives of General Psychiatry, 68*(4), 409–418.

Volkmar, F. R. (2011). Asperger's disorder: Implications for psychoanalysis. *Psychoanalytic Inquiry, 31*(3), 334–344.

Volkmar, F. R., Chawarska, K., Carter, A., & Lord, C. (2007). Diagnosis of autism and related disorders in infants and very young children: Setting a research agenda for DSM-V. In W. E. Narrow (Ed.), *Age and gender considerations in psychiatric diagnosis: A research agenda for DSM-V* (pp. 259–270). Arlington, VA: American Psychiatric Association.

Volkmar, F. R., & Klin, A. (2000). Diagnostic issues in Asperger syndrome. In A. Klin, F. R. Volkmar, & S. S. Sparrow (Eds.), *Asperger syndrome* (pp. 25–71). New York: Guilford Press.

Volkmar, F. R., Klin, A., & Pauls, D. (1998). Nosological and genetic aspects of Asperger syndrome. *Journal of Autism and Developmental Disorders, 28*(5), 457–463.

Volkmar, F. R., Klin, A., Schultz, R., Bronen, R., Marans, W. D., Sparrow, S., et al. (1996). Asperger's syndrome. *Journal of the American Academy of Child and Adolesecent Psychiatry, 35*(1), 118–123.

Volkmar, F. R., Klin, A., Schultz, R. T., Rubin, E., & Bronen, R. (2000). Asperger's disorder. *American Journal of Psychiatry, 157*(2), 262–267.

Volkmar, F. R., Klin, A., Siegel, B., Szatmari, P., Lord, C., Campbell, M., et al. (1994). Field trial for autistic disorder in DSM-IV. *American Journal of Psychiatry, 151*(9), 1361–1367.

Volkmar, F. R., & Reichow, B. (in press). Autism in DSM-5: Progress and challenges. *Molecular Autism, 4*(13).

Volkmar, F. R., & Tsatsanis, K. D. (2005). Asperger syndrome. *Journal of Autism and Developmental Disorders, 35*(2), 259–260.

Volkmar, F. R., & Wiesner, L. (2009). *A practical guide to autism: What every parent, family member, and teacher needs to know.* New York: Wiley.

Volkmar, F. R., & Woolston, J. L. (1997). Comorbidity of psychiatric disorders in children and adolescents. In S. Wetzler & W. C. Sanderson (Eds.), *Treatment strategies for patients with psychiatric comorbidity: An Einstein psychiatry publication, No. 14* (pp. 307–322). New York: Wiley.

Wainwright-Sharp, J. A., & Bryson, S. E. (1996). Visual–spatial orienting in autism. *Journal of Autism and Developmental Disorders, 26*(4), 423–438.

Weintraub, S., Mesulam, M. M., & Kramer, L. (1981). Disturbances in prosody: A right-hemisphere contribution to language. *Archives of Neurology*, 742–744.

Weiss, J. A., & Lunsky, Y. (2010). Group cognitive behaviour therapy for adults with Asperger syndrome and anxiety or mood disorder: A case series. *Clinical Psychology and Psychotherapy, 17*(5), 438–446.

Wendland, J. R., De Guzman, T. B., McMahon, F., Rudnick, G., Detera-Wadleigh, S. D., & Murphy, D. L. (2008). Asperger syndrome and obsessive–compulsive disorder. *Psychiatric Genetics, 18*(1), 31–39.

Williams, D. L., Goldstein, G., Kojkowski, N., & Minshew, N. J. (2008). Do individuals with high-functioning autism have the IQ profile associated with nonverbal learning disability? *Research in Autism Spectrum Disorders, 2*(2), 353–361.

Wilson, C. E. Comparison of ICD-10R, DSM-IV-TR and DSM-5 in an adult autism spectrum disorder diagnostic clinic. *Journal of Autism and Developmental Disorders, 43*(11), 2515–2525.

Wing, L. (1981). Asperger's syndrome: A clinical account. *Psychological Medicine, 11*(1), 115–129.

Wing, L. (2005). Reflections on opening Pandora's box. *Journal of Autism and Developmental Disorders, 35*(2), 197–203.

Wolff, S. (1996). The first account of the syndrome Asperger's described? *European Child and Adolesecent Psychiatry, 5*, 119–132.

Wolff, S. (1998). Schizoid personality in childhood: The links with Asperger syndrome, schizophrenia spectrum disorders, and elective mutism. In E. Schopler & G. B. Mesibov (Eds.), *Asperger syndrome or high-functioning autism?: Current issues in autism* (pp. 123–142). New York: Plenum Press.

Wolff, S. (2004). The history of autism. *European Child and Adolesecent Psychiatry, 13*(4), 201–208.

Wolff, S., & McGuire, R. J. (1995). Schizoid personality in girls: A follow-up study—what are the links with Asperger's syndrome? *Journal of Child Psychology and Psychiatry and Allied Disciplines, 36*(5), 793–817.

Wood, J. J., Drahota, A., Sze, K., Har, K., Chiu, A., & Langer, D. A. (2009). Cognitive behavior therapy for anxiety in children with autism spectrum disorders: A randomized controlled trial. *Journal of Child Psychology and Psychiatry and Allied Disciplines, 50*(3), 224–234.

World Health Organization. (1993). *The ICD-10 classification of mental and behavioral disordedrs: Diagnostic criteria for research.* Geneva: Author.

Woodbury-Smith, M. R., & Volkmar, F. R. (2009). Asperger syndrome. *European Child and Adolesecent Psychiatry, 18*(1), 2–11.

Yu, K. K., Cheung, C., Chua, S. E., & McAlonan, G. M. (2011). Can Asperger's syndrome be distinguished from autism? *Journal of Psychiatry and Neuroscience, 36*(2), 1001–1008.

Ziatas, K., Durkin, K., & Pratt, C. (2003). Differences in assertive speech acts produced by children with autism, Asperger syndrome, specific language impairment, and normal development. *Development and Psychopathology, 15*(1), 73–94.

CHAPTER 2

Evidence-Based Assessment of Asperger Syndrome

A Selective Review of Screening and Diagnostic Instruments

Jonathan M. Campbell
Carrah L. James
Sarah F. Vess

Asperger syndrome (AS) is defined as a developmental disorder characterized by significant impairments in social communication and restricted patterns of interest or behaviors in the presence of generally age-appropriate language acquisition and cognitive functioning (Klin, Volkmar, & Sparrow, 2000). AS was first described by Hans Asperger (1944) and "reintroduced" with Lorna Wing's (1981) description of a series of clinical cases. Interest in AS grew after Wing's clinical account and has culminated in the inclusion of AS into widely used diagnostic classification systems, such as the fourth edition of the *Diagnostic and Statistical Manual of Mental Disorders* (DSM-IV; American Psychiatric Association, 1994) and the 10th edition of the *International Classification of Diseases and Related Health Problems* (ICD-10; World Health Organization, 1993).[1] Diagnosis of AS, especially

---

[1]The fifth edition of the *Diagnostic and Statistical Manual of Mental Disorders* (DSM-5; American Psychiatric Association, 2013) does not identify Asperger's Disorder as a diagnostic category. Currently, the DSM-5 identifies a single Autism Spectrum Disorder diagnostic category whereby individuals with a prior DSM-IV diagnosis of Asperger's Disorders may be classified in the new system.

the differentiation between AS and high-functioning autism (HFA), is complicated, in part, due to differing diagnostic criteria and changing sets of
criteria over time. Various diagnostic definitions of AS show poor agreement (Kopra, von Wendt, Nieminen-von Wendt, & Paavonen, 2008); therefore, research in the area of test validation is limited by the absence of diagnostic consensus. Despite ongoing debate regarding the diagnostic validity
of AS and lack of diagnostic consensus, a number of measures exist for
screening and diagnosis of AS.

The purpose of our chapter is to evaluate instruments and scales
designed for use in detection and diagnosis of individuals with AS. In doing
so, we organize our review and discussion of instruments for AS according
to principles of evidence-based assessment (EBA). We introduce the tenets
of EBA and recently developed operational definitions for EBA classifications. Next, we introduce and critique third-party ratings and self-report
measures designed to screen for or diagnose AS. We describe each measure,
including its format, length, and intended purposes, followed by a review
of each scale's construction and psychometric properties. Each scale is then
evaluated in terms of how well it satisfies EBA criteria according to its
intended purposes.

GUIDING PRINCIPLES AND STANDARDS
FOR EVIDENCE-BASED ASSESSMENT

Analogous to the movement toward empirically supported treatments
(ESTs) and evidence-based medicine, the field of psychological assessment
has begun to develop guidelines for EBA. The basic tenet of the EBA movement is enticing in its simplicity: Clinicians should use assessment measures that are supported by an empirical knowledge base characterized
by carefully conducted research. Of course, the complexity of this goal is
quickly realized when one considers the varied purposes of psychological
assessment, such as screening, diagnosis, treatment planning, prognosis,
and treatment monitoring (Mash & Hunsley, 2005), and that no measure
is designed to respond to all assessment purposes. Further, the seemingly
simplistic goal of establishing standards of technical adequacy for psychological instruments also becomes complex as one considers how to go about
evaluating reliability evidence, validity evidence, and norming techniques.
For example, an assessment measure cannot simply be judged to be valid
or invalid in general terms; rather, a measure can be supported as valid for
specific usages, such as general population screening, differential diagnosis,
or treatment monitoring.

In an ambitious attempt to operationalize the principles of EBA, the
Society of Pediatric Psychology Evidence-Based Assessment Task Force
(EBA-TF) developed standards to classify measures according to degree of
empirical support for their intended usage (Cohen et al., 2008; see Table

2.1). Consistent with defining features from the EST movement, the EBA-TF criteria highlight the importance of standardized procedures to allow for replication of findings across different investigative teams. The EBA-TF criteria also require that "good" psychometric data (i.e., reliability and validity statistics) be published in order for a measure to qualify as "well established." For the purposes of our chapter, we determined that total score internal consistency and temporal stability reliability ≥ .80 was "good" and ≥ .90 was "excellent"; for categorical test–retest reliability and interrater agreement expressed as kappa, we considered .60–.74 "good," and .75–1.00 "excellent" (Cicchetti, 1994). When an instrument featured subscales, we used the same guidelines to evaluate the technical adequacy of subscales using median subscale values. For validity evidence, we summarized different types of data, and in the case of evaluating validity

TABLE 2.1. Society of Pediatric Psychology's Criteria for Evidence-Based Assessments

Category	Criteria
Well-established assessment	The measure must have been presented in at least 2 peer-reviewed articles by different investigators or investigatory teams
	Sufficient detail about the measure to allow critical evaluation and replication (e.g., measure and manual provided or available upon request)
	Detailed (e.g., statistics presented) information indicating good validity and reliability in at least 1 peer-reviewed article
Approaching well-established assessment	The measure must have been presented in at least 2 peer-reviewed articles, which might be by the same investigator or investigatory team
	Sufficient detail about the measure to allow critical evaluation and replication (e.g., measure and manual provided or available upon request)
	Validity and reliability information either presented in vague terms (e.g., no statistics presented) or only moderate values presented
Promising assessment	The measure must have been presented in at least 1 peer-reviewed article
	Sufficient detail about the measure to allow critical evaluation and replication (e.g., measure and manual provided or available upon request)
	Validity and reliability information either presented in vague terms (e.g., no statistics presented) or moderate values presented

Note. From Cohen et al. (2008, p. 913). Copyright 2008 by the Society of Pediatric Psychology.

coefficients (e.g., correlation between the test and similar measures), no specific thresholds were established. Screening for AS and differential diagnosis between AS and other ASDs were of particular interest to us in our review; therefore, we rendered separate EBA decisions based upon these purposes where appropriate (e.g., a test could be "well established" as a screener but only "promising" for diagnosis).

We also calculated readability estimates based on Streiner's (1993) recommendation that rating scales, and by extension self-reports, be comprehensible to lay respondents. For ratings and self-reports, we calculated Flesh Reading Ease (FRE) and Flesh–Kincaid Grade Level (F-KG) readability statistics. FRE rates text on a 100-point scale with higher scores indicating easier comprehension; the F-KG score rates text on a grade-based level (e.g., F-KG score of 7.0 indicates that text is comprehensible for the average seventh grader).

THIRD-PARTY RATING SCALES

Building on Campbell's (2005) review, five third-party rating scales were selected for inclusion in this chapter: (1) Asperger Syndrome Diagnostic Scale (ASDS; Myles, Bock, & Simpson, 2001), (2) Autism Spectrum Screening Questionnaire (ASSQ; Ehlers, Gillberg, & Wing, 1999), (3) Childhood Asperger's Screening Test (CAST; Scott, Baron-Cohen, Bolton, & Brayne, 2002), (4) Gilliam Asperger's Disorder Scale (GADS; Gilliam, 2001), and (5) Krug Asperger's Disorder Index (KADI; Krug & Arick, 2003). We updated Campbell's (2005) review by conducting a literature search for each instrument using Social Science Citation Index and PsycINFO.

Asperger Syndrome Diagnostic Scale

The ASDS is a 50-item norm-referenced scale that requires the respondent to indicate the presence or absence of behaviors indicative of AS. The ASDS contains five subscales: Language, Social, Maladaptive, Cognitive, and Sensorimotor (Table 2.2). Raw scores are summed within domains and yield scaled scores ($M = 10$, $SD = 3$) and percentile ranks for subtests. Items are summed for the entire scale to yield an Asperger Syndrome Quotient (ASQ), which is a standard score ($M = 100$, $SD = 15$) that indicates the probability of AS. The ASDS manual identifies the purposes of the scale as follows: (1) to aid in the identification of persons with AS, (2) to document behavioral progress, (3) to formulate target goals for individualized education programs (IEPs), and (4) for research. Raters can be general education teachers, special education teachers, paraprofessionals, or parents; an appropriate rater should have 2 weeks of sustained contact with the individual being rated and should know the examinee well.

TABLE 2.2. Description of Third-Party Ratings and Self-Report Instruments for Asperger Syndrome

Instrument	Purpose(s)	Ages[a]	Items	Subscales	Readability (RE/GL)[b]
Third-party ratings					
ASDS	Diagnostic aid Monitor behavior Generate IEP goals Research	5–18	50	Language Social Maladaptive Cognitive Sensorimotor	40.5/9.9
ASSQ	Screener Research	6–17	27	Overall score	46.3/8.7
CAST	Screener Research	4–11	37	Overall score	74.9/4.1
GADS	Diagnostic aid Assess behavior Monitor behavior Generate IEP goals	3–22	32	Social Interaction Restricted Behaviors Cognitive Patterns Pragmatic Skills	55.7/8.1
KADI	Screener Generate IEP goals Research	6–21	32	Overall score	51.2/8.2
Self-reports					
AQ	Screener	18–69	50	Social Skill Attention Switching Attention to Detail Communication Imagination	63.4/7.4
EQ	Assess empathy	15–60	60	Overall score	64.1/7.6
RAADS	Diagnostic aid	18–65	78	Social Relatedness Language/ Communication Sensorimotor/ Stereotypies	68.5/7.4

Note. ASDS, Asperger Syndrome Diagnostic Scale; ASSQ, Autism-Spectrum Screening Questionnaire; CAST, Childhood Asperger Syndrome Test; GADS, Gilliam Asperger's Disorder Scale; KADI, Krug Asperger's Disorder Index; AQ, Autism Spectrum Quotient; EQ, Empathy Quotient; RAADS, Ritvo Autism and Asperger's Diagnostic Scale.

[a]Age ranges presented in years.

[b]RE = Reading ease (RE) represented by the Flesch Reading Ease score, which rates text on a 100-point scale, with higher score indicating easier comprehension. Grade level (GL) represented by the Flesch–Kincaid Grade Level score, which rates text on a U.S. grade school level.

Authors selected the 50 ASDS items based on review of diagnostic manuals and a review of the literature on AS. The ASDS was normed using a sample of 115 individuals diagnosed with AS (83% male) ranging in age from 5 to 18 (M = 10.42, SD = 3.44) from 21 states across the United States. The standardization sample was recruited from professionals in school districts (e.g., teachers, psychologists) who were asked to complete the ASDS on students previously diagnosed with AS, and from parents of children with AS recruited through mailings and speaking engagements. Authors did not establish independent diagnosis for the standardization sample. Subtest and ASQ scores were created using cumulative frequency tables collapsed across age groups and gender.

Reliability and Readability

Authors provide evidence for internal consistency reliability and interrater reliability; Cronbach's alpha for the total score is .83, subscale values range from .64 (Cognitive) to .83 (Social) with a median value of .72. Parent and teacher interrater reliability is .93 for the ASQ (14 pairs of raters). No information is provided for temporal stability reliability. Test authors recommend only the interpretation of the ASQ in decision making due to subscale unreliability. The ASDS FRE score is 40.5 and F-KG score is 9.9.

Validity

Test authors report using rational item selection to create the ASDS items, including review of DSM-IV and ICD-10 diagnostic criteria, literature review, and review of Asperger's (1944) report. Test authors cite evidence for criterion validity because the ASQ total score correctly identified 85% of children across five classifications, including AS, autism, behavioral disorder (BD), attention-deficit/hyperactivity disorder (ADHD), and learning disability (LD). Evidence for construct validity includes (1) statistically significant item–total score correlations for the ASDS items, (2) concurrent and divergent validity with total scores and subscales of the Gilliam Autism Rating Scale (GARS), and (3) lack of statistically significant relationship between ASQ scores and age (r = .14). The ASDS and GARS total score correlation for 16 individuals was moderate (r = .46). Boggs, Gross, and Gohm (2006) examined the divergent, convergent, and discriminative validity of the ASDS with a sample of 76 children identified with AS, autism, or no diagnosis. The ASDS produced differences between AS (n = 21; M = 108) and autism (n = 14; M = 93) and classified the AS and autism groups with 72.7% accuracy. Boggs et al. (2006) report that the ASQ strongly correlated with the GARS in the nondiagnosed sample (r = .82) and the sample of children with autism (r = .65); however, ASQ and GARS

TABLE 2.3. Reliability of Instruments for Asperger Syndrome

Instrument	Internal consistency[a]	Test–retest[b]	Interrater reliability[b]
Third-party ratings			
ASDS	.83/.64–.83 *Mdn* = .72 (*n* = 115)	NR	.93/NR (*n* = 14)[c]
ASSQ-T[d]	.89 (Teacher)/NA	.94/NA (*n* = 65)[e]	.34–.79/NA (*n* = 20–3,128)[c]
ASSQ-P[d]	.86 (Parent)/NA	.96/NA (*n* = 86)[f]	NR
CAST[d]	NR	.67–.83; kappa = .41–70 (*n* = 73–136)	NR
GADS	.87/.70–.81 *Mdn* = .77 (*n* = 360)	.93/.71–.77 *Mdn* = .76 (*n* = 10)	.89/.72–.84 *Mdn* = .82 (*n* = 16)[c]
KADI[d]	.93/NA (*n* = 130)	.98/NA (*n* = 25)	90% agreement (*n* = 19 pairs)
Self-Reports			
AQ	.71–.85/.40–.77 *Mdn* = .47–.65	*r* = .7–.87 (*n* = 17–75)	*r* = .71 (*n* = 32; self/parent)
EQ[d]	.81–.92/NA (*n* = 137–410)	*r* = 84–.97 (*n* = 15–36)	NR
RAADS	NR/.60–.86 *Mdn* = .70 (*n* = 94)	NR	NR

Note. AQ, Autism-Spectrum Quotient; ASDS, Asperger Syndrome Diagnostic Scale; ASSQ-P, Autism Spectrum Screening Questionnaire—Parent Respondent; ASSQ-T, Autism Spectrum Screening Questionnaire—Teacher Respondent; CAST, Childhood Asperger Syndrome Test; EQ, Empathy Quotient; GADS, Gilliam Asperger's Disorder Scale; KADI, Krug Asperger's Disorder Index; *Mdn*, Median; NA, not applicable; NR, not reported; RAADS, Ritvo Autism and Asperger's Diagnostic Scale.

[a]Total test score/range of values for subtest scores.

[b]Total test score/range of values for subtest scores.

[c]Parent–teacher agreement.

[d]The ASSQ, CAST, KADI, and EQ do not contain subscales; therefore, subtest values are not applicable (NA).

scores were weakly related ($r = .23$) for the AS sample. Although findings provide initial independent psychometric support for the ASDS, this support is limited by the lack of matching between the AS and autism groups on important variables such as age and cognitive ability. As such, differences between the AS and autism groups may reflect differences in cognitive functioning or age, which replicates limitations from the original validation study.

Evidence-Based Assessment Classification

Perhaps the most significant weakness with the ASDS is the standardization sample with which the diagnosis of AS was not verified. Efforts to establish differential diagnostic validity have not included information about cognitive functioning for the sample of individuals with autism—an important omission, as Cognitive and Language subscales are included in the ASDS. If the autism comparison groups showed cognitive impairment, which is likely, the diagnostic utility of the ASDS would be diminished. Reliability data are variable for the ASDS; the ASQ meets the minimal .80 criterion for internal consistency; however, the median subtest reliability falls below the minimum standard, and no temporal stability data are presented. Overall, the ASDS is considered a "promising" measure for diagnosis of AS, with one peer-reviewed article examining its psychometric properties (Boggs et al., 2006), sufficient detail about the measure provided in the test manual, and moderate psychometric properties presented for the measure.

Autism Spectrum Screening Questionnaire

The ASSQ consists of 27 behavioral descriptions rated on a 3-point scale: Items are summed to yield a total raw score that may range from 0 to 54. Items sample problems in social interaction, communication, restricted and repetitive behavior, motor clumsiness, and associated symptoms such as motor tics. The ASSQ is designed as a screening instrument with items selected based on the authors' clinical experience with autism and on their literature review. The pool of items was selected to reflect symptoms characteristic of AS in children and adolescents. The ASSQ was created and used in Ehlers and Gillberg's (1993) epidemiological investigation and reliability and validity established with a clinical population that consisted of two samples: (1) 110, 6- to 17-year-old children referred to a clinic for evaluation, and (2) 34 children diagnosed with AS (Ehlers et al.). Parent scores of 19 and teacher scores of 22 are recommended screening cutoffs. The ASSQ has been employed in epidemiological studies in Denmark (Petersen, Bilenberg, Hoerder, & Gillberg, 2006), South Wales (Webb et al., 2003), and Norway (Posserud, Lundervold, & Gillberg, 2006).

Reliability and Readability

Ehlers and Gillberg (1993) reported a test–retest reliability coefficient of .90 (n = 139) for ASSQ teacher scores across an 8-month interval. Posserud et al. (2008) reported internal consistency reliability coefficients (Cronbach's alpha) of .89 for teacher ASSQ and .86 for parent ASSQ. In the clinical sample, Ehlers et al. (1999) reported a test–retest reliability coefficient of .94 (n = 65) for teachers and .96 (n = 86) for parents for a 2-week interval. Authors do not report the number or percentage of children rated who were diagnosed with an ASD. Ehlers and Gillberg (1993) reported interrater reliability coefficients for parent–teacher agreement of .79 (n = 139) for typical children and .77 (n = 20) for children with ASD. For the larger clinical sample, parent–teacher agreement was .66 (n = 105). Posserud et al. (2006) found that teacher and parent ratings correlated .48 for boys (n = 3,101) and .34 for girls (n = 3,128). The ASSQ FRE readability score is 46.3 and the F-KG readability score is 8.7.

Validity

Mean scores for the ASSQ significantly differed between ASD, ADHD/BD, and LD diagnostic groups for both parent and teacher reports (Ehlers et al., 1999), although this was not the case for two non-ASD rating scales. Diagnosis for each group was determined via clinical case conference. The ASSQ showed strong relationships with the Rutter and Conners rating scales (r's = .58–.77), indicating undesirable redundancy. Using Norway epidemiological data, Posserud et al. (2008) examined the factor structure and convergent–divergent validity of the ASSQ. Authors found a three-factor structure for both the parent and teacher forms and reported expected relationships between the ASSQ factors and subscales from the Strengths and Difficulties Questionnaire (SDQ). For example, the parent ASSQ "social difficulties" factor correlated .66 with the SDQ Peer Problems scale and –.31 with the SDQ Prosocial Behavior scale.

The ASSQ has shown good specificity in correctly identifying non-AS cases and variable sensitivity for correctly detecting AS cases (Ehlers et al., 1999). Posserud, Lundervold, and Gillberg (2009) examined the validity of the ASSQ as a general population screener for 9,430 children 7–9 years of age. Combined parent and teacher screening at a cut-point of 17 resulted in sensitivity of .91 (21 of 23 children with ASD) and specificity of .86. Positive predictive value (PPV) was 36% whereas negative predictive value (NPV) was 99%. Webb et al. (2003) utilized teacher ASSQ as a second-level screener to determine prevalence of ASDs in a large sample of children in Wales. For 47 children with ASSQ scores ≥ 22 and information sufficient for diagnosis, Webb et al. found that 12 were diagnosed with an ASD (8 with AS/HFA, 4 with PDD-NOS; PPV = .25).

Evidence-Based Assessment Classification

The ASSQ features good to excellent internal consistency, temporal stability, and interrater reliability. The scale has shown evidence of concurrent (i.e., positive correlations with like scales), divergent (i.e., negative correlations with dissimilar scales), and discriminant (i.e., differences between groups of children with ASD and other clinical groups) validity. The scale has also been subjected to independent psychometric examination by groups of researchers in Norway, South Wales, and Denmark. As a screener, the ASSQ shows adequate specificity but poor sensitivity for both the parent and teacher forms. Sensitivity improves when parent and teacher ratings are combined in the screening process. The PPV values reported in the literature (.25–.36) are low but expected when screening for low base-rate disorders such as ASDs. Overall, the ASSQ is considered a "well-established" screening measure to identify school-age children with high-functioning ASD. The ASSQ has been presented in at least two peer-reviewed articles by different investigative teams (e.g., Petersen et al., 2006; Webb et al., 2003), the measure is presented in sufficient detail, and it features good psychometrics in at least one article (e.g., Posserud et al., 2008). There is insufficient support for the ASSQ to differentiate between AS and other variants of autism, such as HFA and PDD-NOS.

Childhood Asperger Syndrome Test/Childhood Autism Spectrum Test

The CAST was designed initially to screen school-age populations for AS and later expanded to screen for higher functioning ASD. The CAST is a 37-item parent-rating scale of behavioral indicators of AS scored as either present or absent; 31 items are summed to yield an overall score, with 6 items sampling general development, which do not contribute to the total score. A CAST cutoff score of 15 or greater indicates the need for further evaluation for AS. CAST items were selected from behavioral descriptions found in ICD-10 and DSM-IV diagnostic manuals relevant to the core features of ASD as well as items from the ASSQ and the Pervasive Developmental Disorders Questionnaire (PDD-Q). The CAST was piloted with a sample of 13 children with AS and 37 typically developing children.

Reliability and Readability

Williams et al. (2006) reported test–retest reliability of .83 (n = 136; 22-day interval), and kappa = .70 agreement for CAST screening results at two time points for a general sample. For a sample of children scoring around the cutoff score, Allison et al. (2007) reported test–retest reliability of .67 (n = 73; 54-day *median* interval) and kappa = .41 agreement for CAST screening results over two time points. We found no reports of internal

TABLE 2.4. Classification Accuracy of Asperger Syndrome Assessment Instruments

Instrument	% correct classification	Sensitivity	Specificity	PPV	NPV
Third-party ratings					
ASDS	73–85%	NR	NR	NR	NR
ASSQ-T	NR	.65–.70	.91	.25	NR
ASSQ-P	NR	.62–.82	.90	NR	NR
ASSQ-C	NR	.91	.86	.36	.99
CAST	NR	.73–1.0	.46–.98	.64–.85	.75
GADS	83%	.85	.74	.93	.67
KADI	90%	.78	.67–.94	.83–.87	.70
Self-reports					
AQ	72–83%	.76–.95	.52–.71	.24–.84	.78–.96
EQ	NR	NR	NR	NR	NR
RAADS	100%	1.0	1.0	1.0	NR

Note. Statistics represent discrimination between AS and no disorder or AS and other disorders. AQ = Autism Spectrum Quotient; ASDS, Asperger Syndrome Diagnostic Scale; ASSQ-C, Autism Spectrum Screening Questionnaire—Combined Teacher and Parent; ASSQ-P, Autism Spectrum Screening Questionnaire—Parent; ASSQ-T, Autism Spectrum Screening Questionnaire—Teacher; CAST, Childhood Asperger Syndrome Test; EQ = Empathy Quotient; GADS = Gilliam Asperger's Disorder Scale; KADI = Krug Asperger's Disorder Index; NPV, negative predictive value; NR, not reported; PPV, positive predictive value; RAADS = Ritvo Autism and Asperger's Diagnostic Scale.

consistency reliability or interrater reliability. The CAST FRE score is 74.9 and the F-KG score is 4.1.

Validity

During initial validation, 50 parents completed the CAST, 13 with children with a prior diagnosis of AS or ASD and 37 with typical children. Parents produced average CAST scores that differed significantly between the AS/ASD ($M = 21.08$, $SD = 5.51$) and typical ($M = 4.73$, $SD = 3.57$) samples. The CAST was later validated with 1,150 children ages 4–11 enrolled in mainstream education. Of the 1,150 parents approached for participation, 199 (17.3%) responded, and 139 children were evaluated for the presence of an ASD. Using a cutoff score of 15, the CAST yielded a sensitivity of

.88 and a PPV of .64 for ASD diagnosis. The CAST yielded a specificity value of .98 at the 15-point cutoff score. Williams et al. (2005) reported sensitivity of 1.0, specificity of .97, and PPV of .50 for a sample of 387 children using gold-standard instruments and clinical consensus diagnosis as criterion. Matson, Dempsey, and Rivet (2008) reported sensitivity of .73, specificity of .46, PPV of .85, and NPV of .75 for AS versus non-AS clinical diagnosis. Providing evidence of concurrent validity, Matson et al. found the CAST to correlate with the GADS ($r = .87$) and KADI ($r = .83$). Williams et al. (2008) found sex differences for the CAST, with boys scoring higher than girls, which is consistent with other measures of ASD symptomatology.

Evidence-Based Assessment Classification

The CAST demonstrates temporal stability that straddles the minimum thresholds set for good reliability (i.e., $r = .67-.83$; kappa = $.41-.70$); there have been no published reports of CAST internal consistency reliability or interrater reliability. The CAST has demonstrated strong correlations with other measures of AS symptomatology, which suggests a high degree of redundancy between the CAST and other measures. The CAST has demonstrated variable sensitivity, variable specificity, and moderate PPV. Support for the CAST as a screening instrument must be tempered by low participation rates for population screening studies, such as 26–29% response rates (Williams et al., 2005, 2008). The CAST meets criteria as a "well-established" screening instrument for school-age children because it has appeared in at least two peer-reviewed articles by different investigative teams (e.g., Matson et al., 2008; Williams et al., 2006), the measure is presented in sufficient detail, and it features good psychometrics in at least one article (Williams et al., 2006). Although the measure meets the EBA-TF "well-established" threshold, the psychometric data are incomplete (e.g., no interrater reliability); therefore, we do not fully endorse its use as a screener.

Gilliam Asperger's Disorder Scale

The GADS is a 32-item norm-referenced scale that assesses frequency of AS-related behaviors in four domains: Social Interaction, Restricted Patterns of Behavior, Cognitive Patterns, and Pragmatic Skills. Raw scores are summed within domains to yield scaled scores ($M = 10$, $SD = 3$) and percentile ranks for subtests. Subtest scaled scores are summed to yield an Asperger's Disorder Quotient (ADQ), which is a standard score ($M = 100$, $SD = 15$), indicating probability of AS. The GADS also includes a Parent Interview Form to document the absence of clinical delays in language and cognitive development, and the presence of adaptive behavior and curiosity about the environment, which are necessary for DSM-IV-TR diagnosis.

The purposes of the scale are fivefold: (1) identify individuals with AS, (2) assess persons who show unique behavioral features, (3) document behavioral progress, (4) target goals for IEPs, and (5) conduct research. Raters can be teachers, teacher aides, parents, psychologists, or psychological associates who have had at least 2 weeks of sustained contact with the individual being rated.

Authors selected GADS items based on review of the DSM-IV-TR and ICD-10, a literature review, and review of instruments designed to assess AS, including the ASSQ. Seventy experimental items were examined and reduced to 32 items; the GADS manual does not describe how the 38 items were discarded or how the 32 items were grouped into subscales. The GADS was normed using a sample of 371 individuals 85% male diagnosed with AS who ranged in age from 3 to 22 ($M = 10$, $SD = 4$) from 46 states across the United States and other countries. As with the ASDS, the test author did not establish independent diagnosis of AS for the GADS standardization sample.

Reliability and Readability

Cronbach's coefficient alpha for the GADS total score is .87, with subscale score coefficient alphas ranging from .70 (Restricted Patterns of Behavior) to .81 (Cognitive Patterns); median subtest internal consistency reliability is .77. Temporal stability reliability is .93 for the ADQ for 10 teachers rating students with AS over a 2-week interval. Test–retest reliability ranged from .71 (Restricted Patterns of Behavior) to .77 (Pragmatic Skills) for GADS subscales. Parent and teacher interrater reliability is reported to be .89 for the ADQ for 16 children, 10 of whom were children with AD. The GADS FRE readability is 55.7 and the F-KG readability is 8.1.

Validity

Content validity is established by referencing DSM-IV-TR and ICD-10 diagnostic criteria when creating test items. The GADS has shown moderate to strong relationship with like subscales and total score of the GARS. Construct validity is addressed by the author's documenting of (1) strong item–subscale correlations; (2) no differences between males and females on GADS scores; (3) lack of statistically significant correlation between age and GADS scores, with the exception of the Restricted Patterns of Behavior subscale; and (4) mean differences on the GADS between AS, autism, other disability groups, and nondisabled groups. The GADS discriminated between AS and a group of children diagnosed with autism and other disabilities, such as ADHD, LD, and intellectual disability (Gilliam, 2001). Matson et al. (2008) found the following screening values for the GADS in discriminating between 14 children with AS versus children with HFA or no ASD: sensitivity (.85), specificity (.74), PPV (.93), and NPV (.67). The

GADS correlated strongly with the CAST ($r = .86$) and KADI ($r = .86$) in a sample of 40 children (Matson et al.).

Evidence-Based Assessment Classification

The GADS features a large ($N = 371$) standardization sample and offers some evidence that this sample is representative of the larger AS population, as evidenced by age-appropriate cognitive functioning in 33 of 371 individuals. ADQ internal consistency reliability falls within the good to excellent range, and the median subtest internal consistency falls below the "good" criterion of .80. Similar to the ASDS, a questionable group was used to create the norms for the GADS, as diagnoses were not verified by the test author. The GADS meets criteria as a "promising" instrument for diagnosing individuals with AS because it has appeared in one peer reviewed article (Matson et al., 2008), the measure is presented in sufficient detail, and it features good psychometrics in at least one article (Matson et al.). Matson et al.'s independent validation study is limited by a small sample size, the use of clinical consensus to establish AS versus HFA diagnosis, and lack of matching on age and IQ variables. In addition, the GADS was administered in interview format with at least some children who fell outside of the age range for the normative sample. It is unclear how modifying the GADS in this manner may have affected the findings of the study.

Krug Asperger's Disorder Index

The KADI is a 32-item norm-referenced rating scale that assesses the presence or absence of AS-related behaviors. Raw scores are weighted and summed to yield a KADI total standard score ($M = 100$, $SD = 15$) that indicates the likelihood for a diagnosis of AS. The KADI consists of two groups of items: a subset of 11 items that are used as an initial screen for AS and the entire set of 32 items that contribute to the KADI total. The KADI also consists of two forms, an elementary form appropriate for ages 6–11 and a secondary form appropriate for ages 12–21. The KADI manual identifies the purposes of the scale as (1) identifying individuals with AS, (2) targeting goals for intervention, and (3) research. Authors identify an appropriate rater as someone at the sixth-grade reading level with regular and daily contact with the individual for at least a few weeks.

An original pool of 106 items was reduced to 32 based upon items' ability to discriminate between AS and typical children, or AS and children with HFA. The KADI was standardized on a sample of 486 individuals, 130 with AS, 162 with autism, and 194 nondiagnosed. Normative scores were calculated using the sample of 130 individuals with AS recruited from 32 states and 10 countries; the normative sample ranged in age from 6 years to 21 years, 11 months. Based on the examiner's manual, authors did not establish independent diagnosis for the normative sample of individuals with AS or the sample of individuals with autism, but rather relied on

TABLE 2.5. Summary Classification for Instruments Based on Evidence-Based Assessment Criteria

Type of measure Test name	Purpose and classification
Third-party ratings	
ASDS	Diagnosis (promising)
ASSQ	Screening (well established)
CAST	Screening (well established, with minor reservations; see text)
GADS	Diagnosis (promising)
KADI	Screening (promising)
Self-reports	
AQ	Adult screening (well established)
EQ	Assessment of empathy (well established)
RAADS	Adult screening (promising)
Other	
AAA System	Diagnosis (promising)

Note. AAA, Adult Asperger Assessment; AQ, Autism Spectrum Quotient; ASDS, Asperger Syndrome Diagnostic Scale; ASSQ, Autism Spectrum Screening Questionnaire; CAST, Childhood Asperger Syndrome Test; EQ, Empathy Quotient; GADS, Gilliam Asperger's Disorder Scale; KADI, Krug Asperger's Disorder Index; RAADS, Ritvo Autism and Asperger's Diagnostic Scale. Data from Cohen, La Greca, Blount, Kazak, Holmbeck, et al. (2008).

diagnosis as reported by others. The final 32 items were those that discriminated between the "normal" sample and the AS sample, i.e., the 11 screening items, and/or discriminated between the AS and autism samples.

Reliability and Readability

Test authors provide evidence for internal consistency reliability, temporal stability, and interrater reliability. Within the standardization sample, Cronbach's alpha for the KADI total is .93, with temporal stability of .98 over a 2-week interval. Percent agreement of 90% is reported for 19 pairs of raters for individuals with AS, with agreement defined as standard scores falling within one standard deviation of each another. The KADI FRE is 51.2 and the F-KG score is 8.2, slightly higher than the authors' requirements that the rater read at a sixth-grade level.

Validity

Authors provide evidence of the KADI's concurrent validity in the test manual. The KADI shows sensitivity of .78, specificity of .94, and PPV of .83 within the standardization sample of 486 individuals. Mean scores also significantly differ between AS, autism, and "normal" groups in the standardization sample. Construct validity for the KADI includes high item–total test correlations, which are not reported in the KADI manual. Matson et al. (2008) reported concurrent validity for the KADI, with correlations of .86 with the GADS and .83 with the CAST. Matson et al. reported sensitivity of .78, specificity of .67, PPP of .87, and NPV of .70 for detecting AS versus non-AS in a sample of 40 children.

Evidence-Based Assessment Classification

The KADI features strong reliability data, although interrater reliability was calculated by percent agreement versus correlation or kappa, which may inflate the KADI's reliability in this area. Similar to the ASDS and GADS, test authors did not confirm diagnoses of AS and autism. The test authors also do not provide data relevant to the cognitive functioning of the autism contrast group, which is of particular importance when differential diagnosis of AS and HFA is required. The vast majority of raters in the AS normative sample were relatives (94%), not teachers; however, the manual indicates that teachers are appropriate raters. Thus, information reported in the KADI manual pertains almost exclusively to ratings made by parents or other relatives. Overall, the KADI meets criteria as a "promising" screening instrument for identifying individuals with AS because it has appeared in one peer-reviewed article (Matson et al., 2008), the measure is presented in sufficient detail, and it features moderate psychometrics in at least one article (Matson et al.). Similar to the information presented for the GADS, Matson et al.'s study involves some children who fall outside of the normative range for the KADI, the administration format of the KADI was modified from third-party rating to an interview; therefore, it is unclear how well the findings may apply to those who consider using the KADI as developed by test authors.

General Comments about Third-Party Rating Scales

The ASSQ and CAST emerged as "well-established" screeners when using the EBA-TF criteria and have been subjected to ongoing validation efforts. The commercially available instruments (i.e., ASDS, GADS, and KADI) were all classified as "promising" instruments. General limitations for the commercial instruments include the (1) lack of information about the cognitive functioning for AS and clinical comparison groups and (2) lack of confirmation of clinical diagnoses. Matching on cognitive functioning is important for differential diagnosis, otherwise differences found between diagnostic groups become tautological as the test merely confirms that groups are different in terms of preexisting cognitive functioning. The ASDS, GADS, and KADI ratings have been normed via mailing and survey methods without independent confirmation of AS diagnosis; therefore, test users have no assurances that the normative samples consist only of individuals diagnosed with AS. Assuming that all survey respondents are, in fact, rating an individual with AS, one has no idea what definition of AS is being used to establish the diagnosis. Independent validation for the ASDS, GADS, and KADI measures has begun (e.g., Boggs et al., 2006; Matson et al., 2008); however, the validation studies have been limited by similar problems, with a lack of specificity regarding diagnostic procedures used to establish criterion groups and a lack of age and IQ matching between diagnostic groups.

SELF-REPORT SCALES

In general, self-report rating scales provide the benefits of efficiency, cost-effectiveness, and nonconfrontational assessment of internal states. General limitations of self-report ratings include the examinee's need for a particular level of reading comprehension, his or her willingness and cognitive ability to accurately report on internal states, and the subjective nature of items and response choices. Specific to the assessment of AS, self-report ratings would seem valuable in differential diagnosis. For example, when assessing adults, third-party raters may be unavailable or, if available, less informed than third-party raters of children due to limited direct supervision.

   There are also potential limitations of self-report ratings in AS. Adults often cannot report on their early language development, the age of which was a key DSM-IV diagnostic criterion for AS and still often guides the differential diagnosis between HFA and AS. Not surprisingly, the self-report rating scales reviewed here have been adapted to overcome this limitation by combining individuals with either AS or HFA diagnoses for purposes of validation and statistical comparison with nondiagnosed or non-ASD groups. A second major concern is whether individuals with suspected ASD can accurately rate their own social behavior. As noted by Baron-Cohen and colleagues (Baron-Cohen, Wheelwright, Skinner, Martin, & Clubley, 2001), however, individuals with AS rate themselves as demonstrating more social and behavioral characteristics of AS than do comparison groups.

Autism-Spectrum Quotient

The Autism-Spectrum Quotient (AQ; Baron-Cohen et al., 2001) is a 50-item scale designed to screen for characteristics of ASD in adults of normal intelligence. Respondents rate items using four options (definitely agree, slightly agree, slightly disagree, or definitely disagree), but scoring is dichotomous such that endorsements consistent with characteristics of ASD receive 1 point and those inconsistent with ASD receive no points. Items are summed to yield a total raw score that may range from 0 to 50. Items assess social skill, attention switching, attention to detail, communication, and imagination (10 items per domain).

AQ items were based on the "triad of autistic symptoms" and "demonstrated areas of cognitive abnormality in autism" (Baron-Cohen et al., 2001, p. 6). Drafts of the scale underwent multiple iterations and pilot testing. Reliability and validity data are reported for the initial study of the instrument (Baron-Cohen et al.) and for a follow-up study specific to AS (Woodbury-Smith, Robinson, Wheelwright, & Baron-Cohen, 2005). In the initial validation study, four groups were assessed: (1) a sample of 58 adults (78% male) diagnosed with HFA or AS, (2) 174 controls (44% male), (3) 840 college students, and (4) 16 Mathematics Olympiad winners. For the HFA/AS group, diagnosis was rendered by psychiatrists using DSM-IV criteria; individuals were recruited from clinics, advertisements in HFA/AS-targeted media, and through the National Autistic Society. Controls were sampled from individuals living in and around East Anglia. Both groups were sent the AQ by mail, and enrollment reflects the returned responses (58 of 63 for HFA/AS and 174 of 500 for controls). Mean age was 31.6 years (SD = 11.4, range: 16.5–58.3) for the HFA/AD group, and 37.0 years (SD = 7.7, range: 18.1–60.0) for the control group. Fifteen individuals from each group were administered four subtests of the Wechsler Adult Intelligence Scale—Revised (WAIS-R), and all earned prorated IQ scores over 85 (HFA/AS group M = 105.8). Based upon differences between the two groups, a cutoff of ≥ 32 was chosen, met by 79.3% of the HFA/AD sample and 2% of the control sample.

Reliability and Readability

Test authors provided Cronbach alphas for each domain: Communication = .65, Social = .77, Imagination = .65, Local Details = .63, and Attention Switching = .67 (Mdn = .65). For a sample of 201 undergraduates, Austin (2005) reported internal consistency reliability of .82 for the AQ total score and subscale reliabilities from .58 (Attention Switching) to .75 (Social); median subscale reliability was .65. In a Japanese sample, Wakabayashi, Baron-Cohen, Wheelwright, and Tojo (2006) found internal consistency as follows: .81 for the AQ total, subscale reliabilities ranging from .51 to .78, and median reliability of .63. In another Japanese sample, Kurita, Koyama, and Osada (2005) found total AQ score internal consistency reliability of .78. Hurst, Mitchell, Kimbrel, Kwapil, and Nelson-Gray (2007) found total AQ internal consistency of .67 and Mdn subtest internal consistency of .47 (n = 1,005 college students). In a Dutch sample, Ketelaars et al. (2008) found internal consistency of .85 for AQ total and average subscale reliability to be .67 for a sample of 15 individuals with ASD. In another Dutch sample, Hoekstra, Bartels, Cath, and Boomsma (2008) modified the AQ scoring rules to allow for 4-point responses per item (range 0–200) and found internal consistency of .81 (n = 961) for a college student sample and

.71 (n = 302) for a general population sample. Subscale reliabilities ranged from .49 to .76 across both groups (Mdn = .63).

Test–retest data (r = .7; 2-week interval) were obtained for college students (n = 17; Baron-Cohen et al., 2001). Kurita et al. (2005) found a test–retest value of .77 for 19 individuals with ASD (7.3-month interval). Wakabayashi et al. (2006) found a temporal stability of .87 for 54 Japanese college students (2- to 3-week interval). Hoekstra et al. (2008) reported test–retest of r = .78 for the AQ total and subtest temporal stabilities ranging from .60 to .87 (Mdn = .69) for 75 individuals (3.9-month interval). Wakabayashi et al. (2006) reported interrater reliability of .71 for self-parent report for 32 adults with HFA/AS diagnoses. The AQ FRE readability is 63.4 and the F-KG readability is 7.4.

Validity

Test authors present discriminant validity evidence in the form of significant differences between HFA/AS (M = 35.8, SD = 6.5) and control groups (M = 16.4, SD = 6.3) for AQ total scores and subscales. Kurita et al. (2005) found AQ total scores to correctly classify 72% of the ASD group, with sensitivity of .76, specificity of .71, PPV of .24, and NPV of .96. Woodbury-Smith et al. (2005) assessed validity of the AQ as a screening instrument for AS in a clinic-referred, adult sample (N = 100; 75% male; Mdn age = 32 years). Of the total sample, 73 individuals were diagnosed with AS, whereas 27 were not. Using a cut-point of 26 for this sample, sensitivity was .95, specificity was .52, PPV was .84, and NPV was .78. Wakabayashi et al. (2006) also found that adults with ASDs produced higher AQ scores than community controls or college students. Hoekstra et al. (2008) found that adults with ASD scored higher on the AQ when compared to the general population, to individuals with obsessive–compulsive disorder, and to individuals with social anxiety disorder. Ketelaars et al. (2008) did not replicate findings for adults with ASD (n = 15) versus no ASD (n = 21) referred to an autism specialty clinic; groups were matched on age and IQ. Austin (2005) found support for a three-factor structure for the AQ versus five domains as proposed by the test authors. Hoekstra et al. (2008) found a hierarchical factor structure with a higher-order factor of Social Interaction, consisting of the Social Skill, Attention Switching, Communication, and Imagination scales, and separate Attention to Detail factor.

Evidence-Based Assessment Classification

The total test score for the AQ consistently, but not always, meets minimum standards for internal consistency reliability and temporal stability; however, AQ subscale internal consistency (Mdn = .47–.65) values typically fall below minimum standards. The scale has been subjected to validation across various samples from several countries, including community-based samples, college student samples, and clinic-referred samples. The AQ has demonstrated adequate sensitivity but poor specificity in a clinic-referred sample. Overall, the AQ meets criteria as a "well-established" adult screening instrument for HFA/AS because it has appeared in at least two peer-reviewed articles from two investigative teams (Austin, 2005; Kurita et al., 2005), the measure is presented in sufficient detail, and it has demonstrated good psychometric properties in at least one study (e.g., Hoekstra et al., 2008).

Adult Asperger Assessment and Empathy Quotient

The Adult Asperger Assessment (AAA; Baron-Cohen, Wheelwright, Robinson, & Woodbury-Smith, 2005) consists of a clinical interview and two self-report screening measures: the AQ and the Empathy Quotient (EQ; Baron-Cohen & Wheelwright, 2004). As such, the AAA is a diagnostic method as opposed to a self-report measure; however, the inclusion of two self-report screeners in the AAA model warrants inclusion in this section, in our opinion. The AAA is based on more stringent criteria for diagnosis of AS than those outlined in the DSM-IV, such that all persons meeting AAA diagnostic criteria for AS would also meet DSM-IV diagnostic criteria. The AAA features assessment of five domains, four of these found in the DSM-IV definition (communication, social impairments, repetitive behavior/restricted interests, and necessary and exclusionary criteria), and the additional category of "impairments in imagination." The interview and scoring process takes approximately 3 hours to complete and does not include administration time for the AQ or EQ, which the authors note can be completed independently prior to the interview. The interviewer uses the responses to the AQ and EQ to guide the interview, specifically noting examples of symptoms in each of the domains. Respondents receive 1 point for each symptom endorsed/confirmed during the interview, for a possible score range of 0–18. Diagnosis requires a score of ≥ 10, which must include at least three out of five symptoms for each of the social, communication, and restricted/stereotyped domains; one out of three symptoms in the imagination domain; and meeting all criteria of the inclusion–exclusion category (e.g., age of onset). The AAA diagnostic method was tested with a group of 42 participants referred to a specialty clinic for evaluation due to suspected AS. Two clinicians interviewed each participant and independently completed/scored the AAA.

The EQ is a 60-item (40 scored; 20 control items) self-report measure of empathy designed for use by adults with normal intelligence that was based on a two-part theory of empathy that includes cognitive and affective domains. The EQ was initially tested in a sample of 90 individuals with HFA or AS and 174 volunteers from the general population (Baron-Cohen & Wheelwright, 2004). EQ scoring is as follows: slight or strong nonendorsement receives zero (0) points, slight endorsement receives one (1), and strong endorsement receives two (2). Items are summed to yield a total raw score that may range from 0 to 80. Higher scores correspond to higher empathy (i.e., AQ and EQ scores correlate negatively). A pilot study of 20 control volunteers was conducted to ensure comprehension and readability of the EQ.

Reliability and Readability

Test authors report EQ internal consistency reliability of .92 ($n = 297$ adult controls; Baron-Cohen & Wheelwright, 2004). Muncer and Ling (2006) reported alpha = .85 for a sample of 362 college students in the United Kingdom. With a Japanese sample, Wakabayashi et al. (2007) found internal consistency reliability of .86 for control participants ($n = 137$). Berthoz, Wessa, Kedia, Wicker, and Grezes (2008) reported Cronbach's alpha = .81 in sample of 410 French college students. Test authors report EQ temporal stability of .97 ($n = 15$ individuals with AS/HFA; 12-month interval); Lawrence, Shaw, Baker, Baron-Cohen, and David (2004) found temporal stability of .84 ($n = 24$ community volunteers; 12-month interval). Berthoz et al. (2008) documented temporal stability of .93 ($n = 36$ community volunteers; 6- to 24-week interval). The EQ FRE readability is 64.1 and the F-KG readability is of 7.6.

For the AAA method, no reliability statistics were provided in the initial validation study (Baron-Cohen, Wheelwright, Robinson, & Woodbury-Smith, 2005), despite two interviewers' independent scoring of the AAA protocol. When utilized in concert in the AAA method, EQ and AQ overall FRE readability is 63.8 and the F-KG is 7.5.

Validity

Test authors report significant differences in EQ scores between the HFA/AS group ($M = 20.4$, $SD = 11.6$) and an age- and sex-matched control group ($n = 90$; $M = 42.1$, $SD = 10.6$; Baron-Cohen & Wheelwright, 2004). Based on cumulative score percentages for each group, a cutoff of ≤ 30 was recommended for detecting HFA/AS. Wakabayashi et al. (2007) reported mean differences between a group of individuals with HFA/AS ($n = 48$; $M = 24.9$; $SD = 8.3$) and both community controls ($n = 137$; $M = 33.9$; $SD = 11.0$) and college students ($n = 1250$; $M = 33.4$; $SD = 10.7$). Berthoz et al. (2008) found that 15 of 16 adults with ASD (93.75%) scored at or below the cutoff score of 30.

Lawrence et al. (2004) examined the factor structure of the EQ and found evidence for a three-factor structure (Cognitive Empathy, Emotional Reactivity, and Social Skills) with 28 of 40 EQ items. Berthoz et al. (2008) found the three-factor structure to be a good fit for French college students; however, Muncer and Ling (2006) found the three-factor structure to be a poor fit and suggested modifications to the scale to improve its measurement properties, proposing that a 15-item shortened form may be appropriate. Lawrence et al. found that the EQ correlated with the Interpersonal Reactivity Index (IRI) in a sample of 28 community volunteers; Berthoz documented good convergent validity for the EQ via correlations with the IRI and another measure of empathy.

For the initial AAA validation study, individuals diagnosed with HFA/AS (n = 34) obtained significantly higher AAA algorithm, AQ, and EQ scores than did the nondiagnosed participants (n = 8). Specifically, AAA-diagnosed group means for the AAA, AQ, and EQ were 14.7 (SD = 1.8), 34.6 (SD = 7.3), and 21.8 (SD = 10.6), respectively, whereas the nondiagnosed group means for the AAA, AQ, and EQ were 4.9 (SD = 2.5), 25.0 (SD = 10.3), and 32.0 (SD = 12.2), respectively. Of the nondiagnosed participants, three met the less stringent DSM-IV criteria for AS. No sensitivity, specificity, or PPV values have been reported for the AAA diagnostic system.

Evidence-Based Assessment Classification

The EQ demonstrates good to excellent internal consistency reliability and temporal stability. There is compelling evidence to support the finding that individuals with HFA/AS produce lower EQ scores when compared to other groups of adults. The factor structure of the EQ continues to be investigated, with evidence that at least some EQ items are not sufficiently correlated with the total score. Overall, the EQ meets criteria as a "well-established" measure of empathy because it has appeared in at least two peer-reviewed articles from two investigative teams (Berthoz et al., 2008; Muncer & Ling, 2006), the measure is presented in sufficient detail, and it has demonstrated good psychometric properties in at least one study (e.g., Berthoz et al.).

Taken together, the AQ and EQ measures both satisfy EBT-TF criteria for "well-established" measures; however, their combined utility to inform diagnostic interviewing procedures featured in the AAA method has yet to be appropriately validated. The authors of the AAA provide no psychometric evidence for the method's reliability and little evidence of its validity. It would also be of interest to learn if the AQ and EQ items fall into four scales, as indicated in the AAA algorithm. As such, the AAA diagnostic method meets "promising" assessment criteria because it has appeared in one peer-reviewed article (Baron-Cohen et al., 2005), the measure is presented in sufficient detail, and it features initial validity data (i.e., discriminant validity) in at least one study (Baron-Cohen et al.).

Ritvo Autism and Asperger's Diagnostic Scale

The Ritvo Autism and Asperger's Diagnostic Scale (RAADS; Ritvo et al., 2008) is a 78-item rating scale of feelings/thoughts and behaviors indicative of autism and AS. The RAADS contains three subscales: Social Related-ness, Language and Communication, and Sensorimotor and Stereotypies; however, instructions for summing only a single total score are provided. Cutoff scores indicating the probability of autism or AS are provided. The RAADS pilot study states that the purpose of the scale is to aid clinicians in diagnosis of autism or AS in adults.

Authors developed the RAADS based on review of DSM-IV-TR and ICD-10 diagnostic criteria for autism and AS. Items were revised or omit-ted based on feedback from expert review and field trials, ultimately result-ing in a reduction from 100 to 78 items. The RAADS was piloted using a small, combined sample of individuals diagnosed with autism or AS and a control sample. Difficulties ascertaining age of language acquisition led to the combining of autism and AS diagnostic groups. The autism/AS sample (n = 37; 59% male) ranged in age from 18 to 65 (M = 37 and 33 for AS and autism). Participants in the autism/AS group were recruited from (1) patients known to the authors, (2) national support groups, (3) referrals from clinicians, and (4) advertisements on AS websites. Independent diag-noses by two psychiatrists were made based on DSM-IV-TR criteria. The control sample (n = 57; 44% male) was also comprised of two groups: 16 individuals with Axis I conditions other than autism/AS and 41 individuals without prior Axis I diagnosis. RAADS cutoff scores were created using the means, standard deviations, and ranges of each group; there was no overlap in total score ranges between the autism/AS group and the control group.

Reliability and Readability

Authors provide evidence for internal consistency reliability for each of the three subscales, but not for the total test. For the entire group of partici-pants, Cronbach's alpha was .86 for Social Relatedness, .60 for Language and Communication, and .70 for Sensorimotor and Stereotypies. No infor-mation is provided for temporal stability. The RAADS FRE score was 68.5 and the F-KG score was 7.4.

Validity

Test authors employed expert review to assess item content. Two field trials were conducted in which extensive feedback on the measure was elicited from individuals with and without autism/AS, leading to removal of several items. Authors provide evidence of criterion validity, as score ranges did not overlap between groups (sensitivity, specificity = 1.0). Additional evi-dence for criterion validity includes significant differences found between the autism/AS group and the comparison group for (1) total test scores, (2) scores on each of the three subscales, and (3) for 77 of the 78 items. The pilot study included no evidence of concurrent or divergent validity.

Evidence-Based Assessment Classification

The authors of the RAADS acknowledge that the measure may benefit from some revision, including removal of three items to increase internal consistency for the Language/Communication and Sensorimotor/Stereotypies scales, and removal of the item that showed no discrimination between the autism/AD group and the comparison group. In addition, several other issues should be addressed prior to clinical use. First, the RAADS should undergo standardization with a larger sample. Second, reliability data are weak and incomplete for the RAADS, as no total score internal consistency coefficient is provided, median subtest reliability fails to meet our .80 criterion for internal consistency, and no temporal stability data are presented. Overall, the RAADS meets criteria as a "promising" assessment for diagnosing adults with autism or AS because the scale has appeared in one peer-reviewed article, the measure is presented in sufficient detail, and it features moderate psychometrics in at least one article (Ritvo et al., 2008).

General Comments about Self-Report Scales

Researchers and diagnosticians have taken notice of the utility of self-report measures for the purposes of screening adult populations for HFA/AS and to aid in the diagnostic assessment of adults suspected to have HFA/AS. The AQ has undergone an impressive amount of validation to date, including cross-cultural validation, and is considered a "well-established" measure according to the EBA-TF criteria. The EQ is not designed as a diagnostic instrument, per se, but shows reasonable psychometric properties as a self-report measure of empathy. Similar to the AQ, the EQ has been validated across cultures.

SUMMARY AND CONCLUSIONS

The field has reached consensus regarding "gold-standard" assessment and diagnosis for autism which is the combination of ADOS and ADI-R. For assessment and diagnosis of AS, the field has not yet reached consensus regarding the appropriate definition of AS vis-á-vis HFA. Well-documented problems with the DSM-IV definition of AS (Mayes, Calhoun, & Crites, 2001) and research findings documenting few, if any, differences between matched groups of individuals with AS and HFA have contributed to the omission of AS in the DSM-5 (American Psychiatric Association, 2013). Due to recent changes to the DSM-5, efforts to develop and validate diagnostic and screening instruments specific to AS will likely cease. If a modified definition of AS were to be re-introduced in subsequent revisions to the DSM system, further efforts to develop and validate measures by the AS will likely reemerge. What has resulted thus far within the AS diagnostic literature is that investigators use different case definitions for AS that have yielded different classification accuracy rates. As such, psychometric research may not cleanly disentangle what accounts for discrepancies across studies: That is, is the predictive validity of the scale or the diagnostic criterion at issue? When wide variation is inherent in the diagnostic definition of a disorder, summative statements about its valid detection and measurement cannot be rendered.

A significant reason that consensus diagnostic criteria do not exist for AS is that no clinical, neuropsychological, or behavioral indicator reliably discriminates between individuals with AS and those with HFA. The search for "phenotypic" differences between AS and HFA has produced contradictory findings in the literature, which are undoubtedly reviewed in the present text. It should not be surprising that the measures presented and reviewed here show significant limitations with respect to discrimination between AS and HFA.

Measurement efforts within the field of ASD have responded to the lack of definitional clarity and phenotypic distinctiveness of AS by expanding criterion groups to include individuals with HFA or AS. This approach is consistent with recent changes to the diagnostic classification system that considers AS within the autism spectrum, rather than as a distinct disorder. Without diagnostic consensus, we cannot nominate any measure as a "gold-standard" instrument for diagnosing AS. Several measures emerged as valid screeners for the larger autism spectrum and showed good ability to discriminate between ASD and non-ASD criterion groups. At this point, however, no measure is well established for rendering a differential diagnosis between HFA and AS.

At a minimum, we hope that we have provided the reader with an organized introduction and critique of several diagnostic and screening measures of AS. It is our intention to stimulate thought and discussion regarding the applicability of EBA tenets and classification procedures within the field of ASD, in general. We realize that our chapter focused on third-party ratings and self-report instruments; however, in our opinion, interviewing methods, observation techniques, and perhaps other assessment procedures also warrant careful evaluation from an EBA perspective. If the value of the EBA movement is acknowledged within the field of ASD and "sticks," which we hope will be the case, finer-grained criteria are worth development and perhaps worthy of a separate contribution, such as a special issue, focused on various purposes of assessment (e.g., treatment planning) across all ASD.

REFERENCES

Allison, C., Williams, J., Scott, F., Stott, C., Bolton, P., Baron-Cohen, S., et al. (2007). The Childhood Asperger Syndrome Test (CAST): Test–retest reliability in a high scoring sample. *Autism, 11,* 173–185.

American Psychiatric Association. (1994). *Diagnostic and statistical manual of mental disorders* (4th ed.). Washington, DC: Author.

American Psychiatric Association. (2013). *Diagnostic and statistical manual of mental disorders* (5th ed.). Arlington, VA: Author.

Asperger, H. (1944). Die "Autistischen Psychopathen" im Kindesalter. *Archiv für Psychiatrie und Nervenkrankheiten, 117,* 76–136.

Austin, E. J. (2005). Personality correlates of the broader autism phenotype as assessed by the Autism Spectrum Quotient (AQ). *Personality and Individual Differences, 38,* 451–460.

Baron-Cohen, S., & Wheelwright, S. (2004). The Empathy Quotient: An investigation of adults with Asperger syndrome or high-functioning autism, and normal sex differences. *Journal of Autism and Developmental Disorders, 34,* 163–175.

Baron-Cohen, S., Wheelwright, S., Robinson, J., & Woodbury-Smith, M. (2005). The Adult Asperger Assessment (AAA): A diagnostic method. *Journal of Autism and Developmental Disorders, 35,* 807–819.

Baron-Cohen, S., Wheelwright, S., Skinner, R., Martin, J., & Clubley, E. (2001). The Autism-Spectrum Quotient (AQ): Evidence from Asperger syndrome/high-functioning autism, males and females, scientists and mathematicians. *Journal of Autism and Developmental Disorders, 31,* 5–17.

Berthoz, S., Wessa, M., Kedia, G., Wicker, B., & Grezes, J. (2008). Cross-cultural validation of the Empathy Quotient in a French-speaking sample. *Canadian Journal of Psychiatry, 53,* 469–477.

Boggs, K. M., Gross, A. M., & Gohm, C. L. (2006). Validity of the Asperger Syndrome Diagnostic Scale. *Journal of Developmental and Physical Disabilities, 18,* 163–182.

Campbell, J. M. (2005). Diagnostic assessment of Asperger's disorder: A review of five third-party rating scales. *Journal of Autism and Developmental Disorders, 35,* 25–35.

Cicchetti, D. V. (1994). Guidelines, criteria, and rules of thumb for evaluating normed and standardized assessment instruments in psychology. *Psychological Assessment, 6,* 284–290.

Cohen, L. L., La Greca, A. M., Blount, R. L., Kazak, A. E., Holmbeck, G. N., & Lemanek, K. L. (2008). Introduction to Special Issue: Evidence-based assessment in pediatric psychology. *Journal of Pediatric Psychology, 33,* 911–915.

Ehlers, S., & Gillberg, C. (1993). The epidemiology of Asperger syndrome: A total population study. *Journal of Child Psychology and Psychiatry, 34,* 1327–1350.

Ehlers, S., Gillberg, C., & Wing, L. (1999). A screening questionnaire for Asperger syndrome and other high-functioning autism spectrum disorders in school age children. *Journal of Autism and Developmental Disorders, 29,* 129–141.

Gilliam, J. E. (2001). *Gilliam Asperger's Disorder Scale.* Austin, TX: PRO-ED.

Hoekstra, R. A., Bartels, M., Cath, D. C., & Boomsma, D. I. (2008). Factor structure, reliability, and criterion validity of the Autism Spectrum Quotient (AQ): A study in Dutch population and patient groups. *Journal of Autism and Developmental Disorders, 38,* 1555–1566.

Hurst, R. M., Mitchell, J. T., Kimbrel, N. A., Kwapil, T. K., & Nelson-Gray, R. O. (2007). Examination of the reliability and factor structure of the Autism Spectrum Quotient in a non-clinical sample. *Personality and Individual Differences, 43,* 1938–1949.

Ketelaars, C., Horwitz, E., Sytema, S., Bos, J., Wiersma, D., Minderaa, R., et al. (2008). Brief report: Adults with mild autism spectrum disorders (ASD): Scores on the Autism Spectrum Quotient (AQ) and comorbid psychopathology. *Journal of Autism and Developmental Disorders, 38,* 176–180.

Klin, A., Volkmar, F. R., & Sparrow, S. S. (Eds.). (2000). *Asperger syndrome.* New York: Guilford Press.

Kopra, K., von Wendt, L., Nieminen-von Wendt, T., & Paavonen, E. J. (2008). Comparison of diagnostic methods for Asperger syndrome. *Journal of Autism and Developmental Disorders, 38,* 1567–1573.

Krug, D. A., & Arick, J. R. (2003). *Krug Asperger's Disorder Index.* Austin, TX: PRO-ED.

Kurita, H., Koyama, T., & Osada, H. (2005). Autism-Spectrum Quotient: Japanese version and its short forms for screening normal intelligence persons with pervasive developmental disorders. *Psychiatry and Clinical Neurosciences, 59,* 490–496.

Lawrence, E. J., Shaw, P., Baker, D., Baron-Cohen, S., & David, A. S. (2004). Measuring empathy: Reliability and validity of the Empathy Quotient. *Psychological Medicine, 24,* 911–924.

Mash, E. J., & Hunsley, J. (2005). Evidence-based assessment of child and adolescent disorders: Issues and challenges. *Journal of Clinical Child and Adolescent Psychology, 34,* 362–379.

Matson, J. L., Dempsey, T., & Rivet, T. (2008). A comparison of Asperger symptom rating scales with children and adolescents. *Research in Autism Spectrum Disorders, 2,* 643–650.

Mayes, S. D., Calhoun, S. L., & Crites, D. L. (2001). Does DSM-IV Asperger's disorder exist? *Journal of Abnormal Child Psychology, 29,* 263–271.

Muncer, S. J., & Ling, J. (2006). Psychometric analysis of the empathy quotient (EQ) scale. *Personality and Individual Differences, 40,* 1111–1119.

Myles, B. S., Bock, S. J., & Simpson, R. L. (2001). *Asperger Syndrome Diagnostic Scale.* Los Angeles, CA: Western Psychological Services.

Petersen, D. J., Bilenberg, N., Hoerder, K., & Gillberg, C. (2006). The population prevalence of child psychiatric disorders in Danish 8- to 9-year-old children. *European Child and Adolescent Psychiatry, 15,* 71–78.

Posserud, B., Lundervold, A. J., & & Gillberg, C. (2006). Autistic features in a total population of 7- to 9-year-old children assessed by the ASSQ (Autism Spectrum Screening Questionnaire). *Journal of Child Psychology and Psychiatry, 47,* 167–175.

Posserud, B., Lundervold, A. J., & Gillberg, C. (2009). Validation of the Autism Spectrum Screening Questionnaire in a total population sample. *Journal of Autism and Developmental Disorders, 39,* 126–134.

Posserud, B., Lundervold, A. J., Steijnen, M. C., Verhoeven, S., Stormark, K. M., & Gillberg, C. (2008). Factor analysis of the Autism Spectrum Screening Questionnaire. *Autism, 12,* 99–112.

Ritvo, R. A., Ritvo, E. R., Guthrie, D., Yuwiler, A., Ritvo, M. J., & Weisbender, L. (2008). A scale to assist the diagnosis of autism and Asperger's disorder in adults (RAADS): A pilot study. *Journal of Autism and Developmental Disorders, 38,* 213–223.

Scott, F. J., Baron-Cohen, S., Bolton, P., & Brayne, C. (2002). The CAST (Childhood Asperger Syndrome Test): Preliminary development of a UK screen for mainstream primary-school age children. *Autism, 6,* 9–31.

Streiner, D. L. (1993). A checklist for evaluating the usefulness of rating scales. *Canadian Journal of Psychiatry, 38,* 140–148.

Wakabayashi, A., Baron-Cohen, S., Uchiyama, T., Yoshida, Y., Kuroda, M., & Wheelwright, S. (2007). Empathizing and systemizing in adults with and without autism spectrum conditions: Cross-cultural stability. *Journal of Autism and Developmental Disorders, 37,* 1823–1832.

Wakabayashi, A., Baron-Cohen, S., Wheelwright, S., & Tojo, Y. (2006). The Autism-Spectrum Quotient (AQ) in Japan: A cross-cultural comparison. *Journal of Autism and Developmental Disorders, 36,* 263–270.

Webb, E., Morey, J., Thompsen, W., Butler, C., Barger, M., & Fraser, W. I. (2003). Prevalence of autistic spectrum disorder in children attending mainstream schools in a Welsh education authority. *Developmental Medicine and Child Neurology, 45,* 377–384.

Williams, J., Allison, C., Scott, F., Stott, C., Bolton, P., Baron-Cohen, S., et al. (2006). The Childhood Asperger Syndrome Test (CAST): Test–retest reliability. *Autism, 10,* 415–427.

Williams, J., Allison, C., Scott, F., Stott, C., Bolton, P., Baron-Cohen, S., et al. (2008). The Childhood Asperger Syndrome Test (CAST): Sex differences. *Journal of Autism and Developmental Disorders, 38,* 1731–1739.

Williams, J., Scott, F., Stott, C., Allison, C., Bolton, P., Baron-Cohen, S., et al. (2005). The Childhood Asperger Syndrome Test (CAST): Test accuracy. *Autism, 9,* 45–68.

Wing, L. (1981). Asperger's syndrome: A clinical account. *Psychological Medicine, 11,* 115–129.

Woodbury-Smith, M. R., Robinson, J., Wheelwright, S., & Baron-Cohen, S. (2005). Screening adults for Asperger syndrome using the AQ: A preliminary study of its diagnostic validity in clinical practice. *Journal of Autism and Developmental Disorders, 35,* 331–335.

World Health Organization. (1993). *International classification of diseases and related health problems* (10th ed.). Geneva, Switzerland: Author.

CHAPTER 3

Neuropsychological Characteristics of Asperger Syndrome

Katherine D. Tsatsanis

In this chapter neuropsychological functioning in Asperger syndrome (AS) is examined. Several social-cognitive and perceptual and learning models have led the field, such as joint attention, theory of mind, central coherence, and enactive mind, that are also sometimes considered as part of the neuropsychological literature on autism spectrum disorders (ASD); however, these areas of research require critical evaluation in their own right and are addressed elsewhere. In the discussion that follows, an effort is made to examine the extant research on core domains of neuropsychological functioning—domains that are typically assessed as part of a comprehensive clinical neuropsychological evaluation. In each section, a brief overview describes how the domain of functioning is assessed, as well as its putative relationship to the behavioral expression of AS. A review of the research on each domain of functioning is followed by a summary of the findings, clinical relevance, and suggestions for future directions.

Before consideration is given to this body of work, several caveats are worth addressing. The research reviewed spans two decades, and in that time the nosological status of AS has been called into question, with variable usage of diagnostic schemas among researchers. This variation limits the extent to which samples are comparable and findings are generalizable; it is not clear whether the composition of AS groups is consistent across studies. Moreover, increasingly investigators have chosen to combine clinical groups, opting to use the term ASD to represent a mixed sample of high-functioning individuals with autism, AS, and/or pervasive developmental disorder not otherwise specified (PDD-NOS). A recurrent methodological issue is that of subject sample size; in the studies examining cognitive processes in AS, it is not uncommon for subject samples to include as few as 8 or 12 participants, limiting power to detect differences, particularly when this is also combined with an age range that spans childhood, adolescence, and in some cases (young) adulthood. It is also the case (with some notable exceptions) that very few studies focus on any one domain of neuropsychological functioning in AS and follow a more comprehensive or intensive path of inquiry. A systematic approach seems warranted to increase understanding and address some of the unanswered questions that remain of interest and relevant to the field.

The findings from the studies reviewed may not be characteristic of, or generalizable to, all individuals with AS, but they are representative of the research to date and provide considerations for clinical management as well as point to opportunities for future directions of research. Both relative assets and deficits are identified in the domains of sensory perception, motor functioning, attention, memory, and executive functioning; although language abilities also fall within the scope of a neuropsychological assessment, this area of functioning is comprehensively addressed in a separate chapter. General cognitive and neuropsychological profiles are also reviewed herein. Each of these domains can be seen to have relevance for how individuals with AS acquire and process information and in turn form an internal representation of the world and respond to its demands.

SENSORY PERCEPTION

Tactile, visual, and auditory perceptual functioning are generally assessed at elementary levels, such as basic sensory perception/imperception, as well as higher levels of perceptual ability, such as finger agnosia and form or coin recognition in the tactile domain. Results from the assessment of the perceptual systems contribute to the formulation of initial hypotheses regarding which side and region of the brain is impaired in its functioning. Also, assessment of the sensory–perceptual systems has particular significance for developmental disorders such as AS that exhibit onset in early childhood. If an individual has basic impairments in one or more sensory–perceptual systems early in life, developmental consequences may ensue over time. The cumulative effects of deficient information processing through a particular sensory modality may result in a lack of the type or amount of stored information needed to readily judge current or incoming information (Rourke, van der Vlugt, & Rourke, 2002). As such, the early templates that serve as a foundation for higher-order skills/processes may not be well formed. In addition, experiences may be fragmented in a very fundamental way if information received through one sensory–perceptual modality must be shared with another modality in order to learn and complete complex tasks. For example, reading involves the translation of visual and auditory information into the other (i.e., graphemes to phonemes), and it seems likely that the social experience at some critical point would require the integration of auditory, visual, and tactile information.

A pattern of atypical sensory responses was noted by Ornitz and Ritvo (1968) very early on in the study of autism, and this pattern was the basis of their theory of perceptual inconstancy. Ornitz and Ritvo documented sensory hypo- and hypersensitivities in over 150 individuals with autism and, based on their observations, hypothesized that people with autism have an inability to regulate their sensory input, manifesting in alternating states of excitement and inhibition. These atypical sensory responses present in a variety of ways. Hypo- and hypersensitive responses include visual fixation on patterns and movement; hyposensitivity to pain, cold, or heat; aversion to specific kinds of tactile input; and hypersensitivity to some sounds but failure to react to others. The repetitive behaviors often seen in autism may involve a sensory stimulation component (e.g., visual fascination with movement, such as spinning objects, hand flapping, rocking, spinning); one perspective is that individuals with autism may engage in these behaviors to seek wanted sensory input.

Asperger's case reports (translated by Frith, 1991; Wing, 1981) also indicated the presence of unusual sensory responses in children with AS. Atypical sensory responses have since been documented in a larger sample of 42 children with AS (Dunn, Myles, & Orr, 2002). Using the Sensory Profile (Dunn, 1999), a questionnaire with 125 items describing responses to sensory events in daily life, the children with AS were reported to differ significantly from their nondisabled peers, selected from the standardization sample, in 22 of the 23 domains examined. The children with AS in this study showed processing difficulties across modalities and difficulties with factors related to both hypo- and hyperresponsiveness. As proposed for children with autism, children with AS appear to show differences in their ability to regulate their responses to sensory information.

The above findings are based on *observation* of behaviors manifest in everyday functioning. Psychophysical studies of tactile perception have also been used to examine whether atypical sensory responses are present in this modality. Two studies have confirmed increased sensitivity to tactile stimulation, specifically vibration, in a small sample of adults with AS (Blakemore et al., 2006) and AS/HFA (Cascio et al., 2008). When rating the *perception* of tactile stimulation, the adults with AS also showed tactile hypersensitivity, rating both externally and self-produced touch as more intense than the control group (Blakemore et al., 2006). The AS group showed a typical perceptual response with regard to attenuation of self- versus externally produced touch. Thresholds for detecting light touch and mild warmth and coolness were found to be similar in the mixed ASD group as compared to controls (Cascio et al., 2008). Sensitivity to thermal pain was increased; that is, thresholds for cold and heat pain sensitivity were lower in the AS/HFA group.

The direct assessment of perceptual processes using traditional neuropsychological instruments is more equivocal as to areas of deficit and/or distinction in the way tactile information is processed. A retrospective review of medical, psychiatric, and assessment records indicated that out of 101 children (91 with a diagnosis of AS), 42 had auditory-perceptual and 36 had tactile-perceptual dysfunction, with 21 children showing combined deficits (Sturm, Fernell, & Gillberg, 2004). In a study of preschool children with AS and HFA, the two clinical groups did not differ in their performance on measures of stereognosis (perception of form/object through touch) and finger localization, but notably 70% of the AS sample scored below the average range on the former and 40% on the latter (Iwanaga, Kawasaki, & Tsuchida, 2000). Performance in this domain of functioning (tactile perception) was not correlated with intelligence scores. This finding was not replicated in a small sample of 8- to 14-year-olds with AS when their performance was compared to a typically developing control group. Measures of tactile perception such as finger agnosia and fingertip writing tasks as well as memory, location, or time to completion on the Tactile Performance Test were not found to discriminate between children with AS and typically developing controls (Ryburn, Anderson, & Wales, 2009).

The visual-perceptual characteristics of individuals with autism have been interpreted to indicate a detail-focused processing bias and a relative challenge seeing the "big picture" or abstracting the gestalt form when processing incoming information for meaning (Frith, 1989; Happé & Frith, 2006; Happé & Booth, 2008). Using simple local–global stimuli (e.g., large number composed of smaller numbers), the visual processing of local versus global information was compared in autism, AS, and controls (Rinehart, Bradshaw, Moss, Brereton, & Tonge, 2000). The results indicated no difference between the clinical groups, with both groups showing disrupted processing of global stimuli when the local information was incongruent, a result not found in the control group. The findings were interpreted to support an "absence of global precedence," as originally proposed by Mottron and Belleville (1993), wherein global processing or apprehension of the *whole* does not take priority over processing of local features or the *parts*. Additionally, it was proposed that the interference effect of local on global processing could be consistent with deficits in inhibition and set shifting associated with dysfunction in the frontal systems, and/or right-hemispheric functioning associated with global processing. Adults with AS and autism were found to show a preference for local features specifically when there was an emphasis on the processing of interelemental spatial relationships (Rondan & Deruelle, 2007). The latter finding supports the notion that enhanced local processing may arise as the demand for configural analysis increases.

A similar conclusion was reached when perceptual organizational processes were analyzed using the Rey–Osterrieth Complex Figure Test (ROCF), a standard neuropsychological test that requires the analysis and reproduction of an unfamiliar, nonmeaningful figure (Tsatsanis et al., 2011). The individuals with ASD appeared to rely on a part-oriented strategy to cope with the complexity of the task; organizational processes affecting whether they perceived the pieces of information as connected to one another appeared to further impact later recall of the features. The ASD group did not show superiority for attending to, copying, and recalling the details of the ROCF figure; rather, they were likely to process complex information by parsing it into its component parts. The latter findings are more consistent with Kanner's (1943) language on this topic, with specific reference to how the individual with ASD may experience the world—that is, as made up of elements, challenged to experience wholes without full attention to the constituent parts.

Different aspects of auditory perception and processing have also been examined in individuals with AS, but often using event-related potential (ERP) methods. Few studies have directly assessed speech–sound discrimination, perhaps because of the relative language preservation in AS. Rather, research on language functioning has typically focused on the pragmatic aspects of language and communication, a characteristically deficit area. In a recent comprehensive investigation of language abilities in school-age children with AS, measures of phonological processing and nonword repetition as well as sentence comprehension in background noise were included in the assessment battery (Saalasti et al., 2008). The results indicated that the AS group did not perform differently than the typically developing (TD) control group on these measures, although there was a trend toward lower performance overall on the phonological processing task. (The AS group did perform significantly more poorly than the controls on a language comprehension task also included in the language battery).

Auditory discrimination and orienting are two components of speech perception that have been investigated using ERP paradigms with children with AS. Lepistö et al. (2006) found a diminished involuntary orienting response to speech pitch and phoneme changes, but not to corresponding changes in nonspeech sounds. Despite the relative preservation of their language development, the children with AS differed from controls and were similar to children with autism in their sound-discrimination and orienting responses at the cortical level as measured through ERP. Consistent with expectations, impairments were specific to the socially relevant versus nonsocial information; neural response to nonspeech changes appeared to be enhanced.

Enhanced cortical processing of pitch-related changes but impairments in discriminating changes in sound duration was reported in this group of children with AS (Lepistö et al., 2006); when examined in adults with AS, auditory hypersensitivity for detection of changes in both pitch and sound durations was identified (Kujala et al., 2007). The findings for enhanced discrimination abilities may be akin to what is reported in the visual realm with regard to a bias toward processing low-level perceptual information. The change in response over time is hypothesized to be related to the complexity of the neural networks involved in duration discrimination, specifically, and to the possibility of improvement with maturation. Additionally, right-hemisphere dominance for sound-discrimination accuracy was found for the AS but not the control group; neural response to speech pitch changes was parietally enhanced (Lepistö et al., 2006). Hemispheric differences may suggest an altered balance in interhemispheric information processing in individuals with AS. Neural responses to affective prosody in children with AS were also reported to be atypical, particularly over the right hemisphere (Korpilahti et al., 2007). Notably, this same atypicality was found in the boys' fathers as well.

In addition to auditory hypo- and hypersensitivities, understanding speech in noisy environments may be problematic for individuals with AS. When assessed using speech reception thresholds, a significant difference was found specifically for background sounds containing temporal or spectrotemporal dips (Alcantara, Weisblatt, Moore, & Bolton, 2004). It was proposed that a reduced ability to integrate information from the fragments present in temporal dips in noise may be a factor contributing to difficulties in understanding speech in noisy environments. Segregation of concurrent stream sounds may also contribute to such challenges; ERP recordings indicated differences for conditions requiring stream segregation but not for simple feature detection for children with AS, compared to their age-matched controls (Lepistö et al., 2009).

In summary, there is evidence from behavioral report, neuropsychological measures, and ERP paradigms for atypical sensory and perceptual processing in AS. When comparisons are made to individuals with autism, few discrepancies are found between the clinical groups. Despite the prevalence of sensory–perceptual differences in AS, this domain of functioning remains understudied in comparison to higher-order levels of cognition, such as executive functioning, and core features of the disorders, such as social and communication impairments. Yet, integrated higher-order functioning generally builds from simple perceptual discrimination to more complex levels of perceptual organization. A better understanding of the role of sensory perception and modulation from earliest development might also help to elucidate whether there are basic impairments in one or more sensory–perceptual systems, with ensuing downstream effects. Although differences between AS and TD groups are a consistent finding, it is not clear what, if any, the association is between the results from behavioral report, performance on neuropsychological measures, and response at the cortical level as measured through ERP. Further study to identify whether atypicalities in the sensory–perceptual domain bear any relationship to arousal, emotional regulation, and reward/salience systems, as well as to core impairments in social functioning, is warranted. As pursued in other domains of functioning, it would also be interesting to examine whether there are differences in sensory–perceptual processing in response to social versus nonsocial stimuli. From a clinical standpoint, sensory disturbances may be associated with regulatory difficulties and parents may express concern when their child encounters everyday stimuli and reacts quite differently from peers or siblings. Additionally, sensory input (e.g., tactile, auditory, olfactory, vestibular) would appear to be an integral part of the social and relational experience from the earliest days of development; impairments and/or atypicalities in this domain could reasonably impact the formation of coherent percepts as well as the ability to plan and coordinate an appropriate social response.

MOTOR FUNCTIONING

As with the sensory–perceptual examination, assessment of motor functioning involves the use of measures ranging from simple to more complex; for many higher-order motor tasks there is involvement of skills not solely motor in nature, but also, for example, the integration of visual and tactile processing. Results are again significant for both overall level of performance and comparative level of performance on the two sides of the body.

Motor clumsiness is a characteristic of many individuals with AS described in Asperger's clinical accounts (Wing, 1981). In addition, motor clumsiness is a feature identified in the DSM-IV-TR description of AS, although not a defining diagnostic feature. Motor impairments are not part of the DSM clinical description of PDD-NOS or autism, although repetitive motor movements do represent a diagnostic feature of autism. The results of studies of motor skills in individuals with AS have been equivocal, specifically as concern differences between AS and autism groups. Questions raised include how to operationalize the definition of *motor clumsiness* and to adequately describe and measure the different components of motor functioning.

Early reports suggestive of impaired motor skills and/or greater relative deficit in children with AS versus autism (Tantam; 1988; Gillberg, 1989; Szatmari, Bartolucci, & Bremner, 1989) were criticized for significant methodological issues (Ghaziuddin, Tsai, & Ghaziuddin, 1992). Subsequent studies reported motor problems but no group differences on standardized measures of motor skills and motor coordination (Ghaziuddin, Butler, Tsai, & Ghaziuddin, 1994; Manjiviona & Prior, 1995; Ghaziuddin & Butler, 1998). Motor impairments may not be a *distinguishing* feature of AS relative to autism, but they do appear to be a frequent part of the clinical picture in individuals with AS.

Although no difference between clinical groups has been found, as many as 50–85% of the AS subject samples showed significant levels of motor impairment (Ghaziuddin et al., 1994; Manjiviona & Prior, 1995;

Miyahara et al., 1997). Green et al. (2002) reported that motor impairment was present for the entire AS group, with 9 of the 11 children scoring below the fifth percentile on a measure of manual dexterity, ball skills, and balance. The children with AS were at least as impaired as the comparison group (children with a specific developmental disorder of motor function; SDD-MF) on this battery and more impaired in the domain of ball skills, specifically, which was relatively spared in the SDD-MF group. Ball skills were also found to be particularly impaired for the children with autism and AS in Manjiviona and Prior's (1995) study and when compared to individuals with learning disabilities (Miyahara et al., 1997). As noted by Green et al., ball skills differ from other tasks in the motor battery for their social component and complexity, requiring a spatial–temporal mental model as well as a sensory–motor map of one's body schema.

Further consideration has been given to the influence of related processes (e.g., sensory, executive) on motor performance. Performance on motor coordination tasks did not differ significantly when compared in a preschool-age sample of children with AS or HFA (Iwanaga et al., 2000). However, in the latter study foundation skills, including items such as "standing balance" and "walks line," were uniformly impaired in the small sample of preschool children with AS, and to a greater extent overall relative to the autism participants. The motor items that were differentially impaired share an equilibrium function. Similarly, when motor functioning in children and adolescents with AS was examined, motor tasks specifically involving proprioception were impaired (e.g., one-leg balance with eyes closed, tandem gait, repetitive finger–thumb apposition), but not motor speed, fine motor control, and visual–motor integration tasks (e.g., as assessed on finger tapping, grooved pegboard, and trail-making tests; Weimer, Schatz, Lincoln, Ballantyne, & Trauner, 2001). In a combined sample of adolescents and adults with HFA or AS, dynamic balance and performance of rapid alternating motor movements (diadochokinesis) were most impaired on a measure involving simple and complex motor tasks (Freitag, Kleser, Schneider, & von Gontard, 2007). Taken together, these results raise the question of whether a sensory problem (e.g., a deficit in the vestibular or proprioceptive system) and/or an *integration* deficit in sensory and motor processes may underlie the motor clumsiness and impairments observed in children with AS.

Rinehart et al. (2006a) questioned whether executive function impairments impact motor performance. Both the HFA and AS groups in this study showed deficits at the motor planning versus motor execution stage for upper-body movement; however, a movement preparation deficit was consistently displayed by the HFA group only relative to controls (Rinehart et al., 2006a, 2006b). The hypothesis of a role for executive dysfunction was not supported, as the motor preparation deficits were found across all planning tasks, regardless of complexity level. There was some evidence for task complexity effects with regard to motor *execution*. The authors proposed that the quantitative differences obtained may generate downstream effects on motor function and produce qualitative differences between the groups (e.g., "abnormal posturing" in autism as compared to "motor clumsiness" in AS).

When gait abnormalities and upper-body posturing were compared, children with autism or AS both showed abnormalities in coordination and smoothness relative to TD controls; the autism group showed greater gait variability and more abnormal arm posturing, whereas the AS group showed significantly more abnormalities in head/trunk posture than controls (Rinehart et al., 2006c). The authors noted that the observed impairments are suggestive of cerebellar involvement but also consistent with basal ganglia, possibly thalamic, and frontal striatal regions. No differences were obtained between children and adolescents with HFA or AS using a neurological measure of motor signs; when the combined group was compared to a nonimpaired control group, the ASD group showed significantly greater difficulty with motor overflow, gait, balance, and speed of repetitive timed movements (Jansiewicz et al., 2006). The wide range of motor abnormalities was considered to implicate frontal and subcortical areas rather than a more focal deficit. Rinehart et al. also eschewed a single-circuit hypotheses accounting for the movement abnormalities that present in ASD and suggested it might be worthwhile to examine how dysfunction in multiple neural systems might combine to compromise motor functioning.

Taken as a whole, there is considerable evidence of motor impairment in AS; distinctions from autism are more equivocal. One set of findings is suggestive of a quantitative difference in motor preparation that may contribute to qualitative differences in gait abnormalities and upper-body posturing, with greater presence of abnormal posturing in autism versus motor clumsiness in AS. Further study is required to elucidate whether and to what extent other processes contribute to the motor impairments found in AS. There is preliminary support for a sensory problem (e.g., a deficit in the vestibular or proprioceptive system) and/or an *integration* deficit in sensory and motor processes contributing to motor clumsiness in AS and the question of a role for EF in motor execution. The wide range of motor deficits observed in AS suggests that multiple regions of the brain are involved rather than a focal deficit or single circuit, with both frontal and subcortical regions implicated. Given the range and frequency of differences in motor functioning in individuals on the spectrum, as compared to their peers, the question arises whether there is a special relationship to the disorder and what it might signify. The clinical significance is wide-ranging, as deficits in this area may impact academic (e.g., constructional tasks requiring visual–motor integration), social (e.g., participation in ball play, sports), and adaptive (e.g., motor coordination required for eating, dressing, writing, driving) functioning.

ATTENTION

Attentional deficits may appear behaviorally as distractibility or impairment in the ability to focus behavior or concentrate on an activity, while ignoring other stimuli. Descriptions of the behavior of individuals with ASD underscore aspects of attention specifically related to the disability, such as an exclusive focus on particular details or unusual features of objects, attention to the nonsalient aspects of the environment with failure to attend to social stimuli, and difficulty shifting attention between activities or environmental stimuli. Although perhaps difficult to isolate, it is important to examine the domain of attention before consideration is given to more complex undertakings and levels of processing. Measures of attention by necessity include a perceptual processing component (e.g., visual, auditory, tactile). The clinical assessment may include specific measures of sustained, selective, and divided attention. In addition, during a comprehensive assessment, an individual is typically required to process information under conditions that tap and tax attentional capacities to different degrees; behavioral observations and results from across a number of heterogeneous tasks can be compared to draw conclusions about the individual's attentional capacities.

Intact sustained attention for simple/rote visual information has been reported in autism (Buchsbaum et al., 1992; Casey, Gordon, Mannheim, & Rumsey, 1993; Garretson, Fein, & Waterhouse, 1990; Johnson et al., 2007; Minshew, Goldstein, & Siegel, 1997; Pascualvaca, Fantie, Papageorgiou, & Mirsky, 1998). In contrast, deficits in attention for more complex tasks requiring filtering of information, selective attention, and shifts in attention are indicated (Ciesielski, Courchesne, & Elmasian, 1990; Casey et al., 1993; Courchesne, Townsend, Akshoomoff, Saitoh, Yeung-Courchesne, et al., 1994; Frazier et al., 2001; McGrath, Joseph, Tadevosyan, Folstein, & Tager-Flusberg, 2002; Townsend, Harris, & Courchesne, 1996; Wainwright-Sharp & Bryson, 1996).

There have been comparatively few studies to assess attention directly or systematically in children with AS, despite the presence of associated behavioral features of inattention and distractibility. In an exploratory study of attention using the Test of Visual Attention (TOVA; Greenberg, 1991), five of the eight children/adolescents with AS showed an attention deficit on this measure (Schatz, Weimer, & Trauner, 2002). The TOVA is a continuous performance test requiring sustained attention and inhibitory control. As compared to the TD control group, the AS group was more likely to perform in the abnormal range; mean global scores revealed a significant difference specifically for "Variability," an index of inconsistency of responding.

Attention deficits were also revealed on a battery of tests used to assess sustained attention, selective attention, and the ability to shift attention (Nydén, Gillberg, Hjelmquist, & Heiman, 1999). For all three clinical groups (AS, ADHD, and reading and writing disorder), performance was significantly lower than that of the TD control group on the majority of measures; no specific marker of attention/executive function deficits emerged to distinguish the three groups. The children with AS made few omission or commission errors but showed lengthier reaction times, particularly in the auditory condition, as well as large variability in response time on the go/no-go tasks and conflict conditions, which were presented as measures of the "sustain" and "focus-execute" components of attention. The AS group did not differ from TD controls on the "shift" dimension, as measured using the Wisconsin Card Sorting Test variables, including number of categories sorted, perseverative errors, and failure to maintain set. When the requirement to shift attention was measured using a task involving moving from processing a detail to a whole (Rinehart, Bradshaw, Moss, Brereton, & Tonge, 2001), the AS group again did not show a deficit; the autism group was significantly slower than controls, a finding that is consistent with other reports of impairment in shifting attention in autism.

Given the limited number of studies, small sample sizes, and variable instruments used, few definitive conclusions can be drawn about attentional processes in AS. That said, the findings are suggestive of areas of deficit as well as an attentional profile that is possibly the opposite of that seen in autism; that is, impairments on measures of sustained attention but not on shifting. The caveat is that the studies are few and constructs across studies not necessarily measured the same way. Nonetheless, this area is worthy of further and more systematic study.

Of the comorbid psychiatric disorders described in individuals with AS, the diagnosis of ADHD is of particular interest; symptoms of inattention and overactivity are identified in the DSM-IV-TR (American Psychiatric Association, 2000) as associated features of AS, and it is noted that an ADHD diagnosis frequently precedes a diagnosis of AS in children. Significant problems with attention, hyperactivity, and/or impulse control in children with AS have been identified on parent-report behavioral measures (Holtmann, Bölte, & Poustka, 2005; Thede & Coolidge, 2007), through retrospective review of medical/psychiatric records (Sturm et al., 2004), and through retrospective self-report by adults with AS (Tani et al., 2006). When rates of comorbidity were examined in children with autism (e.g., Leyfer et al., 2006), high-functioning children with PDD (Sturm et al., 2004), and children with AS specifically (Ehlers & Gillberg, 1993; Ghaziuddin, Weidmer-Mikhail, & Ghaziuddin, 1998), a high rate of comorbid ADHD was found.

Taken together, these findings raise questions as to whether observations of inattention, distractibility, and/or overactivity in children with AS are related to a deficit in attention, emotional processing (anxiety, depression, internal preoccupation), and/or the primary social disability itself. In addition, questions remain whether these difficulties affect all or a subset of individuals with ASD, and whether different patterns present in autism versus AS. More systematic and comprehensive study is needed. The clinical implications are also significant because there is an impact on diagnosis; academic, behavioral, and adaptive functioning; and treatment approach.

MEMORY

Memory is a multidimensional construct; divisions include working, implicit, and explicit memory, with the latter further subdivided into two subsystems, semantic and episodic memory. As with the other domains discussed, memory functioning can be assessed in a variety of modalities (e.g., auditory, visual, auditory–visual, tactile). The profile of memory functioning in AS is interesting, as many individuals with AS present with circumscribed interests, wherein they accumulate a wealth of factual information on a narrow topic. In contrast to lengthy monologues on such subjects of interest, bringing to mind previous events and experiences, in which one is aware of oneself in a particular place at a particular time, is a narrative that, by comparison, often appears to be less well developed. Whereas the latter construct (episodic memory) has been examined in a series of studies (largely by Bowler and colleagues in adults with AS), fewer studies have been devoted to working memory and semantic memory, specifically.

Working memory tasks require the ability to attend to, process, and recall information held in an online state. This area of memory functioning can also be considered within the neuropsychological domain of executive functions. In autism research, studies of working memory suggest intact verbal working memory for basic tasks but deficits in spatial working memory (Goldberg et al., 2005; Steele, Minshew, Luna, & Sweeney, 2007; Williams, Goldstein, Carpenter, & Minshew, 2005; Williams, Goldstein, & Minshew, 2006). A deficit in spatial working memory has also been reported in a small sample of adults with AS (Morris et al., 1999). The deficit was not attributed to strategy formation; errors of the AS group suggested they had difficulty remembering even simple sequences of spatial locations as well as holding successive locations in mind over a longer time period. Adults with AS also performed more poorly than controls on a measure of visual memory involving a visual recognition task (for different types of doors) and visual recall (drawing a visual pattern from memory) (Ambery, Russell, Perry, Morris, & Murphy, 2006).

Implicit memory does not require conscious or intentional recollection of experiences, although they have an effect on current performance. When perceptual processing tasks have been used to examine implicit memory in autism and AS, no evidence of impairment has been found (Bowler, Gaigg, & Gardiner, 1997; Gardiner, Bowler, & Grice, 2003; Renner, Klinger, & Klinger, 2000).

Explicit memory, also referred to as declarative memory, is comprised of two subsystems defined by Tulving (1972) as semantic and episodic memory. *Semantic memory* refers to factual knowledge or knowledge of the world, whereas *episodic memory* refers to the system involved in recollecting particular experiences. On individual subtests of the Wechsler scales, strengths are obtained on measures of factual and lexical knowledge (e.g., Ehlers et al., 1997; Ghaziuddin & Mountain-Kimchi, 2004; Mayes & Calhoun, 2003), which is reminiscent of accounts of exceptional stores of factual information in individuals with AS. Performance is lower on Wechsler subtests involving attention to and mental manipulation of (numerical) information; these results may be consistent with the findings reported above suggestive of inconsistent attentional focus.

On list-learning tasks, individuals with autism generally show a selective deficit for retrieval versus encoding (Bennetto, Pennington, & Rogers, 1996; Goldstein, Johnson, & Minshew, 2001; Lincoln, Allen, & Kilman, 1995; Minshew & Goldstein, 1993; Renner et al., 2000), possibly impacted by deficient organization strategies. When examined in adults with AS, they too did not capitalize on semantic or phonological information to aid free recall to the extent that was seen in the typical control group; cued recall support led to performance at the same level as the control group, but training at the time of learning (to enhance relational encoding) did not (Bowler, Matthews, & Gardiner, 1997; Smith, Gardiner, & Bowler, 2007). The results lead to a similar conclusion as reported in autism: Individuals with AS may be challenged to recall information when they have to develop complex organizing strategies to help in their recall. A subsequent study further indicated that patterns of organization tended not to converge in the adults with AS, suggesting that they did not utilize a shared system of organization but rather may have organized the information in more idiosyncratic ways; convergence was seen in the control participants who likely used a conventional semantic system (Bowler et al., 2008).

Boucher (1981) examined memory for recent events in children with autism, children with intellectual disability, and typically developing controls. The children participated in a series of activities for 1–2 hours and were then asked to recall the session's events. The children with autism recalled significantly fewer events relative to both comparison groups, but recall of the children with autism improved when they were provided with cueing strategies, supporting a deficit in retrieval, not encoding. Boucher and Lewis (1989) also reported that when children with autism and children with learning disabilities were asked to recall events from several months earlier, the children with autism had significantly poorer performance on the free recall condition but more similar performance on the cued recall condition, providing further evidence for the idea that children with autism have intact encoding processes but difficulty with retrieval, particularly independently utilizing a metacognitive or organization strategy for retrieval.

Memory performance in relation to witnessing an everyday experience was examined in a group of children with AS (McCrory, Henry, & Happé,

2007), and similar results were obtained. That is, compared to their peers, the children with AS freely recalled less information, but questioning to cue their recall did yield a similar level of recall as the control group. In addition, the AS group was less likely to mention the most salient or gist elements of the event, and was less focused on a socially salient subscene; again, however, their recall was aided by general questioning, yielding a comparable pattern of recall. Impairment at the level of retrieval was suggested; the authors in turn raised the question of whether organizing strategies or a representational deficit with respect to semantic, relational, and contextual properties accounted for the differences in free recall. Notably, whereas recall performance was significantly positively correlated with performance on two (verbal) executive functioning tasks in the AS group, this relationship was not significant in the peer group. Taken together, the results indicated that the AS group may not have accessed gist-based organizational strategies and rather relied on other more broad-based cognitive processes.

When episodic memory functioning was examined in adults with AS, impairments in source memory as well as greater reliance on *knowing* and less reliance on *remembering* characterized the AS group relative to controls (Bowler, Gardiner, & Grice, 2000; Gardiner et al., 2003). A subsequent study confirmed the hypothesis that with source support or cueing, the performance of individuals with AS was comparable to that of controls (Bowler, Gardiner, & Berthollier, 2004). Individuals with AS may show impairments in episodic memory, but consistent with findings from studies in autism, the deficit appears to be at the level of retrieval versus encoding.

Bowler and colleagues further examined the question of whether episodic remembering in adults with AS is qualitatively similar to normal controls (Bowler, Gardiner, & Gaigg, 2007). A *quantitative* impairment in performance on episodic memory tasks was found, but it was concluded that the performance of the adults with AS was not *qualitatively* different than typical individuals; that is, the capacity for recalling past events in a spatial–temporal context and for recalling the self-referential aspects of the episode was demonstrated, although to a lesser extent.

Adults with AS differed from control participants when required to retrieve a memory of a personal experience in response to a word cue; the AS group generated fewer specific memories in response to positive, negative, and neutral cues (e.g., the word *leisure*), and they were also slower overall to retrieve specific memories to cues (Goddard, Howlin, Dritschel, & Patel, 2007). When presented with a social problem-solving task, they were equally able to access a relevant personal experience as well as categorical information. However, their solutions were less effective, less detailed, and showed less appreciation that some solutions to problems evolve over a time course (vs. a focus on the "here-and-now" solution). Notably, in the AS group, retrieval of specific memories on the *cueing* task was significantly related to problem-solving performance, but memory during problem solving was not; in contrast, whether or not past experiences were retrieved *during* problem solving was related to the problem-solving performance of the TD control group. Individuals with AS may possess a store of past experiences, but not see the relevance of applying these past experiences to solve a particular problem.

In summary, the research to date suggests intact implicit memory, a deficit in spatial working memory, impairments at the level of retrieval versus encoding for new learning, and quantitative (both in amount and speed of retrieval) but not qualitative differences in episodic memory. The profile of memory functioning in AS is similar to that found in autism. Episodic memory, in particular, has been examined comprehensively in AS, although replication with a larger subject sample size and wider age range (the studies have typically employed adults) is suggested. Other divisions of memory, such as semantic and working memory, have been less exhaustively studied in AS specifically; comparisons made across modalities (e.g., tactile, verbal, visual, spatial) are also lacking. The impairments in episodic memory, retrieval, and subjective organization are suggestive of frontal lobe dysfunction. One hypothesis for memory deficit is related to limbic–prefrontal pathways (e.g., Ben-Shalom, 2003), and underconnectivity between perceptual and memory regions is cited evidence from neuroimaging (e.g., Just, Cherkassky, Keller, & Minshew, 2004; Koshino, Carpenter, Minshew, Cherlassky, Keller, et al., 2005). Given the specific deficits in retrieval of information on learning tasks, simple repetition alone cannot be counted on to facilitate recall of new information; rather, the provision of specific context cues is suggested. Consideration should also be given to how information is organized for the person with AS; information may be organized but in an idiosyncratic way. When creating meaning from experiences, individuals with AS may have difficulty connecting past and present experiences to create a structure by which to guide their social behavior. Information about a relevant past event may be stored but not readily applied to solve a problem; individuals with AS may be less likely than their TD peers to call up relevant information from a past experience for problem-solving a current situation. Learning and problem solving may be advanced through direct support for connecting a current learning episode with prior concepts or events.

EXECUTIVE FUNCTIONING

Executive functioning (EF) is comprised of a set of processes that contribute to maintaining an appropriate problem-solving set to guide future behaviors. These processes include inhibition, set shifting, planning, self-monitoring, organization, flexibility, and working memory. There is a great deal of overlap between components of EF and other neuropsychological domains, namely, attention and memory. As such, for this chapter, working memory, which falls under both the memory and executive control domains, was addressed in the memory section above, and attention was also covered in an independent section. Behaviors observed in individuals with ASD are suggestive of executive dysfunction; these include response perseveration, disinhibition, narrow range of interests, concrete thinking, difficulty with flexibly shifting perspectives, as well as challenges with self-monitoring and planning.

The results of several studies in autism indicate deficits in EF, specifically cognitive flexibility and set shifting, as measured by performance relative to controls on traditional EF tasks, such as the Wisconsin Card Sorting Test (WCST; Heaton et al., 1993) (Bennetto et al., 1996; Goldstein et al., 2001; Minshew, Meyer, & Goldstein, 2002; Ozonoff, Rogers, & Pennington, 1991; Ozonoff, Strayer, McMahon, & Filloux, 1994; Szatmari, Tuff, Finlayson, & Bartolucci, 1990; Verté, Geurts, Roeyers, Oosterlaan, & Sergeant, 2006) as well as on the switching conditions within subtests from the Delis–Kaplan Executive Function System (D-KEFS), such as Trails, Color–Word Interference, and Design Fluency (Kleinhans, Akshoomoff, & Delis, 2005). A task from the CANTAB that measures flexibility (Intra-Dimensional/Extra-Dimensional set-shifting task) has provided mixed results (e.g., Goldberg et al., 2005; Ozonoff, South, & Miller, 2000; Ozonoff et al., 2004).

Individuals with autism have also been shown to have deficits in planning, as measured by the traditional Tower of Hanoi or similar versions of the task, which require the individual to problem-solve by planning before acting and to identify the subgoals needed to reach an end goal (Hughes, Russell, & Robbins, 1994; Joseph, McGrath, & Tager-Flusberg, 2005; Ozonoff et al., 1991, 2004; Szatmari et al., 1990), with notable exceptions (e.g., Goldberg et al., 2005). Overall, Ozonoff et al. (2004) and Goldstein et al. (2001) propose that the challenge for individuals with autism on planning-related tasks are planning efficiency and resolving subgoal conflicts.

Lopez, Lincoln, Ozonoff, and Lai (2005) reported impairments in cognitive flexibility and planning in their adult participants with HFA, with similar performance to controls on measures of response inhibition and working memory. A model inclusive of strengths in response inhibition and working memory and deficits in cognitive flexibility accounted for a significant portion of the variance in restricted, repetitive behavior symptoms. Only partial support was found for a relationship between EF performance (again using the WCST as a measure of cognitive flexibility) and repetitive behaviors in children and adolescents (South, Ozonoff, & McMahon, 2007). In school-age children, EF (specifically on the higher-order Tower task) and theory-of-mind abilities were reported to explain significant variance in communication symptoms in children with autism (Joseph & Tager-Flusberg, 2004). No mediating role for EF ability with regard to theory-of-mind task performance was found once the shared effects of nonverbal ability and language level were controlled; the exception was a specific process related to inhibitory control and working memory and the ability to represent epistemic mental states (e.g., knowledge and belief). EF performance (on measures of working memory, working memory and inhibitory control, and planning) was not found to be related to core social interaction or repetitive behavior symptoms once the effects of language were controlled (Joseph & Tager-Flusberg, 2004).

Higher-level EF and a representational understanding of mind appear to be related to severity of communication impairments in autism. Joseph and Tager-Flusberg (2004) hypothesized that social-perceptual skills (e.g., information communicated through eye gaze, facial expressions, vocal intonation) would be more closely related to impairments in social reciprocity. The relationship between language and EF ability was also examined in a subsequent study of school-age children with autism; deficits in EF performance were found in the autism group, but performance was not related to level of language functioning (with nonverbal ability controlled). Language and EF were significantly positively correlated in control participants. The results were interpreted to suggest that executive dysfunction and language impairment are not directly related in autism, with support for the hypothesis that there may instead be a deficit in the use of (internal) language in the service of executive control (Joseph et al., 2005).

EF deficits have been reported in individuals with AS. The EF profile and degree of impairment in children with AS has generally been found to be similar to that of individuals with HFA (Kenworthy et al., 2005; Klin, Volkmar, Sparrow, Cicchetti, & Rourke, 1995; Manjiviona & Prior, 1999; Miller & Ozonoff, 2000; Ozonoff et al., 1991; Verté et al., 2006), with exceptions (e.g., Szatmari et al., 1990) and in mixed samples (e.g., Kaland, Smith, & Mortensen, 2008). In the latter study, differences between the clinical group (mixed AS/HFA) and control participants on the WCST was significant only for ability to maintain set or maintain a consistent sorting strategy (Kaland et al., 2008). The study was limited by a small sample and wide age range, which likely impacted the power to detect differences. That said, given differences in the Wechsler Intelligence Scale for Children—Third Edition (WISC-III) profiles of the two groups, the authors proposed that problems with attention and inhibitory control may have impacted the ASD group's ability to keep the storing strategy in mind.

Employing tests from the Delis–Kaplan Executive Function System (DKEFS) in a small sample of adults with AS or HFA, Kleinhans et al. (2005) found that performance was not impaired for the higher-order conditions involving inhibition or inhibition and switching; rather, the degree of inherent structure was seen as a variable that was relevant to performance across the different tasks. When cognitive switching and initiation of efficient retrieval strategies were required, deficits were found in the verbal domain specifically. A visual scanning deficit was characteristic of the HFA but not the AS group. When inhibitory control was assessed using five task levels increasing in cognitive load, the performance of the AS group did not differ from that of the control participants in any of the conditions; the HFA group showed deficits in inhibitory control as cognitive load increased (e.g., with the addition of a set-shifting component) as well as more response variability than the AS group (Rinehart, Bradshaw, Tonge, Brereton, & Bellgrove, 2002). In a study of adults with AS, impairments in set shifting, word generation and flexibility, but not in response inhibition were found (Ambery et al., 2006).

Hill and Bird (2006) reported no differences between adults with AS and TD controls on traditional measures of inhibition, set shifting, cognitive flexibility, and verbal fluency; rather, the greatest area of impairment overall in their AS group was on measures of response initiation, intentionality, and planning; that is, the ability to engage and disengage actions in the service of overarching goals. Preliminary evidence for an association between these measures of EF and rating measures of autistic symptomatology (Autism-Spectrum Quotient and Communication Checklist) was also presented. Towgood, Meuwese, Gilbert, Turner, and Burgess (2009), using the same measures, found similar deficits for response initiation and suppression but not planning. Slowed processing/motor speed was also characteristic of the AS groups in both studies. Towgood et al. observed that variability in performance was the most defining feature in the AS group. They did not find a relationship between EF performance and autistic symptomatology (as measured by the Autism-Spectrum Quotient) but did report a significant association between the amount of individual variability on the tests and the Social and Communication subscales of the Autism Diagnostic Observation Schedule (ADOS).

Studies of inhibitory control in ASD also include reports of a differential pattern of impairment relative to other clinical groups, most notably ADHD. As compared to ADHD groups, individuals with ASD display deficits in the area of planning and cognitive flexibility, whereas more marked deficits in inhibition are reported in the ADHD comparison groups (Ozonoff & Jensen, 1999; Geurts, Verté, Oosterlan, Roeyers, & Sergeant, 2004; Gioia, Isquith, Kenworthy, & Barton, 2002), with an exception (Goldberg et al., 2005) finding greater impairment on a spatial working memory task in the HFA children versus ADHD group. Happé, Booth, Charlton, and Hughes (2006) reported group differences for the domains of response selection and planning but not flexibility. Specifically, the ADHD group showed marked deficits for response selection/inhibition and planning on a spatial working memory task; the ASD group (mixed AS/HFA, predominantly AS) showed poorer performance on a measure of response selection/monitoring. The older ASD group (11–16 years) performed better than their younger counterparts (8–10 years, 11 months) and showed far less impairment relative to the older ADHD sample, suggesting an age-related improvement in EF in ASD. EF performance was also related to adaptive functioning in the Communication and Socialization domains of the Vineland Adaptive Behavior Scales, and the relationship was stronger in the ASD as compared to the ADHD group.

Ratings on *behavioral* measures of EF also identify significant concerns for this area of functioning. Parental ratings of children and adolescents with AS yielded significantly more behaviors associated with a dysexecutive syndrome than parent ratings for TD controls (Channon, Charman, Heap, Crawford, & Rios, 2001). When HFA and AS groups were compared on a parent-report measure of EF challenges in day-to-day behavior, the overall results indicated more frequent concerns for attention and working memory in the HFA versus AS group (Kenworthy et al., 2005). This finding was interpreted to reflect differences in language abilities and in response to spoken information as there were no differences between the groups on, for example, their measured attention on a visual continuous performance task. Flexibility and planning/organization were pervasive concerns in both groups. On a parent-report neurobehavioral measure, children and adolescents with HFA or AS showed significant elevations on the EF scales relative to controls, but no significant differences between each other (Thede & Coolidge, 2007). The clinical groups were elevated on the EF Deficits scale overall and for the Decision-Making Difficulties, Metacognitive Problems, and Social Inappropriateness subscales. Consistent with the finding obtained using EF performance measures, an association has been reported between behavioral ratings of EF and levels of adaptive functioning in children and adolescents with ASD (Gilotty, Kenworthy, Sirian, Black, & Wagner, 2002). Specifically, deficits in metacognitive skills, particularly in working memory and initiation, were important contributors to adaptive functioning impairments.

In summary, on neuropsychological measures of EF, response inhibition appears to be intact in AS, whereas deficits in the area of cognitive flexibility and planning are reported. When compared across young and old age groups, Happé et al. (2006) report less severe and persistent deficits in individuals with ASD as compared to ADHD with the caveat that the study is cross-sectional in nature. Two studies of adults with AS indicate few differences from TD controls on traditional EF measures of inhibition, set shifting, and cognitive flexibility, and rather identify specific deficits in response initiation and suppression on newer EF tasks. Children with AS have difficulty on measures requiring them to resolve goal/subgoal conflicts and develop effective problem-solving strategies; for adults with AS, the ability to engage and disengage actions in the service of overarching goals appears to be specifically challenging. In both cases, advance preparation and external support may be needed to break down tasks that are more abstract, novel/ambiguous, and/or involve multiple steps, also drawing on any strengths in language abilities to effectively support problem solving and planning.

Behavioral ratings of EF also indicate challenges in day-to-day behavior. The EF profile in AS is not very distinct from autism; flexibility and planning/organization are identified concerns for both AS and HFA groups on behavioral ratings and neuropsychological measures. Exceptions include behavioral ratings of attention and working memory, which are significant for autism alone, and measures of inhibitory control, which suggest a deficit in autism, but not in AS, as cognitive load increases. There is a relationship between EF functioning, as measured through both behavioral ratings and performance on neuropsychological tests, and level of adaptive functioning; EF impairment is associated with adaptive impairment. In autism, EF ability may be associated with communication symptoms but not language impairment; the evidence for an association with repetitive behaviors has been mixed. The mediating role of EF in social, communication, language, and adaptive functioning has not been examined in AS specifically.

GENERAL INTELLECTUAL ABILITY

The intellectual profiles of individuals with AS often show significant scatter and point to better verbal than perceptual organizational skills overall (deBruin, Verheif, & Ferdinand, 2006; Ehlers et al., 1997; Ghaziuddin & Mountain-Kimchi, 2004; Koyama, Tachimori, Osada, & Kurita, 2007; Lincoln, Courchesne, Allen, Hanson, & Ene, 1998; Ozonoff et al., 2000). A particular pattern of neuropsychological assets and deficits, consistent with a nonverbal learning disability (NLD; Rourke, 1989), has been proposed to be characteristic of individuals with AS and potentially to serve as a source of external validity for the syndrome (Klin et al., 1995; Klin & Volkmar, 1997).

The NLD subtype, which emerged from research on children with learning disabilities, represents a distinct profile of neuropsychological functioning characterized by better developed verbal relative to visual, tactile, and complex motor skills, in addition to deficits in novel problem solving and concept formation. In Rourke's (1989) model, it is proposed that this pattern of neuropsychological assets and deficits eventuates in a specific pattern of strengths and weaknesses in academic (e.g., well-developed single-word reading and spelling relative to mechanical arithmetic) and social (e.g., overreliance on language to learn about themselves and the world, and to navigate social situations with less efficient use of nonverbal information) functioning. Individuals with NLD are at risk for internalizing disorders such as depression and anxiety.

The descriptive accounts of individuals with AS show considerable overlap with the clinical manifestations of the NLD syndrome. In addition, an extensive investigation comparing the neuropsychological profiles of well-characterized individuals with AS or HFA offered strong support for a relationship between AS and NLD (Klin et al., 1995). The sample in this study consisted of 19 individuals with HFA and 21 individuals with AS, diagnosed using stringent criteria according to the tenth revision of the

International Classification of Diseases (ICD-10; World Health Organization, 1992). The neuropsychological records of each subject were reviewed and rated according to 22 items: 7 assets and 15 deficits considered to be the defining criteria of NLD. An overwhelming concordance between AS and NLD was obtained (*n* = 18), whereas there was virtually no overlap between HFA and NLD (*n* = 1). Furthermore, 11 of the 22 NLD items discriminated between AS and HFA, of which 9 appeared to be independent of diagnostic criteria. A detailed analysis of the individual criteria revealed that six criteria were predictive of AS and another five criteria were predictive of "not AS." Deficits that were predictive of AS were in the areas of fine motor skills, visual motor integration, visual–spatial perception, nonverbal concept formation, gross motor skills, and visual memory. Deficits that were identified as not predictive of AS included the areas of articulation, verbal output, auditory perception, vocabulary, and verbal memory. These findings were also reflected in the IQ profiles, which revealed a significant verbal–nonverbal split, with higher verbal than nonverbal skills. This discrepancy was not seen in the HFA group.

In light of these findings it was proposed that NLD characterizes the cognitive and neuropsychological profile of individuals with AS. Few subsequent reports have used a comprehensive battery of tests to examine the question of whether the neuropsychological profile in AS is consistent with the NLD profile. Of the two studies that have been conducted, one study examining children and adults with AS found support (Gunter, Ghaziuddin, & Ellis, 2002), whereas the other study of adults with AS did not support the finding of an NLD profile (Ambery et al., 2006).

In the latter study, it was observed that a significant verbal IQ (VIQ)–performance IQ (PIQ) (VIQ–PIQ) discrepancy, irrespective of direction, was more common in the sample of AS adults as compared to the general population. Although the VIQ > PIQ intellectual profile is often considered to typify individuals with AS, a recent report indicated that this profile is also found in children and adults with HFA with some frequency (Williams, Goldstein, Kojkowski, & Minshew, 2007). Joseph, Tager-Flusberg, and Lord (2002) examined the cognitive profiles of children with ASD and also found that large discrepancies in either direction were more frequent in the ASD group relative to controls, although patterns in the cognitive profiles differed between school-age and preschool groups. The direction of the discrepancy was significantly correlated with symptom severity; specifically, enhanced nonverbal abilities were associated with greater severity of autistic symptoms. It was further proposed that this disparity in cognitive abilities may reflect a significant disturbance in brain development and organization. In a subsequent study, Tager-Flusberg and Joseph (2003) found a significant inverse relationship between magnitude of the discrepancy (nonverbal abilities greater than verbal) and both head circumference and brain volume; that is, the subgroup of children with autism who showed discrepantly high nonverbal cognitive abilities also had enlarged head circumference and brain volume. These studies provide evidence that isolating distinct cognitive profiles in ASD is relevant to expression of the disorder and may provide a path to identifying specific neurobiological mechanisms and possibly associated genes.

A high degree of unevenness in the cognitive profiles of individuals with ASD often seems to be the rule rather than the exception clinically and may be the most consistent finding to emerge from the research. As such, the traditional approach to identifying group differences—a comparison of group means—may in fact obscure some important findings. Widely discrepant interindividual as well as intraindividual scores are potentially masked by group averages. Indeed, when both group and single-case study methods were employed in a sample of AS adults, group-level analyses alone inadequately characterized the cognitive profiles (Towgood et al., 2009). As noted above, it was concluded that the most defining characteristic of the ASD group was a pattern of marked variability both within and across individuals. Moreover, the relationship between individual variability on neuropsychological (EF) measures and social communication subscale scores on ADOS was significant, whereas level of test performance was not.

FUTURE DIRECTIONS

The categorical boundaries between autism and AS (and PDD-NOS) are being increasingly blurred and the diagnostic boundaries have been called into question. The use of the term *ASD* has long been widespread in both the lay and scientific literature, and it has been officially embraced in the fifth edition of DSM; researchers are increasingly using mixed clinical groups (e.g., HFA and AS) in their investigations. Initially, competing theories emerged concerning the primacy of one or another particular deficit in explaining these disorders. Most researchers have since eschewed a single-deficit hypothesis and acknowledge that pathogenesis of these disorders is, in all likelihood, multifaceted; multiple genes and gene combinations and different neural pathways are involved. In contrast, the nosological debate as to whether to "lump" or "split" the behavioral expressions of the disorders continues.

Psychiatric nosology is comprised of diagnostic constructs that are descriptive; thus, there is an assumption that such descriptive partitions based on clusters of behavioral symptoms are in some way related to a shared etiological mechanism. AS and the other PDDs are defined in behavioral terms and specifically united by social impairments, problems in social communication and social imagination (Wing), an insistence on sameness (Kanner), or a pattern of restricted and repetitive behaviors (DSM). Clinical presentation is marked by substantial heterogeneity; from a sheer combinatorial standpoint, there is a variety of ways to meet diagnostic criteria based on symptom presentation.

As with previously proposed etiological constructs, there may not be supremacy in either a lump or split approach; rather, there may be a role for both. That is, it may be equally relevant to look for points of convergence as well as points of divergence. At least one of the points of convergence is predefined and thus represents an assumption about homogeneity; diagnostically it has been decided that the core identifying features of ASDs are related to social impairment. The suggestion is that it is the social impairment specifically that profoundly impacts the lives of those so affected. In this case, the point of divergence is from typical development; therefore a fundamental question for this line of research is how does atypical development in ASD relate to typical development?

However, taking this as the point of convergence, it is also the case that there are many ways in which these individuals, so grouped together, also differ from each other (e.g., levels of cognitive and language functioning, neuropsychological profiles, behavioral expressions). The variability appears to lie at both the individual and group levels. Identifying the points of divergence may be relevant to the complexity and diversity of expression of the disorder as well as to uncovering etiological pathways. In this instance, the points of convergence represent the intersection of co-presenting disorders. This might be referred to as comorbidity but is then limited to categorical distinctions; it may be equally important to take a dimensional approach and examine the intersection points of different processes—that is, to determine the implications of covariation among the different dimensions of interest.

Heterogeneity is a fact of these disorders; therefore, it is also reasonable to assume that frequently a particular impairment (or strength) will be characteristic of only a fraction of children. One important implication for research methodology is consideration not only of the group but of individuals within the group. Overall group effects may represent the extreme performance of a subset of children or the average of two extremes. Group means may mask individual differences within the group and also the fact that many children may in fact perform in the "normal" range. This limitation could be addressed simply by reporting (1) the percentage of the sample showing a significant strength or weakness or clinical elevation on a measure, (2) ranges and frequencies of performance levels, and/or (3) comparisons of variance in scores between clinical groups and controls. More sophisticated approaches include the application of, for example, the multiple case series approach employed by Hill and Bird (2006) and Towgood et al. (2009). It may be the case that variability is not only an index by which to separate groups but also the measured variable and construct of interest.

Further research is needed to understand better the neuropsychological phenotype and its relationship to the diagnostic phenotype in ASD, with a shift away from the perspective that a particular neuropsychological construct need be the most important determinant of the diagnostic expression of the syndrome. Rather, it would be of interest to continue to address whether, and in what way, neuropsychological processes contribute to heterogeneous diagnostic subtypes, and neurocognitive subtypes (as defined using neuropsychological measures) contribute to clinical outcome and inform about etiological pathways. There are likely subsets of children with AS who present with significant impairment in a domain of functioning and others who do not, or who present with a particular neuropsychological profile (e.g., NLD) with others who do not, despite sharing the same diagnosis. If so, the question arises, what do these points of divergence signify with regard to expression of the disorder as well as to individuals' adaptive functioning, presence of comorbid affective disorders, differences in regulatory functioning, treatment (e.g., impact of having impairments on one or more dimensions), brain development, and genetic susceptibility? Another approach might be to consider whether there are protective factors (e.g., particular components of functioning) that, if intact, contribute to a positive outcome. Finally, a developmental approach is crucial; by mapping the continuities and discontinuities of the central features of a developmental disability from first detection early in childhood, there is the potential to clarify syndrome expression and diagnostic pathways at the level of developmental processes as well as to disentangle what leads to social disabilities from the effects of having such disabilities. Diagnostic validity depends on finding differences in etiology and identifying meaningful group distinctions. By examining the early dimensions along which diagnostic groups differ, the timing of their emergence, and the contributions of these dimensions to later diagnostic outcome, we may obtain some clues as to the beginning of different developmental pathways for ASD.

REFERENCES

Alcantara, J. I., Weisblatt, E. J. L., Moore, B. C. J., & Bolton, P. F. (2004). Speech-in-noise perception in high-functioning individuals with autism or Asperger's syndrome. *Journal of Child Psychology and Psychiatry, 45,* 1107–1114.

Ambery, F. Z., Russell, A. J., Perry, K., Morris, R., & Murphy, D. G. M. (2006). Neuropsychological functioning in adults with Asperger syndrome. *Autism, 10,* 551–564.

American Psychiatric Association. (2000). *Diagnostic and statistical manual of mental disorders* (4th ed., text rev.). Washington, DC: Author.

Bennetto, L., Pennington, B. F., & Rogers, S. J. (1996). Intact and impaired memory functions in autism. *Child Development, 67,* 1816–1835.

Ben-Shalom, D. (2003). Memory in autism: Review and synthesis. *Cortex, 39,* 1129–1138.

Blakemore, S. J., Tavassoli, T., Calò, S., Thomas, R. M., Catmur, C., Frith, U., et al. (2006). Tactile sensitivity in Asperger syndrome. *Brain and Cognition, 61,* 5–13.

Boucher, J. (1981). Memory for recent events in autistic children. *Journal of Autism and Developmental Disorders, 11,* 293–301.

Boucher, J., & Lewis, V. (1989). Memory impairments and communication in relatively able autistic children. *Journal of Child Psychology and Psychiatry, 30,* 99–122.

Bowler, D. M., Gaigg, S. B., & Gardiner, J. M. (2008). Subjective organisation in the free recall learning of adults with Asperger's syndrome. *Journal of Autism and Developmental Disorders, 38,* 104–113.

Bowler, D. M., Gardiner, J. M., & Berthollier, N. (2004). Source memory in adolescents and adults with Asperger's syndrome. *Journal of Autism and Developmental Disorders, 34,* 533–542.

Bowler, D. M., Gardiner, J. M., & Gaigg, S. B. (2007). Factors affecting conscious awareness in the recollective experience of adults with Asperger's syndrome. *Consciousness and Cognition, 16,* 124–143.

Bowler, D. M., Gardiner, J. M., & Grice, S. J. (2000). Episodic memory and remembering in adults with Asperger syndrome. *Journal of Autism and Developmental Disorders, 30,* 295–304.

Bowler, D. M., Matthews, N. J., & Gardiner, J. M. (1997). Asperger's syndrome and memory: Similarity to autism but not amnesia. *Neuropsychologia, 35,* 65–70.

Buchsbaum, M. S., Siegel, B. V., Jr., Wu, J. C., Hazlett, E., Sicotte, N., & Haier, R. (1992). Brief report: Attention performance in autism and regional brain metabolic rate assessed by positron emission tomography. *Journal of Autism and Developmental Disorders, 22,* 115–125.

Cascio, C., McGlone, F., Folger, S., Tannan, V., Baranek, G., Pelphrey, K. A., et al. (2008). Tactile perception in adults with autism: A multidimensional psychophysical study. *Journal of Autism and Developmental Disorders, 38,* 127–137.

Casey, B. J., Gordon, C. T., Mannheim, G. B., & Rumsey, J. M. (1993). Dysfunctional attention in autistic savants. *Journal of Clinical and Experimental Neuropsychology, 15,* 933–946.

Channon, S., Charman, T., Heap, J., Crawford, S., & Rios, P. (2001). Real-life-type problem-solving in Asperger's syndrome. *Journal of Autism and Developmental Disorders, 31,* 461–469.

Ciesielski, K. T., Courchesne, E., & Elmasian, R. (1990). Effects of focused selective attention tasks on event-related potentials in autistic and normal individuals. *Electroencephalography and Clinical Neurophysiology, 75,* 207–220.

Courchesne, E., Townsend, J., Akshoomoff, N. A., Saitoh, O., Yeung-Courchesne, R., Lincoln, A. J., et al. (1994). Impairment in shifting attention in autistic and cerebellar patients. *Behavioral Neuroscience, 108,* 848–865.

deBruin, E. I., Verheij, F., & Ferdinand, R. F. (2006). WISC-R subtest but not overall VIQ–PIQ difference in Dutch children with PDD-NOS. *Journal of Abnormal Child Psychology, 34,* 263–271.

Dunn, W. (1999). *Sensory profile.* San Antonio, TX: Psychological Corp.

Dunn, W., Myles, B. S., & Orr, S. (2002). Sensory processing issues associated with Aspgerger syndrome: A preliminary investigation. *American Journal of Occupational Therapy, 56*(1), 97–102.

Ehlers, S., & Gillberg, C. (1993). The epidemiology of Asperger syndrome: A total population study. *Journal of Child Psychology and Psychiatry, 34,* 1327–1350.

Ehlers, S., Nydén, A., Gillberg, C., Dahlgren-Sandberg, A., Dahlgren, S.-O.,

Hjelmquist, E., et al. (1997). Asperger syndrome, autism, and attention disorders: A comparative study of the cognitive profiles of 120 children. *Journal of Child Psychology and Psychiatry, 38,* 207–217.

Frazier, J. A., Beiderman, J., Bellordre, C. A., Garfield, S. B., Geller, D. A., Coffey, B. J., et al. (2001). Should the diagnosis of attention deficit/hyperactivity disorder by considered in children with pervasive developmental disorder? *Journal of Attention Disorders, 4,* 203–211.

Freitag, C. M., Kleser, C., Schneider, M., & von Gontard, A. (2007). Quantitative assessment of neuromotor function in adolescents with high-functioning autism and Asperger syndrome. *Journal of Autism and Developmental Disorders, 37,* 948–959.

Frith, U. (1989). *Autism: Explaining the enigma.* Oxford, UK: Blackwell.

Frith, U. (1991). *Autism and Asperger syndrome.* Cambridge, UK: Cambridge University Press.

Gardiner, J. M., Bowler, D. M., & Grice, S. J. (2003). Further evidence of preserved priming and impaired recall in adults with Asperger's syndrome. *Journal of Autism and Developmental Disorders, 33,* 259–269.

Garretson, H. B., Fein, D., & Waterhouse, L. (1990). Sustained attention in children with autism. *Journal of Autism and Developmental Disorders, 20,* 101–114.

Geurts, H. M., Verté, S., Oosterlaan, J., Roeyers, H., & Sergeant, J. A. (2004). How specific are executive functioning deficits in attention deficit hyperactivity disorder and autism? *Journal of Child Psychology and Psychiatry, 45,* 836–854.

Ghaziuddin, M., & Butler, E. (1998). Clumsiness in autism and Asperger syndrome: A further report. *Journal of Intellectual Disability Research, 42,* 43–48.

Ghaziuddin, M., Butler, E., Tsai, L. Y., & Ghaziuddin, N. (1994). Is clumsiness a marker for Asperger syndrome? *Journal of Intellectual Disabilities Research, 38,* 519–527.

Ghaziuddin, M., & Mountain-Kimchi, K. (2004). Defining the intellectual profile of Asperger syndrome: Comparison with high-functioning autism. *Journal of Autism and Developmental Disorders, 34,* 279–284.

Ghaziuddin, M., Tsai, L. Y., & Ghaziuddin, N. (1992). Brief report: A reappraisal of clumsiness as a diagnostic feature of Asperger syndrome. *Journal of Autism and Developmental Disorders, 22,* 651–656.

Ghaziuddin, M., Weidmer-Mikhail, E., & Ghaziuddin, N. (1998). Comorbidity of Asperger syndrome: A preliminary report. *Journal of Intellectual Disability Research, 42,* 279–283.

Gillberg, C. (1989). Asperger syndrome in 23 Swedish children. *Developmental Medicine and Child Neurology, 31,* 520–531.

Gilotty, L., Kenworthy, L., Sirian, L., Black, D. O., & Wagner, A. E. (2002). Adaptive skills and executive function in autism spectrum disorders. *Child Neuropsychology, 8,* 241–248.

Gioia, G. A., Isquith, P. K., Kenworthy, L., & Barton, R. M. (2002). Profiles of everyday executive function in acquired and developmental disorders. *Child Neuropsychology, 8,* 121–137.

Goddard, L., Howlin, P., Dritschel, B., & Patel, T. (2007). Autobiographical memory and social problem-solving in Asperger syndrome. *Journal of Autism and Developmental Disorders, 37,* 291–300.

Goldberg, M. C., Mostofsky, S. H., Cutting, L. E., Mahone, E., M., Astor, B. C., Denkla, M. B., et al. (2005). Subtle executive functioning impairment in children with autism and children with ADHD. *Journal of Autism and Developmental Disorders, 35,* 279–293.

Goldstein, G., Johnson, C. R., & Minshew, N. J. (2001). Attentional processes in autism. *Journal of Autism and Developmental Disorders, 31,* 433–440.

Green, D., Baird, G., Barnett, A. L., Henderson, L., Huber, J., & Henderson, S. E. (2002). The severity and nature of motor impairment in Asperger's syndrome: A comparison with specific developmental disorder of motor function. *Journal of Child Psychology and Psychiatry, 43,* 655–668.

Greenberg, L. M. (1991). *TOVA manual.* Minneapolis, MN: Author.

Gunter, H. L., Ghaziuddin, M., & Ellis, H. D. (2002). Asperger syndrome: Tests of right hemisphere functioning and interhemispheric communication. *Journal of Autism and Developmental Disorders, 32,* 263–281.

Happé, F., & Booth, R. (2008). The power of the positive: Revisiting weak coherence in autism spectrum disorders. *Quarterly Journal of Experimental Psychology, 61,* 50–63.

Happé, F., Booth, R., Charlton, R., & Hughes, C. (2006). Executive function deficits in autism spectrum disorders and attention-deficit/hyperactivity disorder: Examining profiles across domains and ages. *Brain and Cognition, 61,* 25–39.

Happé, F., & Frith, U. (2006). The weak coherence account: Detail-focused cognitive style in autism spectrum disorders. *Journal of Autism and Developmental Disorders, 1,* 5–25.

Heaton, R. K., Chelune, G., Talley, J., Talley, J. L., Kay, G. G., & Curtiss, G. (1993). *Wisconsin card sorting test manual: Revised and expanded.* Odessa, FL: Psychological Assessment Resources.

Hill, E. L., & Bird, C. M. (2006). Executive processes in Asperger syndrome: Patterns of performance in a multiple case series. *Neuropsychologia, 44,* 2822–2835.

Holtmann, M., Bölte, S., & Poustka, F. (2005). ADHD, Asperger syndrome, and high-functioning autism. *Journal of the American Academy of Child and Adolescent Psychiatry, 44,* 1101.

Hughes, C., Russell, J., & Robbins, T. W. (1994). Evidence for executive dysfunction in autism. *Neuropsychologia, 32,* 477–492.

Iwanaga, R., Kawasaki, C., & Tsuchida, R. (2000). Brief report: Comparison of sensory–motor and cognitive function between autism and Asperger syndrome in preschool children. *Journal of Autism and Developmental Disorders, 30,* 169–174.

Jansiewicz, E. M., Goldberg, M. C., Newschaffer, C. J., Denckla, M. B., Landa, R., & Mostofsky, S. H. (2006). Motor signs distinguish children with high functioning autism and Asperger's syndrome from controls. *Journal of Autism and Developmental Disorders, 36,* 613–621.

Joseph, R. M., McGrath, L. M., & Tager-Flusberg, H. (2005). Executive dysfunction and its relation to language ability in verbal school-age children with autism. *Developmental Neuropsychology, 27,* 361–378.

Joseph, R. M., & Tager-Flusberg, H. (2004). The relationship of theory of mind and executive functions to symptom type and severity in children with autism. *Development and Psychopathology, 16,* 137–155.

Joseph, R. M., Tager-Flusberg, H., & Lord, C. (2002). Cognitive profiles and social-communicative functioning in children with autism spectrum disorders. *Journal of Child Psychology and Psychiatry, 43*, 807–821.

Johnson, K. A., Robertson, I. H., Kelly, S., Silk, T., Barry, E., Daibhis, A., et al. (2007). Dissociation in performance of children with ADHD and high-functioning autism on a task of sustained attention. *Neuropsychologia, 45*, 2234–2245.

Just, M. A., Cherkassky, V. L., Keller, T. A., & Minshew, N. J. (2004). Cortical activation and synchronization during sentence comprehension in high-functioning autism: Evidence of underconnectivity. *Brain, 127*, 1811–1821.

Kaland, N., Smith, L., & Mortensen, E. L. (2008). Brief report: Cognitive flexibility and focused attention in children and adolescents with Asperger syndrome or high-functioning autism as measured on the computerized version of the Wisconsin Card Sorting Test. *Journal of Autism and Developmental Disorders, 38*, 1161–1165.

Kanner, L. (1943). Autistic disturbances of affective contact. *Nervous Child, 2*, 217–250.

Kenworthy, L. E., Black, D. O., Wallace, G. L., Ahluvalia, T., Wagner, A. E., & Sirian, L. M. (2005). Disorganization: The forgotten executive dysfunction in high-functioning autism (HFA) spectrum disorders. *Developmental Neuropsychology, 28*, 809–827.

Kleinhans, N., Akshoomoff, N., & Delis, D. C. (2005). Executive functions in autism and Asperger's disorder: Flexibility, fluency, and inhibition. *Developmental Neuropsychology, 27*, 379–401.

Klin, A., & Volkmar, F. R. (1997). Asperger syndrome: In D. J. Cohen & F. R. Volkmar (Eds.), *Handbook of autism and pervasive developmental disorders* (pp. 94–122). New York: Wiley.

Klin, A., Volkmar, F. R., Sparrow, S. S., Cicchetti, D. V., & Rourke, B. P. (1995). Validity and neuropsychological characterization of Asperger syndrome. *Journal of Child Psychology, Psychiatry, and Allied Disciplines, 36*, 1127–1140.

Korpilahti, P., Jansson-Verkasalo, E., Mattila, M.-L., Kuusikko, S., Suominen, K., Rytky, S., et al. (2007). Processing of affective speech prosody is impaired in Asperger syndrome. *Journal of Autism and Developmental Disorders, 37*, 1539–1549.

Koshino, H., Carpenter, P. A., Minshew, N. J., Cherkassky, V. L., Keller, T. A., & Just, M. A. (2005). Functional connectivity in an fMRI working memory task in high-functioning autism. *NeuroImage, 24*, 810–821.

Koyama, T., Tachimori, H., Osada, H., & Kurita, H. (2007). Cognitive and symptom profiles in high-functioning pervasive developmental disorder not otherwise specified and attention-deficit/hyperactivity disorder. *Journal of Autism and Developmental Disorders, 36*, 373–380.

Kujala, T., Aho, E., Lepistö, T., Jannson-Verkasalo, E., Nieminen-von Wendt, T., von Wendt, L., et al. (2007). Atypical pattern of discriminating sound features in adults with Asperger syndrome as reflected by the mismatch negativity. *Biological Psychology, 75*, 109–114.

Lepistö, T., Kuitunen, A., Sussman, E., Saalasti, S., Jansson-Verkasalo, Nieminen-von Wendt, T., et al. (2009). Auditory stream segregation in children with Asperger syndrome. *Biological Psychology, 82*, 301–307.

Lepistö, T., Silokallio, S., Nieminen-von Wendt, T., Alku, P., Naatanen, R., & Kujala, T. (2006). Auditory perception and attention as reflected by the brain event-related potential in children with Asperger syndrome. *Clinical Neurophysiology, 117,* 2161–2171.

Leyfer, O. T., Folstein, S. E., Bacalman, S., Davis, N. O., Dinh, E., Morgan, J., et al. (2006). Comorbid psychiatric disorders in children with autism: Interview development and rates of disorders. *Journal of Autism and Developmental Disorders, 36,* 849–861.

Lincoln, A., Allen, M. H., & Kilman, A. (1995). The assessment and interpretation of intellectual abilities in people with autism. In E. Schopler & G. B. Mesibov (Eds.), *Learning and cognition in autism* (pp. 89–117). New York: Plenum Press.

Lincoln, A., Courchesne, E., Allen, M., Hanson, E., & Ene, M. (1998). Neurobiology of Asperger syndrome: Seven case studies and quantitative magnetic resonance imaging findings. In E. Schopler & G. B. Mesibov (Eds.), *Asperger syndrome or high-functioning autism?: Current issues in autism* (pp. 145–163). New York: Plenum Press.

Lopez, B. R., Lincoln, A. J., Ozonoff, S., & Lai, Z. (2005). Examining the relationship between executive functions and restricted, repetitive symptoms of autistic disorder. *Journal of Autism and Developmental Disorders, 35,* 445–460.

Manjiviona, J., & Prior, M. (1995). Comparison of Asperger syndrome and high-functioning autistic children on a test of motor impairment. *Journal of Autism and Developmental Disorders, 25,* 23–29.

Manjiviona, J., & Prior, M. (1999). Neuropsychological profiles of children with Asperger syndrome and autism. *Autism, 3,* 327–356.

Mayes, S. D., & Calhoun, S. L. (2003). Analysis of WISC-III, Stanford–Binet, IV, and academic achievement test scores in children with autism. *Journal of Autism and Developmental Disorders, 33,* 329–341.

McCrory, E., Henry, L. A., & Happé, F. (2007). Eye-witness memory and suggestibility in children with Asperger syndrome. *Journal of Child Psychology and Psychiatry, 48,* 482–489.

McGrath, L., Joseph, R., Tadevosyan, O., Folstein, S., & Tager-Flusberg, H. (2002, May), *Overlapping ADHD symptoms in autism: Relationship to executive functioning.* Poster presented at the International Meeting for Autism Research, Orlando, Florida.

Miller, J. N., & Ozonoff, S. (2000). The external validity of Asperger disorder: Lack of evidence from the domain of neuropsychology. *Journal of Abnormal Psychology, 109,* 227–238.

Minshew, N. J., & Goldstein, G. (1993). Is autism an amnesic disorder?: Evidence from the California Verbal Learning Test. *Neuropsychology, 7,* 209–216.

Minshew, N. J., Goldstein, G., & Siegel, D. J. (1997). Neuropsychologic functioning in autism: Profile of a complex information processing disorder. *Journal of the International Neuropsychological Society, 3,* 303–316.

Minshew, N. J., Meyer, J., & Goldstein, G. (2002). Abstract reasoning in autism: A dissociation between concept formation and concept identification. *Neuropsychology, 16,* 327–334.

Miyahara, M., Tsuji, M., Hori, M., Nakanishi, K., Kageyama, H., & Sugiyama, T. (1997). Brief report: Motor incoordination in children with Asperger syndrome and learning disabilities. *Journal of Autism and Developmental Disorders, 27,* 595–603.

Morris, R. G., Rowe, A., Fox, N., Feigenbaum, J. D., Miotto, E. C., & Howlin, P.

(1999). Spatial working memory in Asperger's syndrome and in patients with focal frontal and temporal lobe lesions. *Brain and Cognition, 41,* 9–26.

Mottron, L., & Belleville, S. (1993). A study of perceptual analysis in a high-level autistic subject with exceptional graphic abilities. *Brain and Cognition, 23,* 279–309.

Nydén, A., Gillberg, C., Hjelmquist, E., & Heiman, M. (1999). Executive function/attention deficits in boys with Asperger syndrome, attention disorder, and reading/writing disorder. *Autism, 3,* 213–228.

Ornitz, E. M., & Ritvo, E. R. (1968). Neurophysiological mechanisms underlying perceptual inconstancy in autistic and schizophrenic children. *Archives of General Psychiatry, 19,* 22–27.

Ozonoff, S., Cook, I., Coon, H., Dawson, G., Joseph, R. M., Klin, A., et al. (2004). Performance on Cambridge Neuropsychological Test Automated Battery subtests sensitive to frontal lobe function in people with autistic disorder: Evidence from the Collaborative Programs of Excellence in Autism Network. *Journal of Autism and Developmental Disorders, 34,* 139–150.

Ozonoff, S., & Jensen, J. (1999). Brief report: Specific executive function profiles in three neurodevelopmental disorders. *Journal of Autism and Developmental Disorders, 29,* 171–177.

Ozonoff, S., Rogers, S., & Pennington, B. (1991). Asperger's syndrome: Evidence of an empirical distinction. *Journal of Child Psychology and Psychiatry, 32,* 1107–1122.

Ozonoff, S., South, M., & Miller, J. N. (2000). DSM-IV-defined Asperger syndrome: Cognitive, behavioral and early history differentiation from high-functioning autism. *Autism, 4,* 29–46.

Ozonoff, S., Strayer, D. L., McMahon, W. M., & Filloux, F. (1994). Executive function abilities in autism and Tourette syndrome: An information processing approach. *Journal of Child Psychology and Psychiatry, 35,* 1015–1032.

Pascualvaca, D. M., Fantie, B. D., Papageorgiou, M., & Mirsky, A. F. (1998). Attentional capacities in children with autism: Is there a general deficit in shifting focus? *Journal of Autism and Developmental Disorders, 28,* 467–478.

Renner, P., Klinger, L. G., & Klinger, M. R. (2000). Implicit and explicit memory in autism: Is autism an amnesic disorder? *Journal of Autism and Developmental Disorders, 30,* 3–14.

Rinehart, N., Bellgrove, M. A., Tonge, B. J., Brereton, A. V., Howells-Rankin, D., & Bradshaw, J. L. (2006a). An examination of movement kinematics in young people with high-functioning autism and Asperger's disorder: Further evidence for a motor planning deficit. *Journal of Autism and Developmental Disorders, 36,* 757–767.

Rinehart, N., Bradshaw, J. L., Moss, S. A., Brereton, A. V., & Tonge, B. J. (2000). Atypical interference of local detail on global processing in high-functioning autism and Asperger's disorder. *Journal of Child Psychology and Psychiatry, 41,* 769–778.

Rinehart, N., Bradshaw, J. L., Moss, S. A., Brereton, A. V., & Tonge, B. J. (2001). A deficit in shifting attention present in high-functioning autism but not Asperger's disorder. *Autism, 5,* 67–80.

Rinehart, N., Bradshaw, J. L., Tonge, B. J., Brereton, A. V., & Bellgrove, M. A. (2002). A neurobehavioral examination of individuals with high-functioning autism and Asperger's disorder using a fronto-striatal model of dysfunction. *Behavioral and Cognitive Neuroscience Reviews, 1,* 164–177.

Rinehart, N., Tonge, B. J., Bradshaw, J. L., Iansek, R., Enticott, P. G., Johnson, K. A. (2006b). Movement-related potentials in high-functioning autism and Asperger's disorder. *Developmental Medicine and Child Neurology, 48,* 272–277.

Rinehart, N., Tonge, B. J., Bradshaw, J. L., Iansek, R., Enticott, P. G., McGinley, J. (2006c). Gait function in high-functioning autism and Asperger's disorder: Evidence for basal-ganglia and cerebellar involvement? *European Journal of Child and Adolescent Psychiatry, 15,* 256–264.

Rondan, C., & Deruelle, C. (2007). Global and configural visual processing in adults with autism and Asperger syndrome. *Research in Developmental Disabilities, 28,* 197–206.

Rourke, B. P. (1989). *Nonverbal learning disabilities: The syndrome and the model.* New York: Guilford Press.

Rourke, B. P., van der Vlugt, H., & Rourke, S. B. (1992). *Practice of child-clinical neuropsychology: An introduction.* Lisse, The Netherlands: Swets & Zeitlinger.

Rourke, B. P., van der Vlugt, H., & Rourke, S. B. (2002). *Practice of child-clinical neuropsychology: An introduction.* Lisse, The Netherlands: Swets & Zeitlinger.

Ryburn, B., Anderson, V., & Wales, R. (2009). Asperger syndrome: How does it relate to non-verbal learning disability? *Journal of Neuropsychology, 3,* 107–123.

Saalasti, S., Lepistö, T., Toppila, E., Kujala, T., Laakso, M., Nieminen-von Wendt, T., von Wendt, L., et al. (2008). Language abilities of children with Asperger syndrome. *Journal of Autism and Developmental Disorders, 38,* 1574–1580.

Schatz, A. M., Weimer, A. K., & Trauner, D. A. (2002). Brief report: Attention differences in Asperger syndrome. *Journal of Autism and Developmental Disorders, 32,* 333–336.

Smith, B. J., Gardiner, J. M., & Bowler, D. M. (2007). Deficits in free recall persist in Asperger's syndrome despite training in the use of list-appropriate learning strategies. *Journal of Autism and Developmental Disorders, 37,* 445–454.

South, M., Ozonoff, S., & McMahon, W. M. (2007). The relationship between executive functioning, central coherence, and repetitive behaviors in the high-functioning autism spectrum. *Autism, 11,* 437–451.

Steele, S. D., Minshew, N. J., Luna, B., & Sweeney, J. A. (2007). Spatial working memory deficits in autism. *Journal of Autism and Developmental Disorders, 37,* 605–612.

Sturm, H., Fernell, E., & Gillberg, C. (2004). Autism spectrum disorders in children with normal intellectual levels: Associated impairments and subgroups. *Developmental Medicine and Child Neurology, 46,* 444–447.

Szatmari, P., Bartolucci, G., & Bremner, R. (1989). Asperger's syndrome and autism: Comparison of early history and outcome. *Developmental Medicine and Child Neurology, 31,* 709–720.

Szatmari, P., Tuff, L., Finlayson, M. A. J., & Bartolucci, G. (1990). Asperger's syndrome and autism: Neurocognitive aspects. *Journal of the American Academy of Child and Adolescent Psychiatry, 29,* 130–136.

Tager-Flusberg, H., & Joseph, R. M. (2003). Identifying neurocognitive phenotypes in autism. *Philosophical Transactions of the Royal Society B, Biological Sciences, 358,* 303–314.

Tani, P., Lindberg, N., Appelberg, B., Nieminen-von Wendt, T., von Wendt, L., & Porkka-Heiskanen, T. (2006). Childhood inattention and hyperactivity symptoms self-reported by adults with Asperger syndrome. *Psychopathology, 39,* 49–54.

Tantam, D. (1988). Lifelong eccentricity and social isolation: I. Psychiatric, social, and forensic aspects. *British Journal of Psychiatry, 153,* 777–782.

Thede, L. L., & Coolidge, F. L. (2007). Psychological and neurobehavioral comparisons of children with Asperger's disorder versus high-functioning autism. *Journal of Autism and Developmental Disorders, 37,* 847–854.

Towgood, K. J., Meuwese, J. D. I., Gilbert, S. J, Turner, M. S., & Burgess, P. W. (2009). Advantages of the multiple case series approach to the study of cognitive deficits in autism spectrum disorder. *Neuropsychologia, 47,* 2981–2988.

Townsend, J., Harris, N. S., & Courchesne, E. (1996). Visual attention abnormalities in autism: Delayed orienting to location. *Journal of the International Neuropsychological Society, 2,* 541–550.

Tsatsanis, K. D., Noens, I. L. J., Illmann, C. L., Pauls, D. L., Volkmar, F. R., Schultz, R. T., et al. (2011). Managing complexity: Impact of organization and processing style on nonverbal memory in autism spectrum disorders. *Journal of Autism and Developmental Disorders, 41,* 135–147.

Tulving, E. (1972). Episodic and semantic memory. In E. Tulving & W. Donaldson (Eds.) *Organization of memory* (pp. 381–403). New York: Academic Press.

Verté, S., Geurts, H. M., Roeyers, H., Oosterlaan, J., & Sergeant, J. A. (2006). Executive functioning in children with an autism spectrum disorder: Can we differentiate within the spectrum? *Journal of Autism and Developmental Disorders, 36,* 351–372.

Wainwright-Sharp, J. A., & Bryson, S. E. (1996). Visual–spatial orienting in autism. *Journal of Autism and Developmental Disorders, 26,* 423–438.

Weimer, A. K., Schatz, A. M., Lincoln, A., Ballantyne, A., & Trauner, D. A. (2001). "Motor" impairment in Asperger syndrome: Evidence for a deficit in proprioception. *Journal of Developmental and Behavioral Pediatrics, 22,* 92–101.

Williams, D. L., Goldstein, G., Carpenter, P. A., & Minshew, N. (2005). Verbal and spatial working memory in autism. *Journal of Autism and Developmental Disorders, 35,* 747–756.

Williams, D. L., Goldstein, G., Kojkowski, N., & Minshew, N. (2007). Do individuals with high-functioning autism have the IQ profile associated with nonverbal learning disability? *Research in Autism Spectrum Disorders, 1,* 1–9.

Williams, D. L., Goldstein, G., & Minshew, N. J. (2006). Neuropsychologic functioning in children with autism: Further evidence of disordered complex information processing. *Child Neuropsychology, 12,* 279–298.

Wing, L. (1981). Asperger's syndrome: A clinical account. *Psychological Medicine, 11,* 115–129.

World Health Organization. (1992). *International statistical classification of diseases and related health problems* (10th ed.). Geneva, Switzerland: Author.

CHAPTER 4

Communication in Asperger Syndrome

Rhea Paul
Rebecca Landa
Elizabeth Simmons

According to the fifth edition of the *Diagnostic and Statistical Manual of Mental Disorders* (DSM-5; American Psychiatric Association, 2013), intelligent people with ASD, like others on the autism spectrum, receive a diagnosis of ASD, with note taken of their high level of function.

This chapter focuses primarily on the communication skills of speakers with ASD over the age of 5 years. A general picture of communication skills in these children and youth is described. Special attention is paid to the area of pragmatics, or the social uses of language. Finally, we address the issues involved in the assessment and treatment of communication disorders in higher-functioning individuals on the autism spectrum (HFA).

COMMUNICATION SKILLS IN SPEAKERS WITH AUTISM SPECTRUM DISORDERS

Language Form and Meaning

In general, as Tager-Flusberg (1995) discussed, language form and word meaning—that is, the ability to produce sounds (phonology), learn word meanings (semantics), and acquire word and sentence structures (morphology, syntax)—is generally commensurate with mental age (MA) in speakers with ASD. However, more recently Tager-Flusberg and Joseph (2003) identified two patterns of language development among verbal children with autism: one in which children show MA-appropriate linguistic abilities (phonological skills, vocabulary, syntax, and morphology) and the other in which children show both autism *and* disordered language development, similar to the phenotype found in specific language impairment (SLI).

Despite this generality, there are some aspects of basic language form in which speakers with ASD show deficits. Paralinguistic features such as vocal quality, intonation, and stress patterns—often referred to as *prosody*—are frequently noted atypical speech characteristics of these speakers (Rutter & Schopler, 1978). Odd intonation patterns and voice quality seem to be some of the most immediately recognizable clinical signs of the disorder. Paul, Shriberg, et al. (2005) reported that about 50% of individuals with AS showed these kinds of prosodic difficulties. Moreover, the presence of prosodic deficits was negatively related to ratings of social and communicative competence in these subjects. Koning and Magill-Evans (2001) investigated whether adolescents diagnosed with AS were able to use nonverbal cues, including facial expression, body gestures, and prosody, to interpret the feelings of people acting in videotaped scenes. They found that the adolescents with AS were significantly worse than controls in interpreting the emotions of the actors and relied least on prosodic information. Paul, Augustyn, Klin, and Volkmar (2005) also reported deficits in the understanding of prosody in speakers with AS. Other kinds of speech problems are also more prevalent in ASD than in the typical population. Shriberg et al. (2001) found that one-third of speakers with AS retained residual speech distortion errors on sounds such as /r/, /l/, and /s/ into adulthood, whereas the rate of these errors in the general population is 1%.

Abnormal use of words and phrases has been described in ASD for many years (Rutter & Schopler, 1978). In samples of high-functioning adolescents and adults, a significant minority has been found to use words with special meanings (Volden & Lord, 1991; Rumsey, Andreasen, & Rapoport, 1985), or "metaphorical language," as Kanner (1946) termed it. In most cases, these words or phrases were modifications of ordinary word roots or phrases that produced slightly odd-sounding but comprehensible terms such as *cuts and bluesers* for cuts and bruises (Tager-Flusberg, Paul, & Lord, 2005). These constructions, also called *idiosyncratic language*, often reference meaningful aspects of verbal constructs without regard for popular convention, likely reflecting an understanding of semantic content but a lack of appreciation for social custom.

Tager-Flusberg (1992) reported that the speakers with ASD used few mental state words, particularly terms for cognitive states (e.g., *know, think, remember, pretend*) in spontaneous speech. These findings were replicated in research including older children with ASD (Tager-Flusberg & Sullivan, 1994). Other studies suggest that children with ASD have particular difficulty understanding social–emotional terms as measured on vocabulary tests such as the *Peabody Picture Vocabulary Test* (Eskes, Bryson, & McCormick, 1990; Hobson, 1989; van Lancker, Cornelius, & Needleman, 1991). Thus, although vocabulary may be a relative strength in ASD, the acquisition of words for mental states may be specifically impaired.

The scant research on the development of syntax and morphology in ASD (see Tager-Flusberg et al., 2005, for review) suggests that when these children acquire grammatical skills, they follow a more or less typical sequence. Scarborough et al. (1991) compared the relationship between sentence length, which is a general index of grammatical development, and the appearance of specific syntactic structures in children with ASD. The authors found that sentence length tended to significantly overestimate grammatical complexity in this population, suggesting that these speakers made use of a narrower range of sentence constructions, particularly questions. This observation may be linked more closely to pragmatic than to syntactic deficits.

Pragmatics

Impairments in pragmatics are a hallmark of HFA (Asperger, 1944; Kanner, 1943; Dewey & Everard, 1974; Tager-Flusberg, 1981; Volkmar et al., 1987; Baron-Cohen, 1988), and pragmatic impairment represents a stigmatizing and handicapping aspect of these disorders. Unlike most speakers with communication impairments—for whom the more they talk, the more adaptive language is likely to be—for speakers with ASD, unusual aspects of language increase with the amount of speech (Caplan, Guthrie, Shields, & Yudovin, 1994; Volden & Lord, 1991). Individuals with HFA report that their social language vulnerabilities give rise to anxiety, avoidance of some social situations, and self-image challenges and are a source of great concern to them. Adults diagnosed with HFA report having difficulty at jobs and establishing friendships due to their social communication impairment, despite being professionally productive and otherwise quite capable.

Pragmatic language skills can be subdivided into three basic areas: the expression of *communicative intents*, or the reasons for talking; *presupposition*, or the ability to provide the correct amount and type of information, depending on the needs and interests of the listener; and the management of turns and topics in *discourse*. We describe each of these areas, give a brief overview of their typical course of development, and discuss what is known about their acquisition in ASD.

Communicative Intents

Utterances produced by a speaker typically have an intended communicative function (Austin, 1962), and thereby represent what Searle (1975) called a "speech act." According to Dore (1977), even the intentional communicative vocalizations and gestures of preverbal children (which begin at around 9 months of age) can be assigned a function (e.g., greeting, showing, commenting, rejecting, protesting). Speakers may communicate different intentions through the production of a single form and, conversely, may use a variety of forms to express a single intention. For example, the form "Can you walk the dog tonight?" may have intended functions of politely commanding, requesting information, or making a sarcastic comment. The intended communicative function of the sentence will be made clear by the context, including shared information between the speakers (e.g., both parties knowing that the listener has tentative plans for the evening that might affect the dog-walking routine), cues signaled through intonation (vocal pitch and loudness variations), facial and gestural expressions, and environmental cues.

The use of various forms to express one intention is illustrated by the options to use indirect, polite expressions such as "Do you have the time?" when in a somewhat formal situation, or a more direct expression "What time is it?" in less formal situations. For social success, it is important to develop the ability to recognize situations in which intentions should be expressed indirectly (e.g., requesting politely rather than commanding that an action be completed). It is also important to have the linguistic flexibility to select appropriate forms for expressing the intention. Failure to do so could have severe social consequences, including negative perceptions by others, decreased cooperation from others, and academic or vocational failure and isolation.

In typical development, children express a variety of declarative (attention getting, socially oriented) and imperative (efforts to regulate others' behavior) communicative intentions through gestures (including pointing), vocalizations, and facial expressions before words are acquired. They actively check the gaze patterns of their communicative partner to determine whether their intent has been accurately recognized (Bates, O'Connell, & Shore, 1987). During the preschool years, children develop increasing options for expressing their intentions and learn how to frame their messages indirectly. Nevertheless, preschoolers tend to be quite forthright in expressing themselves, sometimes to the embarrassment of their parents. A variety of new intentions appears during the preschool years (e.g., teasing), and most communicative intentions (e.g., negotiation, introductions, clarification requests) are acquired in informal and formal polite forms by 9 years of age (Wiig, 1982). Throughout childhood, there is an increase in the means (grammatical, semantic, integration of paralinguistic signals) of expressing intentions and tailoring them to the interpersonal context.

In ASD, generally, impairment in the development of communicative intentions is characteristic at all levels of functioning. These children show idiosyncratic forms of expressing intentions, a restricted variety of intentions expressed, and limitations in their ability to flexibly control the degree of directness with which some intentions are expressed (Landry &

Loveland, 1988). Atypical nonverbal strategies for making requests involve leading others by the hand to objects of interest rather than using pointing gestures and gaze patterns (Landry & Loveland, 1988). Even when pointing and eye contact are used during requests, they are not coordinated and do not involve the normal pattern of looking from the object of desire to the communicative partner (Mundy, Sigman, Ungerer, & Sherman, 1986). Children with ASD also differ in the types of communicative intentions expressed. Expression of social intentions (e.g., greeting, commenting) are greatly outnumbered by instrumental intentions (having own needs met; Wetherby & Prutting, 1984) in children with ASD.

Two behaviors are typical in the expression of communicative intention in autism are *echolalia* and *pronoun reversal*. Echolalia, or the immediate or delayed imitation of language heard, is often a transitional stage from prelinguistic to linguistic communication in children with autism. Similarly, some children with autism go through a stage of pronoun reversal, substituting *you* for *I* in early phases of spoken language acquisition.

Finally, a dearth of flexibility in the forms of language available to express intentions may result in utterances that are expressed forthrightly rather than in more subtle, socially acceptable ways, leading to impressions of impoliteness, rudeness, or insensitivity. This characteristic poses a particular problem for teenage and adult individuals who express their fondness or desire to be near someone of the opposite sex in an offensively direct way. Understanding the intended meaning of others may also pose a problem for the speaker with ASD, who may interpret indirect expressions literally (Ozonoff & Miller, 1996; Rumsey & Hanahan, 1990). This deficit limits the ability to respond in the socially expected way and sets the stage for communication breakdowns.

Presupposition

Presupposition refers to the knowledge, expectations, and beliefs that a speaker assumes are shared with the conversational partner. When making a presupposition, a speaker assesses what information he or she shares with the communicative partner and uses this information to plan the content and form of the message to be communicated. Other aspects of the situation are also taken into consideration, including physical qualities (e.g., age) and social status of the partner, setting (e.g., formal office setting vs. a picnic), contextual variables (e.g., presence or absence of referent), history of shared experiences, and previous content of the discourse. Accurate judgments about amount and type of shared knowledge may enable the speaker to communicate clearly with only one word (Bates, 1976). An example of a presuppositional error is when a speaker uses informal words and speech patterns (e.g., "Wanna soda?") rather than more formal means (e.g., "Would you like something to drink?") when speaking to an authority figure. Another example would be omitting important background information or details that the partner needs to fully understand the message (e.g., giving too few details in directions to get to the airport when the listener has never driven in that part of town before and does not know that the highway splits, yet both veins are labeled with the same highway number).

Presuppositional ability requires intact attentional mechanisms, an awareness of social rules, and the ability to consider the perspectives of others (Flavell, Botkin, Fry, Wright, & Jarvis, 1968), and the ability to consider alternative ways of phrasing ideas and to have the language skills to do so. Presuppositional skills include knowing when and how to be polite, formal, or colloquial; when to elaborate on an idea or to give a condensed version; how much background information to provide; how complex the words and sentence structures should be; and what topics are taboo in what situations. These judgments affect how receptive, motivated, and successful a partner will be in continuing the conversational interaction. Communicative behavior resulting from these judgments also leaves an impression on the listener about the overall social appropriateness of the speaker and may have substantial consequences in situations such as job interviews.

In typical development, many skills that seem important for building presuppositional abilities are acquired in the first 2 years of life. For example, joint referencing skills (looking in the direction that a partner is looking) are present in an early form at 6 months of age. Joint attention skills are needed to track the changes in referents during conversations, so that inferences about the speaker's intended meaning can be made successfully. Another example is the awareness of saliency that young children develop regarding their environment. They pay attention to what is important. This awareness of saliency is reflected in children's first words, which typically represent important people, objects, and actions—such as *ball, kitty,* or *cookie*—rather than inanimate objects having little relevance in their lives, such as *wall.* This seemingly innate detection of salience sets the stage for identifying referents of others' utterances, detecting salient social cues that guide interpretation of ambiguous linguistic input, and, later, recognizing the main topic of someone's utterance or of text.

By 4 years of age, children recognize differences in listeners' ability to process language input. Four-year-olds speak differently to younger children, age peers, and adults, adjusting the complexity of their grammar to their audience (Shatz & Gelman, 1973). They also adjust their language in consideration of a listener's role or occupation (Bates, 1976; Ervin-Tripp, 1977). They recognize the communicative significance of nonlinguistic cues and of requests for them to clarify ambiguous messages. Strategies for clarifying misunderstood messages increase across the preschool years. Whereas 12- to 24-month-old children clarify messages by repeating them more loudly and with more precise articulation, 3-year-olds are able to substitute, delete, or add words to revise their messages (Gallagher, 1977).

Rules that certain manners of expression and types of topics are taboo in certain contexts are acquired. Thus the preschooler who bluntly comments on a stranger's personal features learns more acceptable speech behavior with age.

In ASD, failure to adjust language production in consideration of the ever-changing interpersonal context is common. Reports of difficulty in making appropriate judgments about how much/little to say in conversational responses (Lord & Schopler, 1989); problems in taking another's perspective in conversation (Loveland et al., 1989), in providing a relevant, adequate response to what the previous speaker said (Baltaxe & D'Angiola, 1992), and in asking appropriate questions in conversation (Hurtig, Ensrud, & Tomblin, 1982) are common in the literature. The tendency to use a pedantic, formal speaking style when a more relaxed or colloquial speech register is more appropriate (Kanner, 1943) is another example of failure to adjust speech style to the social context, and is especially prevalent in HFA (Paul, Orlovski, Marcinko, & Volkmar, 2009).

In part, impaired presuppositional skills may result from impaired comprehension of nonverbal and verbal cues. For example, limited comprehension of affective (Sigman, Yirmiya, & Capps, 1995) and linguistically based intonational cues (Baltaxe & Simmons, 1985; Fine, Bartolucci, Ginsberg, & Szatmari, 1991; Paul et al., 2005) may compromise the speaker's ability to understand marked syntactic boundaries, judge others' degree of social engagement, judge speakers' attitudes, and recognize that an utterance is not meant to be taken literally (e.g., jokes and sarcasm). Such difficulty, in addition to poor comprehension of implied meaning (as expressed in indirect speech acts), contributes to poor recognition that a request for clarification has been presented by a listener. For example, Paul and Cohen (1985) looked at the ability of participants with ASD to understand indirect requests for action (e.g., "Can you color this circle blue?") of varying syntactic complexity. The group with ASD performed similarly to contrast subjects in a context in which the request intent of the utterance was made explicit (e.g., "I'm going to tell you to do some things. Can you . . . ?"). However the ASD group performed significantly worse when the same requests were presented in an unstructured context with no prefacing cue as to the intention of the utterance. The authors concluded that individuals with ASD are impaired in the ability to determine the speaker's intention without explicit cueing, over and above any syntactic comprehension deficit that might be present.

Similarly, Loveland and Tunali (1991) reported that speakers with ASD failed to respond to general inquiries for them to produce additional information, and required specific prompts to clarify their ambiguous utterances. Even once the clarification request had been comprehended, adolescents with HFA reportedly made fewer revisions in their messages compared to controls (Baltaxe, 1977). Paul and Cohen (1984) studied responses to requests for clarification in adults with ASD and found that although the participants did respond to requests for clarification, their answers were less specific than those of contrast subjects with intellectual disability. They were also less likely to add additional information that might be of help to the listener, suggesting that they had difficulty judging which piece of information would be relevant. Baltaxe (1977) further reported that when revisions were made, they reflected the developmentally immature strategy of repetition rather than changing the content of the message.

Impaired recognition of nonverbal and indirect verbal cues is also evident in the tendency of speakers with ASD to repeatedly initiate topics of their special interest without regard for the listener's interest in the topic (Wing & Attwood, 1987). Socially inappropriate topics (e.g., asking a stranger his or her age) may be initiated (Langdell, 1980) and messages may be expressed in an overly direct manner (bluntly). In addition, individuals with ASD display poor awareness of contextual rules for discourse behavior. This is illustrated by the experience of a young woman with ASD who loudly answered her minister's questions during his sermon on Sundays. She did not appreciate the rule that individual members of an audience do not take the role of responder. From her view, she was simply doing the expected by responding to the questions. Like other speakers with ASD, this young woman reported puzzlement at the irritated reactions she sometimes received in response to her social-communicative behaviors. Once a discourse rule is explicitly stated, however, such individuals often follow successfully.

Making inferences about the intended meaning of others may also be disrupted by a difficulty in understanding nonliteral uses of language (e.g., jokes and metaphor) and of how meaning shifts with changes in context. The literature indicates that speakers with ASD show impaired nonliteral language comprehension abilities, in the presence of typical understanding of literal language. Speakers with ASD do recognize general differences in different types of speech acts. For example, they understand the formal requirement that jokes end in a humorous way but that stories may not (Ozonoff & Miller, 1996). Furthermore, they are able to appreciate simple or slapstick humor, though comprehension of more complex humor is a challenge (Van Bourgondien & Mesibov, 1987).

Speakers with ASD not only have problems appreciating socially relevant signals but often fail to provide signals that would permit their listeners to make appropriate presuppositions about them. The ability to signal intended meaning is partly compromised by an impaired use of intonational cues to express special or novel meanings, such as a deadpan delivery of a statement intended to be comical (Fine et al., 1991; Rumsey et al., 1986; Shriberg et al., 2001). Listeners may not know how to "read" what has been said and are then unsure about how to react. Such challenges in the communicative interchange may, again, cause the listener to perceive the speaker with ASD as odd or rude and to avoid frequent contact with him or her.

Discourse Management

Discourse management refers to the organization, by means of turn structure and topic selection, of an ongoing series of utterances that create a "text" or cohesive unit. It may have a hierarchy of topics and subtopics (Bates & MacWhinney, 1987) or a series of topics, with digressions from the main topic. There is a variety of types of discourse genres, only two of which are discussed here: social discourse (conversation) and narrative discourse (storytelling). Both types of discourse have predictable organizational structures and developmental sequences.

Conversation

Social discourse, or conversation, is guided by rules for topic management (i.e., topic initiation, maintenance, and termination) and conversational repair following a communication breakdown. Information is presented in a predictable way, with speakers giving signals that they are about to speak, relinquish a turn, change a topic, add new information to an ongoing topic, and so on. When these tacit rules, such as contributing informative and relevant information in the discourse (Grice, 1975), are broken, the coherence of the discourse is likely to decrease and communication may break down.

The organization of information in discourse typically involves providing background information early on. This principle is also followed at the sentence level, where old information precedes new information, providing a context for interpreting new information. Speakers also use lexical devices to link current information to that presented earlier in the discourse (Halliday & Hassan, 1976). Effective use of cohesion enables conversational partners to avoid confusion about referents. For example, in the two utterances "Tom broke the chair. He felt terrible about it," the cohesive devices *he* and *it* make sense because they refer to words previously presented in the discourse. Using pronouns enables the speaker to avoid redundancy, but if the rules for using cohesive devices are not followed properly, the referent for a pronoun may be difficult to determine and coherence will be compromised.

Cohesion and other strategies are used to maintain topics. Topic maintenance is a complex skill, requiring the ability to flexibly employ grammatical skills, understand and produce meaningful semantic relationships, recognize shared information with conversational partners, notice and interpret the significance of changing contextual cues, and so on.

In typical development, the rudiments of discourse are seen early in infancy. Infants initiate social-communicative interactions as well as respond to and maintain the interactions initiated by others. They engage in reciprocal gaze and affective exchanges (Stern, 1974), setting the stage for later conversational turn taking. The rules for reciprocal verbal turn taking appear to be appreciated very early in development, with rare instances of turn overlap or "interruption" (Ninio & Bruner, 1978). As early as 3 months of age, infants take a vocal turn after being spoken to by their caregivers (Bloom, Russell, & Wassenberg, 1987). Effective verbal turn taking continues once language forms are acquired, as can be observed when 1- and 2-year-olds remain quiet during the conversational turn of their mothers (Schaffer, Collis, & Parsons, 1977). With increasing age, children attend to and recognize signals being sent by multiple conversational partners at once. They become capable of negotiating a three-way conversational exchange by 4 years of age.

Early forms of topic maintenance are observed when infants and their caregivers attend to the same thing at the same time (joint attention). Between 6 and 8 months of age, infants begin to follow their caregiver's line of visual regard (Scaife & Bruner, 1975), setting the stage for later topic maintenance. With the acquisition of words, children become increasingly adept at establishing topics pertaining to themselves and to objects/events outside themselves. At first, adults shoulder the responsibility for developing and maintaining these topics. They do this by building a sort of scaffold (Bruner, 1978) around what the child says. By referring to events, engaging in routines, and using words and sentence structures familiar to children, adults foster their development of mental scripts for events with associated socially and semantically appropriate language (Foster, 1981, 1986; Ervin-Tripp, 1979). This skill acquisition both supports the likelihood that the child will maintain the topic and sets a foundation for later topic maintenance skills. As the ability to integrate verbal (linguistic content) and nonverbal (including intonational cues, shared experiences, setting, body language) cues develops, children become increasingly capable of identifying others' topics. During the primary grades, children become quite facile at identifying the gist, or topic, of an entire discourse text, such as a conversation or story, and making inferences and predictions based on that gist. Recognizing topics and gists is paramount to producing topically contingent responses and contributing to the discourse in a coherent and socially acceptable way.

Strategies for maintaining topics, from repeating part of the partner's utterance to adding new information, increase with development. A repertoire of topic maintenance strategies is developed, enabling the speaker to select a strategy that is well suited to the context. One set of strategies involves the use of cohesive devices (cohesion). Use of cohesive devices to tie segments of the discourse together and make smooth transitions to new topics increases in sophistication with age. By kindergarten, children make semantic ties between current utterances and previous discourse using phrases (e.g., "*Speaking* of games, I learned a new game today") and cohesive devices (substituting pronouns for nouns, etc.; see above). Competent use of cohesive devices is important for discourse to be coherent, but it is not sufficient. Coherent discourse also depends on factors such as well-organized presentation of information and appropriate signaling of how messages are to be interpreted.

In ASD, the early bases of discourse, joint attention, and reciprocal social play are impaired (Mundy & Sigman, 1989; Ungerer & Sigman, 1981). Gaze is not used to determine whether the communicative partner is looking at the referent of the child's communication. Early deficits in reciprocal social-communicative exchanges appear to linger throughout the lifespan, perhaps in more subtle form for the more able individuals with HFA. For example, the communicative value of eye movements and gaze patterns continue to be poorly recognized. This will have an impact on abilities such as establishing co-reference with a partner (leading to topic maintenance difficulties), using eye contact to modulate turn length, and detecting signals (e.g., rolling the eyes) indicating nonliteral language use.

Speakers with ASD exhibit difficulty using signals to modulate discourse. Some typical situations in which they inconsistently or inappropriately use signals in discourse include indicating that they are about to speak, clearly identifying the intended recipient of their message, indicating that they are about to relinquish a turn, and indicating an intended transition in the course of the topic (Langdell, 1980). One major consequence of poor signaling is confusion on the part of the listener; the stage has been set for a faulty exchange of information.

Another difficulty involves maintaining topics of interest to the communicative partner. Individuals with HFA have a reputation for being associative, which may lead them to shift a topic abruptly when the current topic reminds them of something else. Poor maintenance of others' topics stands in stark contrast to their ability to sustain topics of their own special interest for extended periods of time. However, the information shared on these topics tends to be a series of detailed facts rather than a story that leads to a gist or main point. Therefore, conversational partners tend to have difficulty building a reciprocal exchange of information with individuals with HFA. The information imparted by these individuals may be new and interesting to a listener upon the first encounter, but repeated encounters often reveal that the information is stereotyped in nature, with the same facts recounted each time the topic is discussed. Perhaps as a consequence, reduced engagement in turn taking during reciprocal conversations is seen (Ghaziuddin & Gerstein, 1996).

Within a discourse event, speakers with ASD have difficulty using linguistic strategies, such as cohesion, to tie new information to previous discourse (Loveland, McEvoy, Kelley, & Tunali, 1990; Baltaxe & D'Angiola, 1992; Fine, Bartolucci, Szatmari, & Ginsberg, 1994). The precise nature of the types of cohesion errors exhibited by this group is difficult to determine due to differences across studies in comparison groups, in subjects' language functioning and ages, and in type of elicitation task.

Narrative

The ability to understand and a produce a narrative monologue, or a unit of discourse that gives a cohesive account of events or tells a story, is an important aspect of typical pragmatic development and has been shown to be related to academic success (Bishop & Edmundson, 1987; Boudreau, 2007). Like other basic units of language, narratives have a grammar or rule-based form. In mainstream U.S. culture, the grammar of the narrative is characterized by an episode (plot) structure that has several critical parts (Stein & Glenn, 1979), including a problem encountered by the characters, their attempt to resolve the problem, and the outcome of that attempt.

In typical development, children begin attempting to provide accounts of events or retell stories by 2 years of age, although their accounts are usually brief and poorly organized. By 3, they can produce a series of utterances around a theme with some causal connections. Around 6 years of age, children can organize stories to conform to the narrative structure of their culture (Applebee, 1978). However, these early narratives are often sparse and simple. Only during the elementary school years do children acquire the ability to center the story around a pivotal "high point," and it is not until the early teen years that children typically provide rich stories with embedded episodes and literate language style (Hughes et al., 1997).

In ASD, narrative skills are generally found to be commensurate with language ability. These speakers are able to narrate stories and follow simple scripts for common social events, such as a birthday party. Particular difficulties in making causal statements were found in one study (Tager-Flusberg, 1995), but these findings were not replicated in a later study (Capps, Losh, & Thurber, 2000). Loveland, McEvoy, Kelley, and Tunali (1990) reported that the children with ASD in their study were more likely to exhibit pragmatic violations, including bizarre or inappropriate utterances, and were less able to take into consideration the listener's needs than control participants with Down syndrome. Landa, Martin, Minshew, and Goldstein (1995), in a study comparing narrative production in teens and adults with ASD to that of controls matched on age, IQ, and gender, reported subjects' failure to clearly provide sufficient background information and overall coherence, despite more or less complete episode structure in the stories. Norbury and Bishop (2003), however, found few differences between narrative skills of children with ASD and those with specific language impairment, suggesting that difficulties with stories may be common to children with communication impairments.

Summary

Although basic intention to communicate often exists in speakers with ASD, these individuals have impaired skills in communicative activities involving joint reference or shared topics, particularly in using presuppositional skills to judge listener needs and purposes. The strategies used by an individual with ASD to maintain conversation are less advanced than syntactic ability would predict, as is the ability to infer the interlocutor's implicit intentions.

Studies Contrasting High-Functioning Autism and Asperger Syndrome

Recent changes in DSM-5 resulted in the deletion of AS as a diagnostic category. Some of the research that led to this decision is summarized in this section. Szatmari, Archer, Fishman, Streiber, and Wilson (1995) divided school-age children with autism spectrum disorders into two groups based on their preschool history of language development and found no differences between groups on current nonverbal communication function. Eisenmajer et al. (1996) compared groups with clinical diagnoses, based on DSM-IV criteria, of AS and HFA followed to school age. They found few clinical differences between the groups. Mayes, Calhoun, and Crites (2001) studied children with ASD and normal IQ and divided them into two groups based on the presence of early language delay. The researchers found no significant differences on any of a large number of variables analyzed, including autistic symptomatology and current language function. Several other studies (Szatmari et al., 2000; Howlin, 2003; Gilchrist et al., 2001; Mayes & Calhoun, 2001) reported that older individuals with diagnoses of AS based on absence of language delay are indistinguishable from those diagnosed with HFA and early language delay. Freeman, Cronin, and Candela (2002) also reviewed studies that found few differences between groups of children with normal cognition and autistic symptoms, when groups created on the basis of language history were compared. Nonetheless, as Frith (2004) pointed out, children diagnosed with AS do tend to score higher than those with HFA on verbal IQ measures, although studies are not consistent in finding poorer nonverbal scores in AS.

Despite the lack of categorical distinction in the symptom picture of school-age and older individuals diagnosed with AS, when compared to those diagnosed with HFA who were slower to acquire language initially, there have been reports that find between-group differences. Some research has suggested that speakers with AS are more likely to perseverate on obsessive topics in conversation than those with HFA (McPartland & Klin, 2006), but these findings have not been consistently replicated (Cuccaro et al., 2007; Paul et al., 2000; Shriberg et al., 2001). Shriberg et al. (2001) compared a group of young adults diagnosed by a team of experienced clinicians using DSM-IV criteria as having AS with a similar group having HFA. Those with AS were significantly more garrulous, although other aspects of speech studied did not differ.

Paul, Orlovski, Marcinko, and Volkmar (2009) showed that when conversations of youth (12–18 years of age) with AS were compared with those of an HFA group, using a rating scale developed by Landa, Folstein, and Isaacs (1991), both groups showed the largest differences from typically speaking age-mates in nonverbal communication. Both groups also showed significant difficulties in three broad areas of pragmatics: (1) topic management, specifically, the ability to produce a comment pertinent

to the topic introduced by the partner and the ability to introduce topics of shared relevance and interest; (2) information management, specifically, providing the appropriate amount and type of information based on
listener needs; and (3) reciprocity, the ability to produce and respond to
conversational exchanges in both verbal and nonverbal ways. Only two
between-group differences were significant: Significantly more difficulties
with gaze management were observed in the group with HFA, and use of
overly formal, pedantic language style was rated significantly more often
in the group with AS, which replicates an earlier finding (Ghaziuddin &
Gerstein, 1996).

One study has suggested that youth with HFA differ from those with
AS in their pattern of cohesion use. Fine et al. (1994) compared referential
cohesion use in HFA, AS, and nonautistic socially impaired children and
teens. The groups differed in the relative frequency with which they used
different types of cohesive devices. Subjects with HFA referred more often
to the physical environment and less often to previous discourse, making
it difficult to build a reciprocal conversation. The group with AS differed
from the other groups in the production of more unclear references (using
words that have more than one possible referent in the previous discourse
or that have no previous referent). Although the specific types of cohesion
errors were different in the HFA and AS groups, both groups made significantly more errors than did other socially impaired children. Together with
the findings of other studies of cohesion usage by individuals with ASD,
these findings indicate that rules for tying units of discourse together are
not often employed appropriately by individuals on the autism spectrum.
This cohension deficit is likely to result in discourse that is compromised.

Ghaziuddin, Leininger, and Tsai (1995) explored the presence of
thought disorder in adolescents with HFA or AS using the Rorschach Ink-
blot Test to elicit and score samples of language output. Despite considerable
heterogeneity within the AS group, subjects with AS produced responses
that reflected "more active internal lives involving complex fantasies and
cognitive processes compared to persons with HFA" (Ghaziuddin et al.,
1995, p. 316). Subjects with AS were also rated as more introverted than
were subjects with HFA. The authors concluded that the groups differed
in their mechanisms of understanding and processing of new information.
Children with HFA have also been shown to use significantly lower propor-
tions of assertions involving explanations or references to internal states
than children with AS (Ziatas, Durkin, & Pratt, 2003).

Summary

Studies that contrast speakers with ASD who do and do not have histories of apparently normal language development usually fail to find differences in presentation at school age or older in these subjects. Speakers with
AS have been reported to be more likely than those with HFA to use an
overly formal speech style, and some reports suggest that they may be more

likely to perseverate on favorite topics in conversation. Although they do show difficulties in gaze management in conversation, these are less pronounced than in speakers with HFA. These somewhat conflicting reports on the communicative profiles of young people with HFA and AS reinforce the need for more extensive and more detailed research in this area. Frith (2004) suggests that it may be more helpful to think of individuals with AS as showing HFA in the presence of high verbal abilities, rather than relying on the presence of normal language history for making the differential diagnosis. Such suggestions require further field testing and empirical validation prior to their adoption as diagnostic standards. Nonetheless, the differences in communication seen in populations identified as ASDs tend to be subtle, and to have little significance for intervention programs. The current recommendations of DSM-5 have thus moved away from using AS as a distinct diagnostic category.

ASSESSMENT IN SPEAKERS WITH ASD

Generally, speeakers with ASD achieve scores within the normal range on most standardized language tests, which typically focus on grammatical and semantic constructs within linguistic units up to a single sentence in length or, rarely, on comprehension of a short text (story). Such scores often make it difficult for these students to qualify for the services of a speech–language pathologist. Yet these speakers experience severe difficulties in social interactions and conversation, especially when interacting with unfamiliar people, including teachers, peers, and classmates, who are not adept at compensating for their social language vulnerabilities. Because the pragmatic language impairment associated with ASD is one of the most stigmatizing aspects of the disorder, appropriate pragmatic assessment and intervention are central to maximizing the potential of these children for communicative development. However, few measures of pragmatic or conversational skill meet psychometric standards of validity, reliability, sensitivity, and specificity. Valid assessment of pragmatic skills requires observation of an individual in a dynamic social context. For this reason, it is often difficult to assemble data that will allow clinicians and educators to establish eligibility for communicative services as well as provide detailed information about pragmatic strength and needs.

In this section we suggest a two-step strategy for helping clinicians to establish eligibility for speech–language services and design assessments for intervention planning for speakers with ASD. The first step involves documenting a significant discrepancy between skills in language form/meaning and those in pragmatic areas on standardized measures. We review standard assessments that have been shown to provide these data in research studies. The second step involves the use of more informal assessments that can supply the detailed picture of pragmatic abilities and can serve as a basis for the design of an intervention program.

Documenting Pragmatic Deficits with Standard Instruments

Five instruments have been studied in recent literature and shown to have strong psychometric properties for documenting a significant gap between basic language form/meaning and pragmatics. These are reviewed briefly below.

Test of Language Competence—Expanded Edition

The Test of Language Competence—Expanded Edition (TLC-E; Wiig & Secord, 1989) taps abstract language skills such as multiple-meaning words/sentences, formulating sentences with content appropriate to the pictured context, making inferences, and interpreting figures of speech. This test has been shown to differentiate adolescents and adults with HFA from IQ-matched controls (Minshew, Goldstein, & Siegel, 1995). Although speakers with ASD generally score at the low end of the normal range on this measure (with standard scores of 80–90), research by Diakonova, Paul, Klin, and Saulnier (2008) suggests that these scores are significantly lower than scores obtained by the same individuals on other, more traditional measures of basic language performance. Thus, scores obtained on the TLC-E can be compared to those on a more traditional language assessment (see Table 4.1) to identify a significant gap in higher-level language function that can serve as a basis for eligibility of communication services. The TLC-E is going to be replaced by the CELF-5 Metalinguistics (Wiig & Secord, 2014) in the summer of 2014. This assessment has four subtests to measure inference skills, conversation, language with multiple meanings, and figurative language.

Test of Problem Solving—3

The Test of Problem Solving–3 (TOPS-3; Huisingh, Bowers, & LoGiudice, 2005) employs photographs of familiar contexts and associated questions to explore comprehension of key vocabulary and social problem-solving skills. The child must integrate pictured cues to appropriately infer the nature of the situation, and then generate solutions to problems associated with that context. The standardized score provided by this test allows for comparison of a child's performance to that of a normative sample. In addition to this developmental information, the language specialist obtains valuable information from the child's responses to test stimuli, including his or her ability to formulate language in response to a novel question (outside the context of scripted conversational routines); ability to express thoughts in a specific way; perspective-taking skills; perseverative tendencies; ability to focus responses on the question at hand rather than an associated or unrelated topic; ability to monitor the adequacy of responses and appropriately modify responses when prompted to provide additional

TABLE 4.1. A Sample of Traditional Language Assessment Instruments

Test name (author[s]/date/publisher)	Age range	Areas assessed
Clinical Evaluation of Language Fundamentals, Fifth Edition Semel, E., Wiig, E. H., & Secord, W. (2003). San Antonio, TX: Harcourt Assessment.	5–21 yr	Semantics, syntax, memory, receptive and expressive, composite, Pragmatic Activities Checklist and Pragmatic Rating Scale
Communication Abilities Diagnostic Test Johnston, E. B., & Johnston, A. V. (1990). Austin, TX: Pro-Ed.	3–9 yr	Syntax, semantics, pragmatics (e.g., predicting outcomes)
Detroit Tests of Learning Aptitude— Primary 2 Hammill, D. D., & Bryant, B. R. (1991). Austin, TX: Pro-Ed.	3–9:11 yr	Domains: linguistic, cognitive, attentional, motoric
Diagnostic Evaluation of Language Variation (DELV—Criterion Referenced) Seymour, H. N., Roeper, T. W., & de Villiers, J. (2003). San Antonio, TX: Harcourt Assessment.	4–9 yr	Comprehensive speech and language, including pragmatics, syntax, semantics, and phonology
Expressive One-Word Picture Vocabulary Test, Fourth Edition (2010) Brownell, R. (Ed.). (2000). Novato, CA: Academic Therapy.	2–18 yr	Expressive vocabulary
Expressive Vocabulary Test Williams, K. T. (1997). Circle Pines, MN: AGS Publishing.	2:6–90+ yr	Expressive vocabulary and word retrieval
Fullerton Language Test for Adolescents— Second Edition Thorum, A. R. (1986). Austin, TX: Pro-Ed.	11 yr–adult	Auditory synthesis, morphology, oral commands, convergent and divergent production, syllabification, grammar competency, idioms
OWLS-II Listening Comprehension and Oral Expresson Test, Second Edition Carrow-Woolfolk, E. (1996). Circle Pines, MN: American Guidance Service.	3–21 yr	Receptive and expressive language
Patterned Elicitation of Syntax Test (Revised) with Morphophonemic Analysis Young, E. C., & Perachio, J. J. (1993). San Antonio, TX: Harcourt Assessment.	3–7:6 yr	Expressive syntax and morphology

(continued)

TABLE 4.1. *(continued)*

Peabody Picture Vocabulary Test–4 Dunn, L. M., & Dunn, L. M. (2006). Circle Pines, MN: AGS Publishing.	2:6 yr–adult	Receptive vocabulary
Receptive One-Word Picture Vocabulary Test, Fourth Edition (2010) Brownell, R. (Ed.). (2000). Novato, CA: Academic Therapy Publications.	2:11–12 yr	Receptive vocabulary
Structured Photographic Expressive Language Test 3 (SPELT-3) Dawson, J., Eyer, J., & Stout, C. (2003). DeKalb, IL: Janelle.	4–9:11 yr	Syntax and morphology
Test of Adolescent and Adult Language–3 Hammill, D. D., Brown, V. L., Larsen, S. C., & Wiederholt, J. L. (1994). Austin, TX: Pro-Ed.	12–24:11 yr	Receptive and expressive, vocabulary and grammar, reading and writing, auditory comprehension
Test for Auditory Comprehension of Language—3rd Edition (TACL-3) Carrow-Woolfolk, E. (1999). Austin, TX: Pro-Ed.	3–9:11 yr	Auditory comprehension, word classes and relations, grammatical, morphemes, elaborated sentence constructions
Test of Language Development—Primary (TOLD-P:3)/Intermediate (TOLD-I:3) Newcomer, P. L., & Hammill, D. D. (1997). Austin, TX: Pro-Ed.	Primary: 4–8:11 yr Intermediate: 8:6–12:11 yr	Receptive and expressive semantics, syntax
Utah Test of Language Development—4 Mecham, M. J. (2003). Austin, TX: Pro-Ed.	3–9:11 yr	Receptive and expressive language, auditory comprehension
Woodcock Language Proficiency Battery— Revised Woodcock, R. W. (1991). Chicago: Riverside.	2–95 yr	Oral language, vocabulary, antonyms and synonyms, reading and writing

information; ability to speculate on events and outcomes that are within and outside personal life experience; ability to discuss a range of events involving a variety of social settings and different types of people; and impulsivity.

Griswold, Barnhill, Myles, Hagiwara, and Simpson (2002) compared the performance of 21 young men diagnosed with AS on the TOPS with their performance on the Wechsler Individual Achievement Test (WIAT; Weschler, 1991). Results indicated that the participants' average scores on the TOPS were between one and two standard deviations below the mean of 100 (M = 73.52, SD = 17.52). Comparing scores of the subjects on the two tests indicated that there was a significant difference in their performance on the TOPS and the Language Composite of the WIAT; the Language Composite scores for the WIAT fell within the average range, whereas the overall TOPS mean score fell significantly below the norm. The TOPS, too, then appears useful for establishing the gap in pragmatic versus other language skills in students with HFA.

Test of Pragmatic Language–2

The Test of Pragmatic Language–2 (TOPL-2; Phelps-Terasaki & Phelps-Gunn, 2007) focuses on a student's ability to monitor and judge the effectiveness of a response to resolve a social problem situation. The TOPL-2 includes 44 items, each of which establishes a social context by means of a picture. After a verbal prompt from the examiner, who also displays the picture, the student responds to the dilemma shown. Items are divided into six core subcomponents of pragmatic language: physical setting, audience, topic, purpose (speech acts), visual-gestural cues, and abstraction. Young, Diehl, Morris, Hyman, and Bennetto (2005) showed that the TOPL was useful in documenting the pragmatic deficits of 17 speakers with ASD relative to typical peers.

Comprehensive Assessment of Spoken Language

The Comprehensive Assessment of Spoken Language (CASL; Carrow-Woolfolk, 1999) is a norm-referenced assessment used to measure oral language skills in four areas: lexical/semantic, syntactic, supralinguistic, and pragmatic. The CASL was standardized using a large, nationally representative sample and has well-established reliability and validity. Reichow, Salamak, Paul, Volkmar, and Klin (2008) compared scores on subtests within the CASL for 35 speakers with ASD, 11 of whom had AS. The results of this study showed that participants performed at above-average levels on CASL subtests that measured formal aspects of language (lexical/semantic and syntactic areas), but their performances on the Pragmatic Judgment and Inferences subtests were near the bottom of the normal range, and were close to one standard deviation below scores on the other subtests. Statistical comparisons revealed significant differences between lexical/semantic scores and those on the Pragmatic Judgment and Inferences subtests. This significant deviation provides another form of documentation that can be used to support the need for communication services for students with HFA.

Children's Communication Checklist–2

The Children's Communication Checklist–2 (CCC-2; Bishop, 2003) is a 70-item questionnaire completed by a caregiver to screen for communication problems in children ages 4–16 years. It is designed to identify language disorder and/or pragmatic impairment in children with communication problems, and to differentiate pragmatic language impairments from those confined to language form. Scores are provided on 10 subscales (speech, syntax, semantics, coherence, inappropriate initiation, stereotyped language, use of context, nonverbal communication, social relations, and interests). Two composite scores are derived: The General Communication Composite (GCC) is used to identify children likely to have clinically significant communication problems; and the Social Interaction Deviance Composite (SIDC) can assist in identifying children with significant pragmatic deficits. Moreover, the GCC and SIDC can be compared to identify a significant discrepancy between basic language and pragmatic skills. Several studies have shown that the CCC-2 can identify varying patterns of communicative performance. For example, Norbury, Nash, Baird, and Bishop (2004) found that the CCC-2 distinguished children with communication impairments from nonimpaired peers. Furthermore, the SIDC of the CCC-2 identified children with disproportionate pragmatic and social difficulties in relation to their structural language impairments.

Assessing Pragmatic Performance with Informal Instruments for Intervention Planning

Although poor performance on the measures discussed previously is likely to suggest abnormal pragmatic ability and assist in establishing eligibility for communicative services for children with HFA who have average or above-average performance on traditional measures of language performance, the assessment of pragmatic skills is not complete without an evaluation of multiple aspects of performance in socially valid contexts. This information provides the basis for understanding the areas in which the student is having the most difficulty and where relative strengths exist, and thus for developing a plan to improve pragmatic performance.

It is also important to be aware of communication patterns among typical students. Turstra, Ciccia, and Seaton (2003) examined conversational behaviors in typically developing adolescents engaged in 3-minute interactions with peers and found that behaviors occurring at the highest rates were looking at the partner (especially during listening), nodding and showing positive facial expressions, using back-channel responses indicating understanding and agreement (such as "uh-huh" or "yeah"), and giving contingent responses. Behaviors that occurred with very low frequency included expressions of negative emotions, turning away, asking for clarification, and failing to answer questions. These findings suggest that we need to be careful about choosing pragmatic targets. That is, although focusing only on discourse structure and content aspects of conversation is important, these areas should be supplemented by appropriate paralinguistic behaviors in peer interactions. Moreover, we need to help students find ways to express empathy and establish affiliation through conversation. Two methods of conducting informal assessment of pragmatics in HFA are discussed: observational rating systems and questionnaires.

Observational Rating Scales

Observational rating systems can be used to evaluate conversational or narrative skills. These evaluations are usually accomplished by engaging the student in a conversation, interview, or storytelling situation either with an adult or a peer, videotaping the interaction, and analyzing components using the categories listed on the form of interest. Typically, norms for these instruments are not provided; their purpose is not to compare the student to those with typical development, but to identify areas of disordered behavior.

One example of such a system is the Pragmatic Rating Scale (Landa et al., 1992). This instrument was designed specifically to examine the communicative behaviors typically found to be disordered in speakers with ASD, and it is appropriate to use with individuals over the age of 9. It was designed to be used in conjunction with the standard interview administered during the Autism Diagnostic Observation Scale (ADOS; Lord et al., 2000). Using a consistent interview format across subjects strengthens the clinician's ability to interpret subject responses because all subjects will receive the sample "presses," or opportunities to demonstrate pragmatic skills, across the domains of communicative intentions, discourse management, and presupposition. A sample PRS rating form appears in Figure 4.1. A clinician can observe the ADOS interview and rate each behavior listed on the scale from 0 (appropriate) to 2 (inappropriate). Those behaviors rated as inappropriate can be targeted for conversational intervention. Prutting and Kirchner's (1983) Pragmatic Protocol; Damico's (1992) Systematic Observation of Communicative Interaction; Larson and McKinley's (2003) Adolescent Conversational Analysis; Bishop, Chan, Adams, Hartley, and Weir's (2006) Assessment of Language Impaired Children's Conversation; Rice, Sell, and Hadley's (1990) Social Interactive Coding System; Bedrosian's (1985) Discourse Skills Checklist can also be used in this way, although they do not employ a standard interview format and were not designed specifically to assess pragmatic skills in ASD.

Adams (2002) suggested that, although natural conversational sampling is the most ecologically valid method for assessing conversational skill, there may be some critical behaviors that simply fail to appear in natural interactions. Brinton and Fujiki (1992) suggested using probes within the interaction to solve this problem. That is, instead of, or in addition to, observing an unstructured peer-to-peer conversation with the client, the clinician can provide stimuli to examine critical aspects of conversational behavior within the interaction and evaluate the client's response to each probe. Some of the probes suggested by Brinton and Fujiki for adolescent

	0	1	2
Inappropriate or absent greeting	___	___	___
Strikingly candid	___	___	___
Overly direct or blunt	___	___	___
Inappropriately formal	___	___	___
Inappropriately informal	___	___	___
Overly talkative	___	___	___
Irrelevant or inappropriate detail	___	___	___
Content "out of sync" with interlocutor	___	___	___
Confusing accounts	___	___	___
Topic preoccupation/perseveration	___	___	___
Unresponsive to cues	___	___	___
Little reciprocal to-and-fro exchange	___	___	___
Terse	___	___	___
Odd humor	___	___	___
Insufficient background information	___	___	___
Failure to reference pronouns or other terms	___	___	___
Inadequate clarification	___	___	___
Vague accounts	___	___	___
Scripted, stereotyped discourse	___	___	___
Awkward expression of ideas	___	___	___
Indistinct or mispronounced speech	___	___	___
Inappropriate rate of speech	___	___	___
Inappropriate intonation	___	___	___
Inappropriate volume	___	___	___
Excessive pauses, reformulations	___	___	___
Unusual rhythm, fluency	___	___	___
Inappropriate physical distance	___	___	___
Inappropriate gestures	___	___	___
Inappropriate facial expression	___	___	___
Inappropriate use of gaze	___	___	___
Subject's Total Score:			

0 = normal; 1 = moderately inappropriate; 2 = absent or highly inappropriate

FIGURE 4.1. Score form based on Landa et al.'s (1992) Pragmatic Rating Scale. Adapted from Landa et al. (1992). Copyright 1992 by Cambridge University Press. Reprinted by permission.

students appear in Table 4.2. Additional pragmatic assessments that include probes include the Yale in vivo Pragmatic Protocol (Chuba et al., 2003; Paul, 2005) and the Peanut Butter Protocol (Creaghead, 1984), which was designed to assess pragmatics in children 4–7 years of age.

TABLE 4.2. Probes for Eliciting Conversational Behavior in Adolescents

Probe for . . .	Example	Target-elicited behavior	Example
Topic initiation	"By the way, I was at the beach over the weekend."	1. Responsiveness 2. Topic maintenance 3. Relevance	"I went skiing." "My girlfriend went too." "I love weekends!"
Questions	"So how was the dance?"	1. Responsiveness 2. Topic maintenance 3. Relevance 4. Informativeness	"It was OK." "I danced with four or five girls." "I knew most of the dances." "They had a hip-hop group."
Requests for repair	"What kind of group?"	1. Responsiveness 2. Adjustment to listener 3. Repair strategies	"A hip-hop band." "You know, they play rap music." "Do you know what hip-hop is?"
Sources of difficulty	"Can you get that marker for me?" (no marker present)	1. Assertiveness 2. Comprehension monitoring 3. Clarification requests	"There's no marker here." "Did you say *marker*?" "Do you mean a *pen*?"

Narrative skills are an additional area of pragmatics in which students with HFA may benefit from intervention. The Strong Narrative Assessment Procedure (SNAP; Strong, 1998) and the Test of Narrative Language (TNL; Gillam & Pearson, 2004) are commercially available materials that include detailed instructions for administration and scoring, as well as norm-referenced scores. Hughes, McGillivray, and Schmidek (1997), Johnston (1982), McCabe and Rollins (1994), Peterson and McCabe (1983), and Westby (2005) provide additional guidance on less formal assessment of narrative abilities. In addition, Klecan-Aker and Kelty (1990) and Paul, Hernandez, McFarland, and Johnson (1996) provide adaptations of Applebee's (1978) narrative stages that can also be used to rate the maturity of narrative organization. Paul et al.'s schema appears in Figure 4.2.

Questionnaires

As an adjunct to direct observation, parent and teacher ratings provide information that can round out the picture of pragmatic abilities in students with AS. Like the probe measures we discussed above, parent and teacher ratings allow information to be gathered that might not be accessible through the observation of a short interaction. Several well-constructed questionnaires are available to suit this purpose. These are outlined in Table 4.3.

COMMUNICATION INTERVENTION FOR SPEAKERS WITH ASD

Strengthening pragmatic skills in students with ASD will improve their ability to negotiate the social world, which is likely to translate into better long-term adjustment and prognosis (Matson & Swiezy, 1994). Since individuals with high-functioning ASD may not be appropriately diagnosed until late childhood or even adulthood, intervention does not always begin early, as it is increasingly more likely to do in autism. Even when diagnosis does not occur until school age, however, intervention can be beneficial. Numerous clinical researchers have reported the effectiveness of socially based interventions with school-age individuals with ASD (e.g., Mesibov, 1984; Williams, 1989; Ozonoff & Miller, 1995).

Intervention for speakers with ASD will focus primarily on the social uses of language in conversation and narration. Speech–language pathologists will most likely be primary agents of intervention for developing these skills, although psychologists, counselors, and social workers may also be involved in the implementation of social skills groups in which these skills can be learned and generalized.

A variety of conversational pragmatic programs is available commercially, many geared specifically toward working with students on the autism spectrum. Some examples of these appear in Table 4.4. In addition,

---

Stage 1 (Heap Stories)

Heaps consist primarily of labels and descriptions of events or actions. There is no central theme or organization among the propositions. Sentences are usually simple declaratives. Stories at this level are used by normally developing children at 2 or 3 years of age.

Example: "Mercer went out his home. He got to the playground. Then he found a frog. Then he fell off the cliff. Frog is in the water. Doggy pulls on a stick. A boy is mad. Then he called the police. Then he rested. And then he goed in jail."

Stage 2 (Sequence Stories)

Sequences consist of labeling events around a central theme, character, or setting. There is nothing that could be considered a plot; rather, there is a description of what a character has done. One event does not necessarily follow temporally or causally from another. Stories at this level are used by normally developing children at 3 years of age.

Example: "Little boy. Tree, frog. Tree, person, dog, bucket, and tree that he climbing on, bucket and dog. They fell off. Then they ran down the hill and trip down. And then the frog was happy. And then the dog was swimming. Then there was a dog happy. Then there's a frog sitting on the tree. So they went to the tree

that fall into the water where the frog is. And then the boy caught the dog. Lookit, the dog's in the net! And then the dog go."

Stage 3 (Primitive Narratives)

Stories have a core or central person, object, or event. They contain three of the story grammar elements: an initiating event, an attempt or action, and some consequence around the central theme. But there is no real resolution or ending and little evidence of motivation of characters. Stories at this level are used by normally developing children at 4–4½ years of age.

   Example: "Find a frog. He sees a frog. He fell. And the frog hopped. And he catched the dog. Frog hopped again. Then he went away. The boy was angry. And the frog was pretty nervous. Then he followed the foot track."

Stage 4 (Chain Narrative)

Stories show some evidence of cause–effect and temporal relationships, but the plot is not strong and does not build on the attributes and motivations of characters. The ending does not necessarily follow logically from the events and may be very abrupt. Four story grammar elements are present. They usually include those found at the primitive narrative level: initiating event, attempt or action, and some consequence around the central theme. Some notion of plan or character motivation may be present. Stories at this level are used by normally developing children at 4½–5 years of age.

   Example: "A boy went for a walk with his dog to fetch water and catch fish. There was a frog. He caught the frog. The boy fell in because he tripped on the dog. The dog fell in too. The frog hopped onto a lily pad. The frog fell off. And the boy tried to catch the frog. And the boy actually caught the dog. The frog climbed onto a rock. The boy called him. They went away. The frog was sad. The frog followed him. He followed him into his house. And the frog was on the dog's head."

Stage 5 (True Narrative)

Stories have a central theme, character, and plot. They include motivations behind the characters' actions, as well as logical and temporally ordered sequences of events. The stories include at least five story grammar elements, including an initiating event, an attempt or action, and a consequence. The ending indicates a resolution to the problem. Stories at this level are used by normally developing children at 5–7 years of age.

   Example: "There was a little boy. And he wanted to get a frog. And he brought his dog. He saw a frog in the pond. He ran to catch it. But he tripped over a log. And he fell in the water. But the frog jumped over to a log. He told his dog to go try to get the frog. He almost caught the frog. But instead, he caught his dog. When he saw what he caught, he was mad. The little boy, he yelled to the frog. Then the boy went home and left the frog. The frog was sad alone. Then he followed the boy's footprints until he got into the house. Then he kept following them into the bathroom where the little boy took a bath with his dog. 'Hi,' said the frog. Then the frog jumped in the tub. And they were all happy together."

FIGURE 4.2. An adaptation of Applebee's System for scoring narrative stages. Adapted from Paul and Norbury (2012, p. 405). Copyright 2012 by Mosby. Reprinted with permission from Elsevier, Inc.

TABLE 4.3. Social Skills Rating Forms

Instrument	Full citation	Age range	Content
Social Responsiveness Scale, Second Edition (SRS-2)	Constantino, J. (2012). *Social Responsiveness Scale.* Los Angeles: Western Psychological Services.	4–18 yr	Social awareness, social information processing, capacity for reciprocal social communication, social anxiety/avoidance, preoccupations within natural contexts
Social Skills Improvement System (SSIS) Rating Scales	Gresham, F., & Elliot, S. (2008). *Social Skills Improvement System (SSIS) Rating Scales.* Minneapolis, MN: Pearson Assessment.	3–18 yr	Social Skills, Problem Behaviors, and Academic Competence Scales
Pragmatic Language Skills Inventory (PLSI)	Gilliam, J., & Miller, L. (2006). *Pragmatic Language Skills Inventory.* Austin, TX: Pro-Ed.	5–12:11 yr	Personal, social, and classroom interaction skills
Assessment of Social and Communication Skills for Children with Autism (ASCSCA)	Quill, K. (2000). *Do–Watch–Say–Listen: Social and Communication Intervention for Children with Autism.* Baltimore: Brookes.	School age	Social and communicative behavior, motivators, nonverbal interaction, imitation, organization, play, group skills, community social skills, communicative functions, social–emotional skills, conversational skills

several methods have been reported in the research literature as effective in developing basic conversational pragmatic skills in the areas of communicative intent, presupposition, and discourse management. These methods are outlined below.

Communicative Intent

One method that has a considerable amount of research support as a way to develop appropriate expressions of communicative intents is video modeling (Charlop-Christy, Le, & Freeman, 2000). In this method, typical peers are enlisted to act out a common social scene that has been identified as an area of need for the target student. The scene is then videotaped and shown to the student, who watches it with a clinician. The student is asked to verbally rehearse what he or she saw, discuss it with the adult, then reenact it. After several sessions the student may be asked to play out the scene with the peers who made the video and critique his or her own performance.

TABLE 4.4. Examples of Commercially Available Programs for Addressing Conversational Pragmatics

Title	Author	Publisher
"Ask and Answer" Social Skills Games	K. Spieloogle, M. Cullough, & M. DeShang	SuperDuper
Let's Be Better Friends: The Peer Integration Program	M. B. DeLaney, N. Griffin, & K. Fox	Janelle
Maxwell's Manor: A Social Language Game	C. LoGiudice & N. McConnell	LinguiSystems
Positive Pragmatic Games	K. Gill & J. DeNinno	SuperDuper
Promoting Social Communication: Children with Developmental Disabilities from Birth to Adolescence	H. Goldstein, L. A. Kaczmarek, & K. M. English	Alimed Inc.
Ready-to-Use Social Skills Lessons & Activities for Grades PreK–K	R. Weltmann Begun, editor	Jossey-Bass
Ready-to-Use Social Skills Lessons & Activities for Grades 1–3	R. Weltmann Begun, editor	Jossey-Bass
Ready-to-Use Social Skills Lessons & Activities for Grades 4–6	R. Weltmann Begun, editor	Jossey-Bass
Room 14: A Social Language Program	C. Wilson	LinguiSystems
Scripting Junior: Social Skill Role-Plays	L. Miller	Thinking Publications
Social Communication Skills for Children	W. McGam & G. Werven	Pro-Ed
Social Skill Builder Software		Academic Communication Associates
Social Star	N. Gajewski, P. Hirn, & P. Mayo	Thinking Publications
Talk About Activities: Developing Social Communication Skills	A. Kelly	Pro-Ed
Talk About: A Social Communication Skills Package	A. Kelly	Pro-Ed
Talk! Talk! Talk! Tools to Facilitate Language	N. Muir, S. McCaig, K. Gerylo, M. Gompf, T. Burke, & P. Lumsden	Thinking Publications
The Socially Speaking Game	A. Schroeder	SuperDuper

Later, the student may try to act it out on his or her own with new peers and report back to the adult.

The use of graphic organizers and written cues (on cards or posters displayed in the classroom) has also been shown to be effective in helping to generalize newly learned conversational and narrative skills. One method making use of these aids is script fading (Krantz & McClannahan, 1998). Here students are encouraged to learn rote scripts for several communicative rituals, such as greetings or asking for a date. The script is written out and the student rehearses it with an adult by reading it many times, attempting to modify intonation, pace, etc., to maximize effectiveness. Krantz and McClannahan showed that fading these scripts, by gradually cutting off increasingly larger segments of the written form and requiring students to rely on their memory rather than the written script, increased generalization of these procedures to settings outside the therapy context. Eventually, mental state terms (*think, believe, expect*), perspective taking, shifting speech registers (formal, informal), understanding and using multiple-meaning words and figurative language, and so on, can be introduced to these scripts.

Presupposition

Role playing and barrier games can be useful activities for encouraging thinking about others' informational needs. An activity might be used in which the student must plan an "attack" on parents to, for example, persuade them to lift their curfew for a special school event. Before role-playing the argument, the students should plan their strategy, stating explicitly the parent needs they will address (e.g., the need to believe the students are safe and chaperoned), what arguments they will use, and how the arguments will be phrased. Only then will they role-play the situation. After the role play, they can evaluate their performance and list ways it could be improved. Barrier games, in which conversational partners are screened from each others' view and must communicate solely by means of language, can also be helpful in this regard. Students can be asked, for example, to explain to a partner behind a barrier how to build a structure, when they have duplicate sets of materials. Before beginning, they can be coached to think about what the other already knows, needs to know, etc. Then they can check their presuppositions as the activity continues.

Discourse Management

Brinton, Robinson, and Fujiki (2004) reported on a method, outlined below, for improving turn taking and topic management in a student with pragmatic language difficulties:

- Brainstorm a list of topics classmates might want to discuss.
- Write each on a slip of paper.

- Put slips in can.
- Take turns pulling out a topic.
- Start conversation:
  - Think first: What should I say?
  - Say two things about the topic.
  - Ask interlocutor a question about the topic.
  - Listen while interlocutor answers.

Including Peers in Social Skills Programs

Research (summarized by Paul, 2003) suggests that these interventions are most effective when delivered through mediated peer interactions. This finding indicates that effort should be made to include typically developing peers in social skills programs for speakers with ASD. Several peer-mediated programs—in which typically developing peers receive some training (usually a relatively small amount) and incentives to engage with speakers with ASD as social skills group members, peer mentors, or part-time "buddies"—have been shown not only to increase peer interactions within the structured setting, but to facilitate generalization of these skills to more natural situations. Kamps, Leonard, Vernon, Dugan, and Delquadi (1997), for example, conducted daily play sessions in groups of one target and three typical elementary school students. Scripted social skills instruction, including greeting, sharing and taking turns, and helping, was provided to the group for 10 minutes, followed by 10 minutes of play in a planned activity. Increases in social skills, length of interactions, and consistency of responding were found for target students and maintained over time, to some degree.

Roeyers (1995) presented another approach for 5- to 13-year-olds with ASD. Each was paired with a peer who was simply told to stay "on the same level" as his or her partner. Although improvements in rate of interaction were seen, the children with ASD still had difficulty managing social situations. Gunter, Fox, Brady, Shores, and Cavanaugh (1988) taught elementary school students to "prompt and praise" students with ASD while engaging in free-play dyads. Prompts involved simple statements such as "Say hello to _____." Peers were also taught to offer verbal praise to the target student when a prompt elicited the desired reply. A "multiple exemplar approach," in which several peers took turns with each student, proved effective in increasing initiations by students with autism. Some generalization to untrained peers and environments was seen.

Peer networks are another strategy that has been used to increase social acceptance and involvement of children with disabilities. Peer networks require awareness training about disabilities for typical peers and supervised joint activities in which typical peers are taught to initiate and model appropriate social interactions. Kamps et al. (1992) applied this method to secondary students with ASD. Two to five peers served as a support network for each target student during several 10- to 20-minute sessions during the school day, including reading, lunch, and game time. They were taught to structure activities using scripts, prompting, and reinforcement for interaction. Results showed increased interaction time for all target students and generalization to new settings for some.

What we know about speakers with ASD suggests that the methods outlined here, which involve use of verbal rehearsal, written cueing, and metalinguistic discussion, are appropriate for this population, especially when verbal skills are a relative strength and preferred avenue of learning for these individuals. One adult with ASD, writing in *The New Yorker* magazine (Page, 2007), described his delight in reading Emily Post's *Etiquette* for the first time as a teenager, because it provided explicit explanations of the reasons for polite behaviors, which the writer had previously found unfathomable, as well as direct suggestions on how to start a conversation and listen to others' contributions. Thus for speakers with ASD, direct instruction using scripts, verbal explanation, and metalinguistic discussion are likely to be effective both in developing pragmatic skills and in reducing speakers' anxiety and confusion.

Regardless of the particular area of pragmatic skills being targeted, seven crucial elements for social skills instruction, suggested by Larson and McKinley (2003), provide useful guidelines for developing either adult-directed or peer-mediated social skills activities. These include:

1. *Introduction.* Tell the students about the skill, what they will learn, and why it is important to them. Have students share experiences related to the skill.
2. *Guided instruction.* Lay out the steps to be taught. Define the skill and list the steps involved in accomplishing it.
3. *Modeling.* Demonstrate the skill to be learned with role playing or audio or video recordings. Model self-talk about thinking through how/when to apply the skill.
4. *Rehearsal.* Students verbally describe the sequence of actions involved in the skill and then role-play with a group of peers.
5. *Feedback.* Provide encouragement for the use of appropriate behaviors and ask students to describe the successful behavior they used; when giving corrective feedback, use a positive, nonthreatening manner and have students describe the appropriate behavior.
6. *Planning.* Have students discuss how/when/with whom they can use the new skill. Encourage them to use the following formula to help plan future interactions:
   - STOP: Think before talking and use self-control strategies, if necessary.
   - PLOT: Plan ahead and brainstorm options before deciding what to say/do.

- GO: Choose the best option from brainstorming and implement it.
- SO: Evaluate. Encourage students to ask themselves how it went, what they did well, what they might *change next time.*
7. *Generalization.* Encourage students to try their new skill at home with family or in class with friends. Have them report back to the clinician to discuss the outcome. If more help is needed, the clinician can discreetly "sit in" on an interaction in which the student uses the skill with a peer, and give feedback.

In addition, environmental supports (Dalrymple, 1995) for students with HFA will assist them to function in social settings. The goal is to create an atmosphere that promotes growth and, at the same time, reduces the social and cognitive stresses to avoid overwhelming the student. "Safe rooms" or "time-out areas" to which a student may retreat in times of stress can be identified, and students can be given opportunities to choose when to use them. Trusted people within the school setting can also be sought out by the student when anxiety becomes too great. When persistent problems with behavior, mood, anxiety, obsessiveness, and so on occur, psychiatric evaluation should be sought to determine whether counseling or medical intervention is warranted.

CONCLUSION

Despite several decades of study of variations to presentations at the high end of the autism spectrum, controversy about subtyping continues to exist, and clouds our picure of the best ways to help these intelligent individuals optimize their opportunities for integration and personal success. What does seem clear is that speakers with ASD have difficulties that center on their ability to learn and use the pragmatic rules of language use, and to a lesser extent, their ability to master the understanding and use of prosody. And yet, despite the fact that their major deficits are in these areas of communication, words and sentences are a relative strength and an optimal path through which learning occurs. Thus, intervention for speakers with ASD will focus on using language to explain communicative rules and elaborate communicative competence. Typical peers, sensitized and educated about ASD, will be important allies in this effort. As more research on this population emerges, more detailed information on how best to help these individuals will, we hope, become available.

ACKNOWLEDGMENTS

Preparation of this chapter was supported by Research Grant No. P01-03008 funded by the National Institute of Mental Health (NIMH); by National Institutes of Health Research Grant No. U54 MH66494, funded by the NIMH, the National Institute on Deafness and Other Communication Disorders (NIDCD), the National Institute of Environmental Health Sciences, the National Institute of Child Health and Human Development (NICHD), and the National Institute of Neurological Disorders and Stroke; by Research Grant No. RO1 DC07129 from the NIDCD; by a MidCareer Development grant to Rhea Paul (No. K24 HD045576, funded by NIDCD); and by the National Alliance for Autism Research.

REFERENCES

Adams, C. (2002). Practitioner review: The assessment of language pragmatics. *Journal of Child Psychology, Psychiatry, and Allied Sciences, 43*, 973–988.

American Psychiatric Association. (2013). *Diagnostic and statistical manual of mental disorders* (5th ed). Arlington, VA: Author.

Applebee, A. (1978). *The child's concept of a story: Ages 2 to 17.* Chicago: University of Chicago Press.

Asperger, H. (1944). Die "Autistischen psychopathen" im Kindesalter. *Archiv für Psychiatrie und Nervenkrankheiten, 117*, 76–136.

Austin, J. (1962). *How to do things with words.* Cambridge, MA: Harvard University Press.

Baltaxe, C. A. M. (1977). Pragmatic deficits in the language of autistic adolescents. *Journal of Pediatric Psychology, 2*, 176–180.

Baltaxe, C. A. M., & D'Angiola, N. (1992). Cohesion in the discourse interaction of autistic, specifically language-impaired, and normal children. *Journal of Autism and Developmental Disorders, 22*, 1–21.

Baltaxe, C. A. M., & Simmons, J. Q. (1985). Prosodic development in normal and autistic children. In E. Schopler & G. B. Mesibov (Eds.), *Communication problems in autism* (pp. 95–126). New York: Plenum Press.

Baron-Cohen, S. (1988). Social and pragmatic deficits in autism: Cognitive or affective? *Journal of Autism and Developmental Disabilities, 18*, 379–402.

Bates, E. (1976). *Language in context.* New York: Academic Press.

Bates, E., & MacWhinney, B. (1987). Competition, variation, and language learning. In B. MacWhinney (Ed.), *Mechanisms on language acquisition* (pp. 157–194). Hillsdale, NJ: Erlbaum.

Bates, E., O'Connell, B., & Shore, C. (1987). Language and communication in infancy. In J. Osofsky (Ed.), *Handbook of infant development* (2nd ed., pp. 149–203). New York: Wiley.

Bedrosian, J. (1985). An approach to developing conversational competence. In D. Ripich & F. Spinelli (Eds.), *School discourse problems* (pp. 221–256). San Diego, CA: College-Hill Press.

Bishop, D. (2003). *Children's Communicative Checklist–2.* San Antonio, TX: Harcourt Assessment.

Bishop, D., Chan, J., Adams, C., Hartley, J., & Weir, F. (2000). Conversational responsiveness in specific language impairment. *Development and Psychopathology, 12*, 177–199.

Bishop, D., & Edmundson, A. (1987). Language-impaired 4-year-olds: Distinguishing transient from persistent impairment. *Journal of Speech and Hearing Disorders, 52*, 156–173.

Bloom, A., Russell, A., & Wassenberg, K. (1987). Turn-taking affects the quality of infant vocalizations. *Journal of Child Language, 14*, 211–227.

Boudreau, D. (2007). Narrative abilities in children with language impairments. In R. Paul (Ed.), *Child language disorders from a developmental perspective: Essays in honor of Robin Chapman* (pp. 331–356). Mahwah, NJ: Erlbaum.

Brinton, B., & Fujiki, M. (1992). Setting the context for conversational language sampling. In W. Secord (Ed.), *Best practices in school speech–language pathology* (Vol. 2, pp. 9–19). San Antonio, TX: Psychological Corporation, Harcourt, Brace Jovanovich.

Brinton, B., Robinson, L., & Fujiki, M. (2004). Description of a program for social language intervention: "If you can have a conversation, you can have a relationship." *Language, Speech and Hearing Services in Schools, 35*, 283–290."

Bruner, J. (1978). The role of dialogue in language acquisition. In A. Sinclair, R. J. Jarvella, & W. J. M. Levelt (Eds.), *The child's conception of language* (pp. 241–256). Berlin: Springer-Verlag.

Caplan, R., Guthrie, D., Shields, W., & Yudovin, S. (1994). Communication deficits in pediatric complex partial seizure disorder and schizophrenia. *Development and Psychopathology, 6*, 499–517.

Capps, L., Losh, M., & Thurber, C. (2000). "The frog ate the bug and made his mouth sad": Narrative competence in children with autism. *Journal of Abnormal Child Psychology, 28*, 193–204.

Carrow-Woolfolk, E. (1999). *Comprehensive assessment of spoken language.* Circle Pines, MN: American Guidance Service.

Charlop-Christy, M. H., Le, L., & Freeman, K. A. (2000). A comparison of video modeling with in vivo modeling for teaching children with autism. *Journal of Autism and Developmental Disorders, 30*, 537–552.

Chuba, H., Paul, R., Klin, A., & Volkmar, F. (2003, November). *Assessing pragmatic skills in individuals with autism spectrum disorders.* Paper presented at the National Convention of the American Speech–Language–Hearing Association, Chicago.

Creaghead, N. (1984). Strategies for evaluating and targeting pragmatic behaviors in young children. *Seminars in Speech and Language, 5*, 241–252.

Cuccaro, M., Brinkley, J., Abramson, R., Hall, A., Wright, H., Gilbert, J., et al. (2007). Autism in African-American families: Clinical phenotypic findings. *American Journal of Medical Genetics, 144B*, 1022–1026.

Dalrymple, N. J. (1995). Environmental supports to develop flexibility and independence. In K. A. Quill (Ed.), *Teaching children with autism: Strategies to enhance communication and socialization* (pp. 243–264). New York: Delmar.

Damico, J. (1992). Language assessment in adolescents: Addressing clinical issues. *Language, Speeech, and Hearing Services in School, 24*(1), 29–35.

Dewey, M., & Everard, P. (1974). The near normal autistic adolescent. *Journal of Autism and Childhood Schizophrenia, 4*, 348–356.

Diakonova-Curtis, D., Paul, R., Klin, A., & Saulnier, C. (2008, November). *Differences among diagnostic groups on the Test of Language Competence.* Poster presented at the National Convention of the American Speech, Language and Hearing Association, Chicago.

Dore, J. (1977). Children's illocutionary acts. In R. O. Freedle (Ed.), *Discourse production and comprehension* (pp. 227–244). Norwood, NJ: Ablex.

Eisenmajer, R., Prior, M., Leekam, S., Wing, L., Gould, J., Welham, M., et al. (1996). Comparison of clinical symptoms in autism and Asperger's disorder. *Journal of the American Academy of Child and Adolescent Psychiatry, 35,* 1523–1531.

Ervin-Tripp, S. (1977). Wait for me, Roller Skate! In S. Ervin-Tripp & C. Mitchell-Kernan (Eds.), *Child discourse* (pp. 165–188). New York: Academic Press.

Ervin-Tripp, S. (1979). Children's verbal turn-taking. In E. Ochs & B. B. Schieffelin (Eds.), *Developmental pragmatics* (pp. 391–429). New York: Academic Press.

Eskes, G., Bryson, S., & McCormick, T. (1990). Comprehension of concrete and abstract words in autistic children. *Journal of Autism and Developmental Disorders, 20,* 61–73.

Fine, J., Bartolucci, G., Ginsberg, G., & Szatmari, P. (1991). The use of intonation to communicate in subjects with pervasive developmental disorders. *Journal of Child Psychology and Psychiatry, 32,* 771–882.

Fine, J., Bartolucci, G., Szatmari, P., & Ginsberg, G. (1994). Cohesive discourse in pervasive developmental disorders. *Journal of Autism and Developmental Disorders, 14,* 315–329.

Flavell, J., Botkin, P. T., Fry, C. C., Wright, J. W., & Jarvis, P. E. (1968). *The development of role-taking and communication skills in children.* New York: Wiley.

Foster, S. (1981). The emergence of topic type in children under 2;6: A chicken and egg problem. *Papers and Reports on Child Language Development, 20,* 52–60.

Foster, S. (1986). Learning discourse topic management in the preschool years. *Journal of Child Language, 13,* 231–250.

Freeman, B. J., Cronin, P., & Candela, P. (2002). Asperger syndrome or autistic disorder? *Focus on Autism and Other Developmental Disabilities, 17,* 147–152.

Frith, U. (2004). Confusions and controversies about Asperger syndrome. *Journal of Child Psychology and Psychiatry, 45,* 672–686.

Gallagher, T. (1977). Revision behaviors in the speech of developing children. *Journal of Speech and Hearing Research, 20,* 303–318.

Ghaziuddin, M., & Gerstein, L. (1996). Pedantic speaking style differentiates Asperger syndrome for high-functioning autism. *Journal of Autism and Developmental Disorders, 26,* 585–595.

Ghaziuddin, M., Leininger, L., & Tsai, L. Y. (1995). Brief report: Thought disorder in Asperger syndrome: Comparison with high-functioning autism. *Journal of Autism and Developmental Disorders, 25,* 311–317.

Gilchrist, A., Green, J., Cox, A., Burton, D., Rutter, M., & Le Couteur, A. (2001). Development and current functioning in adolescents with Asperger syndrome: A comparative study. *Journal of Child Psychology and Psychiatry, 42,* 227–240.

Gillam, R., & Pearson, N. (2004). *Test of narrative language.* Greenville, SC: SuperDuper.

Grice, H. P. (1975). Logic and conversation. In P. Cole & J. Morgan (Eds.), *Syntax and semantics: Speech acts* (pp. 41–58). New York: Academic Press.

Griswold, D., Barnhill, G., Myles, B., Hagiwara, T., & Simpson, R. (2002). Asperger syndrome and academic achievement. *Focus on Autism and Other Developmental Disabilities, 17,* 94–102.

Gunter, P., Fox, J. J., Brady, M. P., Shores, R. E., & Cavanaugh, K. (1988).

Non-handicapped peers as multiple exemplars: A generalization tactic for promoting autistic students' social skills. *Behavioral Disorders, 14,* 3–14.

Halliday, M. A. K., & Hassan, R. (1976). *Cohesion in English.* London: Longman.

Hobson, R. P. (1989). Beyond cognition: A theory of autism. In G. Dawson (Ed.), *Autism: Nature, diagnosis, and treatment* (pp. 22–48). New York: Guilford Press.

Howlin, P. (2003). Outcome of high-functioning adults with autism with and without early language delays: Implications for the differentiation between autism and Asperger syndrome. *Journal of Autism and Developmental Disorders, 33,* 3–13.

Howlin, P., & Ashgarian, A. (1999). The diagnosis of autism and Asperger syndrome: Findings from a survey of 770 families. *Developmental Medicine and Child Neurology, 441,* 834–839.

Hughes, D., McGillivray, L., & Schmidek, M. (1997). *Guide to narrative language.* Eau Claire, WI: Thinking Publications.

Huisingh, R., Bowers, L., & LoGiudice, C. (2005). *Test of Problem Solving–3.* East Moline, IL: Linguisystems.

Hurtig., R., Ensrud, S., & Tomblin, B. (1982). The communicative function of question production in autistic children. *Journal of Autism and Developmental Disorders, 12,* 57–69.

Johnston, J. (1982). Narratives: A new look at communication problems in older language-disordered children. *Language, Speech, and Hearing Services in Schools, 13,* 144–155.

Kamps, D., Leonard, B., Vernon, S., Dugan, E., & Delquadri, J. (1992). Teaching social skills to students with autism to increase peer interactions in an integrated first grade classroom. *Journal of Applied Behavior Analysis, 25,* 281–288.

Kamps, D., Potucek, J., Lopez, A., Kravits, T., & Kemmerer, K. (1997). The use of peer networks across multiple settings to improve social interaction for students with autism. *Journal of Behavioral Education, 7,* 335–357.

Kanner, L. (1943). Autistic disturbances of affective content. *Nervous Child, 2,* 227–250.

Kanner, L., & Eisenberg, L. (1957). *Early infantile autism, 1945–1955* [psychiatric report]. Washington, DC: American Psychiatric Association.

Klecan-Aker, J., & Kelty, K. (1990). An investigation of the oral narratives of normal and language-learning disavled children. *Journal of Childhood Communication Disorders, 13,* 207–216.

Koning, D., & Magill-Evans, J. (2001). Social and language skills in adolescent boys with Asperger syndrome. *Autism, 5,* 23–36.

Krantz, P., & McClannahan, L. (1998). Social interaction skills for children with autism: A script-fading procedure for beginning readers. *Journal of Applied Behavior Analysis, 31,* 191–202.

Landa, R., Folstein, S. E., & Isaacs, C. (1991). Spontaneous narrative-discourse performance of parents of autistic children. *Journal of Speech and Hearing Research, 34,* 1339–1345.

Landa, R., Martin, M., Minshew, N., & Goldstein, G. (1995, April). *Discourse and abstract language ability in non-retarded individuals with autism.* Paper presented at the Society for Research in Child Development, Indianapolis, IN.

Landa, R., Piven, J., Wzorek, M. M., Gayle, J. O., Chase, G. A., et al. (1992).

Social language use in parents of autistic individuals. *Psychological Medicine, 22*, 245–254.

Landry, S. H., & Loveland, K. A. (1988). Communication behaviors in autism and developmental language delay. *Journal of Child Psychology and Psychiatry, 29*, 621–634.

Langdell, T. (1980, September). *Pragmatic aspects of autism: Or why is "I" a normal word.* Paper presented at the BPS Developmental Psychology Conference, Edinburgh, Scotland.

Larson, V., & McKinley, N. (2003). *Communication solutions for older students: Assessment and intervention strategies.* Eau Claire, WI: Thinking Publications.

Lord, C., & Schopler, C. (1989). Stability of assessment results of autistic and non-autistic language-impaired children from preschool years to early school age. *Journal of Child Psychology and Psychiatry, 30*, 575–590.

Lord, C., Risi, S., Lanbrecht, L., Cook, E., Leventhal, B., DiLavore, P., et al. (2000). The Autism Diagnostic Observation Schedule—Generic: A standard measure of social and communication deficits associated with the spectrum of autism. *Journal of Autism and Developmental Disorders, 30*, 205–223.

Loveland, D., & Tunali, B. (1991). Social scripts for conversational interactions in autism and Down syndrome. *Journal of Autism and Developmental Disorders, 21*, 177–186.

Loveland, D., & Tunali, B., McEvoy, R., & Kelley, M. (1989). Referential communication and response adequacy in autism and Down's syndrome. *Applied Psycholinguistics, 10*, 301–313.

Loveland, K. A., McEvoy, R. E., Kelley, M. L., & Tunali, B. (1990). Narrative storytelling in autism and Down's syndrome. *British Journal of Developmental Psychology, 8*, 923.

Loveland, K. A., & Tunali, B. (1991). Social scripts for conversational interactions in autism and Down's syndrome. *Journal of Autism and Developmental Disorders, 21*, 177–186.

Matson, J. L., & Swiezy, N. (1994). Social skills training with autistic children. In J. L. Matson (Ed.), *Autism in children and adults: Etiology, assessment, and intervention* (pp. 241–260). Pacific Grove, CA: Brooks/Cole.

Mayes, S., & Calhoun, S. (2001). Non-signicance of early speech delay in children with autism and normal intelligence and implications for DSM-IV Asperger's disorder. *Autism, 5*, 81–94.

Mayes, S., Calhoun, S., & Crites, D. (2001). Does DSM-IV Asperger's disorder exist? *Journal of Abnormal Child Psychology, 3*, 263–271.

McCabe, A., & Rollins, P. (1994). Assessment of preschool narrartive skills. *Journal of Speech–Language Pathology, 3*(1), 45–56.

McPartland, J., & Klin, A. (2006). Asperger syndrome. *Adolescent Medical Clinics, 17*, 771–788.

Mesibov, G. B. (1984). Social skills training with verbal autistic adolescents and adults: A program model. *Journal of Autism and Developmental Disorders, 14*, 395–404.

Minshew, N. J., Goldstein, G., & Siegel, D. J. (1995). Speech and language in high-functioning autistic individuals. *Neuropsychology, 9*, 255–261.

Mundy, P., & Sigman, M. (1989). The theoretical implications of joint attention deficits in autism. *Development and Psychopathology, 1*, 173–183.

Mundy, P., Sigman, M., Ungerer, J. A., & Sherman, T. (1986). Defining the social deficits in autism: The contribution of non-verbal communication measures. *Journal of Child Psychology and Psychiatry, 27,* 658–669.

Ninio, A., & Bruner, J. S. (1978). The achievement and antecedents of labelling. *Journal of Child Language, 5,* 1–15.

Norbury, C., & Bishop, D. (2003). Narrative skills of children with communication impairments. *International Journal of Language and Communication Disorders, 38,* 287–313.

Norbury, C., Nash, M., Baird, G., & Bishop, D. (2004). Using a parental checklist to identify diagnostic groups in children with communication impairment: A validation of the *Children's Communication Checklist-2*. *International Journal of Language and Communication Disorders, 39,* 345–364.

Ozonoff, S., & Miller, J. (1995). Teaching theory of mind: A new approach to social skills training for individuals with autism. *Journal of Autism and Developmental Disorders, 25,* 415–433.

Ozonoff, S., & Miller, J. (1996). An exploration of right hemisphere contributions to the pragmatic impairments of autism. *Brain and Language, 52,* 411–434.

Page, T. (2007, August 20). Personal history: Parallel play. *The New Yorker,* pp. 36–45.

Palkowitz, R. W., & Wiesenfeld, A. R. (1980). Differential autonomic responses of autistic and normal children. *Journal of Autism and Developmental Disorders, 10,* 347–360.

Paul, R. (2003). Enhancing social communication in high functioning individuals with autistic spectrum disorders. *Child and Adolescent Psychiatric Clinics of North America, 12,* 87–106.

Paul, R. (2005). Assessing communication in autism. In F. Volkmar, A. Klin, R. Paul, & D. Cohen (Eds.), *Handbook of autism and pervasive developmental disorders* (3rd ed., pp. 799–816). New York: Wiley.

Paul, R., Augustyn, A., Klin, A., & Volkmar, F. (2005). Perception and production of prosody by speakers with autism spectrum disorders. *Journal of Autism and Developmental Disorders, 35,* 201–220.

Paul, R., & Cohen, D. (1984). Responses to contingent queries in adults with mental retardation and pervasive developmental disorders. *Applied Psycholinguistics, 5,* 349–357.

Paul, R., & Cohen, D. (1985). Comprehension of indirect requests in adults with autistic disorders and mental retardation. *Journal of Speech and Hearing Research, 28,* 475–479.

Paul, R., Hernandez, R., McFarland, L., & Johnson, K. (1996). Narrative skills in late talkers. *Journal of Speech and Hearing Research, 39,* 1295–1303.

Paul, R., & Norbury, C. F. (2012). *Language disorders from infancy through adolescence: Listening, speaking, reading, writing, and communicating* (4th ed.). St. Louis, MO: Mosby.

Paul, R., Orlovski, S., Marcinko, H., & Volkmar, F. (2009). Conversational behaviors in youth with high-functioning autism and Asperger syndrome. *Journal of Autism and Developmental Disorders, 39,* 115–125.

Paul, R., Shriberg, L., McSweeney, J., Cicchetti, D., Klin, A., & Volkmar, R. (2005). Relations between prosodic performance and communication and socialization ratings in high functioning speakers with autism spectrum disorders. *Journal of Autism and Developmental Disorders, 35,* 861–869.

Peterson, C., & McCabe, A. (1983). *Developmental psycholinguistics: Three ways of looking at a child's narrative.* New York: Plenum Press.

Phelps-Terasaki, D., & Phelps-Gunn, T. (2007). *Test of Pragmatic Language–2.* Austin, TX: PRO-ED.

Prutting, C. A., & Kirchner, D. (1983). Applied pragmatics. In T. M. Gallagher & C. A. Prutting (Eds.), *Pragmatic assessment and intervention issues in language* (pp. 29–64). San Diego, CA: College-Hill Press.

Reichow, B., Salamak, S., Paul, R., Volkmar, F., & Klin, A. (2008). Pragmatic assessment in autism spectrum disorders: A comparison of a standard measure qith parent report. *Communications Disorders Quarterly, 29,* 169–176.

Rice, M., Sell, M., & Hadley, P. (1990). The social interactive coding system (SICS): An online, clinically relevant descriptive tool. *Language, Speech and Hearing Services in Schools, 21,* 2–14.

Roeyers, H. (1995). A peer-mediated proximity intervention to facilitate the social interactions of children with a pervasive development disorders. *British Journal of Special Education, 22,* 161–164.

Rumsey, J., Andreasen, N. C., & Rapoport, J. (1986). Thought, language, communication, and affective flattening in autistic adults. *Archives of General Psychiatry, 43,* 771–777.

Rumsey, J., & Hanahan, A. P. (1990). Getting it "right": Performance of high-functioning autistic adults on a right hemisphere battery. *Journal of Clinical and Experimental Neuropsychology, 12,* 81.

Rutter, M., Macdonald, H., Le Couteur, A., Harrington, R., Bolton, P., & Bailey, A. (1990). Genetic factors in child psychiatric disorders: II. Empirical findings. *Journal of Child Psychology and Psychiatry, 31,* 39–83.

Rutter, M., & Schopler, E. (1978). *Autism: A reappraisal of concepts and treatment.* New York: Springer.

Scaife, M., & Bruner, J. S. (1975). The capacity for joint visual attention. *Nature, 253,* 265–266.

Scarborough, H., Rescorla, L., Tager-Flusberg, H., Fowler, A., & Sudhalter, V. (1991). The relation of utterance length to grammatical complexity in normal and language-disordered groups. *Applied Psycholinguistics, 12,* 23–46.

Schaffer, H. R., Collis, G. M., & Parsons, G. (1977). Vocal interchange and visual regard in verbal and preverbal children. In H. R. Schaffer (Ed.), *Studies in mother–infant interaction* (pp. 291–324). New York: Academic Press.

Searle, J. R. (1975). A taxonomy of illocutionary acts. In K. Gunderson (Ed.), *Minnesota studies in the philosophy of language* (pp. 344–396). Minneapolis: University of Minnesota Press.

Shatz, M., & Gelman, R. (1973). The development of communication skills: Modifications in the speech of young children as a function of the listener. *Monographs of the Society for Research in Child Development* (5, Serial No, 152).

Shriberg, L., Paul, R., McSweeney, J., Klin, A., Cohen, D., & Volkmar, F. (2001). Speech and prosody characteristics of adolescents and adults with high functioning autism and Asperger syndrome. *Journal of Speech, Language and Hearing Research, 44,* 1097–1115.

Sigman, M. D., Yirmiya, N., & Capps, L. (1995). Social and cognitive understanding in high-functioning children with autism. In E. Schopler & G. Mesibov

(Eds.), *Learning and cognition in autism* (pp. 159–176). New York: Plenum Press.

Stein, N. L., & Glenn, C. G. (1979). An analysis of story comprehension in elementary school children. In R. O. Freedle (Ed.), *New directions in discourse processing* (pp. 53–120). Norwood, NJ: Ablex.

Stern, D. N. (1974). Mother and infant at play: The dyadic interaction involving facial, vocal, and gaze behaviours. In M. Lewis & L. A. Rosenblum (Eds.), *The effect of the infant on its caregiver* (pp. 187–213). New York: Wiley.

Strong, C. (1998). *Strong narrative assessment procedure.* Eau Claire, WI: Thinking Publications.

Szatmari, P., Archer, L., Fishman, S., Streiber, D., & Wilson, F. (1995). Asperger syndrome and autism: Differences in behavior, cognition, and adaptive functioning. *Journal of the American Academy of Child and Adolescent Psychiatry, 34,* 1662–1671.

Szatmari, P., Bryson, S., Streiner, D., Wilson, F., Archer, L., & Ryerse, C. (2000). Two-year outcome of preschool children with autism or Asperger's syndrome. *American Journal of Psychiatry, 157,* 1980–1987.

Tager-Flusberg, H. B. (1981). On the nature of linguistic functioning in early infantile autism. *Journal of Autism and Developmental Disorders, 11,* 45–56.

Tager-Flusberg, H. B. (1992). Autistic children's talk about psychologial states: Deficits in the early acquisition of a theory of mind. *Child Development, 63,* 161–172.

Tager-Flusberg, H. B. (1995). Dissociations in form and function in the acquisition of language in autistic children. In H. B. Tager-Flusberg (Ed.), *Constraints on language acquisition: Studies of atypical children* (pp. 175–194). Hillsdale, NJ: Erlbaum.

Tager-Flusberg, H. B., & Joseph, R. (2003). Identifying neurocognitive phenotypes in autism. *Philosophical Transactions of the Royal Society Series B, 358,* 303–314.

Tager-Flusberg, H. B., Paul, R., & Lord, C. (2005). Communication in autism. In F. Volkmar, A. Klin, R. Paul, & D. Cohen (Eds.), *Handbook of autism and pervasive developmental disorders* (3rd ed., pp. 335–364). New York: Wiley.

Tager-Flusberg, H. B., & Sullivan, K. (1994). Predicting and explaining behavior: A comparison of autistic, mentally retarded and normal children. *Journal of Child Psychology and Psychiatry, 35,* 1059–1075.

Turstra, L., Ciccia, A., & Seaton, C. (2003). Interactive behaviors in adolescent conversation dyads. *Language, Speech, and Hearing Services in Schools, 34,* 117–127.

Ungerer, J., & Sigman, M. (1981). Symbolic play and language comprehension in autistic children. *Journal of the American Academy of Child and Adolescent Psychiatry, 20,* 318–337.

Van Bourgondien, M. E., & Mesibov, G. B. (1987). Humor in high-functioning autistic adults. *Journal of Autism and Developmental Disorder, 17,* 417–424.

Van Lancker, D., Cornelius, C., & Needleman, R. (1991). Comprehension of verbal terms for emotions in normal, autistic, and schizophrenic children. *Developmental Neuropsychology, 7,* 1–18.

Volden, J., & Lord, C. (1991). Neologisms and idiosyncratic language in autistic speakers. *Journal of Autism and Developmental Disorder, 21,* 109–130.

Volkmar, F. R., Sparrow, S. S., Goudrequ, D., Cicchetti, D. V., Paul, R., & Cohen, D. J. (1987). Social deficits in autism: An operational approach using the Vineland Adaptive Behavior Scales. *Journal of the Academy of Child and Adolescent Psychiatry, 26,* 155–161.

Wechsler, D. (1991). *Wechsler Intelligence Scale for Children* (3rd ed.). San Antonio, TX: Psychological Corporation.

Westby, C. (2005). Assessing and facilitating text comprehension problems. In H. Catts & A. Kahmi (Eds.), *Language and reading disabilities* (2nd ed., pp. 157–232). Boston: Allyn & Bacon.

Wetherby, A. M., & Prutting, C. A. (1984). Profiles of communicative and cognitive–social abilities in autistic children. *Journal of Speech and Hearing, 27,* 364–377.

Wiig, E. H. (1982). *Let's talk: Developing prosocial communication skills.* Columbus, OH: Merrill.

Wiig, E. H., & Secord, W. (1989). *Test of Language Competence—Expanded Edition.* San Antonio, TX: Psychological Corporation.

Williams, T. I. (1989). A social skills group for autistic children. *Journal of Autism and Developmental Disorders, 19,* 143–155.

Wing, L., & Attwood, A. (1987). Syndromes of autism and atypical development. In D. J. Cohen & A. M. Donnellan (Eds.), *Handbook of autism and pervasive developmental disorders* (pp. 3–19). New York: Wiley.

Young, E. C., Diehl, J. J., Morris, D., Hyman, S. L., & Bennetto, L. (2005). The use of two language tests to identify pragmatic language problems in children with autism spectrum disorders. *Language, Speech, and Hearing Services in Schools, 36,* 62–72.

Ziatas, K., Durking, K., & Pratt, C. (2003). Differences in assertive speech acts produced by children with autism, Asperger syndrome, specific language disorder and normal development. *Development and Psychopathology, 15,* 73–94.

CHAPTER 5

Treatment and Intervention Guidelines for Asperger Syndrome

Fred R. Volkmar
Ami Klin
James C. McPartland

Most of this volume is concerned with diagnostic, neuropsychological, and neurobiological issues related to Asperger syndrome (AS). Since the first edition of this book, considerable progress has been made in these areas, with a marked increase in the research literature. As described in Chapter 1, enduring debate regarding optimal diagnostic approaches complicates interpretation of this work. Although the publication of DSM-5 eliminates AS as an explicit category, individuals previously carrying a diagnosis of AS and those with characteristics corresponding to DSM-IV-TR diagnoses of AS will continue to require (and benefit) from services. Although this chapter discusses these treatments in the context of AS, interventions for these individuals will, in coming years, occur via the diagnosis of autism spectrum disorder (ASD).

We emphasize that the guidelines for intervention presented here are broadly relevant to treatment programs for individuals with severe social disabilities and relative strengths in cognitive and language functioning. Intervention programs should never be based solely on a given diagnosis; rather, programs should be highly individualized to address a specific child's needs while capitalizing on his or her assets. Therefore, even though

143

treatment programs for individuals with AS do not require the resolution of the vexing questions of diagnosis and etiology, they do require a thorough understanding of the specific individual's profile of skills and deficits in areas important for learning, for communicating and relating with others, and for acquiring independent living skills. We should note that issues of pharmacological treatment are reviewed in Chapter 9, and of course, other chapters in this volume touch on treatment issues.

The aim of this chapter is to provide guidelines for the planning and implementation of intervention programs. We acknowledge that treatment must be tailored to the specifics of a person and situation. We also acknowledge that, although some of the extant work on treatment is peer-reviewed and may qualify as evidence-based (Reichow, Doehring, Cicchetti, & Volkmar, 2011), much is not. Although the literature on interventions for individuals with AS is still less substantial than that for autism, it has grown significantly and provides a wealth of concrete ideas and teaching strategies for individuals with this or similar conditions (e.g., Myles & Simpson, 1998; Quill, 1995; Schopler & Mesibov, 1992; Schopler, Mesibov, & Kunce, 1998; Khouzam, El-Gabalawi, Pirwani, & Priest, 2004; Toth & King, 2008; Reaven & Hepburn, 2003; Browning & Caulfield, 2011; Gould, 2011; Walters, 2010; Tantam & Girgis, 2009). Equally helpful materials can be accessed in the literature of interventions for children with learning disabilities (e.g., Minskoff, 1994; Minskoff & DeMoss, 1994), whose profiles often include a social disability component of varying degrees (Gresham, 1992). In this context, the treatment guidelines outlined by Rourke (1989, 1995) for children with nonverbal learning disabilities (NLD) are of particular relevance, given the convergence in both learning and social style between NLD and AS (Klin, Sparrow, Volkmar, Cicchetti, & Rourke, 1995).

Understandably, the needs of children with autism and the support services available to address these needs—from special education schools to model programs—have become associated with a profile of severe social disability usually accompanied by equally severe cognitive and language limitations and behavioral challenges. As a result, parents of individuals with AS often find it complicated to capitalize upon the considerable resources associated with the term *autism* because their children's needs, challenges, and strengths are quite different. To some extent, service categories based primarily in terms of autism or academic learning disabilities leave AS in ill-defined middle ground. Treatment planning is also complicated by the various diagnoses assigned to many individuals with AS over the lifespan, including social anxiety or generalized anxiety disorder, attention-deficit disorder, learning disability, conduct or impulse control disorder, and obsessive–compulsive disorder. Given these differences between AS and classical autism, the treatment and intervention guidelines discussed here emphasize shared elements and note areas of important difference.

SECURING AND IMPLEMENTING SERVICES

The authorities who decide on entitlement to services are sometimes unaware of the extent and significance of the disabilities involved in AS. Proficient verbal skills, overall IQ within the normal or above-normal range, and a solitary lifestyle often mask outstanding deficiencies observed primarily in novel or otherwise socially demanding situations, thus decreasing others' perception of these children's needs for supportive intervention. Active participation on the part of the clinician, together with parents and possibly an advocate, to forcefully pursue the patient's eligibility for services is often needed. Educational professionals are becoming increasingly more aware of AS because of the extremely effective dissemination of information being carried out by parent support organizations and the expanding clinical and research literature. Also, the apparent increased use of the term *Asperger syndrome* by clinicians has led to an increase in referrals for special education services, forcing educators to pursue further training of their personnel and restructuring of services. Over the last decade, parents are less likely to encounter denial of services because their child is seen as "too bright," "too verbal," or "too academically successful."

In the past, individuals with AS have been identified with different diagnostic concepts, which can frustrate their parents' effort to secure adequate services. For example, many individuals with AS or related conditions have been diagnosed as learning disabled (with the occasional accompanying notes highlighting the presence of some "eccentric features"); this nonpsychiatric diagnostic label is often much less effective in securing services. Laws entitling children to services are idiosyncratic and vary from state to state; in some areas, children with a diagnosis of DSM-IV-TR (American Psychiatric Association, 2000) AS have historically been ineligible for services whereas those with a diagnosis of ASD under DSM-IV-TR were entitled to services, despite the purely semantic difference between these levels of description (with ASD encompassing AS). Parents of children who met criteria for AS but were assigned other diagnoses on the autism spectrum often contended with educational programs designed for lower-functioning children, which failed to address their children's relative strengths and unique disabilities properly.

Another portion of individuals with AS were sometimes characterized as exhibiting "social–emotional maladjustment" (SEM), "social–emotional disturbance" (SED), or as being "emotionally disturbed" (ED)—all educational labels usually associated with conduct problems and willful maladaptive behaviors. Such terms have led to highly inappropriate placement in programs for individuals with conduct problems, allowing for possibly the worst mismatch: the bringing together of individuals with a naïve understanding of social situations and individuals who can and do manipulate social situations to their advantage without the benefit of self-restraint—in other words, the perfect victims placed with the perfect victimizers (see also

Woodbury-Smith, Chapter 12, this volume, on legal issues). In contrast to individuals with primary conduct problems, maladaptive and disruptive behaviors in AS often result from misunderstanding of social phenomena, poor perspective taking, and limited emotional regulation. The maladaptive social behaviors exhibited by individuals with AS should be considered in the context of a thoughtful and comprehensive intervention to address their social disability, not as punishable, willful behaviors. In fact, academic suspensions or other disciplinary measures based upon isolation may (1) mean very little to individuals with AS, (2) punish them for their disability, and (3) only exacerbate their already poor self-esteem.

A child's advocate must communicate with the school authorities to emphasize that the student with AS can behave better or worse depending on the setting in which he or she is observed. Highly structured and routinized or otherwise academically driven situations tend to be the settings in which optimal school adjustment may be observed. Unstructured social situations (particularly with groups of same-age peers) and novel situations requiring intuitive or quick-adjusting social problem-solving skills tend to maximize the visibility of the condition. The same observation applies to the clinicians conducting the evaluation intended to ascertain the need for special services. Such an evaluation should include detailed interviews with parents and professionals knowledgeable of the child in naturalistic settings (e.g., home and school) and, if possible, direct observations of the child in unstructured periods such as recess time or an otherwise unsupervised circumstance.

Finally, it is not uncommon for the focus of educational professionals' concern to center around a child's increasingly challenging behavioral problems, including noncompliance, anxiety, disruptive behaviors such as "talking back," interrupting classroom activities, "bothering" other children, verbal aggression, or otherwise "acting out." Resources are often allocated to address the disruptive behaviors, including the assignment of an aide, disciplinary measures, and behavioral management aimed at extinguishing the problematic behaviors. Equally important is consideration of the behaviors in question as a partial result of the child's social disability. Effective solutions for disruptive behaviors often focus on social disabilities and their impact on the child's capacity to adjust to the demands of everyday life at school.

Fortunately, a range of intervention methods have now been explored, including more behaviorally focused work (Tiger, Fisher, & Bouxsein, 2009; Mrug & Hodgens, 2008), individual psychotherapy (Donoghue, Stallard, & Kucia, 2011; Attwood, 2006; Weiss & Lunsky, 2010b), group therapy (including social skills work; Countryman, 2008; Mitchel, Regehr, Reaume, & Feldman, 2010), and more general psychotherapeutic approaches (see Volkmar, 2011). Work on supporting parents and siblings has also appeared (Kroodsma, 2008; Daly, Bostic, & Martin, 2006; Moyes, 2003; Sofronoff & Farbotko, 2002; Allgood, 2010; Castorina & Negri, 2011).

AN OVERVIEW OF GENERAL INTERVENTION STRATEGIES

Helpful intervention strategies involve modifications in teaching practices and approaches, use of behavioral management techniques, use of strategies for emotional support, and activities intended to foster social and communication competence. Implementation should be thoughtful, consistent (across settings, staff members, and situations), and individualized. Equally important, the utility, or lack thereof, of specific recommendations should be assessed in an empirical fashion (i.e., based on an evaluation of events observed, documented, or charted), with useful strategies being maintained and unhelpful ones discarded.

The following suggestions may be helpful when considering the optimal approaches to be adopted. However, different degrees of concreteness and rigidity, paucity of insight, social awkwardness, and communicative one-sidedness characterize individuals with AS, and these particular circumstances and patterns of strengths and weaknesses all require consideration. Care providers should embrace the wide range of expression and complexity of the disorder, avoiding dogmatism in favor of practical, individualized, and commonsense clinical judgment. Thus, the following general components of intervention strategies require thoughtful, individualized adjustment:

1. General problem-solving skills, concepts, and helpful behavioral routines should be taught in an explicit and sometimes rote fashion, using a parts-to-whole teaching approach couched in verbal instruction and presented and rehearsed in such a way that the verbalized steps are in the correct sequence for the behavior to be effective.

2. Specific problem-solving strategies should be taught for handling the requirements of frequently occurring troublesome situations. Training should also be given to help these youngsters recognize situations as troublesome and to apply learned strategies in discrepant situations.

3. Individuals with AS should be instructed on how to identify a novel situation and to resort to a preplanned, well-rehearsed list of steps to be taken. This list should involve a description of the situation, retrieval of pertinent knowledge, and step-by-step decision making. When the situation permits (another item to be defined explicitly), one of these steps might be reliance on a counselor's, a friend's, or an adult's advice, perhaps via a telephone consultation.

4. Social awareness and perspective taking should be cultivated at every opportunity, focusing on the relevant and essential aspects of given situations and pointing out the marginal or irrelevant aspects contained therein. Discrepancies between the individual's perceptions regarding the situation in question and the perceptions of others should be made explicit. Both individual work and group work (ideally, some combination of both with at least one therapist crossing the two settings) is often indicated.

5. An important yet challenging priority in an intervention program is to foster generalization of learned strategies and social skills (e.g., Gaylord-Ross, Haring, Breen, & Pitts-Conway, 1984; Ihrig & Wolchik, 1988). A great deal of attention and research has been invested in technology to assist in the generalization of behavioral therapies (Powers, 1997), but research to advance understanding of generalization in the crucial areas of social and communication skills training is growing (e.g., Gena, Krantz, McClannahan, & Poulson, 1996; Taylor & Harris, 1995; Hall & Graff, 2011; Palmen, Didden, & Lang, 2012; Wolff, 2011; Mazefsky, Williams, & Minshew, 2008; Gilotty, Kenworthy, Sirian, Black, & Wagner, 2002; Lee & Park, 2007) but in need of further development. Defining generalization explicitly as a treatment objective, from a programming perspective, is also critical.

6. Self-evaluation should be encouraged and facilitated in a concrete and explicit fashion concerning day-to-day behaviors. Awareness should be gained into which situations are easily managed and which are potentially troublesome (e.g., knowing what one doesn't know). This awareness is especially important with respect to perceiving the need to use prelearned strategies in appropriate situations. Self-evaluation should also be used to strengthen self-esteem, but this should be done by way of choosing or restructuring the situations to promote success. The goal here is to teach the children about situations in which they are more likely to present themselves in a position of strength rather than a position of vulnerability or weakness. If self-evaluation is insight-oriented and involves a fundamental reappraisal of oneself, frustration and/or the exacerbation of negative self-feelings may arise in the child. Over time and particularly later in adolescence, this increased self-awareness also has some potential to contribute to depression and anxiety (Walters, 2010; Whitehouse, Durkin, Jaquet, & Ziatas, 2009).

7. The specific link between frustrating or anxiety-provoking experiences and negative feelings should be taught to individuals with AS in a concrete, cause–effect fashion. This understanding will help individuals with AS gradually increase insight into their feelings and gain more control over the situations that usually result in negative feelings or otherwise emotional pressure. In this context, it is also important to promote awareness of the impact of their actions on other people's reactions and feelings to help them gain increased control over the results of their social experiences (Volkmar, 2011).

8. Adaptive skills intended to increase self-sufficiency should be taught explicitly, with no assumption that general explanations might suffice or, as noted, that the children will be able to generalize from one concrete situation to similar ones. For example, rule sequences for shopping and using transportation should be taught verbally and rehearsed repeatedly. There should be constant coordination and communication among all involved

in care provision in order to maximize consistency. A specific list of adaptive behaviors to be taught can be derived from results obtained on the Vineland Adaptive Behavior Scales—Expanded Edition (Sparrow, Balla, & Cicchetti, 1984), which assesses adaptive behavior skills in the areas of Communication, Daily Living (self-help) Skills, Socialization, and Motor Skills. Because the behaviors listed in the Vineland are normed, it is possible to extract from this instrument all skills that the individual should be exhibiting, given his or her cognitive level, and then to incorporate these skills into the child's intervention/treatment program (Volkmar & Wiesner, 2009). The Vineland can also be used to gauge progress in adaptive skill development using a test–retest model after a meaningful period (e.g., at the end of 2 consecutive school years).

   9. Additional teaching guidelines should be derived from the individual's profile of neuropsychological assets and deficits. The major areas of neuropsychological focus should be motor, fine motor, visual–motor coordination (including graphomotor skills), visual–spatial attention, perception, problem-solving and memory skills; auditory and verbal attention, learning, reasoning, and memory; and cross-modal integration of information and executive functions. Care providers should utilize specific intervention techniques aimed at remediating or circumventing the identified difficulties by means of compensatory strategies, usually of a verbal nature. However, the identified difficulties and corresponding goals established should broadly address central aspects of the social disability. For example, if significant motor, sensory integration, or visual–motor deficits are corroborated during an evaluation, the individual with AS should receive physical and occupational therapies designed to remediate these deficits. Additionally, the individual should receive education on visual–spatial concepts (e.g., order, causation, sequencing, and left–right orientation), real-life navigation issues (e.g., how to get somewhere), and time concepts, pairing narratives and verbal self-guidance with the actual physical activity taking place. If needed, promotion of appropriate use of assistive technology is recommended (e.g., computer-based skills; see Volkmar & Wiesner, 2009). Other neuropsychological deficits, such as difficulties in processing visual sequences or in interpreting visual information simultaneously with auditory information, particularly in social situations, should be addressed by promoting increased reliance on verbal mediation (e.g., having a script) and on explicit routines for seeking relevant information (e.g., setting up a stepwise routine to be followed, including looking at the other person's eyes or listening to the person's voice for explicit cues) (Tsatsanis, 2005). Cross-modal integration is of particular importance as, for example, it is important not only to be able to interpret other people's nonverbal behavior correctly but also to interpret what is being said in conjunction with these nonverbal cues (Minskoff, 1980a, 1980b; Rourke, 1989, 1995; Tsatsanis, 2005).

SUPPORTING SCHOOL-AGE CHILDREN IN SCHOOLS

One of the main social policy debates in special education has focused on whether children with special needs such as autism and related conditions should be placed in self-contained (i.e., classrooms composed of special education students) or in mainstream environments (i.e., integrated into classrooms with typically developing peers; Burack, Root, & Zigler, 1997). Most professionals would agree that these children are best provided with a continuum of services built around their individual needs (Harris & Handleman, 1997). The reality of available services in a given region, however, often determines the specific mix of specialized and inclusive experience that is appropriate, if not optimal, for a given child. Whereas self-contained settings may be best equipped to provide the specialized services a socially disabled child needs, these settings often fail to provide adequate exposure to typical peers. Regular school environments and experiences with typical peers allow a socially disabled child to model appropriate behaviors and learn to function in a "real-life" environment, but both the environments and the peers may lack the resources to address specialized needs. Successful intervention can be provided in either setting given that there is an effort to optimize individualized services by expanding, creating, training, monitoring, and empirically evaluating the program over time.

Parents of individuals with AS often ask the question, "Where are the best schools for children with this condition?" Although some schools specifically designed for AS have been developed, the answer to this question is rarely straightforward. It is difficult to provide a complete, specialized educational intervention in segregated settings, with exposure to typical peers becoming especially complicated. It is also important to note that neither private nor public school settings emerge with a clear advantage over the other. The absence of readily identified schools serving bright children with severe social disabilities makes the process of securing an appropriate program quite difficult for both parents and clinicians seeking the right placement. Detailed state registers are often lacking, and the parents and/or clinicians are left to deal with this issue on their own. Quite often, an effective partnership is established between the child's caregivers and the school district authorities, although at times there is mistrust and even litigation. To avoid adversarial relationships, all people involved should make an effort to acquaint themselves with the following factors involved in securing or providing appropriate placement and programming for children with social disabilities:

1. *The range of services available in the region.* Educational managers should have a detailed knowledge of all resources available within their immediate jurisdiction as well as in a wider contiguous region and make this information available to all those involved in the process. Parents should make an attempt to visit the various suggested educational placements and

service providers available to obtain firsthand knowledge and feelings about them, including the physical setting, staffing, adult–student ratio, range of special/support services, mix of children, and so forth.

2. *Knowledge of model programs.* Parents and professionals should make an effort to locate examples of programs (public or private) that are thought to provide high-quality services according to local experts, parent support organizations, or other parents. Regardless of whether the program is an option for the given child, knowledge of such programs may provide all those concerned with a model and criteria with which to judge the appropriateness of the program in discussion for the specific child.

3. *Knowledge of the rights and duties of all those involved in the process leading to educational placement.* It is crucial that parents become acquainted with their legal rights to become effective advocates for their children (Berkman, 1997; Mandlawitz, 2005), and it is equally important that the school authorities establish their own knowledge base of appropriate services so that fringe or otherwise questionable educational practices unsupported by any data are not forcefully introduced into a program because of legal pressure. Discussions likely to produce consensual agreement tend to (a) be based on detailed and individualized knowledge of a child's needs, (b) refrain from ideological statements (e.g., "Treatment *X* is good for *all* children," regardless of the child's profile), and (c) seek to evaluate existing services while not precluding the creation of new ones. An evolving partnership between parents, educational professionals, and specialists within the educational program is needed.

When reviewing the appropriateness of a given program for a bright child with social disabilities, the infrastructure of educational resources should be the focus of discussion, including the available resources that will serve the given child. Although resources may vary in content from place to place, the following specifications are generally thought to be positive and necessary resources:

1. Although a relatively small setting is usually preferable, regardless of the size of the program, the setting should provide ample opportunity for individual attention, individualized approach, and small-group work. At times, a compromise is reached by placing a socially disabled child in a large setting accompanied by a paraprofessional aide. This alternative is only helpful if there is an infrastructure of expertise and support for the child beyond the immediate presence of the aide. The absence of this arrangement places undue responsibility on a less trained person, however gifted he or she might be. As a result, the aide, rather than supporting the child's inclusion in the program, might end up serving as a virtual partition between the child and peers, constantly redirecting, mediating, or otherwise containing the child.

2. The involvement of a communication specialist is a key resource in an adequate educational program. The specialist should have an interest in pragmatics and social skills training, an availability for individual and small-group work, and the ability to integrate communication and social skills training intervention in all school activities, implemented consistently across staff members, settings, and situations. This professional should also act as a resource for the other staff members and as an advocate for the social and communication skills training aspect of the curriculum.

3. There should be opportunities for social interaction and promotion of social relationships in fairly structured and supervised activities. By building social contact around a common interest or activity, the pressure of unstructured social exchange is lessened, making the experience more likely to be successful. There should be opportunities for naturalistic interactions as well. The availability of different configurations of social settings (e.g., individual work, small groups, structured larger-group activities, and large unstructured natural gatherings such as recess time or lunch) makes it possible for these students to practice social skills in one setting and then to apply them in others. It also allows for frequently troublesome situations to be identified in larger settings and then brought into the small therapeutic setting for correction, skill building, practice, and rehearsal.

4. There should be a concerted effort to promote the acquisition of real-life skills in addition to the academic goals. The norm in individuals with AS is to exhibit a significant discrepancy between cognitive potential (i.e., IQ) and their ability to translate this potential into adaptive functioning (i.e., constructive real-life behaviors consistently performed to meet the demands of everyday life; Klin, 1997). Although it is always encouraging to document a child's potential, longer-term goals, the child's prospects for vocational accomplishment and independent living require higher-level adaptive skills than are usually found in this population. Therefore, adaptive skills should be one of the central points of any program for a child with AS.

5. There should be a willingness to adapt the curriculum content and requirements to provide flexible opportunities for success, to foster the acquisition of a more positive self-concept, and to foster an internalized investment in performance and progress. For example, assignments, and projects should be evaluated in terms of their contribution to the child's longer-term educational goals rather than being enchained to inflexible (e.g., credit) requirements. This may mean that the individual with AS is provided with individual challenges in his or her areas of strengths and with individualized programs in his or her areas of weakness. Social situations can be constructed to allow the child opportunities to take leadership positions by explaining, demonstrating, or teaching others about a favored topic. Such situations can help the individual with AS (a) take the perspective of others, (b) follow conversation and social interaction rules,

and (c) follow coherent and less one-sided, goal-directed behaviors and approaches. In addition, by taking the lead in an activity, the individual's self-esteem is likely to be enhanced, and the his or her (usually disadvantageous) position in relation to peers is for once reversed. When this initiative is entertained, however, appropriate preparation is needed, so that the result is not the reverse of the envisioned goal because of undue pressure placed on the child.

6. Children with AS are often overwhelmed by the day-to-day pressures of life at school. To proactively address this issue, a sensitive in-school counselor should be made available to the child. The counselor should focus on the individual's emotional well-being, serve as the "safe address" for the child, coordinate services, and monitor progress. In addition, the in-school counselor should serve as a resource for other staff members and as an effective and supportive liaison with the family.

SUPPORTING ADOLESCENTS AND ADULTS

Although the literature on treatments for adolescents and adults remains comparatively less substantive than that for younger children, it has grown significantly since the first edition of this volume. This literature now includes several review and "overview" papers (Arora, Praharaj, Sarkhel, & Sinha, 2011; Ozdemir & Iseri, 2004; Tantam, 2003; Barnhill, 2007) as well as guides to diagnosis and assessment, including newly developed instruments for diagnosis (Woodbury-Smith, Robinson, Wheelwright, & Baron-Cohen, 2005; Stoesz, Montgomery, Smart, & Hellsten, 2011; Ritvo et al., 2011; Kanai, Iwanami, Ota, Yamasue, Yokoi, et al., 2011). An increasing body of work is available on intervention methods (i.e., "life coaching"); individual and group treatment as well as marital and couples therapy approaches (Attwood, 2004; Beebe & Risi, 2003; Engstrom, Ekstrom, & Emilsson, 2003; Fangmeier et al., 2011; Golan & Baron-Cohen, 2006; Hagland & Webb, 2009; Jantz, 2011; Koegel & LaZebnik, 2009; Lau & Peterson, 2011; Munro, 2010; Patrick, 2008; Weiss & Lunsky, 2010; Volkmar, 2011; Woodbury-Smith & Volkmar, 2009). Other work has centered on aspects of neuropsychological (Ambery, Russell, Perry, Morris, & Murphy, 2006; Bowler, Gardiner, & Berthollier, 2004; Golan, Baron-Cohen, & Hill, 2006; Gowen & Miall, 2005; Harish, Gangadharan, Bhaumik, & Chaturvedi, 2010; Lepistö et al., 2007; Nyden et al., 2010; Rondan & Deruelle, 2007; Sahlander, Mattsson, & Bejerot, 2008) and communicative functioning (Colle, Baron-Cohen, Wheelwright, & van der Lely, 2008; Jolliffe & Baron-Cohen, 1999; Jolliffe & Baron-Cohen, 2000; Kujala et al., 2007; O'Connor, 2007; Pijnacker, Hagoort, Buitelaar, Teunisse, & Geurts, 2009; Rutherford, Baron-Cohen, & Wheelwright, 2002; Shriberg, Paul, McSweeny, Klin, & Cohen, 2001; Spek, Schatorjé, Scholte, &

van Berckelaer-Onnes, 2009). Researchers have also explored issues of co-morbidity and associated behavioral and other mood disorders, including depression, suicidal ideation, anxiety, and sleep difficulties (Allen et al., 2008; Lugnegard, Hallerback, & Gillberg, 2011; Oyane & Bjorvatn, 2005; Perlman, 2000; Shtayermman, 2006, 2008, 2009). Finally, a substantive body of work on supporting vocational independence and continued education (Dillon, 2007; Welkowitz & Baker, 2005; Howlin, Alcock, & Burkin, 2005; Hurlburt, Happé, & Frith, 1994; Matthews, 1996; Mawhood & Howlin, 1999; Muller, Schuler, Burton, & Yates, 2003; Juhel, 2005; Brown, 2010) has begun to develop. The growth of this literature is a testament both to the importance of recognizing the special needs of adults and to the relevance of AS as a diagnostic concept guiding treatment.

SOCIAL AND COMMUNICATION SKILLS TRAINING

Given that the crux of AS is social disability, the most important component of any intervention program is enhancement of communication and social competence (Kaland, Mortensen, & Smith, 2011). This emphasis does not reflect a societal pressure for conformity nor an attempt to stifle individuality and uniqueness; indeed, we consider it important to respect the "culture" of individuals with AS (e.g., "Aspies"). Rather, this emphasis reflects the inclination to make sociability a choice for individuals who might otherwise be rendered loners, an outcome that, when arrived at without choice, often leads to despondency, negativism, or clinical depression. These negative outcomes are a result of individuals' increasing awareness of personal inadequacy in social situations and their repeated experiences of failure to make and/or maintain relationships (Klin & Volkmar, 1997). We also consider *social function* to encompass all aspects of interpersonal interactions in society, whether they be conventionally social (e.g., dinner party conversation) or unconventionally so (e.g., negotiating a crowded bus or an amorphous checkout line in a grocery). In this way, the social elements of intervention in AS address not just personal choice but the ability to function effectively in a society that presumes baseline levels of social intuition and comprehension of societal mores.

In children with AS, the typical limitations of insight and self-reflection in relation to others often preclude spontaneous self-adjustment to social and interpersonal demands. Therefore, there is a need to teach social and communication skills, explicitly, at all times, as an integral part of a program and as a major priority. Training in communication and social skills usually does not imply that the child will eventually acquire communicative or social spontaneity, naturalness, and gracefulness. However, training does better prepare individuals with AS to cope with social and interpersonal expectations, thus enhancing their effectiveness as conversational partners, as potential friends or companions, and as employable professionals. Many adults with this condition are not given an opportunity to exhibit their considerable talents and skills because of failure during the interview stage of job applications. Earlier in life they might be lost in a vicious cycle of misguided attempts to pursue goals that are incompatible with their profile of strengths and weaknesses, leading to repeated experiences of failure and a resultant poor view of themselves. Limited insight might also signify that the person may pursue an irrelevant course of action. For example, after being turned down in several job interviews, talented college graduates might attempt to pursue a manual job that requires considerable eye–hand coordination skills, manual dexterity, improvisation in novel situations, and speed of execution—all skills usually found to be weaknesses in these individuals' profiles. Feeling the burden of failure in what they might see as a "menial" job not commensurate with their educational training, they might pursue an additional degree, only to repeat this cycle the next time they approach the job market. Unless issues of social presentation and competence are adequately addressed, including what to do in specific situations such as lunch or free-time periods, the chances for vocational satisfaction are lessened.

The observation that social and communication skills building is the core intervention component for individuals with AS and related social disabilities is not novel (Mesibov, 1984, 1986). However, this emphasis in the literature has only recently translated into more readily available educational programs and resources (e.g., Minihan, Kinsella, & Honan, 2011; Castorina & Negri, 2011; Stichter et al., 2010; Mitchel et al., 2010; Muller, 2010; Hanley-Hochdorfer, Bray, Kehle, & Elinoff, 2010; Harvey, 2008; Countryman, 2008; Scharfstein, Beidel, Sims, & Rendon Finnell, 2011). Many of these methods also specifically encompass work on pragmatic language and other relevant communication skills.

Despite the existence of educational programs and resources emphasizing social and communication skills and school systems' increasing awareness, access to appropriate services is confounded by the inconsistency with which experienced clinicians are available and by myriad obstacles to appropriate insurance coverage. At present, the professionals at the greatest advantage to play the central role in social and communication skills training are speech and language therapists who have a special interest in pragmatics or conversational skills (although other mental health or educational professionals could be equally proficient). These professionals require training, not only in social and communication skills training, but also in the unique challenges posed by bright individuals with severe social disabilities.

Although more and more prepackaged social skills programs have become available commercially, these have been shown to have a moderate effect, at best (Reichow & Volkmar, 2010). Despite insubstantial empirical evidence, it is important for the special educator to become acquainted with these materials, as some resources can be of great help in specific areas (e.g., in expanding the vocabulary of emotions, in playing cooperative games, in social problem solving). The evidence base for social skills intervention has gradually been improving (Reichow & Volkmar, 2010), and a number of studies is now available (Mitchel et al., 2010; Loudon, 2009; Rao et al., 2008; Macintosh & Dissanayake, 2006; Ozonoff & Miller, 1995; Pierce & Schreibman, 1997; Thorp, Stahmer, & Schreibman, 1995). Excellent reviews of social and communication skills training and behavioral approaches in promoting social development (e.g., Prizant, Schuler, Wetherby, & Rydell, 1997; Quill, 1995; Twachtman, 1995; Reichow & Volkmar, 2010; Matson, Benavidez, Compton, Paclawskyj, & Baglio, 1996) are also available. However, these reviews often focus on principles and general techniques rather than providing a readily applicable and accessible practical approach. As a result, professionals working in direct service often have requested the translation of these principles into a "package," "instruction manual," or an otherwise concrete plan to follow in their effort to serve their clients. Such concrete, adjustable "packages" are becoming available (see Reichow & Volkmar, 2010), and it should be noted that aspects of programs designed for the promotion of social and communication skills in individuals with autism who exhibit significant cognitive and language deficits (Koegel & Koegel, 1995) may be applicable to higher-functioning individuals with social impairments as well. Below we list selected prepackaged programs for social skills development in individuals with AS.

1. *Social Stories.*™ One of the most interesting approaches for social skills training in autism and related conditions is the work of Gray and colleagues (Gray, 1995, 1998; Gray et al., 1993; Gray & Garand, 1993; Hanley-Hochdorfer et al., 2010; Scattone, 2008; Hanley, 2008; Livanis, Solomon, & Ingram, 2007), who use visual and written materials and techniques based on situations from a child's actual experience to teach social skills. The individualization of the instructional process, the use of written and videotaped resources, and the fact that this approach grew from direct school-based work with individuals with social disabilities makes it an attractive option for special educators.

2. *Visual strategies for improving communication.* This approach, which was developed by Hodgdon (1995, 1996), is a compilation of effective visual tools and resources to aid the child in both communicating more effectively and better understanding the communication demands imposed by the surrounding social environment. The method capitalizes on autistic children's typical visual–spatial strengths to compensate for their social and communication deficits. The major resource book (Hodgdon, 1996) provides concrete ideas and examples that can be readily adopted in the classroom. However, these techniques may not be optimal for students whose visual–spatial processing skills are a weakness rather than a strength (see Volkmar & Wiesner, 2009, for a discussion).

3. *Social perception skills training.* Minskoff and colleague (Minskoff, 1987, 1994; Minskoff & DeMoss, 1994) developed two programs focused on social perception skills training for adolescents and adults, with specific emphasis on social skills judged by employers to be critical for job success.

4. *Teaching theory of mind.* The theory-of-mind (ToM) research in autism (Baron-Cohen, Leslie, & Frith, 1985) has informed teaching programs designed to help children learn the underlying social-cognitive principles necessary to infer the mental states of others (e.g., beliefs, intentions, and feelings). Although studies to date have shown that ToM training improves children's performance on experimental tasks, there is little improvement in general social competence (Ozonoff & Miller, 1995) or in communication competence (Hadwin, Baron-Cohen, Howlin, & Hill, 1997). Despite these initial results, the potential of this approach requires further empirical investigation.

There are several core strategic elements in these various approaches and in specialized clinical practices serving children and adolescents with social disabilities. The following strategies are often included in social and communication skills training:

1. Fostering *awareness of conventional pragmatic or conversation rules* is central to every social and communication program, including addressing topic selection, ways of marking topic shifts, and the ability to consistently provide the necessary amount of background information for an unfamiliar listener. These goals can be advanced by helping the child appreciate who is likely to be more interested or familiar with various topics. For example, relatives are more interested in and acquainted with topics related to the family than are strangers; same-age peers are likely to be more interested in and familiar with topics related to movies, games, TV shows, and so on, than are adults. On the other hand, same-age peers are not likely to be interested in discussing more circumscribed topics such as deep-sea marine biology or politics, or any special interest the child with AS may have that is likely to be unusual or eccentric to same-age peers. These unusual topics are more likely to be of interest to adults and teachers. It is helpful to foster the child's awareness of the varying interests of his or her friends by developing a list of preferred topics and less preferred topics for each individual friend. This goal is sometimes facilitated by having the child compose a letter to a friend, to a same-age acquaintance, to a relative, to an unfamiliar adult, to a celebrity, and so on (Davis, Boon, Cihak, & Fore, 2010; Paul, Orlovski, Marcinko, & Volkmar, 2009; Scattone, 2008; Smith, 2008; Adams, Green, Gilchrist, & Cox, 2002).

2. *Appropriate "reading" of social cues* is a necessary precursor for generating appropriate comments, adjusting to social demands, determining the listener's perspective/reactions, and so on, and for maintaining a level of reciprocity without which there is communication breakdown (e.g.,

the listener may leave, become upset, or have unfavorable impressions of the speaker). In addition to the child potentially requiring explicit instructions on how to monitor or anticipate the relative interests of his or her listener, the meaning of eye contact, gaze, and various inflections, as well as tone of voice and facial and hand gestures need to be taught in a fashion not unlike the teaching of a foreign language. All elements should be made verbally explicit and appropriately and repeatedly drilled. The same principles should guide the training of the individual's expressive skills.

Concrete situations should be rehearsed in the therapeutic setting (individually or, preferably, in small groups) and gradually tried out in naturally occurring situations, moving from static to increasingly dynamic and interactive conditions. All those in close contact with the individuals with AS should be made aware of the program so that consistency, monitoring, and contingent reinforcement are maximized. Of particular importance, encounters with unfamiliar people (e.g., making acquaintances) should be rehearsed until the individual is made aware of the impact of his or her behavior on other people's reactions to him or her. Techniques such as practicing in front of a mirror, listening to recorded speech, and watching a video of recorded behavior should be incorporated into this program. Videotaped feedback, in particular, has been found to be a useful medium for advancing this goal, given the potential for pausing the picture and highlighting specific visual cues in a more explicit manner.

Strategies for deciphering the most salient nonverbal dimensions inherent in these situations should be offered and practiced. The following nonverbal social cues should be included in a program:

a. *Setting.* The child needs to be made aware of where the interaction is taking place and what expectations (e.g., volume of voice, style of speech) are associated with that setting (e.g., school playground, church service).

b. *Body proximity.* Individuals with AS need to know how to position themselves when engaged in conversation, the meaning of different postures, and what information can be gained from such cues.

c. *Facial, bodily, and vocal emotional expressions.* Individuals with AS often require explicit instruction on the need to pay attention to affective expressions in all modalities, on how to decode these separately, and even more importantly, on how to integrate this set of cues into a meaningful context.

d. *Nonliteral forms of communication.* Special instruction is often needed about nonverbal cues that provide the context of nonliteral forms of communication, such as teasing, irony, and sarcasm, as well as figures of speech and humor. Other emotional tones of speech (e.g., excitement and anger) may also require instruction (Pijnacker et al., 2009; Loukusa et al., 2007).

3. *Self-monitoring in conversation* often needs to be taught, with a view toward helping the child adjust his or her speech style in terms of

setting (e.g., more or less formal) and volume (e.g., when a loud voice, say, in a sports game, is appropriate and when a whisper, say, in a funeral, is expected), as well as rate and rhythm, inflection modulation, and stress for emphasis. The child may also need to be taught how to adjust speech depending on proximity to the speaker, number of people, and background noise (Kanai, Twanami, Ota, Yamasue, Matsushima, et al., 2011; Shogren, Lang, Machalicek, Rispoli, & O'Reilly, 2011; Volkmar, 2011).

These goals are often advanced in the context of individual, small-group (up to three students) or slightly larger (up to six students) social skills training formats using a range of specific techniques. For example, in Gray's (1995) approach, "comic strip conversations" are used to visually highlight, using color, the feelings and intentions of each speaker (e.g., red for teasing statements and green for friendly statements). By representing the emotional expression of the characters' statements, thoughts, and feelings in various ways the perspective of those individuals becomes more readily apparent. In "topic boxes," another useful strategy, a topic is drawn out of a box for both the socially disabled student and a peer or therapist to discuss while highlighting different opinions about these topics. These specific techniques are organized under the more general rubric of "social review strategies" and include the following steps: (a) identification of a target social situation known to be problematic for the student; (b) gathering information about what the student already knows about that situation (including both helpful knowledge about setting, perceptions, interpretations, expectations, as well as unhelpful knowledge or absence thereof); (c) sharing observations of nonverbal cues, interpretations of a given situation, and so on, with other people in the group, including peers and therapist; (d) practice of newly acquired knowledge and behaviors in the context of one-to-one exchanges, group interaction, watching videotapes, and casual conversation; and (e) generalization of skills to a variety of contexts under some supervision, so that the student's progress can be determined and outstanding or new problematic areas can be identified as situations to be revisited in the small, therapeutic environment.

In summary, the effort to develop the individual's skills in managing social situations and interpersonal interactions should be a priority in any social and communication skills training program. This development should include the following:

- *Topic management,* to expand and elaborate on a range of different topics initiated by others, shifting topics, ending topics appropriately, and feeling comfortable with a range of topics that are typically discussed by same-age peers.
- *Flexibility in social interaction,* to recognize and use a range of different means to interact, mediate, negotiate, persuade, discuss, and disagree through verbal and nonverbal means.

- *Perception of nonverbal social cues*, to attend to and correctly understand the meaning of gaze, gestures, voice, and posture.
- *Appreciation of social expectations associated with a given setting*, to be aware of the implications of where and with whom the social situation is taking place and to correctly derive the appropriate set of behaviors to that setting.
- *Operational knowledge of the language of mental states and related phenomena*, to make inferences, to predict, to explain motivation, and to anticipate multiple outcomes so as to increase the flexibility with which the person both thinks about and uses language with other people.

ORGANIZATIONAL SKILLS

Among the most established neuropsychological findings in studies of individuals with AS is the observation that they present with significant executive function (EF) deficits (Pennington & Ozonoff, 1996; Ozonoff, 1998; McCrimmon, 2011; Hill & Bird, 2006; Kleinhans, Akshoomoff, & Delis, 2005; Stenberg, 2007). EF denotes a range of specific neuropsychological abilities, including, self-inhibition, adjustment of behavior using environmental feedback, extracting rules from experience, selection of essential from nonessential information, and keeping in mind both a desired goal and the various steps required to accomplish it. The deficits in EF directly impact the well-known real-life difficulties that these individuals encounter in organizing their activities, in completing tasks in an efficient manner, in avoiding getting stuck in counterproductive routines, and in learning from their ongoing experiences. Some parents describe their children as being devoid of a "pilot" or "navigator," requiring help with seemingly trivial matters such as shopping and completing homework assignments, despite being otherwise quite bright.

Such difficulties can result in school failure or an inability to achieve a minimal level of community-related independent living skills. A lack of appreciation for these difficulties often saddles these students with long-term, open-ended assignments and other forms of unstructured homework in which they are unable to perform. This inability to complete assignments often occurs because students with AS have problems producing a realistic stepwise plan on how to achieve their goal and then following the various steps to implement the plan. The combination of social and EF difficulties also results in problems with grooming, scheduling, and other fundamental adaptive behavioral skills.

There are at least two forms of treatment and intervention to be considered in regard to these difficulties. The first approach uses computer-based cognitive rehabilitation packages that take the student along a series of exercises promoting each of the EF areas as well as other neuropsychological capacities underlying EF. Although this form of intervention has been shown to have a positive impact on real-life skills in individuals with neurologically based disorders (e.g., Chen, Thomas, Glueckauf, & Bracy, 1997), the data on individuals with autism-related conditions are still scant.

The second approach switches the focus from underlying neuropsychological capacities to the real-life situations in which the organizational skills deficits are most problematic for a given individual. This approach involves the identification of an individual's frequently troublesome situations in which organizational skills are required and the use of an assistive tool or approach to remediate the given problem. Specific remediation strategies include creating lists or scripts detailing a stepwise approach to achieve a given goal, rehearsing with the individual the implementation of that list, and creating pictorial schedules and reminders through assistive technology (see next section). The latter usually provides the student with a readily available tool such as an electronic organizer or laptop computer, which gives the student immediate access to short-term and long-term schedules, homework assignments containing details of steps to be accomplished in the order that they need to be completed for achieving the goal, and writing programs that organize narrative structure and elicit topics to be covered.

ASSISTIVE TECHNOLOGY

Assistive technology (AT) refers to the use of computer-based resources developed for individuals with disabilities. Although traditionally the focus has been on students with sensory and physical impairment, this focus has expanded considerably in the past few years to include individuals with learning disabilities (Bryant & Bryant, 1998; Raskind & Higgins, 1998). AT was recognized by Congress as a viable need for people with disabilities when it passed the Technology-Related Assistance to Individuals with Disabilities Act in 1988 and reauthorized the legislation in 1994 (Bryant & Seay, 1998). This development has resulted in numerous services benefiting a wide range of individuals with disabilities (Lewis, 1998). The legislation mandating accessibility of this technology to students with disabilities has also led to increasing dissemination of these resources in school programs (Smith, 1998).

Unfortunately, there is still very little documentation on the use of AT in the field of autism and related conditions, particularly in regard to more able students who do not require basic enabling devices to operate a computer, or to learn basic language skills. Nevertheless, individuals with AS and related conditions do exhibit many disabilities that can be effectively addressed by computer-based resources. Given the natural affinity with computers that these children often exhibit, this medium can be used to promote learning and adaption in a range of important areas.

First, graphomotor difficulties are often found in AS; sometimes, students cannot complete their written assignments efficiently, or they cannot properly expand their thoughts and learning because they are required to write their work by hand, resulting in a laborious, untidy, and frustrating process. Although handwriting should be addressed in occupational therapy, from a longer-term perspective, in a digital era, it is unnecessary to enchain the student's learning to whatever he or she will be able to handwrite. The various commonplace tools available for grammatically correct writing and the more specialized software capable of eliciting and structuring a student's work, combined with enabling devices such as a special keyboard or mouse, offer a long-term, empowering strategy to deal with writing deficits.

Second, as previously noted, individuals with AS often exhibit significant organizational and self-management deficits. Software designed to provide students with clear schedules, task organizers, ready-made routines (or algorithms) for completion of frequent tasks, and so on, can be of great help.

Third, communication between home and school can be advanced by use of AT. Components of behavioral management programs, such as reinforcement or reward menus, and other elements of the educational intervention can be written or programmed directly onto the student's computer or organizer. Because the device travels with the child, it is a readily available support for the child in various settings and promote transfer of information among the various professionals and family members.

Fourth, proficiency in computer-related skills allows the student to independently access sources of information for general purpose as well as for school use (e.g., using the Internet), to initiate some social contact in a less stressful fashion by communicating with others by means of electronic mail, and to promote self-initiative and self-reliance in the context of the child's own interests. Although there is always a concern that computer-related activities can further exacerbate social isolation, precautionary measures can be taken to encourage inclusion, or the types of computer-related activities that are more likely to produce teamwork and communication can be chosen. For example, classroom-based activities can and should involve several students acting in collaboration with a computer, where group results require the coordination among all the members of the group. For older individuals, computer-based skills may allow them vocational possibilities not otherwise available. For example, some of our adult clients have established their own Internet businesses, whereas others work in this field for a wide range of agencies, from mental health centers to libraries or schools.

Despite the potential of AT for individuals with social disabilities, and the fact that the use of enabling technology is mandated whenever a case can be made for its benefits to a given child with disabilities, there is no comprehensive compilation of resources currently available from the perspective of autism, AS, and related conditions. The number of AT professionals and consultation services is rapidly expanding, with a proliferation of available but inadequately tested options. Therefore, parents, clinicians, and educational professionals are often left to learn on their own about what might be applicable in the case of a given child—a daunting task. Closing the Gap is a well-known agency for dissemination of AT information. Although some promising work in this area is being done (e.g., LaCava, Golan, Baron-Cohen, & Myles, 2007) a comprehensive and current review of the efficacy of AT, its applications, and easily accessible resources remains needed.

ACADEMIC CURRICULA

Despite intact cognitive abilities, students with AS are likely to benefit from modified academic curricula to accommodate their unique learning styles and social disability. The curriculum content should be decided based on long-term goals, so that the usefulness of each item is evaluated in terms of its long-range benefits for the individual's socialization skills, vocational potential, and quality of life. Emphasis should be placed on skills that correspond to relative strengths for the individual as well as skills that may be viewed as central for the person's future vocational life (e.g., writing skills, computer skills, and science). If the individual has an area of special interest that is not so circumscribed and unusual as to prevent its use in prospective employment, such an interest or talent should be cultivated in a systematic fashion, helping the individual to acquire strategies of learning (library, computerized data bases, Internet, etc.). Specific projects can be set as part of the person's credit gathering, and specific (topic-related) mentorships can be established with staff members or individuals in the community.

This approach is necessary to avoid the common situation in which an inflexible school credit system is applied, enforcing the teaching of academic subjects that are only marginally related to the future life of a student with a social disability. Quite often, this inflexible approach leads to a great deal of frustration and eventually to the student's failure and loss of motivation, sacrificing the whole school experience for the sake of complying with irrelevant requirements. Given that motivation, self-initiative, and a positive self-concept are the main goals to be maximized, special modifications of assignments should be seen as a way to enable a student to complete the requirements of a given a class successfully. For example, if the goal of an English class is to teach composition, the actual topic for research should be tailored to the student's intrinsic interests. A student failing an English course because the topic of research is, for example, standard novels may succeed if the topic is shifted to, say, a science-related topic. A number of research studies relevant to this area has now appeared (e.g., Carter, 2005; Church, Alisanski, & Amanullah, 2000; Graetz, 2009; Griswold, Barnhill, Myles, Hagiwara, & Simpson, 2002; Hagiwara, 2001; Myles, Barnhill, Hagiwara, Griswold, & Simpson, 2001; Whitby & Mancil, 2009)

BEHAVIORAL MANAGEMENT

Individuals with AS often exhibit different forms of challenging behavior. It is crucial that these behaviors are not seen as willful or malicious; rather, they should be viewed as connected to the individual's disability and treated as such by means of thoughtful, therapeutic, and educational strategies rather than by simplistic and inconsistent punishment or other disciplinary measures that imply the assumption of deliberate misconduct. Specific problem-solving strategies, usually following a verbal rule or algorithm, can be taught for handling the requirements of frequently occurring, troublesome situations (e.g., involving novelty, intense social demands, or frustration). As noted, training is usually necessary for recognizing situations as troublesome and for selecting the best available learned strategy to use in such situations (Weiss & Lunsky, 2010a). Anxiety management can be an important component of intervention as well and may include both behavioral procedures such as desensitization and rehearsal and psychopharmacological treatment (Farrugia & Hudson, 2006; Sofronoff, Attwood, & Hinton, 2005; Whitehead, 2005).

Data collection procedures necessary for a functional analysis of problematic behaviors, intervention approaches including the use of reward systems, and evaluation protocols to gauge the success of specific approaches should follow the established guidelines of behavioral assessment and therapy (e.g., Powers, 1997). In this process, it is helpful to compile a list of frequent problematic behaviors such as perseverations, obsessions, interrupting behaviors, or any other disruptive behaviors and then to devise specific plans to deal with them whenever they arise. These plans should be discussed with the individual with AS in an explicit, rule-governed fashion. All professionals involved should be aware of the program so that clear expectations are set and consistency across adults, settings, and situations is maintained. Ad hoc approaches are likely to result in improvised reactions to the student's behaviors, reinforcement of maladaptive patterns of behavior and consequent escalation, and insecurity as to how to act on the part of the adults. A proactive approach that makes the management of problematic behaviors an integral component of the general program of intervention is clearly preferable and increases predictability and consistency—two important factors in any behavioral management approach.

VOCATIONAL TRAINING

Adults with AS often fail to meet entry requirements for advanced education or for jobs in their area of training because of their poor interview skills, social disabilities, eccentricities, or anxiety-related vulnerabilities (Muller et al., 2003). Therefore, an important aspect of vocational training involves helping these individuals acquire social skills in all areas included in applying for an advanced educational degree or a job. The skills to be targeted include grooming, presentation, and application letter writing, as well as every aspect of the interview process. Equally important, individuals with AS should be trained for and placed in jobs for which they are not neuropsychologically impaired, and in which they will enjoy a certain degree of support and shelter. The college experience for individuals with AS should be facilitated by individual tutorial systems, wherein a faculty member and perhaps a peer can act as immediate resources for the student, both being available to him or her and seeking frequent, periodic contact in order to monitor the student's progress and well-being (Welkowitz & Baker, 2005; Dillon, 2007; Wolff, Brown, & Bork, 2009). A similar situation should be available in job placement, where individual supervision and support should be provided by a supervisor or coworker who is aware that, at least initially, the guidance required will extend to areas other than the specific work apprenticeship (Juhel, 2005). It is usually preferable that the job does not involve intensive social demands.

As originally emphasized by Asperger (1944), the development of talents and special interests into marketable skills is necessary for individuals with AS. However, this is only part of the task to secure (and maintain) a work placement. Equal attention should be paid to the social demands defined by the nature of the job, including what to do during meal breaks, contact with the public or coworkers, or any other unstructured activity requiring social adjustment or improvisation. Excellent reviews on vocational possibilities and strategies for vocational training are available in the literature (e.g., Gerhardt & Holmes, 1997; Van Bourgondien & Woods, 1992; Muller et al., 2003). However, the number of knowledgeable professionals available as job coaches, as well as the public resources available in this area, are still quite limited. Equally frustrating is the absence of good compilations of appropriate college, vocational training, and independent living programs, all of which are of crucial importance to adults with AS and their families, who are left to find their own way by means of independent research. It is hoped that one of the major priorities of parent support organizations and clinicians alike will be to pool resources and knowledge in an easily accessible medium.

PSYCHOTHERAPY

Although the research literature is limited, it does not appear that typical insight-oriented psychotherapy is usually helpful (Volkmar, 2011). However, it does appear that fairly focused and structured counseling can be quite useful for individuals with AS and related conditions, particularly in the context of alleviating overwhelming experiences of sadness, negativism, or anxiety. This counseling can also facilitate ongoing social adjustment, promote family functioning, and assist in problem-solving specific frustrations in regard to vocational goals and placement (Pope, 1993). The psychotherapeutic relationship can be used to address concrete issues related to the patient's well-being, from practical, independent living problems to self-management and more intimate, interpersonal problems, including sexuality and fantasy life (Volkmar, 2011). A growing body of work on supporting individuals with AS as they develop relationships, including marital relationships, is also now available (Harvey, 2008; Henderson, 2008; Hendrickx, 2008).

SELF-SUPPORT GROUPS

Individuals with AS are usually self-described loners despite an often intense wish to make friends and have a more active social life. Thus, there is a need to facilitate social contact within the context of an activity-oriented group (e.g., church communities, hobby clubs, and self-support groups) (Mesibov, 1992). Although there is little published documentation on the effects of self-support groups, the available information suggests that some individuals with AS enjoy the opportunity to meet others with similar problems (Bradford, 2010; Jantz, 2011), whereas others either prefer to avoid individuals with similar problems or fail to relate to any commonalities among group members and consequently leave the group. In addition, relationships established during group activities may not carry over to other settings, in which the group members themselves, rather than the therapist or group leader, would have to initiate the contact.

CONCLUSION

Individuals with AS and their families must contend with the fact that public understanding of this condition, including its unique disabilities and strengths and the resources available for educational and other services, is still limited. The recent proliferation of parent support groups coalescing around the terms *Asperger syndrome, high-functioning autism,* or *high-functioning pervasive developmental disorders* underscores the fact that, in the past, individuals with AS were offered a choice between insufficient services for students with academically based learning disabilities, services for children with autism who are at a much lower level of general functioning, or (still) services for children with conduct problems, whose needs are totally different and incompatible with AS. These gaps in awareness and in services are slowly being corrected, although there is still much to be done in producing a more research-based body of knowledge on effective interventions and in considerably augmenting the resources available, including training of professionals, restructuring of current educational curricula, and better preparation of students for the demands of independent living. This chapter highlights some core components of any educational and treatment program for individuals with AS. As part of the approach presented here, social and communication skills training and the acquisition of adaptive skills take center stage. This approach advances the principle that our educational and treatment goals should focus on the longer-term goals of promoting increased social opportunities, of better capitalizing on individuals' natural talents, and on vocational satisfaction and independent living skills, as well as on their general emotional well-being.

REFERENCES

Adams, C., Green, J., Gilchrist, A., & Cox, A. (2002). Conversational behaviour of children with Asperger syndrome and conduct disorder. *Journal of Child Psychology and Psychiatry and Allied Disciplines, 43*(5), 679–690.

Allen, D., Evans, C., Hider, A., Hawkins, S., Peckett, H., & Morgan, H. (2008). Offending behaviour in adults with Asperger syndrome. *Journal of Autism and Developmental Disorders, 38*(4), 748–758.

Allgood, N. R. (2010). The perspective of young adult siblings of individuals with Asperger syndrome and high functioning autism: An exploration of grief and implications for developmental transition. *Dissertation Abstracts International Section A: Humanities and Social Sciences, 71*(6-A), 1921.

Ambery, F. Z., Russell, A. J., Perry, K., Morris, R., & Murphy, D. G. (2006). Neuropsychological functioning in adults with Asperger syndrome. *Autism, 10*(6), 551–564.

American Psychiatric Associaion. (2000). *Diagnostic and statistical manual of mental disorders* (4th ed., text rev.). Washington, DC: Author.

Arora, M., Praharaj, S. K., Sarkhel, S., & Sinha, V. K. (2011). Asperger disorder in adults. *Southern Medical Journal, 104*(4), 264–268.

Asperger, H. (1944). Die "Autistischen Psychopathen" im Kindesalter. *Archiv für Psychiatrie und Nervenkrankheiten, 117,* 76–136.

Attwood, A. (1998). *Asperger's syndrome: A guide for parents and professionals.* Philadelphia: Kingsley.

Attwood, T. (2003). Frameworks for behavioral intervention. *Child and Adolescent Psychiatric Clinics of North America, 12,* 65–86.

Attwood, T. (2004). Cognitive behaviour therapy for children and adults with Asperger's syndrome. *Behaviour Change, 21*(3), 147–161.

Attwood, T. (2006). Review of *Autism and Asperger Syndrome: Preparing for adulthood, second edition. Journal of Child Psychology and Psychiatry, 47*(2), 223–224.

Barnhill, G. P. (2007). Outcomes in adults with Asperger syndrome. *Focus on Autism and Other Developmental Disabilities, 22*(2), 116–126.

Baron-Cohen, S., & Howlin, P. (1998). *Teaching children with autism to mind-read: A practical guide for teachers and parents.* New York: Wiley.

Baron-Cohen, S., Leslie, A. M., & Frith, U. (1985). Does the autistic child have a "theory of mind"? *Cognition, 21*(1), 37–46.

Baron-Cohen, S., Tager-Flusberg, H., & Cohen, D. J. (Eds.). (1993). *Understanding other minds: Perspectives from autism.* Oxford, UK: Oxford University Press.

Beebe, D. W., & Risi, S. (2003). Treatment of adolescents and young adults with high-functioning autism or Asperger syndrome. In M. A. Reinecke, F. M. Dattilio, & A. Freeman (Eds.), *Cognitive therapy with children and adolescents: A casebook for clinical practice* (2nd ed., pp. 369–401). New York: Guilford Press.

Berkman, M. (1997). The legal rights of children with disabilities to education and developmental services. In D. J. Cohen & F. R. Volkmar (Eds.), *Handbook of autism and pervasive developmental disorders* (pp. 808–827). New York: Wiley.

Bowler, D. M., Gardiner, J. M., & Berthollier, N. (2004). Source memory in adolescents and adults with Asperger's syndrome. *Journal of Autism and Developmental Disorders, 34*(5), 533–542.

Bradford, K. (2010). Supporting families dealing with autism and Asperger's disorders. *Journal of Family Psychotherapy, 21*(2), 149–156.

Brown, J. T. (2010). Review of *Realizing the college dream with autism or Asperger syndrome. Journal of Autism and Developmental Disorders, 40*(6), 782.

Browning, A., & Caulfield, L. (2011). The prevalence and treatment of people with Asperger's syndrome in the criminal justice system. *Criminology and Criminal Justice: An International Journal, 11*(2), 165–180.

Bryant, B. R., & Seay, P. C. (1998). The Technology-Related Assistance to Individuals with Disabilities Act: Relevance to individuals with learning disabilities and their advocates. *Journal of Learning Disabilities, 31*(1), 4–15.

Bryant, D. P., & Bryant, B. R. (1998). Using assistive technology adaptations to include students with learning disabilities in cooperative learning activities. *Journal of Learning Disabilities, 31*(1), 41–54.

Burack, J. A., Root, R., & Zigler, E. (1997). Inclusive education for students with autism: Reviewing ideological, empirical, and community considerations. In D. J. Cohen & F. R. Volkmar (Eds.), *Handbook of autism and pervasive developmental disorders* (pp. 796–807). New York: Wiley.

Carr, E. G., Levin, L., McConnachie, G., Cappadocia, M., & Weiss, J. A. (2011). Review of social skills training groups for youth with Asperger syndrome and high functioning autism. *Research in Autism Spectrum Disorders, 5*(1), 70–78.

Carter, S. J. (2005). Comparison of children and adolescents with Asperger syndrome to their peers with learning disabilities in adaptive functioning, academic achievement, and victimization. *Dissertation Abstracts International Section A: Humanities and Social Sciences, 66*(1–A), 138.

Castorina, L. L., & Negri, L. M. (2011). The inclusion of siblings in social skills training groups for boys with Asperger syndrome. *Journal of Autism and Developmental Disorders, 41*(1), 73–81.

Chen, S. A., Thomas, J. D., Glueckauf, R. L., & Bracy, O. L. (1997). The effectiveness of computer-assisted cognitive rehabilitation for persons with traumatic brain injury. *Brain Injury, 11*(3), 197–209.

Church, C., Alisanski, S., & Amanullah, S. (2000). The social, behavioral, and academic experiences of children with Asperger syndrome. *Focus on Autism and Other Developmental Disabilities, 15*(1), 12–20.

Colle, L., Baron-Cohen, S., Wheelwright, S., & van der Lely, H. K. (2008).

Narrative discourse in adults with high-functioning autism or Asperger syndrome. *Journal of Autism and Developmental Disorders, 38*(1), 28–40.

Countryman, J. (2008). Social skills groups for Asperger's disorder and pervasive developmental disorder not otherwise specified. *Psychiatry, 5*(1), 42–47.

Daly, P. A., Bostic, J. Q., & Martin, A. (2006). Review of *Asperger's syndrome: Interventing in schools, clinics and communities* and *Asperger's syndrome in young children: A developmental guide for parents and professionals. Journal of the American Academy of Child & Adolescent Psychiatry, 45*(6), 736–761.

Davis, K. M., Boon, R. T., Cihak, D. F., & Fore, C., III. (2010). Power cards to improve conversational skills in adolescents with Asperger syndrome. *Focus on Autism and Other Developmental Disabilities, 25*(1), 12–22.

Dillon, M. R. (2007). Creating supports for college students with Asperger syndrome through collaboration. *College Student Journal, 41*(2), 499–504.

Donoghue, K., Stallard, P., & Kucia, J. (2011). The clinical practice of cognitive behavioural therapy for children and young people with a diagnosis of Asperger's syndrome. *Clinical Child Psychology and Psychiatry, 16*(1), 89–102.

Engstrom, I., Ekstrom, L., & Emilsson, B. (2003). Psychosocial functioning in a group of Swedish adults with Asperger syndrome or high-functioning autism. *Autism, 7*(1), 99–110.

Fangmeier, T., Lichtblau, A., Peters, J., Biscaldi-Schafer, M., Ebert, D., & van Elst, L. (2011). Psychotherapy of Asperger syndrome in adults. *Der Nervenarzt, 82*(5), 628–635.

Farrugia, S., & Hudson, J. (2006). Anxiety in adolescents with Asperger syndrome: Negative thoughts, behavioral problems, and life interference. *Focus on Autism and Other Developmental Disabilities, 21*(1), 25–35.

Gaylord-Ross, R. J., Haring, T. G., Breen, C., & Pitts-Conway, V. (1984). The training and generalization of social interaction skills with autistic youth. *Journal of Applied Behavior Analysis, 17*(2), 229–247.

Gena, A., Krantz, P. J., McClannahan, L. D., & Poulson, C. L. (1996). Training and generalization of affective behavior displayed by youth with autism. *Journal of Applied Behavior Analysis, 29*(3), 291–304.

Gerhardt, P. F., & Holmes, D. L. (1997). Employment: Options and issues for adolescents and adults with autism. In D. J. Cohen & F. R. Volkmar (Eds.), *Handbook of autism and pervasive developmental disorders* (pp. 650–664). New York: Wiley.

Gilotty, L., Kenworthy, L., Sirian, L., Black, D. O., & Wagner, A. E. (2002). Adaptive skills and executive function in autism spectrum disorders. *Child Neuropsychology, 8*(4), 241–248.

Golan, O., & Baron-Cohen, S. (2006). Systemizing empathy: Teaching adults with Asperger syndrome or high-functioning autism to recognize complex emotions using interactive multimedia. *Development and Psychopathology, 18*(2), 591–617.

Golan, O., Baron-Cohen, S., & Hill, J. (2006). The Cambridge Mindreading (CAM) Face–Voice Battery: Testing complex emotion recognition in adults with and without Asperger syndrome. *Journal of Autism and Developmental Disorders, 36*(2), 169–183.

Gould, K. (2011). Fantasy play as the conduit for change in the treatment of a six-year-old boy with Asperger's syndrome. *Psychoanalytic Inquiry, 31*(3), 240–251.

Gowen, E., & Miall, R. C. (2005). Behavioural aspects of cerebellar function in adults with Asperger syndrome. *Cerebellum, 4*(4), 279–289.

Graetz, J. (2009). Effective academic instruction for students with high functioning autism or Asperger's syndrome. In V. Spencer & C. Simpson (Eds.), *Teaching children with autism in the general classroom: Strategies for effective inclusion and instruction in the general education classroom* (pp. 45–74). Waco, TX: Prufrock Press.

Gray, C. A. (1995). Teaching children with autism to "read" social situations. In K. A. Quill (Ed.), *Teaching children with autism: Strategies to enhance communication and socialization* (pp. 219–242). New York: Delmar.

Gray, C. A. (1998). Social Stories and comic strip conversations with students with Asperger syndrome and high-functioning autism. In E. Schopler & G. B. Mesibov (Eds.), *Asperger syndrome or high-functioning autism?: Current issues in autism* (pp. 167–198). New York: Plenum Press.

Gray, C. A., Dutkiexicz, M., Fleck, C., Moore, L., Cain, S. L., Lindrup, A., et al. (1993). *The Social Story book.* Jenison, MI: Jenison Public Schools.

Gray, C. A., & Garand, J. (1993). Social Stories: Improving responses of students with autism with accurate social information. *Focus on Autistic Behavior, 8,* 1–10.

Gresham, F. M. (1992). Social skills and learning disabilities: Causal, concomitant, or correlational? *School Psychology Review, 21*(3), 348–360.

Griswold, D. E., Barnhill, G. P., Myles, B. S., Hagiwara, T., & Simpson, R. L. (2002). Asperger syndrome and academic achievement. *Focus on Autism and Other Developmental Disabilities, 17*(2), 94–102.

Hadwin, J., Baron-Cohen, S., Howlin, P., & Hill, K. (1997). Does teaching theory of mind have an effect on the ability to develop conversation in children with autism? *Journal of Autism and Developmental Disorders, 27*(5), 519–537.

Hagiwara, T. (2001). Academic assessment of children and youth with Asperger syndrome, pervasive developmental disorders-not otherwise specified, and high-functioning autism. *Assessment for Effective Intervention, 27*(1–2), 89–100.

Hagland, C., & Webb, Z. (2009). *Working with adults with Asperger syndrome: A practical toolkit.* London: Jessica Kingsley.

Hall, H. R., & Graff, J. C. (2011). The relationships among adaptive behaviors of children with autism, family support, parenting stress, and coping. *Issues in Comprehensive Pediatric Nursing, 34*(1), 4–25.

Hanley, K. P. (2008). Social Stories to increase verbal initiations to peers in children with autistic disorder and Asperger's disorder. *Dissertation Abstracts International Section A: Humanities and Social Sciences, 69*(3–A), 874.

Hanley-Hochdorfer, K. P., Bray, M. A., Kehle, T. J., & Elinoff, M. J. (2010). Social Stories to increase verbal initiation in children with autism and Asperger's disorder. *School Psychology Review, 39*(3), 484–492.

Harish, T., Gangadharan, S., Bhaumik, S., & Chaturvedi, S. K. (2010). Adults with Asperger syndrome at a neuropsychiatric centre in India. *British Journal of Developmental Disabilities, 56*(111, Pt. 2), 159–165.

Harris, S. L., & Handleman, J. S. (1997). Helping children with autism enter the mainstream. In D. J. Cohen & F. R. Volkmar (Eds.), *Handbook of autism and pervasive developmental disorders* (pp. 665–675). New York: Wiley.

Harvey, G. (2008). *Social relationships for people with Asperger syndrome: How to help people understand Asperger syndrome and social relationships—adults speak out about Asperger syndrome.* London: Jessica Kingsley.

Henderson, A. (2008). Asperger syndrome and social relationships: My experiences and observations. In Asperger syndrome and social relationships: Adults speak out about Asperger syndrome (pp. 147–149). London: Jessica Kingsley.

Hendrickx, S. (2008). *Love, sex and long-term relationships: What people with Asperger syndrome really really want.* London: Jessica Kingsley.

Hill, E. L., & Bird, C. M. (2006). Executive processes in Asperger syndrome: Patterns of performance in a multiple case series. *Neuropsychologia, 44*(14), 2822–2835.

Hodgdon, L. (1995). Solving social-behavioral problems through the use of visually supported communication. In K. A. Quill (Ed.), *Teaching children with autism: Strategies to enhance communication and socialization* (pp. 265–286). New York: Delmar.

Hodgdon, L. (1996). *Visual strategies for improving communication: Vol. 1. Practical supports for school and home.* Troy, MI: QuirkRoberts.

Howlin, P., Alcock, J., & Burkin, C. (2005). An 8 year follow-up of a specialist supported employment service for high-ability adults with autism or Asperger syndrome. *Autism, 9*(5), 533–549.

Hurlburt, R. T., Happé, F., & Frith, U. (1994). Sampling the form of inner experience in three adults with Asperger syndrome. *Psychological Medicine, 24*(2), 385–395.

Ihrig, K., & Wolchik, S. A. (1988). Peer versus adult models and autistic children's learning: Acquisition, generalization, and maintenance. *Journal of Autism and Developmental Disorders, 18*(1), 67–79.

Jantz, K. M. (2011). Support groups for adults with Asperger syndrome. *Focus on Autism and Other Developmental Disabilities, 26*(2), 119–128.

Jolliffe, T., & Baron-Cohen, S. (1999). A test of central coherence theory: Linguistic processing in high-functioning adults with autism or Asperger syndrome—is local coherence impaired? *Cognition, 71*(2), 149–185.

Jolliffe, T., & Baron-Cohen, S. (2000). Linguistic processing in high-functioning adults with autism or Asperger's syndrome: Is global coherence impaired? *Psychological Medicine, 30*(5), 1169–1187.

Juhel, J.-C. (2005). The integration of college students having Asperger's syndrome. *Revue Quebecoise de Psychologie, 26*(3), 239–255.

Kaland, N., Mortensen, E. L., & Smith, L. (2011). Social communication impairments in children and adolescents with Asperger syndrome: Slow response time and the impact of prompting. *Research in Autism Spectrum Disorders, 5*(3), 1129–1137.

Kanai, C., Iwanami, A., Hashimoto, R., Ota, H., Tani, M., Yamada, T., et al. (2011). Clinical characterization of adults with Asperger's syndrome assessed by self-report questionnaires based on depression, anxiety, and personality. *Research in Autism Spectrum Disorders, 5*(4), 1451–1458.

Kanai, C., Iwanami, A., Ota, H., Yamasue, H., Matsushima, E., Yokoi, H., et al. (2011). Clinical characteristics of adults with Asperger's syndrome assessed with self-report questionnaires. *Research in Autism Spectrum Disorders, 5*(1), 185–190.

Khouzam, H. R., El-Gabalawi, F., Pirwani, N., & Priest, F. (2004). Asperger's disorder: A review of its diagnosis and treatment. *Comprehensive Psychiatry, 45*(3), 184–191.

Kleinhans, N., Akshoomoff, N., & Delis, D. C. (2005). Executive functions in autism and Asperger's disorder: Flexibility, fluency, and inhibition. *Developmental Neuropsychology, 27*(3), 379–401.

Klin, A. (1997, October 16). *Asperger's syndrome: Diagnosis and phenomenology.* Paper presented at the 44th annual meeting of the American Academy of Child and Adolescent Psychiatry, Toronto, Ontario, Canada.

Klin, A., Sparrow, S. S., Volkmar, F. R., Cicchetti, D. V., & Rourke, B. P. (1995). Asperger syndrome. In B. P. Rourke (Ed.), *Syndrome of nonverbal learning disabilities: Neurodevelopmental manifestations* (pp. 93–118). New York: Guilford Press.

Klin, A., & Volkmar, F. R. (1997). Asperger's syndrome. In D. J. Cohen & F. R. Volkmar (Eds.), *Handbook of autism and pervasive developmental disorders* (pp. 94–122). New York: Wiley.

Koegel, L. K., & LaZebnik, C. (2009). *Growing up on the spectrum: A guide to life, love, and learning for teens and young adults with autism and Asperger's.* New York: Viking.

Koegel, R. L., & Koegel, L. K. (Eds.). (1995). *Teaching children with autism: Strategies for initiating positive interactions and improving learning opportunities.* Baltimore: Brookes.

Kroodsma, L. (2008). An educational workshop for parents of children with Asperger syndrome. *Dissertation Abstracts International Section B: Sciences and Engineering, 68*(12-B), 8401.

Kujala, T., Aho, E., Lepist, T., Jansson-Verkasalo, E., Xliemen-vonWendt, T., & von Woud, L. (2007). Atypical pattern of discriminating sound features in adults with Asperger syndrome as reflected by the mismatch negativity. *Biological Psychology, 75*(1), 109–114.

LaCava, P. G., Golan, O., Baron-Cohen, S., & Myles, B. S. (2007). Using assistive technology to teach emotion recognition to students with Asperger syndrome: A pilot study. *Remedial and Special Education, 28*(3), 174–181.

Lau, W., & Peterson, C. C. (2011). Adults and children with Asperger syndrome: Exploring adult attachment style, marital satisfaction, and satisfaction with parenthood. *Research in Autism Spectrum Disorders, 5*(1), 392–399.

Lee, H. J., & Park, H. R. (2007). An integrated literature review on the adaptive behavior of individuals with Asperger syndrome. *Remedial and Special Education, 28*(3), 132–139.

Lepistö, T., Nieminen-von Wendt, T., von Wendt, L., Naatanen, R., & Kujala, T. (2007). Auditory cortical change detection in adults with Asperger syndrome. *Neuroscience Letters, 414*(2), 136–140.

Lewis, R. B. (1998). Assistive technology and learning disabilities: Today's realities and tomorrow's promises. *Journal of Learning Disabilities, 31*(1), 16–26.

Livanis, A., Solomon, E. R., & Ingram, D. H. (2007). Guided Social Stories: Group treatment of adolescents with Asperger's disorder in the schools. In R. W. Christner, J. Stewart, & A. Freeman (Eds.), *Handbook of cognitive-behavior group therapy with children and adolescents: Specific settings and presenting problems* (pp. 389–407). New York: Routledge/Taylor & Francis Group.

Loudon, J. L. (2009). Increasing social skills and decreasing anxiety in adolescents with Asperger syndrome. *Dissertation Abstracts International Section A: Humanities and Social Sciences, 69*(11–A), 4245.

Loukusa, S., Leinonen, E., Kuusikko, S., Jussila, K., Mattila, M.-L., Ryder, N., et al. (2007). Use of context in pragmatic language comprehension by children with Asperger syndrome or high-functioning autism. *Journal of Autism and Developmental Disorders, 37*(6), 1049–1059.

Lugnegard, T., Hallerback, M. U., & Gillberg, C. (2011). Psychiatric comorbidity in young adults with a clinical diagnosis of Asperger syndrome. *Research in Developmental Disabilities, 32*(5), 1910–1917.

Macintosh, K., & Dissanayake, C. (2006). Social skills and problem behaviours in school-aged children with high-functioning autism and Asperger's disorder. *Journal of Autism and Developmental Disorders, 36*(8), 1065–1076.

Mandlawitz, M. R. (2005). Educating children with autism: Current legal issues. In F. R. Volkmar, A. Klin, R. Paul, & D. J. Cohen (Eds.), *Handbook of autism and pervasive developmental disorders* (3rd ed., Vol. 2, pp. 1161–1173). Hoboken, NJ: Wiley.

Matson, J. L., Benavidez, D. A., Compton, L. S., Paclawskyj, T., & Baglio, C. (1996). Behavioral treatment of autistic persons: A review of research from 1980 to the present. *Research in Developmental Disabilities, 17*(6), 433–465.

Matthews, A. (1996). *Employment training and the development of a support model within employment for adults who experience Asperger syndrome and autism: The Gloucestershire Group Homes Model.* New York: Cambridge University Press.

Mawhood, L., & Howlin, P. (1999). The outcome of a supported employment scheme for high-functioning adults with autism or Asperger syndrome. *Autism, 3*(3), 229–254.

Mazefsky, C. A., Williams, D. L., & Minshew, N. J. (2008). Variability in adaptive behavior in autism: Evidence for the importance of family history. *Journal of Abnormal Child Psychology, 36*(4), 591–599.

McCrimmon, A. W. (2011). Executive functions in Asperger's disorder: An empirical investigation of verbal and nonverbal skills. *Dissertation Abstracts International Section B: Sciences and Engineering, 71*(8-B), 5135.

Mesibov, G. B. (1984). Social skills training with verbal autistic adolescents and adults: A program model. *Journal of Autism and Developmental Disorders, 14*, 395–404.

Mesibov, G. B. (1986). A cognitive program for teaching social behaviors to verbal autistic adolescents and adults. In E. Schopler & G. B. Mesibov (Eds.), *High-functioning individuals with autism* (pp. 143–156). New York: Plenum Press.

Mesibov, G. B. (1992). Treatment issues with high-functioning adolescents and adults with autism. In E. Schopler & G. B. Mesibov (Eds.), *Social behavior in autism* (pp. 265–303). New York: Plenum Press.

Minihan, A., Kinsella, W., & Honan, R. (2011). Social skills training for adolescents with Asperger's syndrome using a consultation model. *Journal of Research in Special Educational Needs, 11*(1), 55–69.

Minskoff, E. H. (1980a). A teaching approach for developing nonverbal communication skills in students with social perception deficits: Part I. *Journal of Learning Disabilities, 13*, 118–124.

Minskoff, E. H. (1980b). A teaching approach for developing nonverbal communication skills in students with social perception deficits: Part II. *Journal of Learning Disabilities, 13,* 203–208.

Minskoff, E. H. (1987). *Pass Program: Programming appropriate social skills.* Fishersville, VA: Woodrow Wilson Rehabilitation Center.

Minskoff, E. H. (1994). *TRACC Workplace Social Skills Program.* Fishersville, VA: Woodrow Wilson Rehabilitation Center.

Minskoff, E. H., & DeMoss, S. (1994). Workplace social skills and individuals with learning disabilities. *Journal of Vocational Rehabilitation, 4*(2), 113–121.

Mitchel, K., Regehr, K., Reaume, J., & Feldman, M. (2010). Group social skills training for adolescents with Asperger syndrome or high-functioning autism. *Journal of Developmental Disabilities, 16*(2), 52–63.

Moyes, R. (2003). Incorporating social goals in the classroom: A guide for teachers and parents of children with high functioning autism and Asperger syndrome. *British Journal of Educational Psychology, 73*(1), 138–139.

Mrug, S., & Hodgens, J. (2008). Behavioral summer treatment program improves social and behavioral functioning of four children with Asperger's disorder. *Clinical Case Studies, 7*(3), 171–190.

Muller, E., Schuler, A., Burton, B. A., & Yates, G. B. (2003). Meeting the vocational support needs of individuals with Asperger syndrome and other autism spectrum disabilities. *Journal of Vocational Rehabilitation, 18*(3), 163–175.

Muller, R. (2010). Will you play with me?: Improving social skills for children with Asperger syndrome. *International Journal of Disability, Development and Education, 57*(3), 331–334.

Munro, J. (2010). An integrated model of psychotherapy for teens and adults with Asperger syndrome. *Journal of Systemic Therapies, 29*(3), 82–96.

Myles, B. S., Barnhill, G. P., Hagiwara, T., Griswold, D. E., & Simpson, R. L. (2001). A synthesis of studies on the intellectual, academic, social, emotional and sensory characteristics of children and youth with Asperger syndrome. *Education and Training in Mental Retardation and Developmental Disabilities, 36*(3), 304–311.

Myles, B. S., & Simpson, R. L. (1998). *Asperger syndrome: A guide for educators and parents.* Austin, TX: PRO-ED.

Nyden, A., Niklasson, L., Stahlberg, O., Anckarsater, H., Dahlgren-Sandberg, A., Wentz, E., et al. (2010). Adults with Asperger syndrome with and without a cognitive profile associated with "non-verbal learning disability": A brief report. *Research in Autism Spectrum Disorders, 4*(4), 612–618.

O'Connor, K. (2007). Brief report: Impaired identification of discrepancies between expressive faces and voices in adults with Asperger's syndrome. *Journal of Autism and Developmental Disorders, 37*(10), 2008–2013.

Oyane, N. M. F., & Bjorvatn, B. (2005). Sleep disturbances in adolescents and young adults with autism and Asperger syndrome. *Autism, 9*(1), 83–94.

Ozdemir, D. F., & Iseri, E. (2004). Asperger's syndrome in adults: A review. *Klinik Psikiyatri Dergisi: Journal of Clinical Psychiatry, 7*(4), 223–230.

Ozonoff, S. (1998). Assessment and remediation of executive dysfunction in autism and Asperger syndrome. In E. Schopler, G. B. Mesibov, & L. J. Kunce (Eds.), *Asperger syndrome or high-functioning autism?* (pp. 263–289). New York: Plenum Press.

Ozonoff, S., & Miller, J. N. (1995). Teaching theory of mind: A new approach to social skills training for individuals with autism. *Journal of Autism and Developmental Disorders, 25*(4), 415–433.

Palmen, A., Didden, R., & Lang, R. (2012). A systematic review of behavioral intervention research on adaptive skill building in high-functioning young adults with autism spectrum disorder. *Research in Autism Spectrum Disorders, 6*(2), 602–617.

Patrick, N. J. (2008). *Social skills for teenagers and adults with Asperger syndrome: A practical guide to day-to-day life.* London: Jessica Kingsley.

Paul, R., Orlovski, S. M., Marcinko, H. C., & Volkmar, F. (2009). Conversational behaviors in youth with high-functioning ASD and Asperger syndrome. *Journal of Autism and Developmental Disorders, 39*(1), 115–125.

Perlman, L. (2000). Adults with Asperger disorder misdiagnosed as schizophrenic. *Professional Psychology: Research and Practice, 31*(2), 221–225.

Pennington, B. F., & Ozonoff, S. (1996). Executive functions and developmental psychopathology. *Journal of Child Psychology and Psychiatry, 37*(1), 51–87.

Pierce, K., & Schreibman, L. (1997). Multiple peer use of pivotal response training to increase social behaviors of classmates with autism: Results from trained and untrained peers. *Journal of Applied Behavior Analysis, 30*(1), 157–160.

Pijnacker, J., Hagoort, P., Buitelaar, J., Teunisse, J.-P., & Geurts, B. (2009). Pragmatic inferences in high-functioning adults with autism and Asperger syndrome. *Journal of Autism and Developmental Disorders, 39*(4), 607–618.

Pope, K. K. (1993). The pervasive developmental disorder spectrum: A case illustration. *Bulletin of the Menninger Clinic, 57,* 100–117.

Powers, M. D. (1997). Behavioral assessment of individuals with autism. In D. J. Cohen & F. R. Volkmar (Eds.), *Handbook of autism and pervasive developmental disorders* (pp. 448– 459). New York: Wiley.

Prizant, B. M., Schuler, A. L., Wetherby, A., & Rydell, P. (1997). Enhancing language and communication development: Language approaches. In D. J. Cohen & F. R. Volkmar (Eds.), *Handbook of autism and pervasive developmental disorders* (pp. 572–605). New York: Wiley.

Quill, K. A. (Ed.). (1995). *Teaching children with autism: Strategies to enhance communication and socialization.* New York: Delmar.

Rao, P. A., Beidel, D. C., Murray, M. J., Rao, P. A., Beidel, D. C., & Murray, M. J. (2008). Social skills interventions for children with Asperger's syndrome or high-functioning autism: A review and recommendations. *Journal of Autism and Developmental Disorders, 38*(2), 353–361.

Raskind, M. H., & Higgins, E. L. (1998). Assistive technology for postsecondary students with learning disabilities: An overview. *Journal of Learning Disabilities, 31*(1), 27–40.

Reaven, J., & Hepburn, S. (2003). Cognitive-behavioral treatment of obsessive–compulsive disorder in a child with Asperger syndrome: A case report. *Autism, 7*(2), 145–164.

Reichow, B., Doehring, P., Cicchetti, D. V., & Volkmar, F. R. (Eds.). (2011). Evidence-based practices and treatments for children with autism. In *Evidence-based practices and treatments for children with autism.* New York: Springer Science + Business Media.

Reichow, B., & Volkmar, F. R. (2010). Social skills interventions for individuals with autism: Evaluation for evidence-based practices within a best evidence synthesis framework. *Journal of Autism and Developmental Disorders,* *40*(2), 149–166.

Ritvo, R. A., Ritvo, E. R., Guthrie, D., Ritvo, M. J., Hufnagel, D. H., McMahon, W., et al. (2011). The Ritvo Autism Asperger Diagnostic Scale—Revised (RAADS-R): A scale to assist the diagnosis of autism spectrum disorder in adults—an international validation study. *Journal of Autism and Developmental Disorders, 41*(8), 1076–1089.

Rondan, C., & Deruelle, C. (2007). Global and configural visual processing in adults with autism and Asperger syndrome. *Research in Developmental Disabilities, 28*(2), 197–206.

Rourke, B. P. (1989). *Nonverbal learning disabilities: The syndrome and the model.* New York: Guilford Press.

Rourke, B. P. (1995). Treatment program for the child with NLD. In B. P. Rourke (Ed.), *Syndrome of nonverbal learning disabilities: Neurodevelopmental manifestations* (pp. 497–508). New York: Guilford Press.

Rutherford, M., Baron-Cohen, S., & Wheelwright, S. (2002). Reading the mind in the voice: A study with normal adults and adults with Asperger syndrome and high functioning autism. *Journal of Autism and Developmental Disorders, 32*(3), 189–194.

Sahlander, C., Mattsson, M., & Bejerot, S. (2008). Motor function in adults with Asperger's disorder: A comparative study. *Physiotherapy Theory and Practice, 24*(2), 73–81.

Scattone, D. (2008). Enhancing the conversation skills of a boy with Asperger's disorder through Social Stories™ and video modeling. *Journal of Autism and Developmental Disorders, 38*(2), 395–400.

Scharfstein, L. A., Beidel, D. C., Sims, V. K., & Rendon Finnell, L. (2011). Social skills deficits and vocal characteristics of children with social phobia or Asperger's disorder: A comparative study. *Journal of Abnormal Child Psychology, 39*(6), 865–875.

Schopler, E., & Mesibov, G. B. (Eds.). (1992). *High functioning individuals with autism.* New York: Plenum Press.

Schopler, E., Mesibov, G. B., & Kunce, L. J. (Eds.). (1998). *Asperger syndrome or high-functioning autism?* New York: Plenum Press.

Shogren, K. A., Lang, R., Machalicek, W., Rispoli, M. J., & O'Reilly, M. (2011). Self versus teacher management of behavior for elementary school students with asperger syndrome: Impact on classroom behavior. *Journal of Positive Behavior Interventions, 13*(2), 87–96.

Shriberg, L. D., Paul, R., McSweeny, J. L., Klin, A., & Cohen, D. J. (2001). Speech and prosody characteristics of adolescents and adults with high-functioning autism and Asperger syndrome. *Journal of Speech Language and Hearing Research, 44*(5), 1097–1115.

Shtayermman, O. (2006). An exploratory study of suicidal ideation and comorbid disorders in adolescents and young adults with Asperger's syndrome. *Dissertation Abstracts International Section A: Humanities and Social Sciences, 67*(6–A), 2323.

Shtayermman, O. (2008). Suicidal ideation and comorbid disorders in adolescents and young adults diagnosed with Asperger's syndrome: A population at risk. *Journal of Human Behavior in the Social Environment, 18*(3), 301–328.

Shtayermman, O. (2009). An exploratory study of the stigma associated with a diagnosis of Asperger's syndrome: The mental health impact on the adolescents and young adults diagnosed with a disability with a social nature. *Journal of Human Behavior in the Social Environment, 19*(3), 298–313.

Smith, A. D. B. (2008). Effects of a clinic-based conversation skills group training program on children with high functioning autism/Asperger syndrome. *Dissertation Abstracts International Section B: Sciences and Engineering, 68*(8-B), 5183.

Smith, D. C. (1998). Assistive technology: Funding options and strategies. *Mental and Physical Disabilities Law Report, 22*(1), 115–123.

Sofronoff, K., Attwood, T., & Hinton, S. (2005). A randomised controlled trial of a CBT intervention for anxiety in children with Asperger syndrome. *Journal of Child Psychology and Psychiatry, 46*(11), 1152–1160.

Sofronoff, K., & Farbotko, M. (2002). The effectiveness of parent management training to increase self-efficacy in parents of children with Asperger syndrome. *Autism, 6*(3), 271–286.

Sparrow, S. S., Balla, D., & Cicchetti, D. (1984). *Vineland Adaptive Behavior Scales—Expanded Edition.* Circle Pines, MN: American Guidance Service.

Spek, A., Schatorje, T., Scholte, E., & van Berckelaer-Onnes, I. (2009). Verbal fluency in adults with high functioning autism or Asperger syndrome. *Neuropsychologia, 47*(3), 652–656.

Stenberg, N. (2007). Asperger syndrome and executive dysfunction: Implications for treatment. *Tidsskrift for Norsk Psykologforening, 44*(3), 254–260.

Stichter, J. P., Herzog, M. J., Visovsky, K., Schmidt, C., Randolph, J., Schultz, T., et al. (2010). Social competence intervention for youth with Asperger syndrome and high-functioning autism: An initial investigation. *Journal of Autism and Developmental Disorders, 40*(9), 1067–1079.

Stoesz, B. M., Montgomery, J. M., Smart, S. L., & Hellsten, L.-A. M. (2011). Review of five instruments for the assessment of Asperger's disorder in adults. *Clinical Neuropsychologist, 25*(3), 376–401.

Tantam, D. (2003). The challenge of adolescents and adults with Asperger syndrome. *Child and Adolescent Psychiatric Clinics of North America, 12*(1), 143–163, vii–viii.

Tantam, D., & Girgis, S. (2009). Recognition and treatment of Asperger syndrome in the community. *British Medical Bulletin, 89,* 41–62.

Taylor, B. A., & Harris, S. L. (1995). Teaching children with autism to seek information: Acquisition of novel information and generalization of responding. *Journal of Applied Behavior Analysis, 28*(1), 3–14.

Thorp, D. M., Stahmer, A. C., & Schreibman, L. (1995). Effects of sociodramatic play training on children with autism. *Journal of Autism and Developmental Disorders, 25*(3), 265–282.

Tiger, J. H., Fisher, W. W., & Bouxsein, K. J. (2009). Therapist- and self-monitored DRO contingencies as a treatment for the self-injurious skin picking of a young man with Asperger syndrome. *Journal of Applied Behavior Analysis, 42*(2), 315–319.

Toth, K., & King, B. H. (2008). Asperger's syndrome: Diagnosis and treatment. *American Journal of Psychiatry, 165*(8), 958–963.

Tsatsanis, K. D. (2005). Neuropsychological characteristics in autism and related conditions. In F. R. Volkmar, A. Klin, R. Paul, & D. J. Cohen (Eds.),

Handbook of autism and pervasive developmental disorders (3rd ed., Vol. 1, pp. 365–381). Hoboken, NJ: Wiley.

Twachtman, D. D. (1995). Methods to enhance communication in verbal children. In K. A. Quill (Ed.), *Teaching children with autism: Strategies to enhance communication and socialization* (pp. 133–162). New York: Delmar.

Van Bourgondien, M. E., & Woods, A. V. (1992). Vocational possibilities for high-functioning adults with autism. In E. Schopler & G. B. Mesibov (Eds.), *High-functioning individuals with autism* (pp. 227–239). New York: Plenum Press.

Volkmar, F. R. (2011). Asperger's disorder: Implications for psychoanalysis. *Psychoanalytic Inquiry, 31*(3), 334–344.

Volkmar, F. R., & Wiesner, L. A. (2009). *A practical guide to autism: What every parent, family member, and teacher needs to know.* Hoboken, NJ: Wiley.

Walters, J. B. (2010). The occurrence of maltreatment and depression among adjudicated adolescent sexual offenders with high functioning autism or Asperger's disorder. *Dissertation Abstracts International Section B: Sciences and Engineering, 70*(12-B), 7867.

Weiss, J. A., & Lunsky, Y. (2010). Group cognitive behaviour therapy for adults with Asperger syndrome and anxiety or mood disorder: A case series. *Clinical Psychology and Psychotherapy, 17*(5), 438–446.

Welkowitz, L. A., & Baker, L. J. (2005). Supporting college students with Asperger's syndrome. In L. J. Baker & L. A. Welkowitz (Eds.), *Asperger's syndrome: Intervening in schools, clinics, and communities* (pp. 173–187). Mahwah, NJ: Erlbaum.

Whitby, P. J., & Mancil, G. (2009). Academic achievement profiles in children with high functioning autism and Asperger syndrome: A review of the literature. *Education and Training in Developmental Disabilities, 44*(4), 551–560.

Whitehouse, A. J., Durkin, K., Jaquet, E., & Ziatas, K. (2009). Friendship, loneliness and depression in adolescents with Asperger's syndrome. *Journal of Adolescence, 32*(2), 309–322.

Whitehead, J. L. (2005). Treating AD-related anxiety as measured by the BASC in adolescents with Asperger's disorder. *Dissertation Abstracts International Section A: Humanities and Social Sciences, 66*(6-A), 2174.

Wolff, J. J. (2011). An examination of avoidance extinction procedures in treatment of maladaptive higher-order repetitive behavior in autism. [Dissertation]. *Dissertation Abstracts International Section B: Sciences and Engineering, 71*(7-B), 4496.

Wolff, L. E., Brown, J. T., & Bork, G. R. (2009). *Students with Asperger syndrome: A guide for college personnel.* Shawnee Mission, KS: APC.

Woodbury-Smith, M. R., Robinson, J., Wheelwright, S., & Baron-Cohen, S. (2005). Screening adults for Asperger syndrome using the AQ: A preliminary study of its diagnostic validity in clinical practice. *Journal of Autism and Developmental Disorders, 35*(3), 331–335.

Woodbury-Smith, M. R., & Volkmar, F. R. (2009). Asperger syndrome. *European Child and Adolescent Psychiatry, 18*(1), 2–11.

CHAPTER 6

Addressing Social Communication in Asperger Syndrome

Implementing Individualized Supports across Social Partners and Contexts

Emily Rubin

There is a strong correlation between social communicative competence and long-term positive outcomes for individuals with Asperger syndrome (AS) (National Research Council, 2001). Social-communicative competence, in fact, plays a major role in the ability to form relationships and to adapt to the demands of everyday social situations. Although individuals with AS are often considered "high functioning" on the basis of their performance on standardized measures of cognition, outcome studies with this population highlight that cognitive, academic, and even formal language abilities do not ensure an individual's ability to establish and maintain satisfying relationships that contribute to success at school, at home, and in the community (Klin et al., 2007; Tsatsanis, Foley, & Donehower, 2004). Challenges in social communication significantly compromise adaptive social functioning and the ability to achieve longer-term vocational goals (Gilchrist et al., 2001; Little, 2001; Saulnier & Klin, 2006; Tantam, 2000; see also Tsatsanis, 2003). Likewise, these challenges place the individual at risk for mental health conditions such as anxiety and depression

(Tsatsanis et al., 2004). Therefore, when developing an individualized educational and therapeutic program for an individual with AS, addressing social communication is a critical priority.

Social-communicative competence, however, is not achieved solely in isolated teaching contexts such as a social skills group or one-on-one therapy. Rather, it is achieved through an individual's experience of success across social activities, social partners, and social contexts (e.g., home, school, and community). Although a range of social skills programs is available that provides support at specific times of an individual's day, an appropriate program will ensure that supports are embedded throughout an individual's daily routines. Additionally, the importance of partner training is evident, as setting targets for the individual with AS does not always ensure that social partners will modify their communicative style and the environment to accommodate the individual's unique learning style, address family priorities, and facilitate generalization across situations and contexts (Simpson, de Boer-Ott, & Myles, 2003). The National Research Council (2001) recognized these needs for individuals with autism spectrum disorder (ASD) and recommended the development of partner training as part of a comprehensive effort to implement individualized supports across contexts and activities (e.g., family support, personnel preparation, and peer training).

The SCERTS® Model is a multidisciplinary team approach that provides a comprehensive, curriculum-based assessment (Prizant, Wetherby, Rubin, Laurent, & Rydell, 2006). The assessment process was designed to identify goals and objectives that have been shown to address the core challenges that compromise social-communicative competence and, at the same time, to provide a tool for measuring progress across partners, contexts, and activities (Prizant et al., 2006). Progress is documented not only in the individual with the social disability, but also in how social partners interact with that individual and how environmental arrangements have been made to foster more successful social interaction across daily routines. In this approach, the critical role of a partner is emphasized. Goals and objectives are identified not only for the individual with a social disability but also for that individual's social network of family, teachers, therapists, peers, and members of the community.

When partners are responsive needs of the individual with with AS model appropriate social behavior, modify activities to enhance active engagement, and provide learning supports that enhance adaptive social functioning, individuals with AS are more competent social communicators. The ability to provide these supports, however, is often compromised by the transactional nature of the social disability (Prizant, Wetherby, Rubin, & Laurent, 2003). That is, the atypical social and communicative style of individuals with AS will compromise the ability of a communicative partner to provide these supports. Thus, a social skills program that has a sole focus on enhancing the skills of the individual with the disability does not necessarily ensure success across all social partners. Those who interact with the individual often require direct training and support to ensure competent communicative exchanges (Prizant et al., 2006).

This chapter provides an overview of the SCERTS Assessment Process (SAP) as a tool that can be implemented to facilitate the process of selecting appropriate goals and objectives for the individual with AS as well as the process of determining how partners might modify their communicative style and the environment by selecting specific supports that are evidence-based to promote more competent social communication (Prizant et al., 2006). First, curricular priorities in the SCERTS domains of social communication and emotional regulation are reviewed, as these are two areas of vulnerability frequently observed in individuals with AS that impact social-communicative competence. Next, curricular priorities in the SCERTS domains of interpersonal support and learning support are reviewed to facilitate the development and implementation of supports across social activities, partners, and contexts. The final section of this chapter includes descriptions of practical examples of how partners might implement these supports in home, school, and community settings.

DETERMINING PRIORITIES FOR SOCIAL SKILLS DEVELOPMENT

When determining priorities for enhancing social skills development in individuals with AS, outcome research has demonstrated that gains in adaptive social functioning and academic achievement are linked to efforts to ameliorate the core features of the social disability (Nationl Research Council, 2001). Regardless of cognitive abilities or learning style differences, individuals with AS face core challenges in establishing shared attention and thereby predicting the actions of social partners (Volkmar, Lord, Bailey, Schultz, & Klin, 2004). When an individual has difficulty predicting the actions of social partners, the development of social communication and emotional regulation can be compromised. These are two of the primary domains of the SCERTS curriculum-based assessment. Using observational data from everyday social contexts and information gathered directly from everyday social partners, progress related to these core challenges is measured by assessing the generalization of these skills across functional activities.

In the SCERTS Model, a scope and sequence of goals and objectives is provided that follows a development framework progressing through distinct stages of curricula (Prizant et al., 2006). The earliest stage is the *Social Partner Stage*, which provides a curriculum appropriate for individuals learning how to use gestures and concrete objects as a primary means of establishing shared attention and anticipating another's actions within familiar routines. Once children begin to develop symbolic language, the *Language Partner Stage* curriculum becomes appropriate. At this stage, children are learning to use language (e.g., verbalizations, signs, or pictures) as a primary means of communication and are developing a repertoire of single words, multiword combinations, and creative simple sentence structures. The final stage of the curriculum is the *Conversational Partner Stage*, which is appropriate for an individual using creative sentences and conversational-level discourse to communicate, while developing an awareness of social perspectives and an understanding of social conventions. Individuals with AS often demonstrate strengths in the acquisition of early language skills and thus are frequently in the Conversational Partner Stage at the time of initial diagnosis. The focus of this chapter remains on this stage of development and the associated core challenges that compromise social competence.

Social Communication

Difficulties establishing shared attention and predicting the actions of one's social partners can compromise developmental achievements in the capacity for joint attention. Specific challenges in this capacity are frequently noted with respect to (1) monitoring the attentional focus of others, (2) sharing and understanding emotional cues, (3) sharing intentions for more social functions, (4) sharing experiences by initiating and maintaining conversations that relate to a partner's interests, and (5) persisting and repairing communication breakdowns (Prizant et al., 2006). Although individuals with AS may be able to demonstrate an ability to identify facial expressions or other behaviors indicative of emotional states (e.g., a clear smile, a scowling face, a clenched fist) in static images or story books, they experience challenges particularly in natural social interactions (Klin, 2000; Klin, Jones, Schultz, Volkmar, & Cohen, 2002; Yirmiya, Sigman, Kasari, & Mundy, 1992). Eye-tracking research has shown that, in these fast-paced situations, individuals with AS often neglect emotional cues, fixating on the lower half of the face as opposed to the upper half (i.e., the eyes) (Klin et al., 2002). Similarly, challenges in the ability to integrate visual information to derive social meaning was further revealed on tasks such as the social attribution task (SAT; Heider & Simmel, 1944), an animated cartoon that has been used to determine an individual's ability to glean information related to mental states and intentions of others (Klin, 2000). These differences contribute to a limited awareness of causal factors underlying the emotional states of others, limited empathic reactions, and limited use of others' emotions to guide behavior in social interactions (Capps, Yirmiya, & Sigman, 1992). These challenges further compromise the ability to initiate and maintain conversations that are sensitive to the social context and to the interests and emotions of others. Preferred topics often dominate conversations and the relevance of a topic to a conversational partner may not be considered (Lord & Paul, 1997).

Difficulties establishing shared attention and predicting the actions of one's social partners also impact developmental achievements in the capacity for symbol use and language-related cognitive skills (Prizant et al., 2006). Specific challenges in this capacity are frequently noted with respect to (1) learning by imitation, observation, instruction, and collaboration; (2) understanding nonverbal cues and nonliteral meanings; (3) participating conventionally in dramatic play and recreation; (4) using appropriate gestures and nonverbal behavior for the context and partner; (5) understanding and using generative language; and (6) following the rules of conversation. For individuals with AS who demonstrate apparent strengths in verbal language development, difficulties using more sophisticated language as a means to clarify intentions remain common (Volkmar, Klin, Schultz, Rubin, & Bronen, 2000). Although individuals with AS may demonstrate relative strengths in the structural aspects of language and semantics, the use of more sophisticated syntax as a tool for providing background information to social partners is often impaired (Volkmar et al., 2000).

Sample goals and objectives of the SCERTS curriculum-based assessment in the domain of social communication are outlined in Table 6.1 for the Conversational Partner Stage under the components of joint attention and symbol use.

Emotional Regulation

At the core of the disability, individuals with AS have difficulty predicting the actions of their social partners. While these challenges clearly compromise the development of social communication skills, as described above, they also contribute to challenges in emotional regulation, a primary domain in the SCERTS curriculum-based assessment (Prizant et al., 2006). One needs to accurately predict social behavior in others in order to maintain active engagement in social situations, to feel safe, and to confidently "jump into the mix." This challenge, therefore, contributes to increased frustration, social anxiety, and may ultimately contribute to withdrawal and depression (Little, 2001; Tantam, 2000). Emotional regulation challenges can, in fact, provide a significant obstacle toward the achievement of social and communicative competence if not addressed (National Research Council, 2000).

One aspect of emotional regulation involves the capacity for mutual regulation, namely, the ability to respond to or solicit assistance to regulate one's emotional state. Because individuals with AS frequently misinterpret social cues, they may fail to recognize assistance that is offered by social partners (Laurent & Rubin, 2004) and may avoid opportunities to request support from others due to increased social anxiety and/or withdrawal. Likewise, social partners of individuals with AS often miss opportunities to provide support due to the subtle and atypical signals of emotional dysregulation used by this population. Specific challenges in this capacity include (1) expressing a range of emotions, (2) responding to assistance offered by

TABLE 6.1. SCERTS® Curriculum-Based Assessment: Sample Social Communication Goals and Objectives for Individuals with Asperger Syndrome

Social communication at the conversational partner stage

Joint attention

1. The individual will share attention by:
   a. securing attention to oneself prior to expressing intentions,
   b. understanding nonverbal cues of shifts in attentional focus,
   c. modifying language based on a partner's experiences, and
   d. sharing internal thoughts or mental plans with a partner.

2. The individual will share emotion by:
   a. understanding and using early and advanced emotion words,
   b. understanding and using nonverbal cues of emotional expression, and
   c. describing plausible causal factors for emotions of self and others.

3. The individual will share intentions for a variety of purposes by:
   a. sharing intentions for social interaction (e.g., greeting, regulating turns, praising partners, and expressing empathy) and
   b. sharing intentions for joint attention (e.g., commenting and requesting information on immediate, past, and imagined events, expressing feelings and opinions, and planning outcomes of social events).

4. The individual will share experiences in reciprocal interaction by:
   a. initiating a variety of conversational topics,
   b. initiating and maintaining conversations that relate to partner's interests,
   c. providing needed information based on partner's knowledge of topic, and
   d. gauging the length and content of conversational turn based on partner.

5. The individual will persist and repair communication breakdowns by:
   a. modifying communication to repair breakdowns,
   b. recognizing breakdowns in communication and requesting clarification,
   c. modifying language and behavior based upon partner's change in agenda, and
   d. modifying language and behavior based on partner's emotional reaction.

Symbol use

1. The individual will learn by imitation, observation, instruction, and collaboration by:
   a. using behaviors modeled by partners to guide behavior,
   b. using internalized rules modeled by adult instruction to guide behavior, and
   c. collaborating and negotiating with peers in problem solving.

2. The individual will understand nonverbal cues and nonliteral meanings in reciprocal interactions by:
   a. understanding nonverbal cues of turn taking and topic change,
   b. understanding nonverbal cues of emotional expression,
   c. understanding nonverbal cues and nonliteral meanings of humor, and
   d. understanding nonverbal cues of teasing, sarcasm, and deception.

3. The individual will participate conventionally in dramatic play and recreation by:
   a. using logical sequences of play about familiar and less familiar events,
   b. taking on a role and cooperating with peers in dramatic play, and
   c. participating in rule-based group recreation.

(continued)

TABLE 6.1. *(continued)*

4. The individual will use appropriate gestures and nonverbal behavior for the context and partner by:
   a. using appropriate facial expressions,
   b. using appropriate body posture and proximity, and
   c. using appropriate volume and intonation.

5. The individual will understand and use generative language to express meanings by:
   a. understanding and using a variety of sentence constructions and
   b. understanding and using connected sentences in oral and written discourse.

6. The individual will follow rules of conversation by:
   a. following conventions for initiating conversation and taking turns,
   b. following conventions for shifting topics in conversation,
   c. following conventions for ending conversation, and
   d. following conventions for politeness and register.

Note. Adapted from Prizant, B. M., Wetherby, A. M., Rubin, E., Laurent, A. C., & Rydell, P. J. (2006). *The SCERTS® Model: A comprehensive educational approach for children with autism spectrum disorders: Vol. 1. Assessment.* Baltimore: Paul H. Brookes Publishing Co. Adapted by permission.

partners, (3) responding to feedback and guidance regarding behavior, (4) requesting partner's assistance to regulate state, and (5) recovering from extreme dysregulation with the support of partners (Prizant et al., 2006).

The capacity for self-regulation is also compromised in individuals with AS (Laurent & Rubin, 2004). Because using more conventional or acceptable strategies for self-regulation relies on the ability to share an attentional focus to imitate, follow instruction, and consider the perspective of others, behaviors modeled by social partners are often missed. Likewise, an individual with AS may use behaviors that are not considerate of the perspective of others. These behaviors are frequently perceived by the larger social network as "annoying," "disruptive," or simply, "odd." Specific challenges in this capacity include (1) demonstrating availability for learning and interacting, (2) using behavior strategies to regulate arousal during familiar activities, (3) using language strategies to regulate arousal during familiar activities, (4) using metacognitive strategies (i.e., the ability to reflect and plan) to regulate arousal during familiar activities, (5) regulating emotion during new and changing situations, and (6) recovering from extreme dysregulation by oneself (Prizant et al., 2006).

Individuals with AS often continue to use early developing and/or atypical strategies to regulate their emotions and arousal beyond early childhood. Immature behaviors such as insisting on specific routines, hoarding preferred items, and averting gaze may be observed, as well as more intense strategies such as running away from social situations or lashing out at a peer or teacher. An individual who is less able to benefit from the models provided by others may develop language for self-regulation that follows more idiosyncratic patterns. Individuals with AS may initiate topics of special interest to cope with social anxiety and/or may recite the lines of a favorite video when faced with distressful social circumstances (Rydell & Prizant, 1995). When this behavior occurs, social partners may impose punitive measures, leading to increased emotional dysregulation or diminished self-esteem. Unusual patterns in self-regulation can also hasten social isolation, as the negative perception of these behaviors can create barriers to building relationships. Isolation and victimization within a social network can lead to an increased risk for depression (Little, 2001; Tantam, 2000). Thus, as discussed above, the rationale for peer training and education is clear, as fostering a climate of acceptance, in which the individual with AS feels safe and confident, is a crucial aspect of emotional regulation.

Sample goals and objectives of the SCERTS curriculum-based assessment in the domain of emotion regulation are outlined in Table 6.2 for the conversational partner with respect to the curricular components of mutual regulation and self-regulation.

INDIVIDUALIZING SUPPORTS ACROSS SOCIAL PARTNERS AND CONTEXTS

Intervention research has demonstrated a strong correlation between how communicative partners adapt their communicative styles and modify the environment with learning supports and the social-communicative competence of an individual with ASD (American Speech-Language-Hearing Association, 2006; National Research Council, 2001). An individual with AS must experience successful social interactions with partners across a range of social contexts to develop skills in both social communication and emotional regulation. Unfortunately, social partners do not have an easy task in providing these accommodations, as subtle and unconventional bids for communication while emotionally distressed can lead to frequent misinterpretations. For example, an individual with AS might be making a valiant attempt to engage socially with a peer, but have this attempt thwarted by his or her unconventional style of approaching the peer too closely. Although the peer might perceive this behavior as rude or even threatening, the behavior was not intended to send either of these signals but instead was related to core challenges associated with AS (e.g., considering another's perspective). An intervention approach can certainly address the issue of using appropriate proximity with the individual with AS, but empowering the social partners (e.g., peers, family members, and service providers) with the knowledge of why these behaviors are occurring and how to alter their own communicative style to foster success can have a more efficient impact on social exchanges. In these circumstances, social partners can be encouraged to acknowledge the bids from the individual with AS (e.g., "I look forward to talking with you about this . . . ") but to

TABLE 6.2. SCERTS® Curriculum-Based Assessment: Sample Emotional Regulation Goals and Objectives for Individuals with Asperger Syndrome

Emotional regulation at the Conversational Partner Stage

Mutual regulation

1. The individual will express a range of emotions by:
    a. understanding and using graded emotion words (e.g., *bothered, annoyed, furious*) and
    b. changing emotional expression based upon partner feedback.

2. The individual will respond to assistance offered by partners by:
    a. soothing when comforted by partners,
    b. responding to changes in partners' expression of emotion, and
    c. responding to information or strategies offered by partners.

3. The individual will respond to feedback and guidance by:
    a. considering the appropriateness of regulatory strategies and
    b. accepting ideas from partner during negotiation to reach compromise.

4. The individual will request a partner's assistance to regulate state by:
    a. sharing intentions to regulate the behavior of others such as requesting desired objects and activities, requesting help, requesting a break, and protesting/refusing to participate in undesired activities; and
    b. requesting assistance to resolve conflicts and problem-solve situations.

5. The individual will recover from extreme dysregulation with support from partners by:
    a. responding to partners' efforts to assist with recovery from dysregulation by moving away from activity and
    b. decreasing the amount of time to recover from extreme dysregulation.

Self-regulation

1. The individual will demonstrate availability for learning and interacting by:
    a. monitoring the attentional focus of a social partner,
    b. demonstrating an ability to inhibit actions and behaviors, and
    c. persisting during tasks with reasonable demands.

2. The individual will use behavioral strategies to regulate level of arousal by:
    a. using behaviors modeled by partners to regulate arousal level and
    b. using learned behaviors to engage productively in an extended activity.

3. The individual will use language strategies to regulate level of arousal by:
    a. using advanced emotion words,
    b. using graded emotion words,
    c. using language modeled by partners to regulate arousal level and
    d. using language to talk through an extended activity.

4. The individual will use metacognitive strategies to regulate level of arousal by:
    a. using self-monitoring and self-talk to guide behavior,
    b. using emotional memory to assist with regulation, and
    c. identifying and reflecting on strategies to support regulation.

(continued)

TABLE 6.2. (*continued*)

5. The individual will regulate emotion during new and changing situations by:
   a. using behavioral strategies to regulate arousal and
   b. using language strategies to regulate arousal during transitions.

6. The individual will recover from extreme dysregulation by him- or herself by:
   a. removing self from overstimulating or undesired activities and
   b. reengaging in interaction or activity after recovery from extreme
      dysregulation.

Note. Adapted from Prizant, B. M., Wetherby, A. M., Rubin, E., Laurent, A. C., & Rydell, P. J. (2006). *The SCERTS® Model: A comprehensive educational approach for children with autism spectrum disorders: Vol. 1. Assessment.* Baltimore: Paul H. Brookes Publishing Co. Adapted by permission.

also explicitly state the need for more space (e.g., "but let's sit down at the table or go outside where we will have more space").

In a similar manner, unconventional coping strategies, such as initiating a topic of special interest during a boisterous group activity in the classroom, might be perceived as disruptive and disrespectful to the group. However, it may also be a result of that individual's increased anxiety with the task demands and the lack of a clear and predictable end point to the task. Therefore, although a plan might be developed to support the use of more socially conventional coping strategies (e.g., asking for help or a break), training the social partners to recognize signals of distress and to provide support further enhances a climate wherein the individual with AS feels accepted and safe. In this circumstance, service providers could be encouraged to label the individual's emotions (e.g., "I can tell that you're frustrated . . . ") and to model coping strategies (e.g., "Let's write down the steps we need to complete this task").

Whereas a range of strategies is available that focuses on the individual's acquisition of targeted skills in isolated teaching sessions, the SCERTS Model has been designed to ensure that social partners make adjustments and are accountable for these adjustments across natural routines and social contexts (Prizant et al., 2006). In the SCERTS curriculum-based assessment, the domain of transactional support (TS) provides an ongoing assessment of the consistency with which an individual is provided with interpersonal supports and learning supports across partners and contexts (i.e., school, home, and community). *Interpersonal supports* refer to the communicative style adjustments made by social partners and include the ability to (1) respond to the individual's needs, (2) foster initiation, (3) respect the individual's independence and intentions, (4) set the stage for engagement, (5) provide developmental support, (6) adjust language input to an individual's developmental level and arousal state, and (7) model appropriate behaviors. *Learning supports* refer to the modifications that are made to the environment (e.g., visual and organizational structures) and the provision of alternative and augmentative communication (AAC) supports that foster the ability to establish shared attention, attend to relevant social stimuli in the environment, and predict the actions of social partners (Rubin, Laurent, Prizant & Wetherby, 2008). Sample goals and objectives of the SCERTS curriculum-based assessment in the domain of TS are outlined in Table 6.3 for the Conversational Partner Stage under the components of interpersonal support and learning support.

When social partners embed learning supports across natural activities, these accommodations take on different forms based on the unique circumstances and demands of the social setting. Likewise, how these partners adapt their interactive style for an individual should differ based on that individual's unique learning style differences and preferences for modes of instruction (e.g., visual, written, verbal, kinesthetic) (Tsatsanis et al., 2004). Additionally, it is important to note that addressing social skills development for the individual with AS should not take the form of overly simplified methodologies that suggest a one-to-one correspondence between an interpersonal support or learning support and social communication and emotional regulation goals. Rather, it is more likely that the partner will need to make a number of conscious changes in these areas to make a significant impact on a specific aspect of an individual's social communication or emotional regulation profile. As a result, it is important to continually monitor the effectiveness of specific interpersonal and learning supports in different social situations. The following sections provide an illustration of the influence of partner behavior and TS goals on an achievement of social communication and emotional regulation based upon evidence-based practices in the field. This material is not intended to provide specific instructions or guidelines, merely examples of the variables to consider when developing an individualized plan.

THE INFLUENCE OF PARTNER BEHAVIOR ON SOCIAL COMMUNICATION

Joint Attention

Addressing Shared Attention

An individual's ability to establish *shared attention* and achieve related objectives, such as *modifying his or her use of language based on a partner's experiences* (e.g., what he or she has seen or heard), is related to a partner's ability to make accommodations that involve both interpersonal and learning supports. The provision of interpersonal support might include a partner's learning how to more explicitly *share emotions, internal states, and mental plans with the individual*. The provision of learning support might include a partner's learning how to *use augmentative communication support to foster the individual's understanding of language and behavior*. An individual who is developing an ability to modify the amount

TABLE 6.3. SCERTS® Curriculum-Based Assessment: Sample Transactional Support Goals and Objectives

Transactional support at the Conversational Partner Stage

Interpersonal support

1. Partners will be responsive to the individual by:
    a. attuning to the emotion and pace of the individual,
    b. responding to subtle communicative signals,
    c. recognizing signs of dysregulation and offering support, and
    d. providing information or assistance to regulate state.

2. Partners will foster initiation by:
    a. offering choices,
    b. waiting for and encouraging initiation, and
    c. providing a balance between initiated and respondent turns.

3. Partners will respect the independence of the individual by:
    a. allowing the individual to take breaks to move about as needed,
    b. providing time for the individual to solve problems or complete activities at own pace,
    c. interpreting problem behaviors as communicative and/or regulatory, and
    d. honoring protests, rejections, or refusals when appropriate.

4. Partners will set the stage for engagement by:
    a. securing individual's attention prior to communicating,
    b. using appropriate proximity and nonverbal behavior to encourage interaction, and
    c. sharing emotions, internal states, and mental plans.

5. Partners will provide developmental support by:
    a. providing guidance for success in interacting with peers,
    b. attempting to repair breakdowns in communication,
    c. providing guidance on expressing emotions and understanding the cause of emotion, and
    d. providing guidance on interpreting others' feelings and opinions.

6. Partners will adjust language input by:
    a. using nonverbal cues to support understanding,
    b. adjusting complexity of language input to individual's developmental level, and
    c. adjusting complexity of language input to individual's arousal level.

7. Partners will model appropriate behavior by:
    a. modeling appropriate nonverbal communication and emotional expressions,
    b. modeling a range of communicative functions,
    c. modeling appropriate behavior when individual using inappropriate behavior, and
    d. modeling the use of self-talk.

Learning support

1. Partners will structure activities for active participation by:
    a. defining a clear beginning and ending to activity,
    b. providing a predictable sequence to activity, and
    c. offering repeated learning opportunities.

(continued)

TABLE 6.3. (*continued*)

2. Partners will use augmentative communication support to foster development by:
   a. using visual or written support to enhance communication and expressive language,
   b. using visual or written support to enhance understanding of language and social behavior,
   c. using visual or written support to enhance emotional expression, and
   d. using visual or written support to enhance emotional regulation.

3. Partners will use visual and organizational support by:
   a. defining steps within a task,
   b. enhancing smooth transitions between activities, and
   c. enhancing active involvement in group activities.

4. Partners will modify the goals, activities, and learning environment by:
   a. adjusting the social complexity to support organization and interaction,
   b. adjusting task difficulty,
   c. modifying the sensory properties of the environment,
   d. arranging the environment to promote initiation,
   e. infusing motivating and meaningful materials and topics into activities, and
   f. alternating between movement and sedentary activities as needed.

Note. From Prizant, B. M., Wetherby, A. M., Rubin, E., Laurent, A. C., & Rydell, P. J. (2006). *The SCERTS® Model: A comprehensive educational approach for children with autism spectrum disorders: Vol. 1. Assessment.* Baltimore: Paul H. Brookes Publishing Co. Adapted by permission.

of information provided in a conversational exchange may benefit from having peers coached to explicitly and verbally state when they need more information, as their nonverbal social cues (e.g., facial expressions of confusion) can be elusive to the individual with AS (Klin, 2000). Provision of this type of social feedback by training typically developing peers has been shown to lead to increased social skills in the classroom setting (Thiemann & Goldstein, 2004). Additionally, the use of augmentative communication support may further reinforce the individual's ability to modify language based upon knowledge of a partner's unique experiences. For example, the use of a written chart that illustrates critical pieces of information about one's conversational partners (e.g., their favorite topics, what experiences they have had, their favorite activities) could be provided by the social partners (Winner, 2002, p. 40). The individual could then be encouraged to access these supports in a convenient form (e.g., a pocket-sized "conversation starter" book) before interacting with a peer as a means to increase competence in topic selection and topic maintenance across social situations. Charlop-Christy and Kelso (2003) found that these types of written supports can be effective tools that partners can provide to encourage increased topic maintenance and the provision of background information across settings.

Addressing Shared Emotion

An individual's ability to establish *shared emotion* and achieve related objectives, such as *understanding nonverbal cues of emotional expression* and *describing plausible causal factors for the emotions of self and others,* is related to a partner's ability to make accommodations that involve both interpersonal and learning supports. Interpersonal support might include a partner's learning how to more explicitly *provide guidance for interpreting other's feelings and opinions.* The provision of learning support might include a partner's learning how to *use visual or written support to enhance emotion expression.* An individual who is developing an ability to describe plausible causal factors for emotions of self and others may benefit from the guidance and support of a partner in a small-group context who might serve as a "coach" for interpreting other's feelings and opinions. Partners in these contexts might use cognitive picture rehearsal strategies as helpful tools (Groden & LeVasseur, 1995) or a strategy referred to as *comic strip conversations* as a way to visually depict conversations (Gray, 1995; Kerr & Durkin, 2004).

These methods depict an individual's actions and their consequences on others using sequences of pictures sketched on, for example, a dry erase board or a piece of paper. A coach might sketch out the people involved in a social scenario, what they are saying using a "talking balloon," and their potential thoughts using "thought bubbles" to support the individual's ability to make "educated guesses" as to their emotional state and plausible causal factors (Winner, 2002, p. 52). For the individual with strengths in verbal memory, as is often the case in those with AS, the use of verbal mediation and/or written language cues may also be helpful for facilitating the use of a script that encourages breaking down the process of interpreting social cues to derive meaning (Volkmar et al., 2000). Winner (2002) provides guidelines for scripting the essential steps of social thinking and reflection on another's emotions (p. 42). These types of learning supports (e.g., visually depicted conversations and scripts), paired with the provision of the interpersonal support of social coaching, have been found to be effective supports for improving the understanding of another's emotions (Kerr & Durkin, 2004; Parsons & Mitchell, 1999; Wellman et al., 2002).

Addressing Sharing Intentions for a Variety of Purposes

An individual's ability to *share intentions for a variety of purposes* and achieve related objectives, such as *sharing intentions for social interaction—taking turns, praising partners, and expressing empathy—and sharing intentions for joint attention—commenting and requesting information about immediate, past, and future events—*is related to a partner's ability to make accommodations that involve both interpersonal and learning supports. The provision of interpersonal support might include a partner's learning how to *model a range of communicative functions* and *how to provide a balance between initiated and respondent turns.* The provision of learning support might include a partner's learning how to *use augmentative communication support to enhance an individual's communication and expressive language.*

An individual who is learning the function of praising a communicative partner may benefit from having peers trained to provide the interpersonal support of modeling these statements throughout natural activities as well as the learning support of a written model. In an elementary school gym class, for example, the teacher might remind each of the students to praise each other following turns in a given game, and the learning support of a "teamwork banner" on the wall provides the same information in written form (e.g., "Teammates let each other know when they are doing well!"). Additional augmentative communication support could then be added by having the teacher take photographs and/or videos of students displaying targeted behaviors and pairing these visuals with written or verbal models for self-talk (e.g., "We give each other high fives," "We can use our special hand shakes," "We can do the wave"). Video modeling has been used successfully for fostering these types of social interactions and shows nice promise in ensuring that targeted skills generalize across contexts (Charlop-Christy, Le, & Freeman, 2000; Nikopoulous & Keenan, 2004).

An individual who is learning to request information from others in a conversational exchange may benefit from having peers coached to provide the interpersonal support of pausing for an extended period of time following their conversational turn to provide a greater balance of initiated and respondent turns. Likewise, the provision of learning support, such as an augmentative communication support to visually illustrate the balance between comments and questions in a conversational exchange, might be helpful. One side of a laminated board could display the written cue, "I can make a comment," and the other side could display "I can ask a question." As the conversation unfolds, a small visual cue such as a penny could be placed under the "I can make a comment" side of the board to provide visual feedback. Then, with each question posed by the individual, a larger visual cue such as a quarter could be placed under the "I can ask a question" side of the board. These visual aids highlight the notion that asking a question is more "valuable," as one gains information related to partner perspective.

Addressing the Ability to Share Experiences in Reciprocal Interaction

An individual's ability to *share experiences in reciprocal interaction* and achieve related objectives, such as *initiating and maintaining conversations related to a partner's interests,* is related to a partner's ability to make accommodations that involve both interpersonal and learning supports.

The provision of interpersonal support might include a partner's leaning how to *provide guidance for success in interaction with peers*. The provision of learning support might include a partner's learning to *use augmentative communication to enhance an individual's understanding of language and behavior*. An individual who is developing an ability to modify the amount of information provided in a conversational exchange may need explicit guidance from a supportive partner to develop a personal "fact file" on those peers and adults who are frequent conversational partners (McAfee, 2002, p. 100). These types of supports involve the use of simple index cards to keep track of conversational topics that might interest a particular partner. This support could be paired with the learning support of a "conversation starter" chart that may be helpful for illustrating the important steps that are necessary to take prior to starting a conversation. These steps might include identifying what the person knows or enjoys talking about (based on his or her "personal file"), what comments or questions might be relevant to that topic, and whether an initiation is appropriate given the current social context (McAfee, 2002, p. 101). The use of written and verbal scripts has been found to be effective in supporting and fostering increased bids for social engagement (Charlop-Christy & Kelso, 2003; Goldstein & Cisar, 1992).

Addressing Persisting and Repairing Communication Breakdowns

An individual's ability to *persist and repair communication breakdowns* and achieve related objectives, such as *modifying language based on a partner's emotional reaction*, is related to a partner's ability to make accommodations that involve both interpersonal and learning supports. The provision of interpersonal support might include a partner's learning how to more explicitly *share his or her emotions, internal states, and mental plans*. The provision of learning support might include a partner's learning how to *use visual support to foster active engagement in group activities*. Individuals who have difficulty recognizing that their topic of conversation is not being well received, perhaps due to its repetitive nature, would benefit from partners who are willing to rate their interest in a given topic. The individual with AS thereby develops an awareness that not all topics are equally received by a given partner. Adding humor to reduce the impact of negative feedback, the partner might indicate whether a given topic is "like a recipe in that it is predictable and has been heard before," "like a storm in that it is confusing and complicated," or "like a thrill ride in that it is intriguing, novel, and fun." A visual, wallet-sized conversation starter could then be generated to remind the individual with AS how peers have rated given topics so that he or she can select them more appropriately across social settings. Emphasizing peer training and the role of partners in this aspect of development is critical. When peers use more explicit language to indicate their emotional state and their intentions, the individual with the social disability is more successful (see Paul, 2003, for a review of peer-mediated interventions).

Symbol Use

Addressing the Ability to Learn by Imitation, Observation, Instruction, and Collaboration

An individual's ability to *learn by imitation, observation, instruction, and collaboration* and achieve related objectives, such as *using internalized rules modeled by adult instruction to guide behavior*, is related to the ability of a partner to make accommodations that involve both interpersonal and learning supports. The provision of interpersonal support might include, for example, a partner's learning how to *respond to subtle communicative signals* and *model person–perspective language and the use of self-talk*. The provision of learning support might include a partner's learning how to *provide augmentative communication support to enhance emotional regulation*. If an individual with AS is currently using unconventional strategies for specific social functions of communication, peers, partners, and/ or service providers could be trained to understand the function of these behaviors and to model person–perspective language for more adaptive strategies to serve that same function. For example, the individual might be using the strategy of blowing in a peer's ear to solicit attention while a teacher is talking. A trained peer might model the statement, "Remember, I can talk to my friends when my teacher is finished speaking," and a trained instructional assistant might model, "I can refill my pencil leads when I am listening to my teacher." The instructional assistant may also have access to a key ring that provides visual models for these different statements of self-talk. Modeling person–perspective language and the use of self-talk can be an effective strategy for promoting more adaptive social skills (Barry & Burlew, 2004; Gray, 1995).

Addressing an Understanding of Nonverbal Cues and Nonliteral Meanings in Reciprocal Interactions

An individual's ability to *understand nonverbal cues and nonliteral meanings in reciprocal interactions* and achieve related objectives, such as *understanding nonverbal cues of turn taking and topic change*, is related to a partner's ability to make accommodations that involve both interpersonal and learning supports. The provision of interpersonal support might include, for example, a partner's learning how to *model appropriate nonverbal communication and emotional expressions*. The provision of learning support might include a partner's learning how to *use an augmentative communication support to enhance an individual's understanding of language and behavior*.

For an individual who is developing an ability to understand nonverbal cues of turn taking and topic change, a model of peer training can be helpful to ensure that the partner is modeling these cues in a clear and predictable manner. Likewise, the provision of an augmentative communication support such as a "clue chart" for topic change might be helpful. For example, an individual with AS may initially need very explicit and exaggerated cues signaling a desire for topic change as he or she persists about a subject that is of little interest to a particular peer. Peers could be coached to display friendly signals such as leaning on their palm in boredom, tapping on their watches, or looking away with disinterest. Likewise, partners can provide a clue chart with several of these signals illustrated or depicted in writing so the individual with AS has a static guide to refer to during a group conversation. This clue chart could be modified for other social situations. In a classroom lecture, for example, the chart could be posted on the front wall and include pictures of the teacher writing on the board or talking to the class. These photos could be paired with the statement "I can talk later" to remind the individual that these signals indicate it is the teacher's turn in the conversation. A photograph could be included of the teacher pointing toward the class along with the statement "I can raise my hand now," indicating that the turn of conversation is shifting. Providing explicit guidance or verbal mediation for individuals with AS can help to compensate for their difficulties in attributing meaning to visual stimuli (Volkmar et al., 2000).

Addressing the Ability to Participate Conventionally in Dramatic Play and Recreation

An individual's ability to *participate conventionally in dramatic play and recreation* and achieve related objectives, such as *participating in rule-based group recreation,* is related to a partner's ability to make accommodations that involve both interpersonal and learning supports. The provision of interpersonal support might include a partner's learning how to *model appropriate dramatic play and recreation* activities, and the provision of learning support might include a partner's learning how to *provide a predictable sequence to an activity.* Learning the rules of a complex recreational activity within a group setting can pose significant challenges for an individual with AS. Being able to derive the intent of the game, predict the reactions of peers within the game, and predict the steps toward completion involve core challenges in shared attention. These challenges are further intensified in the presence of a large group due to the increased anxiety that often arises in response to complex social stimuli in such settings. The opportunity to have the steps of the game modeled in a small group or with one other individual provides a context for exposure with less emotional dysregulation. Additionally, this support allows for role play in which the peer and the individual with AS can act out mock scenarios to prepare for the various directions the game may turn in the larger group. This practice provides the learning support of ensuring that there is a predictable sequence to follow and "primes" the individual with AS for the actual event. Koegel, Koegel, Frea, and Green-Hopkins (2003) found priming to be an effective learning support for rehearsing academic and social situations in a classroom environment.

Addressing the Use of Gestures and Nonverbal Behavior Appropriate for the Context and Partner

An individual's ability to *use gestures and nonverbal behavior appropriate for the context and partner* and achieve related objectives, such as *using appropriate volume and intonation,* is related to a partner's ability to make accommodations that involve both interpersonal and learning supports. The provision of interpersonal support might include a partner's ability to *model appropriate behavior when the individual uses inappropriate behavior.* The provision of learning support might include a partner's use of *an augmentative communication support to enhance an individual's communication and expressive language.* A partner's modeling of appropriate volume and intonation, coupled with the use of a visual support to cue these gestures and behaviors in different contexts, may facilitate a greater understanding of how and when to use these nonverbal signals (Volkmar et al., 2000). For example, during quiet work time, an adult facilitator could model an appropriate nonverbal strategy for securing another's attention in this context by whispering when calling on students in the class and talking with students. A "voice-volume dial," placed at the front of the class or in close proximity to each student, could visually represent the current volume of an individual's voice and where it should be, depending upon the context, using color codes and a sliding arrow for "too quiet," "just right," and "too loud." If the individual uses a vocal volume judged to be "too loud," a social partner might model the appropriate volume paired with a person–perspective statements such as, "When I need help, I use a quiet voice to talk with my teacher." Using this visual and interpersonal support in varying contexts may help facilitate a more specific understanding of the level of vocal volume expected in different circumstances (e.g., the library vs. the gymnasium).

Addressing the Understanding and Use of Generative Language to Express Meanings

An individual's ability to *understand and use generative language to express meanings* and achieve related objectives, such as *understanding and using sentences in oral and written discourse,* is related to a partner's ability to make accommodations that involve both interpersonal and learning supports. The provision of interpersonal support might include a partner's learning to *adjust the complexity of language input to an individual's developmental level.* The provision of learning support might include a partner's learning to *use an augmentative communication support to enhance an individual's communication and expressive language.* Although individuals with AS often demonstrate strengths in verbal language comprehension and memory, the use of higher-level syntactic conjunctions, such as those used specifically to clarify one's intentions to a listener or, in the case of written discourse, a reader (Volkmar et al., 2000), are typically missing. Essential details are often omitted, such as where an event took place, how the individual was feeling, and when it occurred. An individual who is developing an ability to use sentences in connected oral discourse might benefit from partners who enhance model sentence constructions that are connected with temporal and causal conjunctions (e.g., "The teacher is riding on a school bus with the class *because* they are all going on a field trip. *After* they arrived at the zoo, the class stood in line to pay their admission"). Likewise, the use of augmentative communication support may further reinforce this achievement during narrative activities. For example, a cartoon storyboard may be helpful in illustrating the important pieces of information to include when providing the steps that took place in the narrative as well as the internal plans of the characters and the consequences of their actions on other characters. Comic strip conversations (Gray, 1998) might also be useful for this function, as the inclusion of thought bubbles to illustrate what each character was thinking and the impact of their actions on others might increase the complexity of oral and narrative discourse.

Addressing the Rules of Conversation

An individual's ability to *follow the rules of conversation* and achieve related objectives, such as *following conventions for initiating conversation and taking turns*, is related to a partner's ability to make accommodations that involve both interpersonal and learning supports. The provision of interpersonal support might include a partner's learning how to *model appropriate behavior when an individual uses inappropriate behavior.* The provision of learning support might include a partner's ability to *use a visual support to enhance active engagement in group activities.* An individual who is developing an ability to follow conventions for initiating conversations and taking turns may benefit from opportunities to practice these skills with peers who are able to model them appropriately (Strain & Kohler, 1998). Additionally, a partner's use of augmentative communication support to foster a greater awareness of the subtleties of conversation (e.g., the need to remain on topic, gauge the length of a conversational turn, and limit interruptions) can be beneficial (Charlop-Christy & Kelso, 2003). Winner (2002) describes the use of a visual support, which she refers to as a "Conversation Street." With this support, social conventions are illustrated visually and verbally using the metaphor of driving. For example, if the individual is in the "carpool lane," he or she is sharing the topic with others by asking relevant questions. In contrast, an individual may receive a "speeding ticket" for "talking too fast."

THE INFLUENCE OF PARTNER BEHAVIOR ON EMOTIONAL REGULATION

Mutual Regulation

Addressing the Ability to Express a Range of Emotions

An individual's *ability to express a range of emotions* and achieve related objectives, such as *understanding and using graded emotions*, is related to a partner's ability to make accommodations that involve both interpersonal and learning supports. The provision of interpersonal support might involve a partner's learning how to *recognize signals of dysregulation and offer support* and *modeling person–perspective language and the use of self-talk*. Additionally, the provision of learning support might include a partner's learning how to *use an augmentative communication support to enhance an individual's expression and understanding of emotion*. Individuals with AS may display extremely intense emotional states, appearing to rise quickly from the absence of an emotion to an intense expression of that emotion (Laurent & Rubin, 2004). Facilitating an understanding and use of graded emotions begins as partners are coached to model language for graded emotions (e.g., *bothered, angry,* and *furious*) along with clear descriptions of the vocal volume and nonverbal behaviors that would be expected at these lower to higher intensities. Next, a visual support might be useful for representing the emotion intensity with a color-coded numerical scale (e.g., "I am 2 angry right now" vs. "I am a 5 furious right now!"). McAfee (2002) provides visual illustrations of "emotion scales" and of a "stress thermometer," which allow partners to keep track of signals of stress and possible relaxation techniques (p. 317).

Addressing the Ability to Respond to Assistance Offered by Partners

An individual's *ability to respond to assistance offered by partners* and achieve related objectives, such as *responding to information or strategies offered by partners*, is related to a partner's ability to make accommodations that involve both interpersonal and learning supports. The provision of interpersonal support might include a partner's learning how to *recognize signs of dysregulation and offer support*. The provision of learning support might include a partner's *use of augmentative communication support to enhance an individual's understanding of language and behavior*. As noted above, an individual with AS may have difficulty with accepting mutual regulation secondary to challenges in predicting the actions of others and the resulting anxiety that these challenges create for that individual. Thus, partners are faced with the challenging task of attempting to build trust by becoming a predictable source of emotional support for that individual. Developing a chart of the individual's subtle signals of emotional distress (e.g., averting gaze, biting fingernails, rubbing bits of eraser between one's fingers) paired with a list of possible coping strategies might be a useful starting point to ensure that partners are providing consistent responses to these subtle and unconventional signals. Next, the use of supports such as Social Stories™ (Gray, 1995) might be helpful for providing language to indicate possible strategies for emotional regulation (e.g., "When I am feeling frustrated, I can ask for help"). Because individuals learn more conventional strategies for self-regulation through mutual regulation, this goal can be critical for achieving positive long-term outcomes in emotional regulation (Laurent & Rubin, 2004).

Addressing the Ability to Respond to Feedback and Guidance Regarding Behavior

An individual's *ability to respond to feedback and guidance regarding behavior* and achieve related objectives, such as *accepting ideas from partners during negotiation to reach compromise,* is related to a partner's ability to make accommodations that involve both interpersonal and learning supports. The provision of interpersonal support might include a partner's learning how to *provide guidance for interpreting others' feelings and opinions.* The provision of learning support might include a partner's *use of augmentative communication support to enhance an individual's emotional regulation.* The use of comic strip conversations (as described above) has shown promise as a technique for helping individuals with AS compensate for their difficulties in comprehending the intentions of others (Gray, 1995; Kerr & Durkin, 2004). This strategy, implemented on a dry erase board, can be used to illustrate the different ideas of partners during a negotiation. A multiple-choice list of strategies to achieve compromise can be presented, and, once selected by the individual and his or her partners, the thought bubbles could be erased and modified to illustrate the concept of persuasion—that is, a discussion can lead to a change in perspective.

Addressing the Ability to Request Partner's Assistance to Regulate State

An individual's ability to *request a partner's assistance to regulate state* and achieve related objectives, such as *sharing intentions to regulate the behavior of others (e.g., requesting desired objects and activities, requesting help, requesting a break),* is related to a partner's ability to make accommodations that involve both interpersonal and learning supports. The provision of interpersonal support might involve a partner's learning of how to *model person–perspective language and the use of self talk*. The provision of learning support might involve a partner's *using augmentative communication support to enhance an individual's emotional regulation*. As individuals with AS have difficulty predicting the actions of others, the ability to predict that a social partner might provide assistance when distressed can be compromised. These individuals often benefit from partners who model a variety of self-talk strategies (e.g., "If I'm frustrated, I can ask an adult for help"), as well as provide the individual with written cues that may help to trigger the use of these self-talk strategies across the day. A teacher may wear a lanyard attached to a series of index cards listing a range of emotions on one side and a variety of possible requests for assistance on the reverse.

Addressing the Ability to Recover from Extreme Dysregulation with Support from Partners

An individual's ability to *recover from extreme dysregulation with support from partners* and achieve related objectives, such as *responding to partners' efforts to assist with recovery from dysregulation by moving away from the activity,* is related to a partner's ability to make accommodations that involve both interpersonal and learning supports. The provision of interpersonal support might include a partner's learning to *recognize signs of dysregulation, to offer coping strategies*, and when to *allow the individual to take breaks to move about as needed.* The provision of learning support might include a partner's learning how to *modify the sensory properties of the environment.* An individual learning to recover from extreme dysregulation might benefit from partners who modify the environment to include a safe area for "escaping" that is always available throughout the day. For an individual in school settings, this might involve developing an arrangement with a staff member such as a school counselor, nurse, or even librarian, who might be willing to provide a quiet room with minimal consequences. Interpersonal supports are also critical for reinforcing this achievement, as staff members may benefit from training to pick up on the early signals of emotional dysregulation so that they can quickly and proactively recommend taking a break before an individual has reached extreme dysregulation.

Self-Regulation

Addressing Availability for Learning and Interacting

An individual's overall *availability for learning and interacting* and ability to achieve related objectives, such as *persisting during tasks with reasonable demands,* is related to a partner's ability to make accommodations that involve both interpersonal and learning supports. The provision of interpersonal support might include a partner's learning to *provide information or assistance to support self-regulation*. The provision of learning support might then include a partner's learning how to *infuse motivating and meaningful materials and topics into activities*. For example, an individual with AS might have difficulty coping with academic tasks that are more rote in nature, as the ability to derive meaning as to the purpose of this task and when it may be useful in the future may be compromised. Thus, individuals in these scenarios might be either agitated or bored when presented with an assignment with rote elements. Rather than imposing punitive measures, the individual with AS might benefit from the provision of explicit verbal guidance for expressing emotion (e.g., "This is boring . . . ") and explicit verbal guidance for stating coping strategies (e.g., "When I am bored, I can ask whether a preferred activity is coming and how many items are left"). In order to develop persistence with a range of tasks, infusing motivating and meaningful materials and topics into less desirable tasks/activities will likely ensure more active engagement (American Speech-Language-Hearing Association, 2006, p. 26).

Addressing the Use of Behavioral Strategies to Regulate Arousal during Familiar Activities

An individual's ability to use *behavioral strategies to regulate their level of arousal during familiar activities* and achieve related objectives such as *using behavioral strategies modeled by partners to regulate arousal level*, is related to a partner's ability to make accommodations that involve both interpersonal and learning supports. The provision of interpersonal support might include a partner's learning to *interpret problem behavior as communicative and/or regulatory*. The provision of learning support might include a partner's ability to *use augmentative communication support to enhance the individual's emotional regulation*. Partners play a critical role in modeling more conventional and appropriate behaviors to self-regulate (Laurent & Rubin, 2004). This role, however, is most effective when partners recognize the function of idiosyncratic behaviors used by the individual with AS for these self-regulatory functions. Examples might include humming to oneself to block out the sounds of peers talking in a loud classroom, walking on one's toes to calm an agitated nervous system, and chewing on one's clothing when underaroused or bored by a task. In the case of this latter example of chewing on one's clothing, a partner's recognition of the regulatory function enables a response such as "I can tell you are bored; when I'm bored, I can ask if it is all right to get a cold drink of water to wake up, run an errand, or go for a brisk walk." These strategies should be highly individualized, based on the individual's learning style and educational setting (e.g., elementary vs. high school settings). A visual support could also be made available with written reminders of these types of alternative coping strategies.

Addressing Language Strategies to Regulate Arousal during Familiar Activities

An individual's ability to *use language strategies to regulate level of arousal during familiar activities* and achieve related objectives, such as *understanding and using advanced emotion words,* is related to a partner's ability to make accommodations that involve both interpersonal and learning supports. The provision of interpersonal support might include a partner's learning how to *provide information to support self-regulation.* The provision of learning support might include the partner's ability to *use an augmentative communication support to enhance the individual's expression and understanding of emotion.* An individual may develop an ability to use advanced emotion words as a result of a partner's use of an augmentative communication support such as the *Feelings Book* (Rubin & Laurent, 2002). This tool facilitates an individual's ability to identify both positive and negative emotional states in natural social contexts while also providing written language models for person–perspective language for emotional expression (e.g., "I feel frustrated when . . . ") and models for person–perspective language for emotional regulation (e.g., "When I'm frustrated, I can go for a walk").

Addressing the Use of Metacognitive Strategies to Regulate Arousal during Familiar Activities

An individual's ability to *use metacognitive strategies to regulate level of arousal during familiar activities* and achieve related objectives, such as *using self-monitoring and self-talk to guide behavior,* is related to a partner's ability to make accommodations that involve both interpersonal and learning supports. The provision of interpersonal support might include a partner's ability to *model the use of person–perspective language and self-talk.* The provision of learning support might include *organizing segments of time across the day* and the *use of visual and organizational support to define steps within a task.* An individual developing the ability to use self-monitoring and self-talk to guide behavior might benefit from a partner's creation of a "check-off system" by listing all the steps required before completion of an activity. Provision of this support might enhance an individual's use of language to independently talk through the steps of a task for him- or herself (Bryan & Gast, 2000; Laurent & Rubin, 2004; Pierce & Schreibman, 1994).

Addressing the Ability to Regulate Emotion during New and Changing Situations

An individual's ability to *regulate emotion during new and changing situations* and achieve related objectives, such as *using language strategies to regulate arousal during transitions,* is related to a partner's ability to make accommodations that involve both interpersonal and learning supports.

The provision of interpersonal support might include a partner's learning how to *recognize signs of dysregulation and offer support* and to *model appropriate behavior when the individual uses inappropriate behavior.* The provision of learning support might include the *use of an augmentative communication support to enhance an individual's emotional regulation* and *the use of support to organize segments of time across the day.* For example, an individual's ability to use language strategies to regulate arousal during transitions may be influenced by the consistency with which partners are able to read signals of dysregulation and offer support by modeling self-talk (e.g., "If I'm angry, I can . . . " or "If I'm tired, I can . . . "). In addition, the individual's partners may spend time reviewing a written list of the day's activities prior to the daily routines in an effort to help the individual anticipate transitions (Laurent & Rubin, 2004).

Addressing the Ability to Recover from Extreme Dysregulation by Self

An individual's *ability to recover from extreme dysregulation* and achieve related objectives, such as *reengaging in interaction or activity after recovery from extreme dysregulation,* is related to a partner's ability to make accommodations that involve both interpersonal and learning supports. The provision of interpersonal support might include a partner's willingness to *allow the individual to take breaks and move about as needed* and for the partner to *interpret problem behavior as communicative and/ or regulatory.* The provision of learning support may include a partner's ability to *adjust the social complexity to support organization and interaction.* For example, facilitating an individual's ability to reengage in an interaction after recovering from extreme dysregulation relies on a partner's ability to recognize that the individual's behavior (e.g., leaving the classroom, drawing on his or her desk, putting his or her head down on the table) may have been a result of emotional dysregulation and not simply a lack of cooperation. This interpersonal support, followed by the provision of adequate time to "regroup," is likely to have a positive influence on the individual by fostering his or her trust in the interpersonal environment. Likewise, environmental arrangements such as providing a "safety zone" that an individual can access independently may enhance his or her success with reengaging in a social activity after being extremely distressed.

FUTURE RESEARCH

Because social-communicative competence is correlated with positive long-term outcomes for individuals with AS and remains one of the most vulnerable aspects of development for this population, addressing this core challenge is an essential part of addressing social skills development (National Research Council, 2001; Tsatsanis et al., 2004). The SCERTS curriculum-based assessment has been derived from descriptive group research studies indicating that developmental achievements in the domains of social communication and emotional regulation are predictive of gains in language development, adaptive social functioning, and academic achievement—all critical areas that foster social competence (Prizant et al., 2006). Within this assessment process, gains related to social-communicative competence must be observable across social partners and social contexts, and partners are held accountable for the provision of supports in these contexts. Furthermore, the assessment provides a measure of partner behavior that can ensure fidelity across partners and contexts. Future research is needed to ensure that the SCERTS curriculum-based assessment provides a reliable measure of progress for the individual with AS as well as a reliable indicator of fidelity across social partners and settings. Next steps might include exploring the relative impact of the presence or absence of specific interpersonal supports or learning supports on specific social communication and emotional regulation abilities.

ACKNOWLEDGMENTS

I would like to extend appreciation to colleagues Barry M. Prizant, PhD, Amy M. Wetherby, PhD, and Amy C. Laurent, EdM, OTR/L.

REFERENCES

American Speech-Language-Hearing Association. (2006). *Guidelines for speech–language pathologists in diagnosis, assessment, and treatment of autism spectrum disorders across the life span.* Retrieved December 23, 2007, from *www.asha.org/NR/rdonlyres/8D2CE221-E7E6-4B60-AAF4-76C13BD8B6A6/0/v3GL_autismLSpan.pdf.*

Barry, L. M., & Burlew, S. B. (2004). Using Social Stories to teach choice and play skills to children with autism. *Focus on Autism and Other Developmental Disabilities, 19,* 45–51.

Bryan, L. C., & Gast, D. L. (2000). Teaching on-task and on-schedule behaviors to higher functioning children with autism via picture activity schedules. *Journal of Autism and Developmental Disorders, 30,* 553–567.

Capps, L., Yirmiya, N., & Sigman, M. D. (1992). Understanding of simple and complex emotions in non-retarded children with autism. *Journal of Child Psychology and Psychiatry, 33,* 1169–1182.

Charlop-Christy, M. H., & Kelso, S. E. (2003). Teaching children with autism conversational speech using a cue card/written script program. *Education and Treatment of Children, 26,* 103–127.

Charlop-Christy, M. H., Le, L., & Freeman, K. A. (2000). A comparison of video modeling with in vivo modeling for teaching children with autism. *Journal of Autism and Developmental Disorders, 30,* 537–552.

Gilchrist, A., Green, J., Cox, A., Burton, D., Rutter, M., & Le Couteur, A. (2001). Development and current functioning in adolescents with Asperger syndrome:

A comparative study. *Journal of Child Psychology, Psychiatry, and Allied Disciplines, 42*(2), 227–240.

Goldstein, H., & Cisar, C. L. (1992). Promoting interaction during sociodramatic play: Teaching scripts to typical preschoolers and classmates with disabilities. *Journal of Applied Behavior Analysis, 25,* 265–280.

Gray, C. A. (1995). Teaching children with autism to "read" social situations. In K. Quill (Ed.), *Teaching children with autism: Strategies to enhance communication and socialization* (pp. 219–241). Albany, NY: Delmar.

Gray, C. A. (1998). Social Stories and comic strip conversations with students with Asperger syndrome and high-functioning autism. In E. Schoper, G. B. Mesibov, & L. Kunce (Eds.), *Asperger syndrome or high-functioning autism* (pp. 167–199). New York: Plenum Press.

Groden, J., & LeVasseur, P. (1995). Cognitive picture rehearsal: A system to teach self-control. In K. A. Quill (Ed.), *Teaching children with autism: Strategies to enhance communication and socialization* (pp. 287–305). Albany, NY: Delmar.

Heider, F., & Simmel, M. (1944). An experimental study of apparent behavior. *American Journal of Psychology, 57*(2), 243–259.

Kerr, S., & Durkin, K. (2004). Understanding of thought bubbles as mental representations in children with autism: Implications for theory of mind. *Journal of Autism and Developmental Disorders, 34,* 637–648.

Klin, A. (2000). Attributing social meaning to ambiguous visual stimuli in higher functioning autism and Asperger syndrome: The social attribution task. *Journal of Child Psychology and Psychiatry, 41,* 831–846.

Klin, A., Jones, W., Schultz, R., Volkmar, F. R., & Cohen, D. J. (2002). Visual fixation patterns during viewing of naturalistic social situations as predictors of social competence in individuals with autism. *Archives of General Psychiatry, 59,* 809–816.

Klin, A., Saulnier, C. A., Sparrow, S. S., Cicchetti, D. V., Volkmar, F. R., & Lord, C. (2007). Social and communication abilities and disabilities in higher functioning individuals with autism spectrum disorders. *Journal of Autism and Developmental Disorders, 37*(4), 748–759.

Koegel, L. K., Koegel, R. L., Frea, W., & Green-Hopkins, I. (2003). Priming as a method of coordinating educational services for students with autism. *Language, Speech, and Hearing Services in Schools, 34,* 228–235.

Laurent, A. C., & Rubin, E. (2004). Emotional regulation challenges in Asperger's syndrome and high functioning autism. *Topics in Language Disorders, 24,* 4.

Little, L. (2001). Peer victimization of children with Asperger spectrum disorders. *Journal of the American Academy of Child and Adolescent Psychiatry, 40*(9), 995–996.

Lord, C., & Paul, R. (1997). Language and communication in autism. In D. J. Cohen & F. R. Volkmar (Eds.), *Handbook of autism and pervasive developmental disorders* (2nd ed., pp. 195–225). New York: Wiley.

McAfee, J. L. (2002). *Navigating the social world: A curriculum for individuals with Asperger's syndrome, high functioning autism, and related disorders.* Arlington, TX: Future Horizons.

National Research Council. (2000). *From neurons to neighborhoods.* Washington, DC: National Academy Press.

National Research Council. (2001). *Educating children with autism.* Washington,

DC: National Academy Press, Committee on Educational Interventions for Children with Autism, Division of Behavioral and Social Sciences and Education.

Nikopoulous, C. K., & Keenan, M. (2004). Effects of video modeling on social initiations by children with autism. *Journal of Applied Behavior Analysis, 34,* 93–96.

Parsons, S., & Mitchell, P. (1999). What children with autism understand about thoughts and thought bubbles. *Autism, 3,* 17–38.

Paul, R. (2003). Promoting social communication in high functioning individuals with autistic spectrum disorders. *Child and Adolescent Psychiatric Clinics of North America, 12,* 87–106.

Pierce, K., & Schreibman, L. (1994). Teaching daily living skills to children with autism in unsupervised settings through pictorial self-management. *Journal of Applied Behavior Analysis, 27,* 471–482.

Prizant, B. M., Wetherby, A. M., Rubin, E., & Laurent, A. C (2003). The SCERTS® Model: A transactional, family-centered approach to enhancing communication and socioemotional abilities of children with autism spectrum disorder. *Infants and Young Children, 16*(4), 296–316.

Prizant, B., Wetherby, A., Rubin, E., Laurent, A., & Rydell, P. (2006). *The SCERTS® Model: A comprehensive educational approach for children with autism spectrum disorders* (Vols. 1 & II). Baltimore, MD: Brookes.

Rubin, E., & Laurent, A.C. (2002). *The feelings book.* Carmel, CA: Communication Crossroads.

Rubin, E., & Laurent, A. C. (2004). Implementing a curriculum-based assessment to prioritize learning objectives in Asperger syndrome and high functioning autism. *Topics in Language Disorders, 24,* 4.

Rubin, E., Laurent, A. C., Prizant, B.M., & Wetherby, A.M. (2008). AAC and the SCERTS® Model: Incorporating AAC within a comprehensive, multidisciplinary educational program. In P. Mirenda & T. Iacono (Eds.), *Autism and augmentative and alternative communication (AAC).* Baltimore: Brookes.

Rydell, P., & Prizant, B. (1995). Assessment and intervention strategies for children who use echolalia. In K. Quill (Ed.), *Teaching children with autism: Strategies to enhance communication and socialization* (pp. 105–129). Albany, NY: Delmar.

Saulnier, C. A., & Klin, A. (2006). Brief report: Social and communication abilities and disabilities in higher functioning individuals with autism and Asperger syndrome. *Journal of Autism and Developmental Disorders, 37*(4), 788–793.

Simpson, R. L., de Boer-Ott, S. R., & Myles, B. S. (2003). Inclusion of learners with autism spectrum disorders in general education settings. *Topics in Language Disorders, 23*(2), 116–133.

Strain, P. S., & Kohler, F. (1998). Peer-mediated social interventions for young children with autism. *Seminars in Speech and Language, 19,* 391–405.

Tantam, D. (2000). Adolescence and adulthood of individuals with Asperger syndrome. In A. Klin, F. R. Volkmar, & S. S. Sparrow (Eds.), *Asperger syndrome* (pp. 367–399). New York: Guilford Press.

Thiemann, K., & Goldstein, H. (2004). Effects of peer training and written-text cueing on social communication of school-age children with pervasive developmental disorder. *Journal of Speech, Language, and Hearing Research, 47,* 126–144.

Tsatsanis, K. D. (2003). Outcome research in Asperger syndrome and autism. *Child and Adolescent Psychiatric Clinics of North America, 12*, 45–63.

Tsatsanis, K. D. (2004). Heterogeneity in learning style in Asperger syndrome and high functioning autism. *Topics in Language Disorders, 24*(4), 260–270.

Tsatsanis, K. D., Foley, C., & Donehower, C. (2004). Contemporary outcome research and programming guidelines for Asperger syndrome and high functioning autism. *Topics in Language Disorders, 24*(4), 249–259.

Volkmar, F. R., Klin, A., Schultz, R., Rubin, E., & Bronen, R. (2000). Clinical case conference: Asperger's disorder. *American Journal of Psychiatry, 157*(2), 262–267.

Volkmar, F. R., Lord, C., Bailey, A., Schultz, R. T., & Klin, A. (2004). Autism and pervasive developmental disorders. *Journal of Child Psychology and Psychiatry, 45*, 145–170.

Wellman, H., Baron-Cohen, S., Caswell, R., Gomez, J. C., Swettenham, J., Toye, E., et al. (2002). Thought bubbles help children with autism acquire an alternative to theory of mind. *Autism, 6*, 343–363.

Winner, M. G. (2002). *Thinking about you thinking about me.* San Jose, CA: Author.

Yirmiya, N., Sigman, M. D., Kasari, C., & Mundy, P. (1992). Empathy and cognition in high-functioning children with autism. *Child Development, 63*, 150–160.

CHAPTER 7

Behavioral Treatments for Asperger Syndrome

Brenda Smith Myles
Kai-Chien Tien
Hyo Jung Lee
Yu-Chi Chou
Sheila M. Smith

Behavioral issues are one of the most common and problematic areas for individuals with Asperger syndrome (AS). This pervasive disorder affects various domains of daily life, including social relationships and academic performance (Horner, Carr, Strain, Todd, & Reed, 2002). Behavioral issues, therefore, should be a primary concern when planning appropriate programs for individuals with AS. This chapter provides a description of the behavioral challenges exhibited by individuals with AS and discusses interventions targeting those challenges. Specifically, this chapter discusses (1) behaviors related to AS; (2) functional assessment of behavior; (3) the cycle of tantrums, rage, and meltdowns; and (4) targeted interventions.

BEHAVIORS RELATED TO ASPERGER SYNDROME

The behavioral issues experienced by individuals with AS are diverse and multifaceted, including difficulties with internalizing as well as externalizing

209

behavior. Problems of conduct, aggression, hyperactivity, and other externalizing behaviors may be combined with internalizing problems, such as withdrawal, in the individual with AS. Layered within these behaviors in many individuals are problematic sensory- and regulation-related behaviors, including sensitivities to noise, touch, and smell; and meltdowns, respectively. In addition, individuals with AS do not perceive themselves as having problems in these areas, making intervention a complex task as well (Barnhill et al., 2000b).

Externalizing Behaviors

The behavioral profile for many children and youth with AS includes externalizing behaviors; that is, behaviors that can be readily observed, such as aggression, hyperactivity, conduct problems, and other "undercontrolled" behaviors (Achenbach & Edelbrock, 1978; Reynolds & Kamphaus, 1992). The frequency and intensity of these "acting-out" behaviors are as unique as the individuals themselves and can have varied causes, including internal issues such as anxiety or stress. Some of these aggressive and oppositional-like behavior problems are often referred to by educational professionals as "tantrums, rage, and meltdowns" (Myles & Southwick, 2005). Extreme symptoms of behavior may arise from a myriad of reasons, including a desire for social relationships (Macintosh & Dissanayake, 2006; Tonge, Brereton, Gray, & Einfeld, 1999).

Research has documented that both children and adolescents with AS can present with high levels of clinically significant behavioral and emotional disturbance, characterizing their personal conduct as disruptive and antisocial (cf. Tonge, Brereton, Gray, & Einfeld, 1999). Researchers and practitioners have also described individuals with AS as having a tendency to be extremely active (Barnhill et al., 2000b; Macintosh & Dissanayake, 2006; Tonge et al., 1999). For example, Myles et al. (2005) found that parents of adolescents with AS reported that their children were at risk for hyperactive behavior and 49% of the children were prescribed central nervous system stimulants to address overactivity.

This is not the case for all individuals with AS, though. It is important to remember that within externalized behaviors, there is a spectrum. Causes vary across individuals, and individuals with AS may not recognize that any issues are present. In the Myles et al. (2005) study, the adolescents with AS did not acknowledge any difficulties with overactivity.

Internalized Behaviors

Internalized behavior is referred to as "overcontrolled" behavior not shown via acting out (Achenbach & Edelbrock, 1978). According to Reynolds and Kamphaus (1992), anxiety, depression, and somatization are the subdomains of internalized behavior problems. Since Asperger's (1944) introduction of the disability that carries his name, several studies have shown that individuals with AS have problems in these areas, with anxiety and depression occurring most frequently (MacNeil, Lopes, & Minnes, 2009; Myles, 2003; Russell & Sofronoff, 2005). These internalized problems are often triggered by or result directly from environmental stressors, such as difficulty in predicting outcomes, a sense of loss of control, misperceptions of social events, and so on (Barnhill, 2001; Barnhill et al., 2000b; Barnhill & Myles, 2001).

For example, Tantam (2000) reported a significant risk of depression in individuals with AS, with up to 15% of adults with this disability experiencing a period of depression. Further, Kim, Szatmari, Bryson, Streiner, and Wilson (2000) reported that one-fifth of their sample size of 168 had "clinically relevant" levels of depression, and the group had substantially higher levels of anxiety than children of a similar age. A 2005 investigation of the comorbid characteristics of 156 adolescents with AS revealed that 20% were diagnosed with depression and/or anxiety disorder and 63% were prescribed medications for these issues (Myles et al.). In fact, among adolescents and adults with AS, depression and anxiety are the most frequently reported secondary diagnoses, more common than obsessive–compulsive disorder (OCD), alcohol and drug abuse, eating disorders, bipolar disorder, schizophrenia and isolated psychotic episodes, catatonia, and suicidal thoughts and acts (Ghaziuddin, Weidmer-Mikhail, & Ghaziuddin, 1998; Tonge et al., 1999). Thus, the common comorbid psychiatric symptoms in the AS population include anxiety and depression, which are conceptualized as "internalizing problems."

According to Attwood (1998), anxiety arises in individuals with AS over a range of issues, including changes in routines and expectations, apprehension in social situations, and minor environmental changes. Barnhill and Myles (2001), investigating attribution styles of adolescents with AS, found that individuals who reported more depressive symptoms were also more likely to exhibit "cognitive errors in thinking" associated with a perception of having little control over negative life events (p. 176).

The manifestation of internalized behaviors may also include withdrawal, lack of social interaction with peers, self-abusive behaviors, compulsive and obsessive behaviors, and inattention (Kim et al., 2000; Todis, Severson, & Walker 1990). Some are oversensitive to criticism and suspicious of other people. As they grow older, many individuals with AS become aware of their differences and show their emotional vulnerability (Church, Alisanski, & Amanulla, 2000; Macintosh & Dissanayake, 2006; Wing, 1981).

Despite agreement as to the presence of internalizing problems within the AS population, the factors giving rise to these internalizing problems remain unclear (Attwood, 1998). Furthermore, the relationship between a number of presenting characteristics of AS and internalizing problems needs to be clarified.

Behavior Problems Related to Sensory Issues

Some investigations have suggested sensory issues as an underlying characteristic of AS (Dunn, Myles, & Orr, 2002; Myles et al., 2004; Myles, Barnhill, Hagiwara, Griswold, & Simpson, 2001; Pfeiffer, Kinnealey, Reed, & Herzberg, 2005). Even though the specific relationship between sensory issues and behavioral characteristics has not yet been identified, there is an assumption in the literature that individuals with AS might be more likely to have behavioral problems related to sensory-processing challenges because of their hypo- or hypersensitivities. For example, Myles et al. (2004) found a significant difference between children with AS and children with autism in the area of (1) emotional/social responses, (2) emotional reactivity, and (3) inattention/distractibility. Church et al. (2000) also reported that most of children with AS had sensory issues and became very anxious or showed inappropriate behaviors to avoid or to seek certain sensory input. Even though further research is required to define the relationship between sensory issues and behaviors evident in those with AS, there are recommendations to consider sensory issues when developing interventions.

FUNCTIONAL BEHAVIORAL ASSESSMENT

Because individuals with AS evidence myriad challenges, manifested as internalized or externalized behaviors, it is essential that a process be in place to address these concerns. One effective means of targeting these issues is a functional behavioral assessment (FBA). Mandated by the Individuals with Disabilities Education Act (2004), this process typically includes (1) identifying and describing student behavior, (2) describing setting demands and antecedents, (3) collecting baseline data and/or work samples, (4) completing assessment measures and developing a hypothesis, (5) developing and implementing a behavioral intervention plan, (6) collecting data, and (7) conducting follow-up procedures to analyze the effectiveness of the plan (O'Neill et al., 1997).

An FBA is pivotal in developing effective programs for students with AS. In fact, this process has been empirically linked to intervention success. That is, functional assessment increases the likelihood that intervention strategies are effective in decreasing inappropriate and increasing appropriate behavior (Carr et al., 1999; Ellingson, Miltenberger, Stricker, Galensky, & Garlinghouse, 2000). Traditional functional assessment often targets conditions hypothesized to be associated with problem behavior, such as (1) escape/avoidance; (2) attention from peers or adults; (3) anger or stress expression; (4) emotional state, such as depression, frustration, or confusion; (5) power/control; (6) intimidation; (7) sensory stimulation; (8) fear or relief of fear; (9) request or obtain something (e.g., food, activity, object, comfort, routine, social interaction); or (10) expression of internal stimulation (e.g., sinus pain, skin irritation, hunger) (Durand & Crimmins, 1992; Janzen, 2003; Kern, Dunlap, Clarke, & Childs, 1994; Lewis, Scott, & Sugai, 1994; O'Neill et al., 1997). Although these behavioral functions may be significant, one might question whether identification of these attributes and related interventions leads to long-term and generalized behavior change.

For example, John, a 12-year-old student with AS, is experiencing behavioral issues in his general education classroom. His teacher has observed that he does not attend to and follow directions. After consulting with other staff, he determined that the function of John's behavior is related to attention span, a reasonable assumption given that John's first diagnosis was attention-deficit/hyperactivity disorder (ADHD). This hypothesis was verified by the school's behavior specialist. Yet, ADHD is not John's only diagnosis. The team should be aware of the characteristics of AS.

Using their hypothesis regarding attention span, the teacher and the behavior specialist planned an intervention that included using visual supports. A visual cue was placed on John's desk to remind him to attend and a social narrative about how to use the visual support was provided.

This intervention might provide a temporary solution to the problem, but most likely will not result in long-term or generalized change. Although the intervention was designed to address attentions span, the underlying characteristics of AS were not addressed, so a potential by-product of the intervention could be John's anxiety or confusion. For example, researchers have found that children and youth with high-functioning autism (HFA) or AS focus on people's mouths in social situations—a profile uniquely dissimilar to individuals who are neurotypical (cf. Grossman, Klin, Carter, & Volkmar, 2000). If John's teacher and the behavior specialist were aware of this underlying characteristic, they could have included visual orientation to interpret social interactions when planning the intervention. An intervention that would match John's manifestation of AS would include (1) teaching John to focus on another's entire face in a social situation and (2) providing instruction on interpreting nonverbal cues. Thus, perhaps the FBA should include an analysis of the characteristics inherent in AS so that interventions could better match student need.

Using the Ziggurat Model to Assess Behavioral Issues

One model of functional assessment, the Ziggurat model (Aspy & Grossman, 2011), combines a modified version of Schopler's (1994) use of an iceberg analogy and an instrument known as the Underlying Characteristics Checklist (UCC; Aspy & Grossman, 2007). Schopler's analogy is used to represent observed behaviors as the tip of the iceberg while the unseen causes lie beneath the surface of the water. Thus, interventions based on this concept are designed to address core deficits that underlie the behaviors experienced by individuals with ASD.

Schopler's representation, however, provides an isolated glimpse of a child's behavior without taking into account critical elements of a functional assessment: the antecedent and consequence. The ABC (antecedent–behavior–consequence) iceberg (Aspy & Grossman, 2011), a modified version of Schopler's work, begins to provide a more comprehensive understanding of behavior by illustrating that behavior does not occur in isolation. And although these aspects are imperative to the analysis of behavior, an additional step is needed. According to Aspy and Grossman (2011):

> There are several routes to determining the underlying factors of a behavior. Knowledge of underlying factors comes from formal and informal assessment and awareness of the characteristics of AS. With experience and training, it is often possible to begin to theorize about underlying factors without in-depth assessment. . . . The iceberg analogy, while emphasizing the underlying characteristics of AS, fails to include an analysis of patterns of behavior; therefore, it is limited in its usefulness for addressing specific behavior concerns. A more structured assessment will help to identify additional underlying factors. The Ziggurat Model incorporates a special assessment—the Underlying Characteristics Checklist (UCC)—to accomplish this task. (p. 47)

The UCC is an informal assessment tool comprised of 90 items designed to identify characteristics across eight empirically valid domains. The first three are Social; Restricted Patterns of Behavior, Interests, and Activities; and Communication. The next five characteristic areas are also associated with AS: Sensory Differences (Dunn et al., 2002; Myles et al., 2004; Volkmar, Cohen, & Paul, 1986), Cognitive Differences (Barnhill, Hagiwara, Myles, & Simpson, 2000a; Reitzel & Szatmari, 2003); Motor Differences (Dunn et al., 2002; Myles et al., 2004), Emotional Vulnerability (Barnhill et al., 2000; Barnhill & Myles, 2001; Ghaziuddin, Ghaziuddin, & Greden, 2002), and Medical and Other Biological Factors (Ghazziuddin, 2002; Kim et al., 2000; Polemini, Richdale, & Francis, 2005). The form described here is titled UCC-HF to indicate that it is intended for individuals who are *high functioning*. It is to be completed by parents, educational professionals, mental health professionals, and others who develop educational and behavioral programs for students with AS. A sample of items under each category appears in Table 7.1.

To use the UCC-HF a rater simply places a checkmark next to each item that describes the characteristics or behaviors of an individual with HFA/AS. A "Notes" column provides a space to describe how a given characteristic is expressed in an individual. Thus, the UCC-HF provides a snapshot of the autism in an individual. The Notes section helps to bring clarity to this picture and to facilitate communication with others involved in developing interventions; it thus becomes a basis for follow-up.

Figure 7.1 provides an example of the ABC iceberg and the UCC-HF as it applies to a student who is experiencing disruptive behavior. These

TABLE 7.1. Sample Items on the Underlying Characteristics Checklist—High Functioning

Areas	Sample items
Social	Has difficulty recognizing the feelings and thoughts of others
	Lacks tact or appears rude
Restricted Patterns	Seems to be unmotivated by customary rewards
	Has problems handling transition and change
Communication	Makes up new words or creates alternate meanings for words or phrases
	Fails to initiate or respond to social greetings
Sensory	Responds in an unusual manner to pain
	Seeks activities that provide touch, pressure, or movement
Cognitive	Displays poor problem-solving skills
	Has poor organizational skills
Motor	Writes slowly
	Has difficulty starting or completing activity
Emotional Vulnerability	Has difficulty identifying, quantifying, expressing, and/or controlling emotions
	Is easily stressed; worries obsessively
Medical or Biological	*Items to be identified by team*

documents provide a starting point in identifying and describing both externalized and internalized behavior. Insertion of identified antecedents and consequences into the iceberg further clarifies the function of the behavior (Aspy & Grossman, 2011). This forms the basis of the student's functional assessment (see Figure 7.1) and is instrumental in the completion of the aforementioned FBA steps: (3) collecting baseline data and/or work samples, (4) completing assessment measures and developing a hypothesis, (5) developing and implementing a behavioral intervention plan, (6) collecting data, and (7) conducting follow-up procedures to analyze the effectiveness of the plan (O'Neill et al., 1997).

Using the Ziggurat Model to Decrease Inappropriate and Increase Appropriate Behavior

Using a five-level pyramid, the Ziggurat model supports the premise that the complexity of needs for individuals with autism spectrum disorders (ASD) requires multifaceted instruction. Following the administration of the UCC-HF and identification of the student's need areas, interventions are planned for each of the Ziggurat levels: (1) sensory, (2) reinforcement, (3) visual/tactile support and structure, (4) task demands, and (5) skills to teach. These interventions then become the basis for development of the

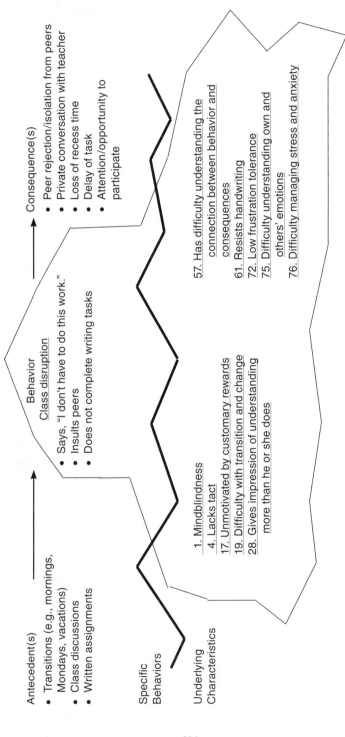

FIGURE 7.1. ABC-I model applied to disrputive behavior.

Antecedent(s)
- Transitions (e.g., mornings, Mondays, vacations)
- Class discussions
- Written assignments

Behavior
Class disruption
- Says, "I don't have to do this work."
- Insults peers
- Does not complete writing tasks

Consequence(s)
- Peer rejection/isolation from peers
- Private conversation with teacher
- Loss of recess time
- Delay of task
- Attention/opportunity to participate

Specific Behaviors

Underlying Characteristics
1. Mindblindness
4. Lacks tact
17. Unmotivated by customary rewards
19. Difficulty with transition and change
28. Gives impression of understanding more than he or she does

57. Has difficulty understanding the connection between behavior and consequences
61. Resists handwriting
72. Low frustration tolerance
75. Difficulty understanding own and others' emotions
76. Difficulty managing stress and anxiety

student's program. Figure 7.2 provides an example of a completed Ziggurat worksheet for disruptive behavior.

THE CYCLE OF TANTRUMS, RAGE, AND MELTDOWNS

Although FBA, including the UCC-HF and Ziggurat, can be effective in addressing behavior issues, children and youth may exhibit tantrums, rage, and meltdowns (terms that are used interchangeably), which often occur due to the combination of innate stress and anxiety and inability to detect personal emotional reactivity. Meltdowns, which typically occur in three stages, can be of variable length. These stages are (1) the rumbling stage, (2) the rage stage, and (3) the recovery stage (adapted from Albert, 1989; Beck, 1985).

Rumbling Stage

The rumbling stage is the initial stage of a tantrum, rage, or meltdown. During this stage, children and youth with AS exhibit specific behavioral changes that may not appear to be directly related to a meltdown. The behaviors may appear to be minor. Individuals with AS may clear their throats, lower their voices, tense their muscles, tap a foot, grimace, or otherwise indicate general discontent. Further somatic complaints may occur during the rumbling stage. Students may also engage in behaviors that are more obvious, such as emotional or physical withdrawal or verbally or physically offending somebody. For example, the student may challenge the classroom structure or authority by attempting to engage in a power struggle.

During this stage, it is imperative that an adult intervene without becoming part of a struggle. Interventions that occur during this stage often fall under the realm of surface behavior management (Long, Morse, & Newman, 1976): antiseptic bouncing (removal from the environment in a nonpunitive manner), proximity control, signal interference, support from routine, or "just walk and don't talk." Other strategies used during this stage that do not belong to the category of surface management but are similar in that they are therapeutic, nonpunitive, and designed to support child success include relocating to a home base and acknowledging student difficulties. All of these strategies can be effective in stopping the cycle of tantrums, rage, and meltdowns and are invaluable in that they can help the child regain control with minimal adult support (Myles & Southwick, 2005). Table 7.2 provides descriptions of these strategies.

When selecting a strategy or an intervention during the rumbling stage, it is important to know the student, as the wrong technique can escalate, rather than deescalate, a behavior problem. Further, although interventions at this stage do not require extensive time, it is advisable that adults

BEHAVIOR/AREAS OF CONCERN	FOR SPECIFIC INTERVENTION PLAN	SELECTED UCC ITEMS	CHECK ALL THAT APPLY.		
			A	B	C
Class disruption	Says, "I don't have to do this work." • Insults peers • Does not complete writing tasks	• Mindblindness • Lacks tact • Unmotivated by customary rewards • Difficulty with transition and change • Gives false impression of understanding more than she actually does • Has difficulty understanding the connection between behavior and consequences. • Resists handwriting • Low frustration tolerance • Difficulty understanding own and others' emotions • Difficulty managing stress and anxiety	✓	✓	
Sensory/Biological Needs	Sensory/ Biological Intervention:	• Seek occupational therapist consult to assess handwriting, including sensory factors and hand fatigue. • Provide student with a sensory diet with direction of an OT to help address anxious or agitated behaviors. • Provide a calming sensory activity prior to giving lengthy writing task. • Teach student to recognize body cues that indicate stress or frustration. • Teach student strategies to address stress and frustration (e.g., engage in sensory calming strategy, ask for help, take slow, deep breaths).			
	Underlying Characteristics Addressed:	• Low frustration tolerance • Difficulty managing stress and anxiety • Resists handwriting • Difficulty understanding own and others' emotions			
Reinforcement	Reinforcement Intervention:	• Develop a positive plan to address social skills and work completion. Have student help to select items for a reinforcer menu. Allow student frequent opportunities to "cash in" by selecting reinforcers from her menu. • Reinforce student for being able to categorize statements as "rude" or "kind." • With the assistance of a speech therapist, develop a card that has rules for class discussion. During a class discussion, give student a card—one side green (with rules for appropriate class discussion—e.g., no insults, on-topic remark) and the other side red (with a list of	✓	✓	✓

				✓	✓
			✓		

appropriate listening behaviors). Begin each class discussion with green side up. Turn card to red if student makes an inappropriate contribution. Remove card at the end of class discussion. Reinforce student for following the rules on either side of the card.

- Provide reinforcement for initiating work on a writing assignment without negative comments. Also reinforce for working for an increasing amount of time.
- Develop a token reinforcement system to address transitioning to school. Use alligator or other favorite animal stamps in student's token reinforcer system. Make the last item on the checklist a school task (e.g., put backpack away). Reinforce student at school for following checklist/schedule. Provide additional reinforcement for following the schedule independently.

Underlying Characteristics Addressed:

- Lacks tact
- Unmotivated by customary rewards
- Difficulties with transition and change
- Resists handwriting
- Low frustration tolerance

Structure/Visual Support Intervention:

- Create visual chart "Rude versus Kind Words." Update as kind/unkind words occur and keep a copy at home and in school.
- Videotape a same-age class during discussion time. Prior to taping, remind all students of behavioral expectations. Show student the tape—stopping to view specific skills (e.g., raising hand, refraining from negative comments when peers answer incorrectly) and to explore facial expressions and gestures of the peer models. Practice skills with student and reinforce. Provide student with a visual reminder of class discussion rules and reinforce for successfully following them.
- Create a visual chart for tracking student's progress on earning rewards. For example, use a drawing of a bug. Let Student color in a segment each time hed or she earns a reinforcer for being on-task or making appropriate comments in class. Student selects a reinforcer from the menu when the drawing is completely colored.
- Use a comic strip conversation to help illustrate the thoughts and feelings of others in the context of a problem situation. For example, teach student to recognize the response of others to his or her comments.
- Parents will provide student with a visual checklist/schedule for the morning routine and transition to school. (see Reinforcement level for description).
- Provide student with a weekly schedule to increase predictability.

Structure & Visual Supports

FIGURE 7.2. (continued)

Task Demands	Underlying Characteristics Addressed:	• Has difficulty understanding the connection between behavior and consequences • Mindblindness • Lacks tact • Unmotivated by customary rewards • Difficulty with transition and change • Difficulty understanding own and others' emotions		
	Task Demand Intervention:	• Use red–green class discussion card (see Reinforcement level for description). The card will explicitly list the steps for discussion for student to use as a guide/reminder. • Provide student with list of sentence starters he or she can use when writing. • Teacher can shorten some lengthy writing assignments or allow student to type or respond orally.	✓	✓
Skills to Be Taught	Underlying Characteristics Addressed:	• Mindblindness • Difficulty understanding the connection between behavior and consequences • Resists handwriting		
	Skill Intervention:	• Teach student strategies to address his or her stress and frustration (see Sensory/Biological Needs level for description). • Use red–green class discussion card (see Reinforcement level for description). • Teach student to recognize the response of others to her comments using comic strip conversations (see Structure & Visual Supports level for description), role play, and actual situations. • Create a Social Story to teach student that some comments may not be polite even though they may be true. The story will assist him or her in learning social consequences of her disruptive, disrespectful comments. • Teach student keyboarding skills.	✓	✓
	Underlying Characteristics Addressed:	• Mindblindness • Resists handwriting • Low frustration tolerance • Lacks tact		

FIGURE 7.2. Completed Ziggurat worksheet for disruptive behavior. Data from Aspy and Grossman (2011).

TABLE 7.2. Interventions during the Rumbling Stage

Antiseptic bouncing

Antiseptic bouncing involves removing a student, in a nonpunitive fashion, from the environment in which he or she is experiencing difficulty. At school, the child may be sent on an errand. At home, the child may be asked to retrieve an object for a parent. During this time, the student has an opportunity to regain a sense of calm. When he or she returns, the problem has typically diminished in magnitude and the adult is on hand for support, if needed.

Proximity control

Rather than calling attention to the behavior, the teacher moves near the student who is engaged in the target behavior. Parents using proximity control move near their child. Often something as simple as standing next to a child is calming. This can easily be accomplished without interrupting an ongoing activity. For example, the teacher who circulates through the classroom during a lesson is using proximity control.

Signal interference

When the child with AS begins to exhibit a precursor behavior, such as clearing throat or pacing, the teacher uses a nonverbal signal to let the student know that he or she is aware of the situation. For example, the teacher can place him- or herself in a position where eye contact with the student can be achieved. Or an agreed-upon "secret" signal, such as tapping on a desk, may be used to alert the child that he or she is under stress. Signal interference may be followed by an in-seat destressor, prescribed by an occupational therapist, such as squeezing a stress ball. In the home or community, parents may develop a signal (i.e., a slight hand movement) with their child that is used when the child is in the rumbling stage. Often this strategy precedes antiseptic bouncing.

Support from routine

Displaying a chart or visual schedule of expectations and events can provide security to children and youth with AS who typically need predictability. This technique can also be used as advance preparation for a change in routine. Informing students of schedule changes can prevent anxiety and reduce the likelihood of tantrums, rage, and meltdowns. For example, the student who is signaling frustration by tapping a foot may be directed to look at the schedule to make him or her aware that after completing two more problems, he or she gets to work on a topic of special interest with a peer. While running errands, parents can use support from routine by alerting the child in the rumbling stage that their next stop in the shopping trip will be at a store the child enjoys.

Home base

A home base is a place in the school or home where an individual can escape stress. The home base should be quiet with few visual or activity distractions. While in home base, the individual can continue with activities, but these should be selected carefully to ensure that they are calming rather than alerting. In school, resource rooms or counselors' offices can serve as a home base. The structure of the room supercedes its location. At home, the home base may be the child's room or an isolated area in the house. But regardless of its location, it is essential that the home base is viewed as a positive environment. Home base is not timeout or an escape from classroom tasks or chores. The student takes class work to home base, and at home, chores are completed after a brief respite in the home base.

(continued)

TABLE 7.2. *(continued)*

Home base may be used at other times than during the rumbling stage. For example, at the beginning of the day, a home base can serve to preview the day's schedule, introduce changes in the typical routine, ensure that the student's materials are organized, or prime for specific subjects. At other times it can be used to help the student gain control after a meltdown (see recovery stage).

Redirecting

Redirecting can be used to direct an individual away from an activity or task that appears to be contributing to a behavioral issue. This technique can be particularly effective when an individual is beginning the rumbling stage and involves helping the student focus on something other than the task or activity that appears to be upsetting. One type of redirection that often works well when the source of the behavior is a lack of understanding is telling the child that he or she and you can make a cartoon of the situation in order to figure out what to do. Sometimes cartooning can be briefly postponed; at other times, the student may need to have the cartoon immediately.

Acknowledging student difficulties

This technique is effective when the student is in the midst of the rumbling stage because of a difficult task, and the parent or educator thinks that the student can complete the activity with support. The parent or teacher offers a brief acknowledgment that supports the verbalizations of the child and helps him or her complete the task. For example, when working on a math problem the student begins to say, "This is too hard." Knowing the student is able to complete the problem, the teacher refocuses the student's attention by saying, "Yes, the problem is difficult. Let's start with number one." This brief direction and support may prevent the student from moving past the rumbling stage.

Just walk and don't talk

The adult using this technique merely walks with the student without talking. The adult's silence is important because a child with AS in the rumbling stage will likely react emotively to any adult statement, misinterpreting it or rephrasing it beyond recognition. On this walk the child can say whatever he or she wishes without fear of discipline or logical argument. In the meantime, the adult should be calm, show as little reaction as possible, and never be confrontational.

understand the events that precipitate the target behaviors so that they can (1) be ready to intervene early or (2) teach children and youth strategies to maintain behavioral control during these times.

It is important to understand that interventions at this stage are merely bandages. They do not teach students to recognize their own frustration or teach self-management skills. Techniques to accomplish these goals are discussed later in this chapter.

Rage Stage

If behavior is not diffused during the rumbling stage, the child or adolescent may move to the rage stage. At this point, the student is disinhibited and acts impulsively, emotionally, and sometimes explosively. These behaviors may be externalized (e.g., screaming, biting, hitting, kicking, destroying property or self-injury) or internalized (e.g., withdrawal). Meltdowns are not purposeful, and once the rage stage begins, it most often must run its course.

During this stage, emphasis should be placed on child, peer, and adult safety as well as protection of school, home, or personal property. The best way to cope with a tantrum, rage, or meltdown is to get the child to home base. As mentioned, this room is not viewed as a reward or disciplinary room, but is seen as a place where the student can regain self-control.

Of importance here is helping the individual with AS regain control and preserve dignity. To that end, adults should have developed plans for (1) obtaining assistance from educators such as a crisis teacher or principal, (2) removing other students from the area, or (3) providing therapeutic restraint, if necessary.

Recovery Stage

Following a meltdown, children with AS may have contrite feelings and often cannot fully remember what occurred during the rage stage. Some may become sullen, withdraw, or deny that inappropriate behavior occurred; others are so physically exhausted that they need to sleep.

It is imperative that interventions are implemented at a time when the student can accept them and in a manner the student can accept and understand. Otherwise, the result is most often a reignition of the cycle, this time usually advancing more rapidly to the rage stage. During the recovery stage, children are often not ready to learn. Thus, it is important that adults work with them to once again become a part of the routine. This is often best accomplished by directing the youth to a highly motivating task that can be easily accomplished, such as activity related to a special interest.

Summary

Students with AS experiencing stress may react by having a tantrum, rage, or meltdown. Behaviors do not occur in isolation or randomly; they are most often associated with a reason or cause. The student who engages in an inappropriate behavior is attempting to communicate. Before selecting an intervention to be used during the rage cycle or to prevent the cycle from occurring, it is important to understand the function or role the target behavior plays.

INTERVENTIONS

Although research on interventions for individual with AS in still in its infancy, some treatments have been identified as effective or potentially effective. These include, but are not limited to, priming, social narratives, visual supports, SODA (Stop, Observe, Deliberate, and Act), video instruction, self-regulation instruction, and Circle of Friends.

Priming

Priming involves providing a preview of upcoming events, academic activities, task procedures, or source materials. It is a preparation for actual instruction or participation in activities, but does not involve teaching or correction. The purpose of priming is to prevent disruptive behaviors, to improve academic performance, and to decrease anxiety (Boettcher, Koegel, McNerney, & Koegel, 2003; Koegel, Koegel, Frea, & Green-Hopkins, 2003). Priming activities provide an expectation of what is going to happen during actual class participation and addresses appropriate or expected behaviors.

Wilde, Koegel, and Koegel (1992) developed a general guideline for implementing priming, whose components include (1) collaboration, (2) communication, (3) priming, and (4) feedback. The first step is to determine the primer and priming activities. Priming can be a collaborative process involving multiple staff, although one staff member should be designated as the primer. Together, staff members decide what materials to use and what activities to do during the priming intervention. The second step involves communication. Staff plans activities, prepares materials for priming, and decides priming procedures. Also, during the priming, teachers and the primer address behaviors with which the child may have trouble, in order to prevent disruptive behaviors. The third step is the priming itself. It is the time when the primer interacts with the student about the materials, activities, and class expectations, introducing them to the student prior to actual teaching and class participation. Reinforcement is utilized to increase the student's confidence and decrease anxiety and stress. The final step is feedback. Teachers and the primer assess the efficiency of the priming intervention by comparing the priming process with the results of instructional activities. In addition, teachers and the primer use this time to brainstorm better strategies to improve appropriate behaviors and academic performance.

Social Narratives

Social narratives can be a powerful intervention for individuals with AS. Specifically, social narratives can be used to shape and increase appropriate behaviors by promoting self-awareness, self-calming, and self-management. In addition, they can support individuals with AS in social interactions by describing desired social behaviors across settings, times, and people.

Social narratives can be written by educators, related professionals, or parents who know the student well. Myles and Southwick (2005) suggested the following guidelines for writing social narratives:

1. Identify a social situation for intervention and select the target behavior.
2. Define the target behavior for data collection.
3. Collect baseline data on the target behavior to determine frequency or duration as well as trend.
4. Write a social narrative using language at the child's level.
5. Choose the number of sentences per page according to the student's functioning level.
6. Use visual cues such as photographs, hand-drawn pictures, or pictorial icons.
7. Read the social narrative to the student and model the desired behavior.
8. Collect intervention data.
9. Review findings and modify the narrative, if needed.
10. Program for maintenance and generalization.

The most widely used social narratives are Social Stories™ and scripts.

Social Stories™

One of the most frequently used and effective social narratives are Social Stories; these are brief, individualized stories often supported by simple pictures that reflect an individual's perspective on a certain subject (Gray, 1995, 2000; Gray & Gerand, 1993). The primary purpose of this intervention is to improve social understanding. Each story has a theme or title and describes a situation with which the individual experiences difficulty. It also includes appropriate responses, such as desirable behaviors or expressions.

Since their introduction, more than a dozen studies have reported the effectiveness of Social Stories as a behavioral intervention for aggressive and disruptive behaviors, inappropriate table manners, and crying (cf. Sansosti, Powell-Smith, & Kincaid, 2004; Scattone, Tingstrom, & Wilczynski, 2006). Many of these investigations included adaptations of the intervention's format across problem behaviors, settings, or disabilities (cf. Brownell, 2002; Ivey, Heflin, & Alberto, 2004; Moore, 2004). In addition, several studies have combined Social Stories with other interventions, such as visual or verbal cues, role play and cartooning, or with technological supports such as a computer-based format and video feedback (cf. Hagiwara & Myles, 1999; Thiemann & Goldstein, 2004).

Scripts

Most people have developed shared rules based on situations that they face in daily life. Through various experiences, people formulate general rules and sequences for each activity. These rules or sequences are known as "scripts" (Volden & Johnston, 1999). The script model, based on cognitive psychology, provides a cognitive context that represents familiar experiences and that is operational for an individual at any given time (Trillingsgaard, 1999). The format of scripts can be varied: Sentences or paragraphs or audio or videotaped scenarios can support social skills instruction (Sarokoff, Taylor, & Poulson, 2001).

Visual Supports

Individuals with ASD, including those with AS, learn in a variety of different ways, but research has shown that they demonstrate strength in visual learning (cf. Just, Cherkassky, Keller, & Minshew, 2004). To support this strength, parents and professionals have developed visual supports for individuals with ASD. Put simply, visual supports make auditory information visual. Visual supports organize a sequence of events, enhancing the student's ability to understand, anticipate, and participate in those events. Visual supports supplement verbal instruction, clarifying the information for the student and increasing comprehension. Visual supports can be used to cue communication, providing reminders of what to do and say in a situation. Research shows that when individuals with AS are given the opportunity to learn with visual supports or cues, they:

- Complete more tasks independently.
- Learn more rapidly.
- Demonstrate decreased levels of frustration, anxiety, and aggression related to task completion.
- Adjust more readily to changes in their environments (cf. Odom et al., 2003; Wheeler, Baggett, Fox, & Blevins, 2006).

Visual supports can be important tools in addressing resistance, withdrawal, and meltdowns by providing visual information that allow individuals to better comprehend what is happening around them (Cardon, 2007) and further reduce environmental stressors. Further, Myles and Adreon (2001) asserted that visual supports are essential for individuals with AS because they help them focus on the task at hand by clarifying, reminding, and directing.

Numerous types of visual supports have been used with individuals with AS. Myles (2005) suggested the following guidelines in developing visual supports:

- Present information in a concise manner.
- Include a minimal amount of visual stimuli.
- Include words, pictures, or a combination of both.
- Make all components durable by using lamination, thick paper, etc.
- Make extra copies of all components in anticipation of lost or damaged materials.
- Involve the individual in making his or her visual supports.

Visual Schedules

Visual schedules take an abstract concept, such as time, and present it in a more concrete and manageable form. Schedules allow individuals to anticipate upcoming events and activities and develop an understanding of time. They facilitate the prediction of change, thereby accommodating the need for predictability and decreasing anxiety about the unknown. Visual schedules can be created to present a range of information, from individual steps in a task, to an entire day's activities. Decisions regarding schedule content and presentation should be based on the specific individual's characteristics and preferences.

Lists/Timelines

Lists and timelines are valuable ways to present information to individuals with AS. Lists might include information that would typically be presented only verbally, such as instructions, steps for handing in homework, or tasks that need to be completed. Timelines might be used to help break down a task, structure or organize completion of an assignment, or help a student visualize when an activity might take place. Because individuals with AS often have difficulty getting started when presented with a complex task, they may need additional structure or assistance to break it into manageable parts. Other individuals with AS simply have difficulty with the concept of time; for example, many students with AS may think they can read a book and write a 10-page reflection paper the night before it is due. As a result, meltdowns may occur as timelines near.

Lists and timelines provide individuals with AS with a solid representation of the information needed to complete a task. Lists and timelines can be written in a variety of formats. These are examples of information that can be usefully presented in the form of a list or timeline:

- Steps to complete a task, or a portion of a task, such as solving math problems that involve fractions with denominators
- Reminders, such as what items to bring to school or when to start an assignment and finish it to meet the deadline
- Routines, such as the routine for taking a bus or handing in assignments
- Choices, such as which activities a student may select once finished with his or her social studies in-class assignment

Stop, Observe, Deliberate, and Act Strategy

SODA is a social-behavioral learning strategy developed by Bock (2001) to enhance social interaction skills of children and adolescents with AS. The purpose of this strategy is to help youth become aware of social cues, process the cues with meaning and relevance, and enact appropriate social skills in novel social interactions (Bock, 2001). SODA incorporates visual icons with three to five self-talk questions and statements (Bock, 2001). To represent the questions and statements, the visual strategy could be changed to meet the individual needs. SODA strategy could be implemented in groups or in individual settings with direct instruction. SODA focuses on the difficulties the children and adolescents have during daily social interaction (Bock, 2007a, 2007b).

SODA uses the think-aloud, think-along model (Andrews & Mason, 1991) that encompasses four components: Stop, Observe, Deliberate, and Act (Bock, 2001). In the first component, Stop, students learn to develop an organizational schema for social interaction events. At this stage, students identify the nature of the activities and learn their sequence using self-questioning. Using the second component, Observe, students learn the social cues people use to form appropriate social interactions. When observing conversations, for example, students are guided to attend to social cues, such as the length of conversation, the tone of communicators, the strategies related to initiating and terminating conversations, and the use of appropriate nonverbal communication. In the third component, Deliberate, students create a plan for social interaction within the activity. At this stage, they have to select appropriate strategies to perform the actions in new situations. Based on the observation of the social cues people use, students plan how they are going to implement those skills in their actions and analyze their thoughts. Using the fourth component, Action, students actively participate in social interaction by using appropriate skills they have planned in advance. At this stage, students generalize the skills they have observed and planned. Two studies support the use of this strategy with adolescents with AS (Bock, 2007a, 2007b).

Video Instruction

Video instruction that provides visual cues and information can be a very helpful strategy for individuals with AS. In fact, video instruction is considered an evidence-based practice for individuals with ASD. Several studies have shown that video instruction, such as video modeling, video monitoring, and video priming, are effective in teaching various skills across settings and populations (cf. Bellini & Akullian, 2007; Ayres & Langone, 2005).

Video Modeling

Bandura (1977) described the power of social modeling and the learning of new skills by observing and imitating others. Since then, modeling has been used widely as an effective intervention strategy (Dowrick, 1999). Video modeling is an intervention that uses video technology to demonstrate desired behaviors that the learner can imitate and generalize.

Video Monitoring/Feedback

Video monitoring uses video to teach a skill. While the student watches video, the teacher provides verbal instruction. One of the benefits of video instruction is that the instructor or the learner can pause and replay a scene repeatedly. This can be helpful to the learner with AS who might have difficulty identifying an important concept while watching the video.

Video Priming

Viewing a videotape of an event prior to its occurrence can reduce the level of anxiety experienced by an individual with AS. Because video priming prepares the individual for upcoming situations and provides an explanation of expectations, it may also be helpful in reducing disruptive behaviors (Schreibman, Whalen, & Stahmer, 2000).

Self-Regulation Instruction

Karoly (1993) defined self-regulation as

> those processes, internal and/or transactional, that enable an individual to guide his/her goal-directed activities over time and across changing circumstances (contexts). Regulation implies modulation of thought, affect, behavior, or attention via deliberate or automated use of specific mechanisms and supportive metaskills. The processes of self-regulation are initiated when reutilized activity is impeded or when goal-directedness is otherwise made salient (e.g. the appearance of a challenge, the failure of habitual action patterns, etc.). (p. 25)

Self-regulation is the ability to establish and maintain the level of arousal/alertness, attention, activity, and affect (or emotion) that is appropriate for the situation at hand. In other words, self-regulation allows individuals to monitor and manage their own behavior (Fouse & Wheeler, 1997). Further, Fouse and Wheeler (1997) noted that "the ultimate goal is for individuals to be aware of their triggers and early reactions that lead to inappropriate behaviors in order to control the behavior that follows" (p. 146).

Individuals with AS experience varying degrees of ability to understand their own feelings (cf. Barnhill, 2001; Ozonoff, Rogers, & Pennington, 1991). They often have difficulty interpreting their emotions and social well-being (Myles, 2005). In fact, research has shown that individuals with AS are not reliable reporters of personal stress, anxiety, or depression (Barnhill et al., 2000b; Myles, Lee, Smith, Tien, et al., 2005). Furthermore, individuals with AS often endure the entire three-stage cycle of tantrums, rage, and meltdown, whereas most people may recognize and react to the potential for behavioral outbursts early in the cycle (Myles, 2003). Individuals with AS generally do not want to engage in the cycle of tantrums, rage, and meltdowns; nevertheless, it may be the only way they know how to express stress, cope with problems, and exhibit a host of other emotions to which they see no other solution (Myles, 2003; Myles & Southwick, 2005).

It is important and beneficial to provide individuals with this kind of exceptionality with self-regulation strategies that will help them understand their emotions and react to them in an appropriate manner (Myles, 2003, 2005). Fouse and Wheeller (1997) noted that teaching self-regulation strategies to individuals is advantageous when it (1) promotes independence, (2) promotes autonomy, (3) assists with increasing prosocial behaviors, (4) increases self-initiation of behaviors, (5) promotes responsibility, (6) decreases time demands on caretakers, and (7) decreases acting out behaviors, "shutdowns," or meltdowns. Altogether, alternative self-regulation skills such as the ability to express emotional state, alternative stress reduction strategies, self-calming skills, and so on, are needed by individuals with AS as a means of preventing or decreasing the severity of behavioral problems.

Two of the instructional strategies that have been developed to address this topic are overviewed here. The first was developed by McAfee (2002). It works well with older individuals with AS and educators who have substantial time to help students develop these skills. The second one is created by Buron and Curtis (2003). It is a streamlined version of strategies for younger individuals with AS to use at home and in school. A discussion of each instructional strategy follows.

McAfee (2002) has developed a visually based curriculum that is designed to assist students in decreasing stress by recognizing emotions and redirecting themselves to a calming or mood-lifting activity when stressed. Through the use of (1) a Stress Tracking Chart, (2) a Summary of Stress Signals Worksheet, and (3) a Stress Thermometer, students with AS learn the following:

- To identify and label their emotions using nonverbal and situational cues
- To assign appropriate values to different degrees of emotion, such as anger
- To redirect negative thoughts
- To identify environmental stressors and common reactions to them
- To recognize the early signs of stress
- To select realization techniques that match student needs

Buron and Curts (2003) created the Incredible 5-Point Scale to help young individuals with AS understand themselves. Individuals with AS are taught to recognize the levels of their specific behavioral challenges and learn a method to self-calm at each level. The scale is unique in that it can not only be used as an anger, feeling, or pain rater but also as an obsessional index, a stress scale, a meltdown or anxiety monitor, a voice volume indicator, and so on.

In addition to those two instructional strategies described above, Faherty (2000) created similar activities in her self-awareness and life lesson workbook to help individuals with AS learn about themselves and facilitate self-awareness though a series of exercises.

Circle of Friends

A "Circle of Friends" was defined by Falvey, Forest, Pearpoint, and Roseberg (1997) as a group of people gathering around a person who has become excluded or isolated. It has also been referred to as a *circle*, a *circle of support*, a *peer network*, and a *friendship circle* (Falvey et al.). The Circle of Friends approach is a strategy aimed at promoting the inclusion of students with disabilities into general education classrooms (Whitaker, Barratt, Joy, Potter, & Thomas, 1998). It was originally developed to support the process of including (1) people with disabilities in local communities where they had previously lived in institutions, and (2) students who experienced special educational needs in mainstream schools where they had previously been educated in separate special schools (Forester & Lusthaus, 1989; Snow & Forest, 1987). This approach also has been adapted to support children experiencing emotional, behavioral, and social difficulties in an educational setting (Frederickson & Turner, 2003; Newton, Taylor, & Wilson, 1996; Pearpoint & Forest, 1992; Taylor, 1996, 1997).

Newton and colleagues (1996) defined the Circle of Friends approach as "a systemic approach that recognizes the power of the peer group— and thereby of pupil culture—to be a positive as well as a constraining or exacerbating influence on individual behavior" (p. 42). Taylor (1997) succinctly described the process of establishing the Circle of Friends to assist students who have emotional and behavioral difficulties in the following steps:

1. *Establishing prerequisites.* The commitment of the school is secured to provide the staff resources needed (30–40 minutes of teacher time to facilitate a small circle group meeting per week). Then the parents and the focus students are approached. Informed consent and support from the students and their parents are obtained.

2. *Holding a class discussion.* The discussion is usually facilitated by an outsider who is familiar with the approach, such as an educational psychologist, and the classroom teacher is present. The focus student usually is not present; nevertheless, his or her strengths and difficulties are described, and the class members are invited to empathize with him or her and to build on their own experiences of friendships. Links with the focus student's behavior are drawn and suggestions are generated for assisting the

child and improving the situation. Volunteers to form a circle are sought at the end of the meeting.

3. *Establishing a circle.* A group of six to eight volunteers are selected to form the Circle of Friends and then meet with the focus student and an adult facilitator. The initial meeting of Circle of Friends generally takes place immediately after the class discussion. The class discussion is summarized for the focus student, and he or she is centrally involved in identifying target goals to be worked on and strategies to be implemented by the focus student and the Circle of Friends in the coming week. A collaborative approach to problems solving and practical arrangements are established.

4. *Conducting weekly meetings of the Circle of Friends.* Weekly meetings are typically held over a period of 6–10 weeks. The students and the school staff member (e.g., class teacher, educational psychologist) meet weekly to review progress, identify difficulties, and plan practical steps to solve problems for the focus student. The meetings are carefully managed to be a positive, supportive experience for all the students.

Based on the procedure delineated above, the Circle of Friends approach addresses every aspect of Dodge, Pettit, McClasky, and Brown's (1986) model of social competence in children, in which they hypothesized that an individual's social behavior is consequentially affected by others' perceptions/judgments and social behaviors (Frederickson & Turner, 2003). In addition, this approach incorporates peers and other people whom the student encounters everyday, such as teachers, and focuses on behaviors valued in everyday settings. Emphasis is placed on reinforcing, as naturally as possible, the application of skills to new and appropriate situations when they occur there (Frederickson & Turner, 2003).

Although the term *Circle of Friends* was not used, Attwood (1998) suggested the use of the same system of circles to help children with AS develop appropriate social behaviors. In spite of no specific data available on individuals with AS, the Circle of Friends has been reported as beneficial for students with moderate to severe disabilities at a variety of age levels, with individuals with ASD and moderate intellectual disability included in the samples (Collins, Ault, Hemmeter, & Doyle, 1996; Hughes et al., 1999; Haring & Breen, 1992; Taylor, 1997; Whitaker et al., 1998). Miller, Cooke, Test, and White (2003) also supported the Circle of Friends as an effective approach in improving social interactions of elementary-age students with mild disabilities.

Schlieder (2004) recommended that when using this strategy with an individual with AS, individuals who make up the Circle of Friends should be (1) high-status peers (e.g., cheerleaders, drill team members, athletes), (2) generally compliant with school rules, (3) socially astute, and (4) genuinely interested in (and, hopefully, like) the student with AS. Moreover, those who participate in the Circle of Friends must value the individual with AS, not merely placate and direct him or her (Myles & Simpson, 2001).

SUMMARY

Individuals with AS exhibit a series of complex behaviors that impact their ability to function successfully across environments. These behaviors must be addressed in a comprehensive manner that includes (1) recognizing that specific behaviors may be related to the individual's AS, (2) conducting an FBA that identifies why the behavior occurs, and (3) designing and implementing treatments that address the behavior's function and target areas of strength. These interventions often include priming, social narratives, visual supports, video instruction, and self-regulation strategies. A myriad of interventions may be needed to address multiple behaviors seen in AS.

REFERENCES

Achenbach, T. M., & Edelbrock, C. S. (1978). Classification of child psychopathology: A review and analysis of empirical efforts. *Psychological Bulletin, 85,* 1275–1301.

Albert, L. (1989). *A teacher's guide to cooperative discipline: How to manage your classroom and promote self-esteem.* Circle Pines, MN: American Guidance Service.

Andrews, J. F., & Mason, J. M. (1991). Strategy usage among deaf and hearing readers. *Exceptional Children, 57,* 536–545.

Asperger, H. (1944). Die "Autistischen Psychopathen" in Kindersalter. *Archives für psychiatrie and Nervenkrankheiten, 117,* 76–136.

Aspy, R., & Grossman, B. G. (2011). *The Ziggurat model: A framework for designing comprehensive interventions for high-functioning individuals with autism spectrum disorders* (2nd ed.). Shawnee Mission, KS: Autism Asperger Publishing Company.

Attwood, T. (1998). *Asperger's syndrome: A guide for parents and professionals.* London: Jessica Kingsley.

Ayres, K. M., & Langone, J. (2005). Intervention and instruction with video for students with autism: A review of the literature. *Education and Training in Developmental Disabilities, 40,* 183–196.

Bandura, A. (1977). *Self-efficacy: The exercise of control.* New York: Freeman.

Barnhill, G. P. (2001). Social attributions and depression in adolescents with Asperger syndrome. *Focus on Autism and Other Developmental Disabilities, 16,* 46–53.

Barnhill, G. P., Hagiwara, T., Myles, B. S., & Simpson, R. L. (2000a). Asperger syndrome: A study of the cognitive profiles of 37 children and adolescents. *Focus on Autism and Other Developmental Disabilities, 15,* 146–153.

Barnhill, G. P., Hagiwara, T., Myles, B. S., Simpson, R. L., Brick, M. L., & Griswold, D. E. (2000b). Parent, teacher, and self-report of problem and adaptive behaviors in children and adolescents with Asperger syndrome. *Diagnostique, 25*(2), 147–167.

Barnhill, G. P., & Myles, B. S. (2001). Attributional style and depression in adolescents with Asperger syndrome. *Journal of Positive Behavior Interventions, 3,* 175–183.

Beck, M. (1985). Understanding and managing the acting-out child. *The Pointer* 29(2), 27–29.

Bellini, S., & Akullian, J. (2007). A meta-analysis of video modeling and video self-modeling interventions for children and adolescents with autism spectrum disorders. *Exceptional Children, 73,* 264–287.

Bock, M. A. (2001). SODA strategy: Enhancing the social interaction skills of youngsters with Asperger syndrome. *Intervention in School and Clinic, 36,* 272–278.

Bock, M. A. (2007a). A social-behavioral learning strategy intervention for a child with Asperger syndrome: Brief report. *Remedial and Special Education, 28,* 258–265.

Bock, M. A. (2007b). The impact of social-behavioral learning strategy training on the social interaction skills of four students with Asperger Syndrome. *Focus on Autism and Other Developmental Disabilities, 22,* 88–95.

Boettcher, M., Koegel, R. L., McNerney, E. K., & Koegel, L. K. (2003). A family-centered prevention approach to PBS in a time of crisis. *Journal of Positive Behavior Interventions, 5*(1), 55–59.

Brownell, M. D. (2002). Musically adapted Social Stories to modify behaviors in students with autism: Four case studies. *Journal of Music Therapy, 39,* 117–144.

Buron, K. D., & Curtis, M. (2003). *The Incredible 5-Point Scale: Assisting students with autism spectrum disorders in understanding social interactions and controlling their emotional responses.* Shawnee Mission, KS: Autism Asperger Publishing Company.

Cardon, T. (2007). *Initiations and interactions: Early intervention techniques for parents of children with autism spectrum disorders.* Shawnee Mission, KS: Autism Asperger Publishing Company.

Carr, E. G., Horner, R. H., Turnbull, A. P., Marquis, J. G., Magito-McLaughlin, D., McAtee, M. L., et al. (1999). *Positive behavior support for people with developmental disabilities: A research synthesis.* Washington, DC: American Association on Mental Retardation.

Church, C., Alisanski, S., & Amanullah, S. (2000). The social, behavioral, and academic experiences of children with Asperger syndrome. *Focus on Autism and Other Developmental Disabilities, 15,* 12–20.

Collins, B., Ault, M., Hemmeter, M., & Doyle, P. (1996). Come play! *Teaching Exceptional Children, 29,* 16–21.

Dodge, K. A., Pettit, C. S., McClasky, C. J., & Brown, M. M. (1986). Social competence in children. *Monographs of the Society for Research in Child Development, 51*(2, Serial No. 213).

Dowrick, P. (1999). A review of self-modeling and related interventions. *Applied and Preventive Psychology, 8,* 23–39.

Dunn, W., Myles, B. S., & Orr, S. (2002). Sensory processing issues associated with Asperger syndrome: A preliminary investigation. *American Journal of Occupational Therapy, 56*(1), 97–102.

Durand, V. M., & Crimmins, D. (1992). *Motivation Assessment Scale.* Topeka, KS: Monaco.

Ellingson, S. A., Miltenberger, R. G., Stricker, J., Galensky, T. L., & Garlinghouse, M. (2000). Functional assessment and intervention for challenging behaviors in the classroom by general classroom teachers. *Journal of Positive Behavior Interventions, 2,* 85–97.

Faherty, C. (2000). *What does it mean to me?* Arlington, TX: Future Horizons.

Falvey, M., Forest, M., Pearpoint, M., & Rosenberg, R. (1997). *All my life's a circle.* Toronto, Canada: Inclusion Press.

Forester, M., & Lusthaus, E. (1989). Prompting education equality for all students: Circles and maps. In S. Stainback, W. Stainback, & M. Forest (Eds.), *Educating all students in the mainstream of regular education* (pp. 43–57). Baltimore: Brookes.

Fouse, B., & Wheeler, M. (1997). *A treasure chest of behavioral strategies for individuals with autism.* Arlington, TX: Future Horizons.

Frederickson, N., & Turner, J. (2003). Utilizing the classroom peer group to address children's social needs: An evaluation of the Circle of Friends intervention approach. *Journal of Special Education, 36,* 234–245.

Ghaziuddin, M. (2002). Asperger syndrome: Associated psychiatric and medical conditions. *Focus on Autism and Other Developmental Disabilities, 17*(3), 138–144.

Ghaziuddin, M., Ghaziuddin, N., & Greden, J. (2002). Depression in persons with autism: Implications for research and clinical care. *Journal of Autism and Developmental Disorders, 32,* 299–306.

Ghaziuddin, M., Weidmer-Mikhail, E., & Ghazziuddin, N. (1998). Comorbidity of Asperger syndrome: A preliminary report. *Journal of Intellectual Disability Research, 42,* 279–283.

Gray, C. (1995). *Social Stories unlimited: Social Stories and comic strip conversations.* Jenison, MI: Jenison Public Schools.

Gray, C. (2000). *Writing Social Stories with Carol Cray.* Arlington, TX: Future Horizons.

Gray, C., A., & Gerand, J. D. (1993). Social Stories: Improving responses of students with autism with accurate social information. *Focus on Autistic Behavior, 8,* 1–10.

Grossman, J. B., Klin, A., Carter, A. S., & Volkmar, F. R. (2000). Verbal bias in recognition of facial emotions in children with Asperger syndrome. *Journal of Child Psychology and Psychiatry and Allied Disciplines, 41,* 369–379.

Hagiwara, T., & Myles, B. S. (1999). A multimedia Social Story intervention: Teaching skills to children with autism. *Focus on Autism and Other Developmental Disabilities, 14,* 82–95.

Haring, T., & Breen, C. (1992). A peer-mediated social network intervention to enhance the social integration of persons with moderate and severe disabilities. *Journal of Applied Behavior Analysis, 25,* 319–333.

Horner, R. H., Carr, E. G., Strain, P. S., Todd, A. W., & Reed, H. K. (2002). Problem behavior interventions for young children with autism: A research synthesis. *Journal of Autism and Developmental Disorders, 32,* 423–446.

Hughes, C., Guth, C., Hall, S., Presley, J., Dye, M., & Byers, C. (1999). "They are my best friends": Peer buddies promote inclusion in high school. *Teaching Exceptional Children, 31,* 32–37.

Individuals with Disabilities Education Act. (2004). *Individuals with Disabilities Education Act Amendments of 2004.*

Ivey, M. L., Heflin, L. J., & Alberto, P. (2004). The use of Social Stories to promote independence behaviors in novel events for children with PDD-NOS. *Focus on Autism and Other Developmental Disabilities, 19,* 164–176.

Janzen, J. (2003). *Understanding the nature of autism: A guide to autism spectrum disorders* (2nd ed.). San Antonio, TX: Therapy Skill Builders.

Just, M. A., Cherkassky, V. L., Keller, T. A., & Minshew, N. J. (2004). Cortical activation and synchronization during sentence comprehension in high-functioning autism: Evidence of underconnectivity. *Brain, 127,* 1811–1821.

Karoly, P. (1993). Mechanisms of self-regulation: A system view. *Annual Review of Psychology, 44,* 23–52.

Kern, L., Dunlap, G., Clarke, S., & Childs, K. (1994). Student-assisted functional assessment interview. *Diagnostique, 19*(2–3), 29–39.

Kim, J. A., Szatmari, P., Bryson, S. E., Streiner, D. L., & Wilson, F. J. (2000). The prevalence of anxiety and mood problems among children with autism and Asperger syndrome. *Autism, 4,* 117–132.

Koegel, L. K., Koegel, R. L., Frea, W., & Green-Hopkins, I. (2003). Priming as a method of coordinating educational services for students with autism. *Language, Speech, and Hearing Services in Schools, 34,* 228–235.

Lewis, T. J., Scott, T. M., & Sugai, G. (1994). The Problem Behavior Questionnaire: A teacher-based instrument to develop functional hypotheses of problem behavior in general education classrooms. *Diagnostique, 19*(2–3), 103–115.

Long, N. J., Morse, W. C., & Newman, R. G. (1976). *Conflict in the classroom: The educational children with problems* (3rd ed.). Belmont, CA: Wadsworth.

Macintosh, K., & Dissanayake, C. (2006). Social skills and problem behaviours in school-aged children with high-functioning autism and Asperger's disorder. *Journal of Autism Developmental Disorders, 36,* 1065–1076.

MacNeil, B. M., Lopes, V. A., & Minnes, P. M. (2009). Anxiety in children and adolescents with autism spectrum disorders. *Reearch in Autism Spectrum Disorders, 3,* 1–21.

McAfee, J. (2002). *Navigating the social world: A curriculum for individuals with Asperger's syndrome, high-functioning autism, and related disorders.* Arlington, TX: Future Horizons.

Miller, M. C., Cooke, N. L., Test, D. W., & White, R. (2003). Effects of friendship circles on the social interactions of elementary age students with mild disabilities. *Journal of Behavioral Education, 12,* 167–184.

Moore, P. S. (2004). The use of Social Stories in a psychology service for children with learning disabilities: A case study of a sleep problem. *British Journal of Learning Disabilities, 32,* 133–138.

Myles, B. S. (2003). Behavioral forms of stress management for individuals with Asperger syndrome. *Child and Adolescent Psychiatric Clinics, 12,* 123–141.

Myles, B. S. (2005). *Children and youth with Asperger syndrome: Strategies for success in inclusive settings.* Thousand Oaks, CA: Corwin Press.

Myles, B. S., & Adreon, D. (2001). *Asperger syndrome and adolescence: Practical solutions for school success.* Shawnee Mission, KS: Autism Asperger Publishing Company.

Myles, B. S., Barnhill, G. P., Hagiwara, T., Griswold, D. E., & Simpson, R. L. (2001). A synthesis of studies on the intellectual, academic, social/emotional, and sensory characteristics of children and youth with Asperger syndrome. *Education and Training in Mental Retardation and Developmental Disabilities, 36,* 304–311.

Myles, B. S., Hagiwara, T., Dunn, W., Rinner, L., Reese, M., Huggins, A., et al. (2004). Sensory issues in children with Asperger syndrome and autism. *Education and Training in Developmental Disabilities, 3,* 283–290.

Myles, B. S., Lee, H., Smith, S. M., Tien, C., Chou, A., & Hudson, J. (2005). A large-scale study of the characteristics of Asperger syndrome. *Education and Training for Developmental Disabilities, 42*(4), 448–459.

Myles, B. S., & Simpson, R. L. (2001). *Asperger syndrome: A guide for educators and parents* (2nd ed.). Austin, TX: PRO-ED.

Myles, B. S., & Simpson, R. L. (2002). Students with Asperger syndrome: Implications for counselors. *Counseling and Human Development, 34*(7), 1–14.

Myles, B. S., & Southwick, J. (2005). *Asperger syndrome and difficult moments: Practical solutions for tantrums, rage, and meltdowns* (2nd ed.). Shawnee Mission, KS: Autism Asperger Publishing Company.

Newton, C., Taylor, G., & Wilson, D. (1996). Circle of Friends: An inclusive approach to meeting emotional and behavioral needs. *Educational Psychology in Practice, 11,* 4.

Odom, S. L., Brown, W. H., Frey, T., Karasu, N., Smith-Cantor, L. L., & Strain, P. (2003). Evidence-based practices for young children with autism: Contributions for single-subject design research. *Focus on Autism and Other Developmental Disabilities, 18,* 166–175.

O'Neill, R. E., Horner, R. H., Albin, R. W., Sprague, J. R., Storey, K., & Newton, J. S. (1997). *Functional assessment and program development for problem behavior: A practical handbook* (2nd ed.). Albany, NY: Brooks/Cole.

Ozonoff, S., Rogers, S., & Pennington, B. (1991). Asperger's syndrome: Evidence of an empirical distinction from high-functioning autism. *Journal of Child Psychology and Psychiatry, 32,* 1107–1122.

Pearpoint, J., & Forest, M. (1992). Kick 'em out or keep 'em in: Exclusion or inclusion. In J. Pearpoint, M. Forest, & K. Snow (Eds.), *The inclusion paper* (pp. 80–88). Toronto, Canada: Inclusion Press.

Pfeiffer, B., Kinnealey, M., Reed, C., & Herzberg, G. (2005). Sensory modulation and affective disorders in children and adolescents with Asperger's disorder. *American Journal of Occupational Therapy, 59,* 335–345.

Polemini, M. A., Richdale, A. L., & Francis, A. J. P. (2005). A survey of sleep problems in autism, Asperger's disorder, and typically developing children. *Journal of Intellectual Disability Research, 49,* 260–268.

Reitzel, J., & Szatmari, P. (2003). Cognitive and academic problems. In M. Prior (Ed.), *Learning and behavior problems in Asperger syndrome* (pp. 35–54). New York: Guilford Press.

Reynolds, C. R., & Kamphaus, R. W. (1992). *Behavior Assessment System for Children.* Circle Pines, MN: American Guidance Services.

Russell, E., & Sofronoff, K. (2005). Anxiety and social worries in children with Asperger syndrome. *Australian and New Zealand Journal of Psychiatry, 39,* 633–628.

Sansosti, F. J., Powell-Smith, K. A., & Kincaid, D. (2004). A research synthesis of Social Story interventions for children with autism spectrum disorders. *Focus on Autism and Other Developmental Disabilities, 19*(4), 194–204.

Sarokoff, R. A., Taylor, B. A., & Poulson, C. L. (2001). Teaching children with autism to engage in conversational exchanges: Script fading with embedded textual stimuli. *Journal of Applied Behavior Analysis, 34,* 81–84.

Scattone, D., Tingstrom, D. H., & Wilczynski, S. M. (2006). Increasing appropriate social interactions of children with autism spectrum disorders using Social Stories™. *Focus on Autism and Other Developmental Disabilities, 21,* 211–222.

Schlieder, M. (2004). *With open arms: Creating school communities of support for kids with social challenges using Circle of Friends, extracurricular activities, and learning teams.* Shawnee Mission, KS: Autism Asperger Publishing Company.

Schreibman, L., Whalen, C., & Stahmer, A. C. (2000). The use of video priming to reduce disruptive transition behavior in children with autism. *Journal of Positive Behavior Intervention, 2,* 3–11.

Schopler, E. (1994). Behavioral priorities for autism and related developmental disorders. In E. Schopler & G. B. Mesibov (Eds.), *Behavioral issues in autism* (pp. 55–75). New York: Plenum Press.

Snow, J., & Forest, M. (1987). Circles. In M. Forest (Ed.), *More education integration* (pp. 169–176). Downsview, Ontario, Canada: G. Allan Roeher Institute.

Tantam, D. (2000). Psychological disorder in adolescents and adults with Asperger syndrome. *Autism, 4,* 47–62.

Taylor, G. (1996). Creating a Circle of Friends: A case study. In H. Cowie & S. Sharp (Eds.), *Peer counseling in school* (pp. 73–86). London: David Fulton.

Taylor, G. (1997). Community building in school: Developing a Circle of Friends. *Educational and Child Psychology, 14,* 45–50.

Thiemann, K. S., & Goldstein, H. (2004). Effects of peer training and written text cueing on social communication of school-age children with pervasive developmental disorder. *Journal of Speech, Language, and Hearing Research, 47,* 126–144.

Todis, B., Severson, H. H., & Walker, H. M. (1990). The critical events scale: Behavioral profiles of students with externalizing and internalizing behavior disorders. *Behavioral Disorders, 15,* 75–86.

Tonge, B. J., Brereton, A. V., Gray, K. M., & Einfeld, S. L. (1999). Behavioural and emotional disturbance in high-functioning autism and Asperger syndrome. *Autism, 3,* 117–130.

Trillingsgaard, A. (1999). The script model in relation to autism. *European Child and Adolescent Psychiatry, 8,* 45–49.

Volden, J., & Johnston, J. (1999). Cognitive scripts in autistic children and adolescents. *Journal of Autism and Developmental Disorders, 29,* 203–211.

Volkmar, F. R., Cohen, D., & Paul, R. (1986). An evaluation of DSM-III criteria for infantile autism. *Journal of the American Academy of Child and Adolescent Psychiatry, 25,* 190–197.

Wheeler, J. J., Baggett, B. A., Fox, J., & Blevins, L. (2006). Treatment integrity: A review of intervention studies conducted with autism. *Focus on Autism and Other Developmental Disabilities, 21,* 45–55.

Whitaker, P., Barratt, P., Joy, H., Potter, M., & Thomas, G. (1998). Children with autism and peer group support: Using "Circle of Friends." *British Journal of Special Education, 25,* 60–64.

Wilde, L. D., Koegel, L. K., & Koegel, R. L. (1992). *Increasing success in school through priming: A training manual.* Santa Barbara: University of California.

Wing, L. (1981). Asperger's syndrome: A clinical account. *Psychological Medicine, 11,* 115–129.

CHAPTER 8

Frameworks for Behavioral Interventions to Improve Peer Relationships and the Management of Emotions in Asperger Syndrome

Tony Attwood

An essential characteristic of Autism Spectrum Disorder Level 1 (Asperger's Syndrome) acccording to the fifth edition of the *Diagnostic and Statistical Manual of Mental Disorders* (DSM-5; American Psychiatric Association, 2013) is persistent deficits in social communication and social interaction, which includes difficulties in making friends and reduced sharing of interests, emotions, or affect and poorly integrated verbal and nonverbal communication. This chapter provides a developmental framework to improve friendship abilities and the understanding and expression of emotions using cognitive-behavioral therapy.

At present, we do not have standardized tests of social interaction abilities and especially of peer relationships to produce a "friendship quotient" for a child or adult with AS. The observation, assessment, and interpretation of various aspects of social interaction skills are primarily a matter of subjective clinical judgments. An assessment of peer relationships is usually achieved by (1) identifying the person's friends; (2) evaluating the quality, stability, depth, and maturity of the friendships; and (3) observing and participating with the person in a social interaction. This interaction format can range from playing with a young child to having a conversation about friendship and social situations with an adult.

FRIENDSHIP CHARACTERISTICS OF ASPERGER SYNDROME

Friendship in children and adults with AS is a relatively neglected area of research (Bauminger et al., 2008a). However, we do know that children with AS have a concept and expression of friendship that is immature in comparison with their intellectual peers (Attwood, 2007; Botroff, Bartak, Langford, Page, & Tong, 1995). The child has fewer friends and plays with other children less often and for a shorter duration (Bauminger & Kasari, 2000; Bauminger, Shulman, & Agam, 2003; Bauminger & Shulman, 2003). The actual friendships may be unusual in that the child may choose to play with younger children, prefer the company of adults, or choose to be alone in the playground. Research has indicated that children who have AS are more likely to be rejected by peers, and have fewer reciprocal friendships and are more often on the periphery of social networks and unengaged in the school playground. They are also increasingly less connected with peers with increasing grade levels at elementary school (Kasari, Locke, Gulsrud, & Rotheram-Fuller, 2011; Rotheram-Fuller, Kasari, Chamberlain, & Locke, 2010). When playing with other children, his or her behavior can be perceived by peers as immature, intrusive, irritating or dominating. The child may not recognize the boundaries of personal space, cope with changes in activities or conversation, or recognize when an interaction has ended. An adult may perceive the behavior with peers as rude and uncooperative (Church, Alisanski, & Amanullah, 2000). Adolescents with AS are also less likely to see friends out of school and be invited to parties and social gatherings of peers (Shattuck, Orsmond, Wagner, & Cooper, 2011).

From early childhood to the adult years there can be changes in the motivation of individuals with AS to seek friends. Very young children with AS may not be interested in the activities of their peers or in making friends. They are usually more interested in understanding the physical rather than the social world, and may enter the kindergarten playground to explore the drainage or plumbing system of the school, or to search for insects and rocks. The social games of peers are perceived as boring, with incomprehensible social rules. These children are content with solitude or may be motivated to interact with adults who can answer questions beyond the knowledge of their peers; or they may seek refuge from the noisy and chaotic playground in the quiet and safe sanctuary of the school library to read about interesting topics such as volcanoes, meteorology, and transport systems.

In the early elementary school years, children with AS often notice that their age peers are having fun socializing, and they actually want to be included in the social games to experience the obvious enjoyment. However, despite intellectual ability, their level of social maturity is usually at least 2 years behind that of their peers, and they may have conspicuous difficulties with the degree of reciprocal and cooperative play expected by other children. These children are unable to accurately read social situations and therefore act inappropriately, to the annoyance of their peers. Such children can also be ridiculed as well as rejected for not being as socially mature as their peers. In general, girls and some boys with AS cope with their difficulties in making friends by the strategy of imitation. They can astutely observe the interactions and games of their peers, making a mental note of what to do and say, and when participating in a game or activity, imitate their peers while not knowing intuitively what to do or why. This strategy can camouflage from adults the children's difficulties with reciprocal interaction with peers and lead to a delay in diagnosis.

In the middle school years children with AS may achieve genuine friendships but have a tendency to be too dominant or to have too rigid a view of what to do together. The shared creativity, flexibility, and spontaneity of typical peers may be missing. These children expect an ordered interaction with set rules. Such children may "wear out their welcome." However, some typical children who are naturally kind and understanding may perceive children with AS as genuine friends and be tolerant of their behavior, forging friendships that last for several years or more.

Sometimes the friendship is not with a compassionate, socially competent and confident child, but with a similarly socially isolated child who shares the same interests but not necessarily the diagnosis. The friendship tends to be functional and practical, exchanging items and knowledge of mutual interest, and may extend beyond a dyad to a small group of like-minded children with a similar level of social competence and popularity. They can be members of a chess club or collect the latest game cards from Japan. A friendship may develop with a child recently enrolled at the school or someone from a different culture who also feels marginalized. However, the friendship may be transitory as the other child eventually finds peers who are more in tune with his or her interests and social maturity. In mid-adolescence, the teenager with AS may start to identify with those on the fringes of adolescent society, characters who may not be good role models but will accept someone who is considered "weird." Being accepted and included by anyone may be of great importance to the adolescent with AS, though parents may be concerned about the nature of the association and the values and morality of the "friends."

In late adolescence, teenagers with AS may seek more than a superficial friendship and express a longing for a boyfriend or girlfriend and eventually a partner. The adolescent boy with AS may ask his parents forlornly, "How do I get a girlfriend?" Attempts to develop a relationship beyond platonic friendship can lead to exclusion, ridicule, and a misinterpretation of intentions with accusations of stalking. The adolescent with AS can feel extremely confused and isolated socially, alone in the crowd. Some adolescents with AS have different value systems and interests to those of their peers, as explained by Caroline, who said of her teenage years, "It was as though I was a generation ahead of the other students."

Typical adolescents compare themselves with their peers to find their own status in the social hierarchy of high school, and feedback from peers can make or break self-esteem. Adolescents with AS frequently report that their peers are very critical, often humiliating and tormenting them and rejecting their requests to participate in a conversation or activity. This treatment has a devastating effect on self-esteem and contributes to feelings of alienation and depression. Eventually, perhaps when emotionally and socially more mature as a young adult, the person with AS can experience an intimate relationship, and some do achieve a lifetime relationship. However, both partners would probably benefit from relationship counseling to identify and encourage the adjustments needed to make an unconventional relationship successful for both. We now have considerable literature on relationship counseling for couples in which one partner has AS (Aston, 2003, 2009; Edmonds & Worton, 2005; Hendrickx, 2008; Jacobs, 2003; Lawson, 2005; Rodman, 2003; Slater-Walker & Slater-Walker, 2002; Stanford, 2003; Thompson, 2008).

Clinicians are becoming more aware that the social and friendship profile of girls who have AS can be different from the profile of boys. Girls can be more creative in their coping and camouflaging mechanisms in friendship situations. They are more likely than the boys to carefully observe and analyze the social play and friendship skills of their peers and subsequently imitate those behaviors to create a superficial sociability. However, there is a lack of social identity and confidence in social situations.

The girl who has AS may also have a single close friend who provides guidance and security in social situations with peers or she may prefer to have animals as substitute friends. She is likely to be described by adults as quiet, shy and sensitive, and unlikely to be of concern to teachers with regard to friendship skills in the elementary school years. Thus, in early childhood, her social and friendship difficulties are almost invisible. In contrast, the social demands in the middle school, and especially the high school years, become more complex and less observable, and at this stage, the girl who has AS may become more conspicuously different from her peers and clearly need programs designed to improve friendship abilities for adolescents who have AS (Attwood, 2007).

Over the last few years there has been an increasing number of training programs published that are specifically designed to encourage boys and girls who have an ASD to improve social and friendship skills (Carter & Santomauro, 2010; Cook O'Toole, 2013; Crooke & Garcia Winner, 2011; Densmore, 2007; Diamond, 2011; Garcia Winner & Crooke, 2011; Kiker Painter, 2006; McAfee, 2002; Ordetx, 2012; Timms, 2011; Williams White, 2011). We also now have interactive DVD training programs, such as *Secret Agent Society* which are specifically designed to improve the friendship and social skills of 8- to 12-year-old children who have AS (Beaumont & Sofronoff, 2008). several research studies have evaluated specific manualized programs with positive results (De Rosier, Swick, Ornstein Davis, McMillen, & Matthews, 2011; Laugeson, Frankel, Gantman, Dillon, & Mogil, 2012; Lopata, Thomeer, Volker, Toomey, Nida, et al., 2010). A recent review of social skills training programs suggests that there is preliminary evidence for the value of group-based social skills interventions for children and adolescents who have AS (Cappadocia & Weiss, 2011).

A DEVELOPMENTAL FRAMEWORK TO IMPROVE FRIENDSHIP ABILITIES

For typical children, the acquisition of friendship skills is based on an innate ability that develops throughout childhood in association with progressive changes in social cognition and the modifications and maturity that occur through social experiences. Unfortunately, children with AS are not able to rely on intuitive abilities in social interactions and must rely more on their intellectual abilities and experiences. They have difficulty in complex social situations that have not been rehearsed or for which they have not prepared. Thus, it is essential that such children receive tuition and guided practice in making and keeping friends and that their friendship experiences are constructive and encouraging. The optimum environment to develop reciprocal play with peers is the classroom and the playground rather than at home or in a clinic. Schools and teachers will need to be aware of the importance of designing a friendship curriculum for children with AS, including staff training and resources. The curriculum should teach social cognition as well as discrete social skills (Crook, Hendrix, & Rachman, 2008). The following suggestions are designed for implementation by teachers and parents, using as a framework the developmental stages of friendship that occur in typical children and that can be applied to children with AS.

Friendship from 3 to 6 Years

Typical children from the ages of 3 to 6 years have a functional and egocentric conceptualization of friendship. When asked why a particular child is his or her friend, a typical child's reply is usually based on possessions (the other child has toys that the child admires or wants to use), proximity (lives next door, sits at same table), and egocentricity (he helps me or she likes me). Sharing toys and playing together are the focus of friendship, and the child gradually moves from engaging primarily in parallel play to recognizing that some games and activities cannot happen unless there is an element of sharing and turn taking.

Very young children with AS usually have a clear end product in mind when playing with toys, especially construction activities; however, they may fail to effectively communicate this goal to a friend or to tolerate or incorporate the other child's suggestions, as this would produce an unanticipated outcome. For example, the child with AS may have the mental image of the completed structure in mind when playing with construction blocks, and become extremely agitated when another child places a brick where, according to this mental image, there shouldn't be a brick. The typical child, meanwhile, does not understand why his or her act of cooperation is rejected. Children with AS often seek predictability and control in play activities, whereas their age peers seek spontaneity, flexibility, and collaboration. For a child with AS, sharing means having to lose control.

An Adult Acting as a Friend

For the young child with AS who is probably not interested in playing with peers, but who may be motivated to interact with adults, reciprocal play can be taught by an adult who "plays the part" of an age peer. The adult "friend" will need to adjust his or her abilities and language to resemble that of the child's peers. The intention is to model and encourage reciprocal play between equals, with neither friend being dominant. A class teacher has a designated and relatively fixed role as an adult not a friend. However, an adult paraprofessional, who provides support to facilitate integration into the kindergarten, can sometimes act the role of friend or mentor, giving guidance and encouragement. It is important that adults, especially parents, observe the natural play of the child's peers, noting the games, equipment, rules, and language. The strategy is for the parent to play with the child using "child speak"—the typical utterances of children of that age—and to be equal and reciprocal in terms of ability, interests, and cooperation. The adult can demonstrate specific social cues and momentarily stop to encourage the child to see or listen to the cue, explaining what the cue means and how he or she is expected to respond. It is important that the adult role-plays examples of being a good friend and also orchestrates situations that illustrate unfriendly actions, such as being autocratic and critical. Appropriate and inappropriate responses can be enacted by the adult to provide the child with a range of responses, and guidance offered to determine which response is friendly and why.

Video Recordings of Children Playing

Children with AS often enjoy watching the same movie many times. Rewatching movies is also a pleasurable activity for typical children, but children with AS may be unusual in terms of the number of times they watch the film or program. Parents can be concerned that watching the same program so many times is a waste of time; however, the problem may not be what the child with AS is doing, but what he or she is watching. Video recordings can be made of the real-life friendship activities and experiences of the child with AS—for example, his or her peers playing in the sandpit or play house, or "show and tell" time in class. The child can then replay, perhaps many times, the "friendship documentary" to better understand the social cues, responses, sequence of activities, actions of peers, and the child's own role as a friend. An adult can use the freeze-frame and replay facility to focus on a specific social cue, identify friendly behavior, and point out what the child with AS did that was appropriate.

Pretend Games

Typical young children often enjoy make-believe, pretend, or dressing-up games based on popular characters and stories from books, television programs, and films. The play of the child with AS can also be based on characters and events in fiction, but may be qualitatively different in that it is usually a solitary rather than shared activity and an exact reenactment with little variation or creativity. The reenactment may include other children, but only if they follow the directions of the child with AS and do not change the script or outcome. The child will need to be encouraged to be more flexible in his or her "imaginative" play with age peers. The principle is to learn that something is not wrong if it is different.

Activities to encourage pretend play can include games in which the objective is to invent as many uses as possible for a given object; that is, to think beyond the most obvious, functional use. For example, how many uses can be imagined for a brick, a paper clip, a section of toy train track? An adult can explain that a section of train track could become the wings of an airplane, a sword, or a ladder, for example. This will encourage the ability to "break set" and feel more comfortable when involved in pretend play with other children. The adult can act as a friend in make-believe games, using the phrase "Let's pretend that . . . ," thus encouraging flexible thinking and creativity. Children with AS can be very rule-bound and need to learn that when playing with a friend, it is possible sometimes to change the rules and be inventive, yet still have an enjoyable experience, and that this is not necessarily a cause for anxiety. Pretend games also encourage flexible thinking for problem solving. Because children with AS have impaired executive function, especially in the area of flexible thinking, "let's pretend" activities can improve social and cognitive development, especially flexibility in problem solving (Attwood, 2007).

Encouragement for Being Friendly

When discussing their childhood social experiences, adults with AS often describe the criticism of teachers and parents when they made social mistakes but note that there was rarely any praise for appropriate behaviors, a common response being, "You should have known what to do." There can be a conspicuous absence of positive feedback. Children with AS often assume that at the end of an interaction, a lack of criticism, sarcasm, or derisory laughter means that the interaction was successful, yet they have no idea what they did that was socially appropriate. When an adult, peer, or friend is interacting with a young child with AS, a conscious effort should be made to point out and comment on what the child did that was friendly. Many children with AS have a pathological fear of failure, especially in a social context, which can contribute to increased social withdrawal or reticence to participate. Conversely, there can be enormous relief and delight when they achieve success, which will encourage further participation.

Friendship from 6 to 9 Years

At this stage in the development of friendships, typical children accept and incorporate the influences, preferences, and goals of their friends in their play with a greater degree of reciprocity. They become more aware of the thoughts and feelings of their peers and how their actions and comments can hurt a friend emotionally. The child is prepared to inhibit some actions and thoughts, to "think it, not say it," or to tell a "white lie" in order not to hurt a friend's feelings. There is the expectation of greater cooperation and mutual assistance. A friendship may develop because both children have similar interests, and aspects of a friend's character, rather than his or her possessions, are recognized ("He's fun to be with," "She has great play ideas," "We laugh together," "We look after each other"), with the genuine sharing of resources and fairness and reliability in games becoming increasingly important.

Role-Play Activities

Supervised role play with peers provides practice in aspects of cooperative play such as giving and receiving compliments, accepting suggestions, working toward a common goal, being aware of personal body space, coping with and giving criticism, recognizing signs of boredom and embarrassment, and knowing when and how to interrupt. The role play and modeling of aspects of friendship such as giving compliments can be recorded on video to provide practice and constructive feedback (Apple, Billingsley, & Schwartz, 2005). Video self-modeling can also be used to teach classroom social rules (Lang et al., 2008) This is also the age at which the child may benefit from a social skills group (see Rubin, Chapter 6, this volume) and guidance from a speech pathologist in the pragmatic aspects of language to facilitate friendships (see Paul et al., Chapter 4, this volume).

   Children with AS can be perceived by peers as being less fun to play with, aloof or authoritarian, and less likely to be helpful or to express positive affect (Attwood, 2007; Bauminger et al., 2008b). A strategy to improve the quality of reciprocal interaction is to use the construction toy Lego, which is very popular with all children but especially with those who have AS. Building a Lego model as a team can be a way of encouraging cooperative play (Owens, Granader, Humphrey, & Baron-Cohen, 2008). Children in the group can be designated specific roles such as the supplier, engineer, or builder. Encouragement from a supervising adult is given for behaviors such as collaboration, assistance, managing potential conflict, and appreciation. The adult can point out examples of problems in cooperation and ask the children to suggest and apply interpersonal solutions.

Young children with AS are usually brutally honest and speak their mind. Their allegiance is to the truth, not to people's feelings. Although honesty is a virtue, peers at this stage are starting to tell white lies so as not to hurt friends' feelings, or to express solidarity and allegiance to a friendship by not informing an adult of the misbehavior of a friend. Such behavior may appear immoral and illogical to children with AS, who are willing to tell the teacher "who did it," or tell a friend that he or she has made a stupid mistake. They may have to learn not to tell the truth all the time.

A Paraprofessional in the Classroom and Playground

To facilitate successful social inclusion and friendships in the classroom and playground, the child with AS will probably need a designated support staff member at school. A paraprofessional can observe the child's social interaction abilities, particularly behaviors indicative of age-appropriate friendship skills, and provide immediate positive feedback and guidance. The paraprofessional has a number of functions, including:

- Helping the child identify the relevant social cues and responses.
- Providing individual tuition using specific activities or games, role play, rehearsal, and writing Social Stories™ (see later section) with the child.
- Encouraging other children to successfully include the child with AS in their play.
- Providing guidance in managing potential conflict between the child with AS and peers.
- Providing positive feedback for the child.

A child with AS is trying to understand the social play of his or her peers in much the same way as an anthropologist who has discovered a new tribe will want to study its people and customs. The anthropologist will need someone from that culture to explain the customs and language. A paraprofessional assigned to the child with AS can take the role of a guide to explain this new culture or civilization. The process is one of discovery and explanation of the reasons for particular customs or friendship rules and expectations to a child whose problem is a lack of knowledge, rather than deliberate rudeness or provocation.

Programs for Peers

Typical children will know that the child with AS does not play or interact with them in the same way as other children, and peers may have a greater influence on successful inclusion of children with AS than the teacher (Bauminger & Kasari, 2000; Humphrey & Lewis, 2008). The reaction to the child with AS can be rejection and ridicule rather than acceptance and inclusion. As much as we have programs to help the child with AS integrate with his or her peers, the other children will need their own guidance and encouragement. They will need to know how to respond appropriately to behaviors that appear unfriendly and how to encourage abilities that facilitate friendships. The class teacher will need to be a good role model of what to do when interacting with the child with AS and should commend other children who adapt to, welcome, and support the child.

Friendship from 9 to 13 Years

During the third stage in the development of friendships there is a distinct gender split in the choice of friends, and a friend is defined not simply as someone who helps but as someone who is carefully chosen because of specific personality attributes. A friend is someone who genuinely cares and who has complementary attitudes, ideas, and values. There is a growing need for companionship, enjoyment of being in a particular friend's company, and a greater selectivity and durability in the friendship alliances. There is a strong desire to be accepted and liked by peers, and a mutual sharing of experiences with lengthy conversations sharing thoughts rather than toys. With an increase in self-disclosure there is the recognition of the importance of being trustworthy and a tendency to seek advice not only for practical problems but also for interpersonal and emotional issues. Friends support each other in terms of repairing each other's feelings. When pre-adolescents are sad, angry, or anxious, friends will cheer them up, calm them down, or provide reassurance.

Same-Gender Friendships

In this developmental stage of friendship, there is usually a clear gender preference in the choice of friends and associates. The activities and interests of boys, who may, for example, be playing ballgames as a team, will be considered of little interest to boys with AS, who often do not understand the rules of team games and are clumsy with ball skills, which require motor planning, dexterity, and coordination (Attwood, 2007). The boy with AS knows that he is probably the last person chosen for a team and can be actively shunned by and alienated from potential male friends.

When the boy with AS is alone on the playground, he is likely to be approached by one of two groups: the predatory males who seek someone socially isolated, vulnerable, and gullible to tease and torment; or girls who feel sorry for the boy because of his apparent loneliness, and offer inclusion and support in their activities and games. Whereas other boys at this age would usually shun girls, a boy with AS can be willingly recruited into the play of girls and actively welcomed. If the boy with AS is unsure what to do, his female friends are more likely to be supportive than critical ("He's a boy, so he wouldn't understand, and I'll help him"). There can be the development of genuine friendships with girls rather than boys.

Girls with AS at this stage of friendship development may reject the companionship of same-gender friends. They may be critical of their female peers, considering girls to be obsessed by "who likes who" for reasons that seem to be illogical or unfriendly. The in- and out-group members and rapidly changing friendship cliques are confusing, as is peer pressure between girls, which can often focus on what is viewed as "cool" in the way of appearance, clothing, and accessories. The girl with AS can have considerable difficulty understanding these new dimensions of friendships; she tends to prioritize honesty and fidelity in friendships and prefers to wear clothing that is comfortable rather than fashionable. The most comfortable clothing can be male clothing. Hair may be worn very long to create a curtain or wall behind which the girl can "hide," or very short for convenience, with no desire to appear "feminine." While the activities of other girls can be confusing and illogical, the activities of boys may be perceived as interesting and based on physical activities rather than conversations and emotions. A girl with AS may be interested in, and then "adopted" or recruited by, a group of boys. She then becomes known as a "tomboy," with male friends who are more tolerant of someone who has "come over to their side"; and once again, if she is unsure what to do in a social situation, she is likely to experience support, not ridicule ("She's a girl, she wouldn't understand—but that's OK, we don't mind"). The child with AS, boy or girl, needs a balance of same- and opposite-gender friends and associates, and some social engineering may be necessary to ensure acceptance by same-gender groups. Teachers will need to monitor group inclusion and exclusion and actively encourage children of the same gender to allow and support the acceptance and integration of the child with AS.

Drama Classes

Another option to help the young adolescent develop friendship skills is to adapt drama classes to focus on the real-life social experiences and difficulties of adolescents with AS. Liane Holliday Willey (1999), in her book *Pretending to Be Normal*, describes how she improved her social understanding by observation, imitation and acting. The teenager with AS can learn and practice aspects of adolescent interaction such as conversation topics popular with peers, being a good listener, expressing affection for someone he or she likes, and how to react to being teased or bullied. Drama activities can teach appropriate body language, facial expressions, and tone of voice, and provide an opportunity for the young person with AS to act and rehearse a potential script to respond to specific situations. We now have resource material for drama therapy specifically for adolescents with AS (Schneider, 2006), relevant publications in the psychodrama literature (Kirk & Dutton, 2006), and research studies (Lerner, Mikami, & Levine, 2011; Portman Minne & Semrud-Clikeman, 2012).

Friendship from 13 Years to Adult

In the previous stage of friendship for typical adolescents, there may be a small core of close friends, but in next developmental stage, the number of friends and the breadth and depth of friendship increase. There can be different friends for different needs, such as a need for comfort, humor, or practical or confidential advice. A friend is defined as someone who "accepts me for who I am" or "thinks the same way I do about things." A friend provides a sense of personal identity and is compatible with one's own personality. There are less concrete and more abstract definitions of friendship, with what may be described as autonomous interdependence.

Teenagers with AS often feel victimized and isolated from their peers at high school. They experience fewer social interactions during and between classes and especially during the lunch break, with fewer, if any, genuine friends (Wainscott, Naylor, Sutcliffe, Tantam, & Williams, 2008). The socially isolated adolescent with AS may retreat after school and at weekends to his or her bedroom, preferring not to venture out to meet teenage peers. Due to past experience, he or she expects to be ridiculed and victimized and have attempts at friendship rejected. Home is perceived as a safe haven or castle, with parents having considerable difficulty encouraging the adolescent to join the family or leave the house for social occasions. This self-imposed isolation can be a significant problem when the adolescent graduates from high school. Unless employment or further education is arranged almost immediately after graduation, the fear of failure in social situations can lead the adolescent to be extremely reluctant to venture out of the house for months or even years.

Internet Friends

The Internet has become the modern equivalent of the dance hall in that it provides an opportunity for young people to meet and make friends. The great advantage of this form of interaction and communication to the person with AS is that he or she often has a greater eloquence in disclosing and expressing thoughts and feelings through typing than in face-to-face conversation. In social gatherings the person is expected to be able to listen to and process the other person's speech, often against a background of other conversations; simultaneously analyze nonverbal cues such as gestures, facial expression, and tone of voice; and immediately reply. When using the computer and keyboard, the person with AS can concentrate on the social exchange without being overwhelmed by so many social signals and background sensory experiences. The Internet provides an opportunity to meet like-minded individuals who accept other people because of their knowledge rather than their social persona and appearance. Internet "friends" can share experiences, thoughts, and knowledge using chat lines, web pages and message boards dedicated to people with AS.

Interactive Internet games can be an alternative world through which to develop friendships. Dean described how the games have clear rules, personas, abilities, and consistent consequences, all of which is a contrast to his real-life experiences with his peers. Friendships can develop between the game players. An intriguing adaptation of virtual world technology is the creation of virtual interaction environments to actually teach social understanding and interaction skills to young adults with AS (Mitchell, Parsons, & Leonard, 2008).

Support Groups

Adults with AS have formed mutual support groups with regular meetings to discuss topics that range from employment issues to personal relationships. Social occasions can be arranged for participants, such as excursions to the train museum or the cinema to see the latest science fiction film. Friendships can develop between like-minded individuals who share similar experiences and circumstances. There is a variety of ways that support groups can begin. For example, a group may initially be formed by parents of young adults with AS or by individuals with AS who originally met each in group counseling or therapy sessions and wanted to maintain contact. Older adults with AS who want to help others who share the same diagnosis and difficulties may form support groups. Groups can be started by final-year college students wanting to help newly enrolled students with AS, or by someone who used to belong to and benefit from a support group, who moves to another town and wants to start a support group locally. Some mature adults with AS have acquired very competent social interaction skills and have written guide books for young adults with AS (Edmonds & Beardon, 2008; Grandin & Barron, 2005).

Information on Relationships

Teenagers with AS may be keen to understand and experience the social and relationship world of their peers, including sexual experiences, but there can be some concerns regarding their source of information on relationships. If the teenager with AS has few friends with whom he or she can discuss personal topics, such as romantic or sexual feelings for someone, the source of information on relationships for girls may typically be television programs ("soap operas" and situation comedies, in particular) and pornography for boys. Another source of information on relationships can be same-age peers who may recognize that the person with AS is naïve, gullible, and vulnerable. Peer advisors with cruel intent can provide information and make suggestions that cause the person with AS to be ridiculed, or encourage others to assume malevolent intentions. The person with AS can easily be "set up" and suffer the consequences of deliberately misleading suggestions. There is invariably a lack of knowledge of the codes of courtship or dating and a likelihood of misinterpreting intentions. The adolescent with AS may attribute a deeper meaning to a simple act of kindness or friendship which can then lead to accusations of stalking and harassment (Stokes, Newton, & Kaur, 2007).

Previously socially isolated teenage girls with AS may feel flattered by the attention of boys after the physical changes that occur at puberty. Due to their naïvety, they do not realize that the interest is sexual, and not simply an appreciation of their conversation and company. When the teenage girl lacks female friends to provide advice on dating and intimacy, concern may arise with regard to promiscuity and sexual experiences. Teenage girls with AS are often not "streetwise" or able to identify sexual predators, and may become vulnerable to sexual exploitation in their desperate bid to be popular with peers. It is important that the teenage boy or girl with AS has access to accurate information on relationships and sexuality, especially when a friendship becomes more intimate. We now have educational literature on puberty and relationships specifically written for teenagers with AS and their parents (Attwood, 2008; Jackson, 2002) and programs to guide professional support staff in ways to explain aspects of sexuality (Hénault, 2005).

The Duration of Socializing

We each have a limited capacity for the duration of social contact. Some typical individuals have a large social capacity "bucket" that can take some time to fill, whereas the person with AS has a social capacity "cup" that becomes full relatively quickly. Conventional social occasions can last too long for those with AS, especially given that these individuals achieve social success by intellectual effort rather than natural intuition. Socializing can be exhausting. Yeshe, a woman who has a diagnosis of AS explained: "I describe my social life with this analogy. Swimming in the water is nice at first, but if it goes on for too long, or too often, I start to drown." The person with AS is more comfortable if social interactions are brief and purposeful. It is important that others are not offended by an abrupt ending to a conversation or social gathering, as offense was not intended.

Teasing and Bullying

The programs and activities described in this chapter are designed to increase the social knowledge and integration of children and adolescents with AS in order to facilitate successful peer relationships. Parents and teachers hope that the integration and friendship will be enjoyable, but whereas some children will be welcoming, "maternal," and kind to the child with AS, some will be "predatory" and consider the child an easy target for teasing and bullying. A few comments designed to confuse, tease, or infuriate can have lifelong implications for the child with AS (Attwood, 2004a). School may not be a safe environment. The child with AS may become extremely anxious in school, with the potential for school refusal, and episodes of anger when retaliating to acts of bullying and teasing can lead to school exclusion. Thus, bullying of children with AS can lead to significant mental health problems (Cappadocia, Weiss, & Peplar, 2012).

A study of the prevalence and frequency of bullying in a sample of more than 400 children with AS, between 4 and 17 years of age found the reported rate of bullying to be at least four times higher than for their peers (Little, 2002). More than 90% of mothers of children with AS who completed the survey reported that their children had been the target of some form of bullying within the previous year. The pattern of bullying was different from that in the general population, with a higher-than-expected level of shunning; and, in the teenage years, 1 in 10 adolescents with AS was a victim of peer gang attack. Unfortunately, this prevalence study by Little may be a conservative estimate of bullying experiences, as targeted children may be reluctant to report acts of bullying to their parents (Hay, Payne, & Chadwick, 2004).

It is essential to create a team approach to reduce the frequency of bullying. The team includes the targeted student of the bullying, school administration, teachers, parents, a child psychologist, other children, and the child who engages in acts of bullying (Gray, 2004a; Heinrichs, 2003; Olweus, 1992). It is important that schools develop and implement a code of conduct that specifically defines bullying and ways to stop it. The definition should be broad and not restricted to acts of intimidation and injury. Staff education is needed, and consensus and consistency in determining what are bullying actions and what are appropriate consequences are essential. Carol Gray (2004a) recommends creating a map of the child's world and identifying places where the child is vulnerable to, or safe from, acts of bullying. Some areas will need more supervision, and more safe-havens can be created. One of the problems with a prevention program that relies primarily on staff surveillance is that acts of bullying are usually covert, with around only 15% of such actions observed by a teacher in the classroom and only 5% on the playground (Pepler & Craig, 1999). However, other children often witness acts of bullying and they will need to be key participants in the program.

Student bystanders, who generally find it disturbing to witness acts of bullying, will need new strategies and encouragement to constructively respond to such acts. Their previous responses may have included relief that they are not the target; feeling immobilized by fear of being a target themselves if they intervene; having a diffused sense of responsibility by being in the majority group; not being sure what to do; being advised not to get involved; and adherence to a code of silence, with peer pressure not to report what is happening. Unfortunately, some bystanders can perceive the event as humorous or deserved by the target, which provides overt encouragement for the child committing the bullying act. Student bystanders can be taught to state clearly that what is happening is wrong, that it must stop, and that if it does not stop it will be reported. This may mean stepping between the perpetrator and the target. Some children among the silent majority invariably have a high social status, a strong sense of social justice, and natural assertiveness. These children can be personally encouraged, and can be highly successful in intervening, to stop bullying. Their high social status may also encourage other children to express their disapproval. Peer pressure can reduce bullying.

The child who is the target of a bullying act can implement various strategies such as trying to avoid potentially vulnerable situations. A child with AS may try to find a socially isolated sanctuary, but this can be one of the most vulnerable situations. Safety is in numbers. The best place to "hide" is among a group of children, or at least near them. It is important that children with AS are welcomed into, or nearby, a group of children when predators are approaching a potential target. That welcome will need to be part of the class code on bullying. Other options can be the provision of activities in a supervized classroom during break times, such as a chess club; or an opportunity for like-minded individuals to meet as a group in the playground.

Should bullying occur, the child must respond in some way, but what should he or she say or do? The general advice is for such children to try to stay calm, maintain their self-esteem, and respond in an assertive and constructive way. Staying calm and maintaining self-esteem are difficult for children with AS, but self-talk strategies can be used to help them maintain self-control. Children who are a target need to know and remember that they are not at fault, they do not deserve these comments or actions, and that the people who need to change their behavior are those who are committing the bullying acts. Gray (2004a) recommends the creation of one simple spoken response that is true and used consistently. Examples are "I don't deserve this, stop it" and "I don't like that, stop it." It is advisable to avoid telling a lie (e.g., to say "I don't care"). In any case, lying would be difficult for children with AS, who are known for their reluctance to lie. There are many programs on the prevention of bullying in schools for typical children, and some of the activities in these programs can be used with children with AS (Rigby, 2002). In addition, there are school-based programs on bullying that are specifically designed by specialists in AS (Attwood, 2004b; Etherington, 2007; Gray, 2004a; Heinrichs, 2003). Parents of children with AS should request that schools implement these programs.

Social Stories™

An evidence-based strategy for learning the relevant social cues, thoughts, feelings, and behavioral script in a reciprocal interaction and friendship is to write Social Stories, which were originally developed by Carol Gray (1998). Preparing Social Stories also enables adults and peers to understand the perspective of the child with AS and why his or her social behavior can appear confused, anxious, aggressive, or disobedient. A Social Story describes a situation, skill, or concept in terms of relevant social cues, perspectives, and common responses in a specifically defined style and format. The intention is to share accurate social and emotional information in a reassuring and informative manner that is easily understood by the child (or adult) with AS. To avoid the problem of Social Stories being associated only with ignorance or failure, the first Social Story, and at least 50% of subsequent Social Stories, should describe, affirm, and consolidate existing abilities and knowledge and what the child does well. Social Stories can also be written as a means of recording achievements in using new knowledge and strategies.

Gray (2004b) has recently revised the criteria and guidelines for writing a Social Story. Her original work on Social Stories has now been examined by many research studies and found to be remarkably effective in improving social understanding and social behavior in children with autism and AS (Crozier & Tincani, 2007; Hagiwara & Myles, 1999; Ivey, Heflin, & Alberto, 2004; Lorimer, 2002; Norris & Dattilo, 1999; Ozdemir, 2008; Rogers & Myles, 2001; Rowe, 1999; Santosi, Powell Smith, & Kincaid, 2004; Scattone, Wilczynski, Edwards, & Rabian, 2002; Scattone, 2008; Smith, 2001; Swaggart et al., 1995; Tarnai & Wolfe, 2008; Thiemann & Goldstein, 2001). A recent systematic review of Social Stories confirms statistically significant benefits for a variety of outcomes (Karkhaneh, Clark, Ospina, Seida, Smith, & Hartling, 2010).

THE UNDERSTANDING AND EXPRESSION OF EMOTIONS

A qualitative difference in the understanding and expression of emotions that was originally described by Hans Asperger (1944) is acknowledged in the diagnostic criteria of the DSM-5 (American Psychiatric Association,

2013) description of Autism Spectrum Disorder, which refers to deficits in emotional reciprocity and nonverbal communication behaviors and reduced sharing of emotions and affect and the development of additional anxiety and depressive disorders (Dickerson Mayes, Calhoun, Murray, Ahuja, et al., 2011; Joshi, Petty, Wozniak, Henin, Fried, et al., 2010; Lopata, Toomey, Fox, Volker, Chow, et al., 2010; Mattila, Hurtig, Haapsamo, Jussila, Kuusikko-Gauffin et al., 2010; van Steensel, Bogels, & Perrin, 2011). Research has also indicated a greater risk of developing bipolar disorder (DeLong & Dwyer, 1988; Frazier, Doyle, Chiu, & Coyle, 2002; Munesue Ono, Mutoh, Shimoda, Nakatani, et al., 2008), and there is evidence to suggest an association with delusional disorders (Kurita, 1999), paranoia (Blackshaw, Kinderman, Hare, & Hatton, 2001), conduct disorders and oppositional defiant disorder (Gadow, De Vincent & Drabick, 2008; Green, Gilcrest, Burton, & Cox, 2000; Tantam, 2000) and an eating disorder such as anorexia nervosa (Zucker et al., 2007). For teenagers with AS, an additional mood disorder is the rule rather than the exception.

The theoretical models of autism developed in cognitive psychology and research in neuropsychology and neuroimaging provide an explanation as to why children and adults with AS are prone to secondary mood disorders. The extensive research on theory-of-mind skills confirms that people with AS have considerable difficulty identifying and conceptualizing the thoughts and feelings of other people and themselves. This deficit will affect the ability of such people to monitor and manage emotions, both within themselves and with others through self-reflection (i.e., thinking about one's own thoughts, or metacognition), leading to a lack of insight into their own problems and to discrepancies between clinician and patient ratings of problems (Rydén & Bejerot, 2008). Children with AS also seem less aware of their own emotions, are less able to acknowledge different emotional perspectives and have fewer coping strategies to deal with negative emotions (Rieffe, Oosterveld, Terwogt, Mootz, Leeuwn, et al., 2011).

Research on executive function and AS suggests characteristics of disinhibition and impulsivity, with a relative lack of insight that affects general cognitive functioning (Eisenmajer et al., 1996; Nyden, Gillberg, Hjelmquist, & Heiman, 1999; Ozonoff, South, & Miller, 2000; Pennington & Ozonoff, 1996). Impaired executive function can also affect the cognitive control of emotions. Clinical experience indicates there is a tendency for children with AS to react to emotional cues without thinking. A fast and impulsive retaliation can lead an adult to conclude that the child with AS has a conduct disorder or a problem with anger management.

Research using neuroimaging technology with people who have autism or AS has also identified structural and functional abnormalities of the amygdala, a part of the brain associated with the recognition and regulation of emotions (Adolphs, Sears, & Piven, 2001; Baron Cohen et al., 1999; Corden, Chilvers, & Skuse, 2008; Critchely et al., 2000; Fine, Lumsden, & Blair, 2001). The amygdala is known to regulate a range of emotions, including anger, anxiety, and sadness. Thus, we also have neuroanatomical evidence that indicates a likelihood of problems with the perception and regulation of emotions.

Anxiety, Depression, Anger, and Love

The assessment of the understanding and expression of emotions of some-one with AS should include the construction of a list of behavioral indica-tors of mood changes. The indicators can include changes in the character-istics associated with AS: for example, an increase in time spent in solitude or in the special interest; increased rigidity in thought processes or behavior intended to impose control over other people to avoid anxiety-provoking situations in the person's daily life. These are in addition to conventional indicators such as panic attacks, comments indicating low self-worth, and episodes of anger.

Several self-rating scales of depression, anxiety, or anger that have been designed for use with typical children and adults can also be adminis-tered to children and adults with AS. However, specific modifications may be needed for someone with AS. He or she may be better able to accurately quantify an emotional experience or response using a numerical represen-tation of the gradation in experience and expression of emotions. People with AS often lack a vocabulary of words to describe subtle or complex emotions, but the concept of an emotion "thermometer," bar graph, or a "volume" scale with numbers to represent the depth of emotion can be extremely useful. These analogue measures can be explained in the emo-tion education component of cognitive-behavioral therapy.

Anxiety

Perhaps the most common secondary mood disorder is an anxiety disor-der (De Bruin, Ferdinand, Meester, de Nijs, & Verheij, 2007; Ghaziuddin, Wieder-Mikhail & Ghaziuddin, 1998; Gillot, Furniss, & Walter, 2001; Green et al., 2000; Kim et al., 2000; Konstantareas, 2005; Kuusikko et al., 2008; Lopata, Toomey, Fox, Volker, Chow, et al., 2010; MacNeil, Lopes, & Minnes, 2009; Mattila, Hurtig, Haapsamo, Jussila, Kuusikko-Gauffin, et al., 2010; Russell & Sofronoff, 2004; Sukhodolsky et al., 2007; Tantam, 2000; Tonge, Brereton, Gray, & Einfeld, 1999). Many children and adults with AS appear to be prone to anxious feelings for much of their day or to be extremely anxious about a specific event. The late Marc Segar had AS and in his essay "The Battles of the Autistic Thinker" he wrote that one emotion autistic people are often good at is worrying. Many adults with AS say that they cannot think of a time in their lives when they did not feel anxious, even in very early childhood. This chronic anxiety may be a con-stitutional feature of AS or a result of excessive stress from trying to social-ize and cope with the unpredictability and sensory experiences of daily life.

There can also be quite unusual fears associated with AS, for example gelo-tophobia, or fear of being laughed at (Samson, Huber, & Ruch, 2011) and fear of mechanical objects such as vacuum cleaners, elevators, and toilets (Dickerson Mayes, Calhoun, Aggarwal, Baker, Mathapati, et al., 2013).

About 25% of adults with AS have the clear clinical signs of obsessive–compulsive disorder (Russell, Mataix Cols, Anson, & Murphy, 2005), and almost 1 in 10 children and adolescents with OCD have characteristics of AS (Ivarsson & Melin, 2008). The vulnerable times to develop OCD for those with AS are between 10 and 12 years and the early adult years (Ghaziuddin, 2005). In OCD, the person has intrusive thoughts that he or she does not want to think about: the thoughts are described as *egodystonic,* as distress-ing and unpleasant. Sometimes parents describe their son's or daughter's special interest as an "obsession," which could suggest an additional diag-nosis of OCD, but there is a distinct qualitative difference between a special interest and an obsession. The person with AS clearly enjoys the interest: it is ego*syn*tonic, not egodystonic, and therefore not necessarily indicative of OCD (Attwood, 2003; Baron-Cohen, 1990). In typical people the intrusive thoughts are often about cleanliness, aggression, religion, or sex. Clinical experience and research studies indicate that the obsessive thoughts of chil-dren and adults with AS are much more likely to be about cleanliness, bul-lying, teasing, making a mistake, and being criticized (McDougle, Kresch, Goodman, & Naylor, 1995).

Depression

People with AS appear vulnerable to feeling depressed, with about one in three children and adults having a clinical depression (Clarke, Baxter, Perry, & Presher, 1999; Ghaziuddin et al., 1998; Ghaziuddin & Zafar, 2008; Gil-lot et al., 2001; Green et al., 2000; Kim et al., 2000; Konstantareas, 2005; Rydén & Bejerot, 2008; Sterling, Dawson, Estes, & Greenson, 2008; Tan-tam, 1988; Vickerstaff, Heriot, Wong, Lopes, & Dosseter, 2007; Wing, 1981). There is evidence to suggest that the rate of depression rises with age (Sterling et al., 2008). There are many reasons for people with AS to feel depressed, including the long-term consequences on self-esteem of feel-ing unaccepted and misunderstood (Humphrey & Lewis, 2008); the men-tal exhaustion from trying to succeed socially; feelings of loneliness; the anguish and humiliation of being tormented, teased, bullied, and ridiculed by peers (Shtayermman, 2007); insight into being different and subsequent assumptions of being defective (Vickerstaff et al., 2007; Williamson, Craig, & Slinger, 2008); and a cognitive style that is pessimistic and focuses on errors and what could go wrong. The depression can lead to a severe with-drawal from social contact and thoughts that, without social success, there is no point in life. There is a serious risk of suicide in this population.

Some of the characteristics of AS can prolong the duration and increase the intensity of depression. The person with AS may not disclose his or her inner feelings, preferring to retreat into solitude, avoiding conversation (especially when the conversation is about feelings and experiences), and trying to resolve the depression by subjective thought. Typical people are better at, and more confident about, disclosing feelings and knowing that another person may provide a more objective opinion and act as an emotional restorative. Family and friends of a typical person may be able to temporarily halt, and to a certain extent alleviate, the mood by words and gestures of reassurance and affection. They may be able to distract the person who is depressed by initiating enjoyable experiences or using humor. These emotional rescue strategies are sometimes less effective for people with AS, who try to solve personal and practical issues by themselves and for whom affection and compassion may not be such effective emotional restoratives.

Anger

We do not know how common anger management problems are with children and adults with AS, but we do know that when problems with the expression of anger occur, the person with AS and family members are very keen to reduce its frequency, intensity, and consequences. The rapidity and intensity of anger, often in response to a relatively trivial event, can be extreme. When feeling angry, the person with AS does not appear to be able to pause and think of alternative strategies to resolve the situation; there is often an instantaneous physical response without careful thought. When the anger is intense, the person with AS may be in a "blind rage" and unable to see the signals indicating that it would be appropriate to stop (see Myles, Tien, Lee, Chou, & Smith, Chapter 7, this volume).

Love

When a person with AS is referred for the treatment of a mood disorder, the referral is almost invariably resulting from concerns regarding feelings of anxiety, sadness, and anger. However, from my extensive clinical experience with children and adults with AS, I would suggest that there is a fourth emotion that is of concern to individuals with AS in terms of their understanding and expression: love.

Typical children enjoy and seek affection from their parents; they are able to read the signals when someone expects affection from them and recognize when to give affection to communicate reciprocal feelings of love or to repair someone's feelings. Children less than 2 years old know that words and gestures of affection are perhaps the most effective emotional restorative for themselves and for someone who is sad. However, the person with AS may not understand why typical people are so obsessed with expressing reciprocal love and affection. For a young person with AS a hug can be experienced as an uncomfortable squeeze, and he or she may soon learn not to cry so as not to elicit a squeeze from someone.

Cognitive-Behavioral Therapy

When a mood disorder is diagnosed in a child or adult with AS, the clinical psychologist or psychiatrist will need to know how to modify psychological treatments for mood disorders to accommodate the unusual ability profile of people with AS (Attwood & Scarpa, 2013). The primary psychological treatment for mood disorders is cognitive-behavioral therapy (CBT), which has been developed and refined over several decades. Research studies have established that CBT is an effective treatment to change the way a person thinks about and responds to emotions such as anxiety, sadness, and anger (Graham, 1998; Grave & Blissett, 2004; Kendall, 2000). CBT focuses on the maturity, complexity, subtlety, and vocabulary of emotions as well as dysfunctional or illogical thinking and incorrect assumptions. Thus, it has direct applicability to children and adults with AS who have impaired or delayed theory-of-mind abilities and difficulty understanding, expressing, and managing emotions. We now have published case studies and objective scientific evidence that CBT does significantly reduce mood disorders in children and adults with AS (Bauminger, 2002; Chalfant, Rapee, & Carroll 2007; Fitzpatrick, 2004; Gaus, 2007; Hare, 1997; Lehmkuhl, Storch, Bodfish, & Geffken, 2008; Nadeau, Sulkowski, Ung, Wood, Lewin, et al., 2011; Puleo & Kendall, 2011; Reaven, Blakely-Smith, Culhane-Shelburne, & Hepburn, 2012; Reaven & Hepburn, 2003; Reaven et al., in press; Scarpa & Reyes, 2011; Sofronoff, Attwood, & Hinton, 2005; Sofronoff, Attwood, Hinton, & Levin, 2008; Sung, Ooi, Goh, Pathy, Fung, et al., 2011; Sze & Wood, 2007; White, Ollendick, Albano, Oswald, Johnson, et al., 2013; Wood et al., 2009).

CBT has four components or stages, the first being an assessment of the nature and degree of the mood disorder using self-report scales and a clinical interview. The subsequent component is affective education to increase the person's knowledge of emotions. Discussion and activities explore the connection among thoughts, emotions, and behavior, and identify the way in which the person conceptualizes emotions and perceives various situations. The more someone understands emotions, the more he or she is able to express and control them appropriately. The third stage of CBT is cognitive restructuring to correct distorted conceptualizations and dysfunctional beliefs and to constructively manage emotions. The last stage is a schedule of activities to practice new cognitive skills for managing emotions in real-life situations (Scarpa, Williams White, & Attwood, 2013).

Affective Education

In the affective education component of CBT the person learns about the advantages and disadvantages of emotions and how to identify the different levels of expression in words and actions, within the person him- or herself and in others (Attwood, Callesen, & Moller Nielsen, 2008). For children with AS, this component can be undertaken as a science project. A basic principle is to explore one emotion at a time, starting with a positive emotion such as happiness before moving on to an emotion of clinical concern. The following are activities and strategies that can be included in the affective education component of CBT.

Creation of an Emotions Scrapbook

One of the affective education activities is to create a scrapbook that illustrates an emotion. This can include pictures or representations that have a personal association for the person with AS: For example, if the emotion is happiness or pleasure, the book can include a photograph of a rare fossil for the person who has a special interest in palaeontology. It is important to remember that the scrapbook illustrates the pleasures in the person's life, which may not always be those more conventional pleasures of typical children or adults. The pictures are usually of objects, scenes, and animals without the presence of family members.

The affective education program also explores the sensations associated with the feeling, such as aromas, tastes, and textures. These should be recorded in the scrapbook, which can also be used as a diary to include compliments that the person has received, records of achievement such as certificates, and memorabilia associated with enjoyable occasions. The scrapbook is regularly updated and can be used at a later stage in CBT to help change a particular mood and encourage confidence and self-esteem.

Perception of Emotional States

An important component of affective education is to enable the person with AS to discover the salient internal cues (e.g., sensations, behavior, thoughts) that indicate a particular level of emotion. These sensations and thoughts can act as early warning signs of an impending escalation of emotion. In part, affective education is designed to improve the function of the amygdala in informing the frontal lobes of the brain about increasing stress levels and emotional arousal. Technology in the form of biofeedback instruments, such as auditory electromyography (EMG) and galvanic skin response (GSR) machines can be used to identify internal cues. The intention is to encourage the person to be more consciously aware of his or her own emotional state and to be able to manage an emotion before its intensity becomes extreme and there is loss of cognitive control.

Affective education includes information on the facial expression, tone of voice, and body language that indicate the feelings of another person. The typical errors of children and adults with AS include not identifying which cues are relevant or redundant, and misinterpreting cues. The CBT therapist uses a range of games and resources to "spot the message" and to explain the multiple meanings of specific cues; for example, a furrowed brow can mean anger, bewilderment, or be a sign of aging skin; a loud voice does not automatically mean that the person is angry. Although people with AS can learn the cues that indicate a specific emotion, there can be difficulties processing such information at speed in real-life situations (Montgomery et al., 2008). The amount of nonverbal information in an interaction can be perceived as overwhelming, especially when facial expressions are fleeting and the person needs more time to intellectually, rather than intuitively, process such information. Slowing down facial expressions and corresponding vocalizations can lead to greater understanding (Tardif, Lainé, Rodriguez, & Gepner, 2007).

There can be an erroneous assumption that people with AS lack empathy and do not care about how someone is feeling. The problem is not a lack of empathy, but rather a problem of reading the signals indicating that a specific response is expected (Dziobek et al., 2008; Rogers, Dziobek, Hassenstab, Wolf, & Convit, 2007), and knowing what would be the appropriate response. People with AS can be extremely caring and concerned about the welfare of others but may not intuitively know when a sympathetic facial expression or gesture and words of compassion using a "warm" voice are expected.

A component of affective education is to constructively use the young child's interest in vehicles and television programs to teach emotion recognition. The television series *Thomas the Tank Engine* is extremely popular with children who have AS in the United Kingdom and Australia. One feature of the program is the animated facial expressions on the front of the locomotives. For the child who is confused about the meanings of facial expressions, these stylized expressions can be linked to specific events, thoughts, and feelings that occur in the storyline. Under the guidance of Simon Baron-Cohen at Cambridge University, a team has created and evaluated a children's television program, *The Transporters,* which uses actors' faces on the front of vehicles. The storyline and script were specifically designed to explain and portray simple and complex emotions to children with an autism spectrum disorder (ASD; Golan et al., 2010).

People with AS often experience great enjoyment playing computer games. A DVD has therefore been designed specifically for those with an ASD as an interactive game that is an electronic encyclopedia of emotions (Baron-Cohen, 2002). The interactive DVD is entitled *Mind Reading: The Interactive Guide to Emotions.* The researchers identified words to describe 412 human emotions and examined the age at which children understand the meaning of each word. They developed a taxonomy that assigned all the distinct emotions into one of 24 different groups. A multimedia company subsequently developed interactive software that was designed for children and adults with an ASD to learn what someone may be thinking or feeling. Actors demonstrate facial expressions, body language, and speech qualities associated with a specific emotion. The DVD also includes audio recordings that illustrate aspects of prosody, filmed scenes with actors, and stories to read that illustrate the circumstances and contexts for each emotion. There is an emotions library, a learning center, and a games zone. An alternative interactive DVD and computer games to provide affective education have been developed in Australia (Beaumont & Sofronoff, 2008).

Measuring the Intensity of Emotion

Once the cues that indicate a particular emotion have been identified, it is important to use a measuring instrument to determine the degree of intensity. The CBT therapist can use a representation of a thermometer, gauge, or volume control and a range of activities to define the level of expression. For example, a series of pictures of faces expressing varying degrees of happiness can be placed at the appropriate point on the instrument. Alternatively, a variety of words that define different levels of happiness can be placed appropriately on the gauge.

During CBT for emotion management, it is important to ensure that the child or adult with AS has the same definition of a word to describe an emotion as the therapist, and to clarify any semantic confusion. Clinical experience has indicated that some children and adolescents with AS tend to use extreme statements when agitated. Affective education increases the person's vocabulary of emotional expression to ensure greater precision and accuracy in verbal expression, thereby avoiding extreme or offensive expressions. This activity is particularly useful for exploring how the words and actions of others affect the feelings of the person with AS, and vice versa.

Resource Material

Many books and games can be used as part of the affective education component of CBT (Attwood, 2007), and CBT manuals for professionals and parents to reduce anxiety and anger in children with AS are available (Attwood, 2004b, 2004c; McNally Keehn, Lincoln, Brown, & Chavira, 2013; Reaven, Blakely-Smith, Nichols, & Hepburn, 2011; Scarpa, Wells, & Attwood, 2013). A new CBT resource is the Cognitive Affective Training program, or CAT-kit, developed in Denmark and recently translated into English (Callesen, Moller Nielsen, & Attwood, 2008). The resources in the CAT-kit include a thermometer to measure the intensity of emotion, words and facial expressions for nine basic emotions, and resources with which to identify the inner or body signals for a particular emotion. There is also a timeline with which to structure emotional experiences during the day and over longer periods; activities that help the individual organize and interpret social relations and friendship; behavior organizers; and different ways of visualizing emotions, behavior, and self-identity. The CAT-kit also includes a representation of a toolbox, a strategy that can be used in cognitive restructuring. We also noww have CBT manuals for children who have AS to learn how to express and enjoy affection with family and friends (Andrews, Attwood, & Sofronoff, 2013; Attwood & Garnett, 2013a, 2013b).

Cognitive Restructuring

Using two of the recognized qualities of a person with AS, namely, logic and intelligence, the cognitive restructuring component of CBT enables the person to change the thinking that contributes to or increases emotions such as anxiety and anger or feelings of low self-esteem. The first stage is to establish the evidence for a particular thought or belief. People with AS can make false assumptions about their circumstances and the intentions of others due to impaired or delayed theory-of-mind abilities. They also have a tendency to make literal interpretations, and a casual comment may be taken out of context or to the extreme.

Comic Strip Conversations

To explain alternative perspectives or to correct errors or assumptions, comic strip conversations, developed by Carol Gray (1998), can help the child or adult determine the thoughts, beliefs, knowledge, and intentions of the participants in a particular situation. The strategy is to draw an event or sequence of events in storyboard form, using stick figures to represent each participant and speech and thought bubbles to represent each participants' words and thoughts. The child and therapist use an assortment of fiber-tipped colored pens, with each color representing an emotion. As the child writes in the speech or thought bubbles, the choice of color indicates his or her perception of the emotion and thoughts conveyed or intended. This concrete representation can clarify the child's interpretation of events and the rationale for his or her thoughts and response. This technique can help the child identify and correct any misperceptions and consider how alternative responses might affect the participants' thoughts and feelings. Although originally developed for children, comic strip conversations can also be used with adults.

An Emotional Toolbox

The concept of an emotional toolbox has proved an extremely successful metaphor for cognitive restructuring in the CBT treatment of anxiety and anger in children with AS (Sofronoff et al., 2005, 2008). The strategy is to identify different types of "tools" to fix problems in expressing anxiety, anger, and sadness. The range of tools can be divided into those that (1) quickly and constructively release, or (2) slowly reduce, emotional energy, and (3) those that improve thinking. The CBT therapist works with the child or adult with AS and the family to identify different tools that help fix the feeling, as well as some tools that can make the emotions or consequences worse. Together they use paper and pens during a brainstorming session in which they draw a toolbox and depict and write descriptions of different types of tools and activities that can encourage constructive emotional repair.

Physical Tools. The emotion management for children and adults with AS can be conceptualized as a problem with "energy management," namely, an excessive amount of emotional energy and difficulty controlling and releasing the energy constructively. These individuals appear less able to slowly release emotional energy by means of relaxation and reflection, and usually prefer to fix or release the feeling by an energetic action. A hammer can represent tools or actions that physically release emotional energy through a constructive activity. A picture of a hammer is drawn on a large sheet of paper and the person with AS and the therapist devise a list of safe and appropriate activities that release physical energy. For young children, this can include bouncing on the trampoline or going on a swing. For older children and adults, going for a run, sports practice, or dancing may be used to "let off steam" or release emotional energy. Other activities may include cycling, swimming, or playing the drums. Some household activities can provide a satisfying release of energy: for example, squeezing oranges to make fresh orange juice, pounding meat in the kitchen, gardening, or diving into household renovations.

Relaxation Tools. Relaxation tools help to calm the person, lower the heart rate, and gradually release emotional energy. Perhaps a picture of a paintbrush could be used to illustrate this category of tools for emotional repair. Relaxation tools or activities could include drawing, reading, or listening to calming music to slowly "unwind" thoughts and fears. People with AS often find that solitude is a very effective means of relaxing. Caroline, a woman with AS, explained, "I relished isolation and solitude and when I was by myself I thoroughly enjoyed the company of an empty room." The child or adult with AS may need to retreat to a quiet, secluded sanctuary as an effective mechanism of emotional repair. There will need to be an emotionally restoring sanctuary at home—perhaps the child's bedroom; and a sanctuary at school—perhaps a secluded area of the classroom or a secluded area of the playground that is safe from predatory children. One of the complaints of children with AS is that they have great difficulty finding somewhere at school to be alone and feel safe from predatory children. Ron, an adult with AS, explained that he finds opportunities where he can be effectively alone yet give the appearance of being engaged and suitably occupied, and that he only feels safe and relaxed when he is alone.
Adolescents and adults with AS may use alcohol and marijuana as a

relaxant, especially as these mood-altering substances are often available at social gatherings. Youngsters who are chronically and severely anxious can discover that drinking alcohol or smoking marijuana can induce an almost never-before-experienced state of relaxation. This discovery can lead to major problems of addiction to mood-altering substances (Tinsley & Hendrickx, 2008). If drugs are used to reduce anxiety, it is important that they are prescription rather than recreational or illegal drugs.

Social Tools. This category of tools uses other people or animals as a means of managing emotions. The strategy is to find and be with someone, or an animal, that can help repair the mood. The social activity will need to be enjoyable and without the stress that can sometimes be associated with social interaction, especially when the interaction involves more than one other person. The supportive social contact needs to be someone who genuinely admires or loves the child, gives compliments (not criticism), and manages to say the right words to repair feelings. Sometimes the best friend may be a pet. Despite the negative mood or stressful events of the day, dogs are delighted to see their owner, show unconditional adoration, and clearly enjoy the person's company, as demonstrated by the wagging tail. The best friend may be a cat, and it is worth noting that cats often behave in ways associated with autism (Hoopmann, 2006). Pets are the best nonjudgmental listeners and more forgiving than humans.

Thinking Tools. The child or adult can nominate another type of implement, such as a screwdriver or wrench, to represent a category of tools that can be used to change thinking or knowledge. The person is encouraged to use his or her intellectual strength to control feelings via a variety of techniques such as an internal dialogue or self-talk. The person is encouraged to use "inner speech" such as "I *can* control my feelings" or "I *can* stay calm" when under stress. The words are reassuring and encourage self-esteem. Another thinking tool is to use a reality check, to put the event in perspective. The approach is to apply logic and facts through a series of questions such as, "Is there another shop where I could buy that computer game?" or "Will children teasing me about my interest in astronomy prevent me from being an astronomer?"

Putting the Emotional Toolbox into Practice. Once the child has a list of emotional repair tools, the CBT therapist can make a replica tool box as provided in the CAT-kit (Callesen et al., 2008). As the therapy evolves, new tools can be discovered and added to the list. A parent may place the emotion thermometer on the fridge door to be easily accessible. In this way, the child can point to the degree of emotion or stress he or she is experiencing, for example, when returning home from school in the afternoon, and decide which tools are first choice to lower the emotional "temperature."

The next stage is to start practicing the emotional repair strategies in a graduated sequence of assignments. The therapist can model the appropriate thinking and actions in role plays with the child or adult with AS, vocalizing thoughts to monitor cognitive processes. A form of graduated practice in real life is used, starting with situations associated with a relatively mild level of distress or agitation. A list of situations or "triggers" that precipitate specific emotions is created, with each situation written on a small card. The child or adult uses the thermometer or measuring instrument originally used in the affective education activities to determine the hierarchy or rank order of situations. The most distressing are placed at the upper level of the thermometer. Strategies to cope with situations associated with a relatively low level of anxiety, anger, or low self-esteem are discussed, enacted, and applied in real-life situations first. As the therapy progresses, the person works through the hierarchy to manage more intense emotions. Successful exposure exercises are an essential aspect of CBT. The therapist will need to communicate and coordinate with those who will be supporting the person in everyday circumstances. After each practical experience there is a subsequent discussion of the degree of success, using activities such as comic strip conversations to debrief and providing reinforcement for achievements, such as a certificate of achievement, and a "boasting book" or the writing of a Social Story to record emotion management success.

THE PROGNOSIS FOR ACQUIRING FRIENDS AND MANAGING EMOTIONS

Children and adults with AS will need guidance and encouragement in acquiring the specific social understanding needed to achieve and maintain friendships. Gradually the person with AS can build a mental library of positive friendship experiences and learn the social rules. The process is similar to learning a foreign language with all the problems of exceptions to the rule for pronunciation and grammar. Some people with AS are eventually able to socialize reasonably well, with typical people unaware of the mental energy, support, understanding, and education that was required to achieve such success.

Although people with AS clearly have problems understanding emotions in themselves and in others, as well as expressing emotions at an appropriate level for the situation, we now have strategies such as CBT to successfully treat secondary mood disorders. Typical people can only imagine what it must be like to live in a world that is socially and emotionally confusing, but when you do understand the world experiences of someone with AS, you achieve greater compassion that can significantly improve that person's quality of life.

REFERENCES

Adolphs, R., Sears, L., & Piven, J. (2001). Abnormal processing of social information from faces in autism. *Journal of Cognitive Neuroscience 13,* 232–240.

American Psychiatric Association. (2000). *Diagnostic and statistical manual of mental disorders* (4th ed., text rev.). Washington, DC: Author.

American Psychiatric Association. (2013). *Diagnostic and statistical manual of mental disorders* (5th ed.). Arlington, VA: Author.

Andrews, L., Attwood, T., & Sofronoff, K. (2013). Increasing the appropriate demonstration of affection behaviour, in children with Asperger syndrome, high functioning autism, and PDD-NOS: A randomized controlled trial. *Research in Autism Spectrum Disorders, 7,* 1568–1578.

Apple, A., Billingsley, F., & Schwartz, I. (2005). Effects of video modelling alone and with self-management on compliment-giving behaviours of children with high-functioning ASD. *Journal of Positive Behaviour Interventions 7,* 33–46.

Asperger, H. (1944). Die autistischen psychopathen im kindesalter. *Archiv für Psychiatrie und Nervenkrankheiten, 177,* 76–137.

Aston, M. (2003). *Aspergers in love: Couple relationships and family affairs.* London: Jessica Kingsley.

Aston, M. (2009). *The Asperger couple's workbook: Practical advice and activities for couples and counsellors.* London: Jessica Kingsley.

Attwood, S. (2008). *Making sense of sex: A forthright guide to puberty, sex and relationships for people with Asperger's syndrome.* London: Jessica Kingsley.

Attwood, T. (2003). Understanding and managing circumscribed interests. In M. Prior (Ed.), *Learning and behavior problems in Asperger syndrome* (pp. 126–147). New York: Guilford Press.

Attwood, T. (2004a). Strategies to reduce the bullying of young children with Asperger syndrome. *Australian Journal of Early Childhood, 29,* 15–23.

Attwood, T. (2004b). *Exploring feelings: Cognitive behaviour therapy to manage anxiety.* Arlington, TX: Future Horizons.

Attwood, T. (2004c). *Exploring feelings: Cognitive behaviour therapy to manage anger.* Arlington, TX: Future Horizons.

Attwood, T. (2007). *The complete guide to Asperger's syndrome.* London: Jessica Kingsley.

Attwood, T., Callesen, K., & Moller Nielsen, A. (2008). *The CAT-kit: Cognitive affective training.* Arlington, TX: Future Horizons.

Attwood, T., & Garnett, M. (2013a). *From like to love for young people with Asperger's syndrome.* London: Jessica Kingsley.

Attwood, T., & Garnett, M. (2013b). *CBT to help young people with Asperger's syndrome (autism spectrum disorder) to understand and express affection.* London: Jessica Kingsley.

Attwood, T., & Scarpa, A. (2013). Modifications of cognitive behavioral therapy for children and adolescents with high-functioning ASD and their common difficulties. In A. Scarpa, S. Williams White, & T. Atwood (Eds.), *CBT for children and adolescents with high-functioning autism spectrum disorders* (pp. 27–44). New York: Guilford Press.

Baron-Cohen, S. (1990). Do autistic children have obsessions and compulsions? *British Journal of Clinical Psychology, 28,* 193–200.

Baron-Cohen, S. (2002). *Mind reading: The interactive guide to emotions.* London: Jessica Kingsley.

Baron-Cohen, S., Ring, H. A., Wheelwright, S., Bullmore, E. T., Brammer, M. J., Simmons, A., et al. (1999). Social intelligence in the normal autistic brain: An fMRI study. *European Journal of Neuroscience, 11,* 1891–1898.

Bauminger, N. (2002). The facilitation of social–emotional understanding and social interaction in high-functioning children with autism: Intervention outcomes. *Journal of Autism and Developmental Disorders, 31,* 461–469.

Bauminger, N., & Kasari, C. (2000). Loneliness and friendship in high-functioning children with autism. *Child Development, 71,* 447–456.

Bauminger, N., & Shulman, C. (2003). The development and maintenance of friendship in high-functioning children with autism. *Autism, 7,* 81–97.

Bauminger, N., Shulman, C., & Agam, G. (2003). Peer interaction and loneliness in high-functioning children with autism. *Journal of Autism and Developmental Disorders, 33,* 489–506.

Bauminger, N., Solomon, M., Aviezer, A., Heung, K., Brown, J., & Rogers, S. (2008a). Friendship in high-functioning children with autism spectrum disorder: Mixed and non-mixed dyads. *Journal of Autism and Developmental Disorders, 38,* 1211–1229.

Bauminger, N., Solomon, M., Aviezer, A., Heung, K., Gazit, L., Brown, J., et al. (2008b). Children with autism and their friends: A multidimensional study of friendship in high-functioning autism spectrum disorder. *Journal of Abnormal Child Psychology, 36,* 135–150.

Bauminger-Zviely, N. (2013). *Social and academic abilities in children with high-functioning autism spectrum disorders.* New York: Guilford Press.

Beaumont, R., & Sofronoff, K. (2008). A multi-component social skills intervention for children with Asperger syndrome: The Junior Detective Training Program. *Journal of Child Psychology and Psychiatry, 49,* 743–753.

Blackshaw, A. J., Kinderman, P., Hare, D. J., & Hatton, C. (2001). Theory of mind, causal attribution and paranoia in Asperger syndrome. *Autism, 5,* 147–163.

Botroff, V., Bartak, L., Langford, P., Page, M., & Tong, B. (1995). *Social cognitive skills and implications for social skills training in adolescents with autism.* Paper presented at the Australian Autism Conference, Flinders University, Adelaide, Australia.

Brown, D. (2012). *The aspie girls guide to being safe with men.* London: Jessica Kingsley.

Callesen, K., Moller-Nielsen, A., & Attwood, T. (2008). *The CAT-kit: Cognitive affective training.* Arlington, TX: Future Horizons.

Cappadocia, M. C., & Weiss, J. A. (2011). Review of social skills training groups for youth with Asperger syndrome and high functioning autism. *Research in Autism Spectrum Disorders, 5,* 70–78.

Cappadocia, M. C., Weiss, J. A., & Pepler, D. (2012). Bullying experiences among children and youth with autism spectrum disorders. *Journal of Autism and Developmental Disorders, 42,* 266–277.

Carter, M. A., & Santomauro, J. (2010). *Friendly facts: A fun, interactive resource to help children explore the complexities of friends and friendship.* Shawnee, KS: Autism Asperger Publishing Company.

Chalfant, A., Rapee, R., & Carroll, L. (2007). Treating anxiety disorders in children with high functioning autism spectrum disorders: A controlled trial. *Journal of Autism and Developmental Disorders, 38,* 1842–1857.

Chasen, L. R. (2011). *Social skills, emotional growth and drama therapy: Inspiring connection on the autism spectrum.* London: Jessica Kingsley.

Church, C., Alisanski, S., & Amanullah, S. (2000). The social, behavioural and academic experiences of children with Asperger disorder. *Focus on Autism and Other Developmental Disabilities, 15,* 12–20.

Clarke, D., Baxter, M., Perry, D., & Prasher, V. (1999). Affective and psychotic disorders in adults with autism: Seven case reports. *Autism, 3,* 149–164.

Cook O'Toole, J. (2013). *The asperkid's secret book of social rules.* London: Jessica Kingsley.

Corden, B., Chilvers, R., & Skuse, D. (2008). Emotional modulation of perception in Asperger's syndrome. *Journal of Autism and Developmental Disorders, 38,* 1072–1080.

Critchley, H. D., Daly, E. M., Bullmore, E. T., Williams, S. C. R., Van Amelsvoort, T., Robertson, D. M., et al. (2000). The functional neuroanatomy of social behavior. *Brain, 123,* 2203–2212.

Crooke, P., & Garcia Winner, M. (2011). *Social fortune or social fate?: A social thinking graphic novel map for social quest seekers.* Great Barrington, MA: Think Social Publishing.

Crooke, P., Hendrix, R., & Rachman, J. (2008). Brief report: Measuring the effectiveness of teaching social thinking to children with Asperger syndrome (AS) and high functioning autism (HFA). *Journal of Autism and Developmental Disorders, 38,* 581–591.

Crozier, S., & Tincani, M. (2007). Effects of Social Stories on prosocial behavior of preschool children with autism spectrum disorders. *Journal of Autism and Developmental Disorders, 37,* 1803–1814.

De Bruin, E., Ferdinand, R., Meester, S., de Nijs, P., & Verheij, F. (2007). High rates of psychiatric co-morbidity in PDD-NOS. *Journal of Autism and Developmental Disorders, 37,* 877–886.

DeLong, G., & Dwyer, J. (1988). Correlation of family history with specific autistic subgroups: Asperger's syndrome and bipolar affective disease. *Journal of Autism and Developmental Disorders, 18,* 593–600.

Densmore, A. E. (2007). *Helping children with autism become more social.* Westport, CT: Praeger.

DeRosier, M. E., Swick, D. C., Ornstein Davis, N., McMillen, J. S., & Matthews, R. (2011). The efficacy of a social skills group intervention for improving social behaviors in children with high functioning autism spectrum disorders. *Journal of Autism and Developmental Disorders, 41,* 1033–1043.

Diamond, S. (2011). *Social rules for kids.* Shawnee, KS: Autism Asperger Publishing Company.

Dickerson Mayes, S., Calhoun, S. L., Aggarwal, R., Baker, C., Mathapati, S., Molitoris, S., et al. (2013).Unusual fears in children with autism. *Research in Autism Spectrum Duisorders, 7,* 151–158.

Dickerson Mayes, S., Calhoun, S. L., Murray, M. J., Ahuja, M., & Smith, L. A. (2011). Anxiety, depression and irritability in children with autism relative to other neuropsychiatric disorders and typical development. *Research in Autism Spectrum Disorders, 5,* 474–485.

Dubin, N. (2007). *Asperger syndrome and bullying: Strategies and solutions.* London: Jessica Kingsley.

Dziobek, I., Rogers, K., Fleck, S., Bahnemann, M., Heekeren, H., Wolf, O., et al. (2008). Dissociation of cognitive and emotional empathy in adults with Asperger syndrome using the Multifaceted Empathy Test (MET). *Journal of Autism and Developmental Disorders, 38,* 464–473.

Edmonds, G., & Beardon, L. (2008). *Asperger syndrome and social relationships: Adults speak out about Asperger syndrome.* London: Jessica Kingsley.

Edmonds, G., & Worton, D. (2005). *The Asperger love guide: A practical guide for adults with Asperger's syndrome to seeking, establishing and maintaining successful relationships.* London: Sage.

Eisenmajer, R., Prior, M., Leekman, S., Wing, L., Gould, J., Welham, M., et al. (1996). Comparison of clinical symptoms in autism and Asperger's syndrome. *Journal of the American Academy of Child and Adolescent Psychiatry, 35,* 1523–1531.

Etherington, A. (2007). Bullying and teasing and helping children with ASD: What can we do? *Good Autism Practice, 8,* 37–44.

Fine, C., Lumsden, J., & Blair, R. J. R. (2001). Dissociation between theory of mind and executive functions in a patient with early left amygdala damage. *Brain Journal of Neurology, 124,* 287–298.

Fitzpatrick, E. (2004). The use of cognitive behavioural strategies in the management of anger in a child with an autistic disorder: An evaluation. *Good Autism Practice, 5,* 3–17.

Frazier, J., Doyle, R., Chiu, S., & Coyle, J. (2002). Treating a child with Asperger's disorder and comorbid bipolar disorder. *American Journal of Psychiatry, 159,* 13–21.

Gadow, K., DeVincent, C., & Drabick, D. (2008). Oppositional defiant disorder as a clinical phenotype in children with autism spectrum disorder. *Journal of Autism and Developmental Disorders, 38,* 1302–1310.

Garcia Winner, M., & Cooke, P. (2009). *Socially curious and curiously social.* Great Barrington, MA: Think Social Publishing.

Gaus, V. (2007). *Cognitive-behavioral therapy for adult Asperger syndrome.* New York: Guilford Press.

Ghaziuddin, M. (2005). *Mental health aspects of autism and Asperger syndrome.* London: Jessica Kingsley.

Ghaziuddin, M., Wieder-Mikhail, W., & Ghaziuddin, N. (1998). Comorbidity of Asperger syndrome: A preliminary report. *Journal of Intellectual Disability Research 42,* 279–283.

Ghaziuddin, M., & Zafar, S. (2008). Psychiatric comorbidity of adults with autism spectrum disorders. *Clinical Neuropsychiatry, 5,* 9–12.

Gillot, A., Furniss, F., & Walter, A. (2001). Anxiety in high-functioning children with autism. *Autism, 5,* 277–286.

Golan, O., Ashwin, E., Granader, Y., McClintock, S., Day, K., Legett, V., et al. (2010). Enhancing emotion recognition in children with autism spectrum conditions: An intervention using animated vehicles with real emotional faces. *Journal of Autism and Developmental Disorders, 40,* 269–279.

Golan, O., Baron-Cohen, S., Ashwin, E., Granader, Y., McClintock, S., Day, K., et al. (2010). Enhancing emotion recognition in children with autism spectrum conditions: An intervention using animated vehicles with real emotional faces. *Journal of Autism and Developmental Disorders, 40,* 269–279.

Graham, P. (1998). *Cognitive behaviour therapy for children and families.* Cambridge, UK: Cambridge University Press.

Grandin, T., & Barron, S. (2005). *Unwritten rules of social relationships: Decoding social mysteries through the unique perspectives of autism.* Arlington, TX: Future Horizons.

Grave, J., & Blissett, J. (2004). Is cognitive behavior therapy developmentally appropriate for young children?: Review of the evidence. *Clinical Psychology Review, 24,* 399–420.

Gray, C. (1998). Social Stories and comic strip conversations with students with Asperger syndrome and high-functioning autism. In E. Schopler, G. Mesibov, & L. J. Kunce (Eds.), *Asperger's syndrome or high-functioning autism?* New York: Plenum Press.

Gray, C. (2004a). Gray's guide to bullying Parts I–III. *The Morning News, 16,* 1–60.

Gray, C. (2004b). Social Stories 10.0. *Jenison Autism Journal, 15,* 2–21.

Gray, C. (2010). *The new Social Story book.* Arlington, TX: Future Horizons.

Green, J., Gilchrist, A., Burton, D., & Cox, A. (2000). Social and psychiatric functioning in adolescents with Asperger syndrome compared with conduct disorder. *Journal of Autism and Developmental Disorders, 30,* 279–293.

Hagiwara, T., & Myles, B. S. (1999). A multimedia Social Story intervention: Teaching skills to children with autism. *Focus on Autism and Other Developmental Disabilities, 14,* 82–95.

Hare, D. J. (1997). The use of cognitive-behavioural therapy with people with Asperger syndrome: A case study. *Autism, 1,* 215–225.

Hay, D., Payne, A., & Chadwick, A. (2004). Peer relations in childhood. *Journal of Child Psychology and Psychiatry, 45,* 84–108.

Heinrichs, R. (2003). *Perfect targets: Asperger syndrome and bullying—practical solutions for surviving the social world.* Shawnee, KS: Autism Asperger Publishing Company.

Hénault, I. (2005) *Asperger's syndrome and sexuality: From adolescence through adulthood.* London: Jessica Kingsley.

Hendrickx, S. (2008). *Love, sex and long-term relationships: What people with Asperger syndrome really want.* London: Jessica Kingsley.

Holliday-Willey, L. (2011). *Safety skills for Asperger women.* London: Jessica Kingsley.

Hoopmann, K. (2006). *All cats have Asperger syndrome.* London: Jessica Kingsley.

Humphrey, N., & Lewis, S. (2008). "Make me normal": The views and experiences of pupils on the autistic spectrum in mainstream secondary schools. *Autism, 12,* 23–46.

Ivarsson, T., & Melin, K. (2008). Autism spectrum traits in children and adolescents with obsessive–compulsive disorder (OCD). *Journal of Anxiety Disorders, 22,* 969–978.

Ivey, M., Heflin, L., & Alberto, P. (2004). The use of Social Stories to promote independent behaviors in novel events for children with PDD-NOS. *Focus on Autism and Other Developmental Disabilities, 19,* 164–176.

Jackson, L. (2002). *Freaks, geeks and Asperger syndrome: A user guide to adolescence.* London: Jessica Kingsley.

Jacobs, B. (2003). *Loving Mr. Spock: The story of a different kind of love.* Arlington, TX: Future Horizons.

Joshi, G., Petty, C., Wozniak, J., Henin, A., Fried, R., Galdo, M., et al. (2010). The heavy burden of psychiatric comorbidity in youth with autism spectrum disorders: A large comparative study of a psychiatrically referred population. *Journal of Autism and Developmental Disorders, 40,* 1361–1370.

Karkhaneh, M., Clark, B., Ospina, M. B., Seida, J. C., Smith, V., & Hartling, L. (2010). Social Stories to improve social skills in children with autism spectrum disorder: A systematic review. *Autism, 14,* 641–662.

Kasari, C., Locke, J., Gulsrud, A., & Rotheram-Fuller, E. (2011). Social networks and friendships at school: Comparing children with and without ASD. *Journal of Autism and Developmental Disorders, 41,* 533–544.

Kendall, P. C. (2000). *Child and adolescent therapy: Cognitive-behavioural therapy procedures.* New York: Guilford Press.

Kiker Painter, K. (2006). *Social skills groups for children and adolescents with Asperger's syndrome.* London: Jessica Kingsley.

Kim, J., Lyoo, I. K., Esres, A. M., Renshaw, P., Shaw, D., Friedman, S. D., et al. (2010). Laterobasal amygdalar enlargement in 6- to 7-year-old children with autism spectrum disorder. *Archive of General Psychiatry, 67,* 1187–1197.

Kim, J. A., Szatmari, P., Bryson, S. E., Streiner, D. L., & Wilson, F. (2000). The prevalence of anxiety and mood problems among children with autism and Asperger syndrome. *Autism, 4,* 117–132.

Kirk, K., & Dutton, C. (2006). "Nobody nowhere" to "somebody somewhere": Researching the effectiveness of psychodrama with young people with Asperger's syndrome. *British Journal of Psychodrama and Sociodrama, 21,* 31–53.

Konstantareas, M. (2005). Anxiety and depression in children and adolescents with Asperger syndrome. In K. Stoddart (Ed.), *Children, youth and adults with Asperger syndrome: Integrating multiple perspectives.* London: Jessica Kingsley.

Kurita, H. (1999). Brief report: Delusional disorder in a male adolescent with high-functioning PDDNOS. *Journal of Autism and Developmental Disorders, 29,* 419–423.

Kuusikko, S., Pollock-Wurman, R., Jussila, K., Carter, A., Mattila, M., Ebeling, H., et al. (2008). Social anxiety in high-functioning children and adolescents with autism and Asperger syndrome. *Journal of Autism and Developmental Disorders, 38,* 1697–1709.

Lang, R., Shogren, K., Machalicek, W., Rispoli, M., O'Reilly, M., Baker, S., et al. (2008). Video self-modeling to teach classroom rules to two students with Asperger's. *Research in Autism Spectrum Disorders, 3,* 483–488.

Laugeson, E, A., Frankel, F., Gantman, A., Dillon, A. R., & Mogil, C. (2012). Evidence-based social skills training for adolescents with autism spectrum disorders: The UCLA PEERS program. *Journal of Autism and Developmental Disorders, 42,* 1025–1036.

Lawson, W. (2005). *Sex, sexuality and the autism spectrum.* London: Jessica Kingsley.

Lehmkuhl, H., Storch, E., Bodfish, J., & Geffken, G. (2008). Brief report: Exposure and response prevention for obsessive compulsive disorder in a 12-year-old with autism. *Journal of Autism and Developmental Disorders, 38*, 977–981.

Lerner, M. D., Mikami, A. Y., & Levine, K. (2011). Socio-dramatic affective relational intervention for adolescents with Aperger syndrome and high functioning autism: Pilot study. *Autism, 15*, 21–42.

Little, L. (2002). Middle-class mothers' perceptions of peer and sibling victimization among children with Asperger syndrome and non-verbal learning disorders. *Issues in Comprehensive Pediatric Nursing, 25*, 43–57.

Lopata, C., Thomeer, M. L., Volker, M., Toomey, J. A., Nida, R. E., Lee, G. K. (2010). RCT of a manualized social treatment for high-functioning autism spectrum disorders. *Journal of Autism and Developmental Disorders, 40*, 1297–1310.

Lopata, C., Toomey, J. A., Fox, J. D., Volker, M., Chow, S. Y., & Thomeer, M. L. (2010). Anxiety and depression in children with high-functioning autism spectrum disorders: Symptom levels and source differences. *Journal of Abnormal Child Psychology, 38*, 765–776.

Lorimer, P. A. (2002). The use of Social Stories as a preventative behavioral intervention in a home setting with a child with autism. *Journal of Positive Behavior Interventions, 4*, 53–60.

MacNeil, B., Lopes, V., & Minnes, P. (2009). Anxiety in children and adolescents with autism spectrum disorders. *Research in Autism Spectrum Disorders, 3*, 1–21.

Mattila, M. L., Hurtig, T., Haapsamo, H., Jussila, K., Kuusikko-Gauffin, S., Kielinen, M., et al. (2010). Comorbid psychiatric disorders associated with Asperger syndrome/high-functioning autism: A community and clinic based study. *Journal of Autism and Developmental Disorders, 40*, 1080–1093.

McAfee, J. L. (2002). *Navigating the social world: A curriculum for individuals with Asperger's syndrome, high functioning autism and related disorders.* Arlington, TX: Future Horizons.

McDougle, C., Kresch, L., Goodman, W., & Naylor, S. (1995). A case controlled study of repetitive thoughts and behavior in adults with autistic disorder and obsessive compulsive disorder. *American Journal of Psychiatry, 152*, 772–777.

McNally Keehn, R. H., Lincoln, A. J., Brown, M. Z., & Chavira, D. A. (2013). The Coping Cat program for children with anxiety and autism spectrum disorder: A randomized controlled trial. *Journal of Autism and Developmental Disorders, 43*, 57–67.

Mills Schuman, C., Carter Barnes, C., Lord, C., & Courchesne, E. (2009). Amygdala enlargement in toddlers with autism related to severity of social and communication impairments. *Biological Psychiatry, 66*, 942–949.

Mitchell, P., Parsons, S., & Leonard, A. (2008). Using virtual environments for teaching social understanding to 6 adolescents with autistic spectrum disorders. *Journal of Autism and Developmental Disorders, 38*, 589–600.

Montgomery, J., Schwean, V., Burt, J., Dyke, D., Thorne, K., Hindes, Y., et al. (2008). Emotional intelligence and resiliency in young adults with Asperger's disorder. *Canadian Journal of School Psychology, 23*, 70–93.

Moreno, S., Wheeler, M., & Parkinson, K. (2012). *The partner's guide to Asperger syndrome.* London: Jessica Kingsley.

Munesue, T., Ono, Y., Mutoh, K., Shimoda, K., Nakatani, H., & Kikuchi, M. (2008). High prevalence of bipolar disorder comorbidity in adolescents and young adults with high-functioning autism spectrum disorder: A preliminary study of 44 outpatients. *Journal of Affective Disorders, 111*, 170–175.

Nadeau, J., Sulkowski, M., Ung, D., Wood, J., Lewein, A. B., Murphy, T., et al. (2011). Treatment of comorbid anxiety and autism spectrum disorders. *Neuropsychiatry, 1*, 567–578.

Norris, C., & Dattilo, J. (1999). Evaluating effects of a social story intervention on a young girl with autism. *Focus on Autism and Other Developmental Disabilities, 14*, 180–186.

Nyden, A., Gillberg, C., Hjelmquist, E., & Heiman, M. (1999). Executive function/attention deficits in boys with Asperger syndrome, attention disorder, and reading/writing disorder. *Autism, 3*, 213–228.

Olweus, D. (1992). Victimization by peers: Antecedents and long-term outcomes. In K. H. Rubin & J. B. Asenddorf (Eds.), *Social withdrawal, inhibition, and shyness in childhood*. Hillsdale, NJ: Erlbaum.

Ordetx, K. (2012). *Teaching theory of mind: A curriculum for children with high functioning autism, Asperger's syndrome, and related social challenges*. London: Jessica Kingsley.

Owens, G., Granader, Y., Humphrey, A., & Baron-Cohen, S. (2008). LEGO® therapy and the social use of language programme: An evaluation of two social skills interventions for children with high functioning autism and Asperger syndrome. *Journal of Autism and Developmental Disorders, 38*, 1944–1957.

Ozdemir, S. (2008). The effectiveness of Social Stories on decreasing disruptive behaviors of children with autism: Three case studies. *Journal of Autism and Developmental Disorders, 38*, 1689–1696.

Ozonoff, S., South, M., & Miller, J. (2000). DSM-IV defined Asperger syndrome: Cognitive behavioral and early history differentiation from high-functioning autism. *Autism, 4*, 29–46.

Pennington, B. F., & Ozonoff, S. (1996). Executive functions and developmental psychopathology. *Journal of Child Psychology and Psychiatry Annual Research Review, 37*, 51–87.

Pepler, D., & Craig, W. (1999). What should we do about bullying?: Research into practice. *Peacebuilder, 2*, 9–10.

Portman Minne, E., & Semrud-Clikeman, M. (2012). A social competence intervention for young children with high functioning autism and Asperger syndrome: A pilot study. *Autism, 16*, 586–602.

Puleo, C. M., & Kendall, P. C. (2011). Anxiety disorders in typically developing youth: Autism spectrum symptoms as a predictor of cognitive-behavioral treatment. *Journal of Autism and Developmental Disorders, 41*, 275–286.

Reaven, J., Blakeley-Smith, A., Nichols, S., Dasari, M., Flanigan, E., & Hepburn, S. (2008). Cognitive-behavioral group treatment for anxiety symptoms in children with high-functioning autism spectrum disorders. *Focus on Autism and Other Developmental Disabilities, 24*, 27–37.

Reaven, J., Blakeley-Smith, A., Culhane-Shelburne, K., & Hepburn, S. (2012). Group cognitive behavior therapy for children with high-functioning autism spectrum dfisorders and anxiety: A randomized trial. *Journal of Child Psychology and Psychiatry, 53*, 410–419.

Reaven, J., Blakeley-Smith, A., Nichols, S., & Hepburn, S. (2011). *Facing your fears: Group therapy for managing anxiety in children with high-functioning autism spectrum disorders*. Baltimore: Brookes.

Reaven, J., & Hepburn, S. (2003). Cognitive-behavioural treatment of obsessive–compulsive disorder in a child with Asperger syndrome: A case report.
Autism, 7, 145–164.

Rieffe, C., Oosterveld, P., Terwogt, M. M., Mootz, S., Leeuwn, E. V., & Stocvk-
mann, L. (2011). Emotion regulation and internalizing symptoms in childrern
with autism spectrum disorders. *Autism, 15,* 655–670.

Rieffe, C., Terwogt, M., & Kotronopoulou, K. (2007). Awareness of single and
multiple emotions in high-functioning children with autism. *Journal of
Autism and Developmental Disorders, 37,* 455–465.

Rigby, K. (2002). *New Perspectives on bullying.* London: Jessica Kingsley.

Rodman, K. (2003). *Asperger's syndrome and adults . . . is anyone listening?:
Essays and poems by partners, parents and family members of adults with
Asperger's syndrome.* London: Jessica Kingsley.

Rogers, K., Dziobek, I., Hassenstab, J., Wolf, O., & Convit, A. (2007). Who cares?:
Revisiting empathy in Asperger syndrome. *Journal of Autism and Developmental Disorders, 37,* 709–715.

Rogers, M. F., & Myles, B. S. (2001). Using Social Stories and comic strip conversations to interpret social situations for an adolescent with Asperger's syndrome. *Intervention in School and Clinic, 38,* 310–313.

Rotheram-Fuller, E., Kasari, C., Chamberlain, B., & Locke, J. (2010). Social
involvement of children with autism spectrum disorders in elementary
school classrooms. *Journal of Child Psychology and Psychiatry, 51,* 1227–
1234.

Rowe, C. (1999). Do Social Stories benefit children with autism in mainstream
primary school? *British Journal of Special Education, 26,* 12–14.

Russell, A., Mataix Cols, D., Anson, M., & Murphy, D. (2005). Obsessions and
compulsions in Asperger syndrome and high functioning autism. *British Journal of Psychiatry, 186,* 525–528.

Russell, E., & Sofronoff, K. (2004). Anxiety and social worries in children with
Asperger syndrome. *Australian and New Zealand Journal of Psychiatry, 39,*
633–638.

Rydén, E., & Bejerot, S. (2008). Autism spectrum disorders in an adult psychiatric
population: A naturalistic cross-sectional controlled study. *Clinical Neuropsychiatry, 5,* 13–21.

Samson, A. C., Huber, O., & Ruch, W. (2011). Teasing, ridiculing and the relation
to the fear of being laughed at in individuals with Asperger's syndrome. *Journal of Autism and Developmental Disorders, 41,* 475–483.

Santosi, F., Powell Smith, K., & Kincaid, D. (2004). A research synthesis of Social
Story interventions for children with autism spectrum disorders. *Focus on
Autism and Other Developmental Disabilities, 19,* 194–204.

Scarpa, A., & Reyes, N. M. (2011). Improving emotion regulation with CBT in
young children with high functioning autism spectrum disorders: A pilot
study. *Behavioural and Cognitive Psychotherapy, 39,* 495–500.

Scarpa, A., Wells, A., & Attwood, T. (2013). *Exploring feelings for young children
with high-functioning autism or Asperger's disorder: The STAMP treatment
model.* London: Jessica Kingsley.

Scarpa, A., Williams White, S., & Attwood, T. (Eds.). (2013). *CBT for children
and adolescents with high-functioning autism spectrum disorders.* New
York: Guilford Press.

Scattone, D. (2008). Enhancing the conversation skills of a boy with Asperger's disorder through Social Stories™ and video modeling. *Journal of Autism and Developmental Disorders, 38*, 395–400.

Scattone, D., Wilczynski, S. M., Edwards, R. P., & Rabian, B. (2002). Decreasing disruptive behaviors of children with autism using Social Stories. *Journal of Autism and Developmental Disorders, 32*, 535–543.

Schneider, C. (2006). *Acting antics: A theatrical approach to teaching social understanding to kids with Asperger syndrome.* London: Jessica Kingsley.

Shattuck, P. T., Orsmond, G. I., Wagner, M., & Cooper, B. P. (2011). Participation in social activities among adolescents with an autism spectrum disorder. *PLoS ONE, 6*(11).

Shtayermman, O. (2007). Peer victimization in adolescents and young adults diagnosed with Asperger's syndrome: A link to depressive symptomatology, anxiety symptomatology, and suicidal ideation. *Issues in Comprehensive Pediatric Nursing, 30*, 87–107.

Simone, R. (2010). *Aspergirls: Empowering females with Asperger's syndrome.* London: Jessica Kingsley.

Simone, R. (2012). *22 things a woman with Asperger's syndrome wants her partner to know.* London: Jessica Kingsley.

Slater-Walker, G., & Slater-Walker, C. (2002). *An Asperger marriage.* London: Jessica Kingsley.

Smith, C. (2001). Using Social Stories with children with autistic spectrum disorders: An evaluation. *Good Autism Practice, 2*, 16–23.

Sofronoff, K., Attwood, T., & Hinton, S. (2005). A randomized controlled trial of a CBT intervention for anxiety in children with Asperger syndrome. *Journal of Child Psychology and Psychiatry, 46*, 1143–1151.

Sofronoff, K., Attwood, T., Hinton, S., & Levin, I. (2008). A randomized controlled trial of a cognitive behavioural intervention for anger management in children diagnosed with Asperger syndrome. *Journal of Autism and Developmental Disorders, 38*, 1203–1214.

Stanford, A. (2003). *Asperger syndrome and long-term relationships.* London: Jessica Kingsley.

Sterling, L., Dawson, G., Estes, A., & Greenson, J. (2008). Characteristics associated with presence of depressive symptoms in adults with autism spectrum disorder. *Journal of Autism and Developmental Disorders, 38*, 1011–1018.

Stokes, M., Newton, N., & Kaur, A. (2008). Stalking, and social and romantic functioning among adolescents and adults with autism spectrum disorder. *Journal of Autism and Developmental Disorders, 38*, 1969–1986.

Sukhodolsky, D., Scahill, L., Gadow, K., Arnold, L., Aman, M., McDougle, C., et al. (2007). Parent-rated anxiety symptoms in children with pervasive developmental disorders: Frequency and association with core autism symptoms and cognitive functioning. *Journal of Abnormal Child Psychology, 36*, 117–128.

Sung, M., Ooi, Y., Goh, T., Pathy, P., Fung, D., Ang, R., et al. (2011). Effects of cognitive-behavioral therapy on anxiety in children with autism spectrum disorders: A randomized controlled trial. *Child Psychiatry and Human Development, 42*, 634–649.

Swaggart, B. L., Gagnon, E., Bock, S. J., Earles, T. L., Quinn, C., Myles, B. S., et al. (1995). Using Social Stories to teach social and behavioral skills to children with autism. *Focus on Autistic Behavior, 10*, 1–16.

Sze, K., & Wood, J. (2007). Cognitive behavioral treatment of comorbid anxiety disorders and social difficulties in children with high-functioning autism: A case report. *Journal of Contemporary Psychotherapy, 37*, 133–143.

Tantam, D. (1988). Asperger's syndrome. *Journal of Child Psychology and Psychiatry, 29*, 245–253.

Tantam, D. (2000). Psychological disorder in adolescents and adults with Asperger disorder. *Autism, 4*, 47–62.

Tardif, C., Lainé, F., Rodriguez, M., & Gepner, B. (2007). Slowing down presentation of facial movements and vocal sounds enhances facial expression recognition and induces facial–vocal imitation in children with autism. *Journal of Autism and Developmental Disorders, 37*, 1469–1484.

Tarnai, B., & Wolfe, P. (2008). Social Stories for sexuality education for persons with autism/pervasive developmental disorder. *Sexuality and Disability, 26*, 29–36.

Thiemann, K. S., & Goldstein, H. (2001). Social Stories, written text cues, and video feedback: Effects on social communication of children with autism. *Journal of Applied Behavior Analysis, 34*, 425–446.

Thompson, B. (2008). *Counselling for Asperger couples*. London: Jessica Kingsley.

Timms, L. A. (2011). *60 social situations and discussion starters to help teens on the autism spectrum deal with friendships, feelings, conflict and more*. London: Jessica Kingsley.

Tinsley, M., & Hendrickx, S. (2008). *Asperger syndrome and alcohol: Drinking to cope?* London: Jessica Kingsley.

Tonge, B., Brereton, A., Gray, K., & Einfeld, S. (1999). Behavioral and emotional disturbance in high-functioning autism and Asperger syndrome. *Autism, 3*, 117–130.

Uhlenkamp, J. (2009). *The guide to dating for teenagers with Asperger syndrome*. Shawnee, KS: Autism Asperger Publishing Company.

van Steensel, F., Bogels, S. M., & Perrin, S. (2011). Anxiety disorders in children and adolescents with autism spectrum disorders: A meta-analysis. *Clinical Child and Family Psychological Review, 14*, 302–317.

Vickerstaff, S., Heriot, S., Wong, M., Lopes, A., & Dossetor, D. (2007). Intellectual ability, self-perceived social competence, and depressive symptomatology in children with high-functioning autistic spectrum disorders. *Journal of Autism and Developmental Disorders, 37*, 1647–1664.

Wainscot, J., Naylor, P., Sutcliffe, P., Tantam, D., & Williams, J. (2008). Relationships with peers and use of the school environment of mainstream secondary school pupils with Asperger syndrome (high-functioning autism): A case-control study. *International Journal of Psychology and Psychological Therapy, 8*, 25–38.

Weston, L. (2010). *Connecting with your Asperger partner, negotiating the maze of intimacy*. London: Jessica Kingsley.

White, S. W., Ollendick, T., Albano, A. M., Oswald, D., Johnson, C., Southam-Gerow, M. A., et al. (2013). Randomized controlled trial: Multimodal anxiety and social skills intervention for adolescents with autism spectrum disorder. *Journal of Autism and Developmental Disorders, 43*, 382–394.

Willey, L. H. (1999). *Pretending to be normal*. London: Jessica Kingsley.

Williamson, S., Craig, J., & Slinger, R. (2008). Exploring the relationship between measures of self-esteem and psychological adjustment among adolescents with Asperger syndrome. *Autism, 12,* 391–402.

Williams-White, S. (2011). *Social skills training for children with Asperger syndrome and high-functioning autism.* New York: Guilford Press.

Wing, L. (1981). Asperger's syndrome: A clinical account. *Psychological Medicine, 11,* 115–130.

Wood, J., Drahota, A., Sze, K., Har, K., Chiu, A., & Langer, D. (2009). Cognitive behavioral therapy for anxiety in children with autism spectrum disorders: A randomized, controlled trial. *Journal of Child Psychology and Psychiatry, 50,* 224–234.

Zucker, N., Losh, M., Bulik, C., LaBar, K., Piven, J., & Pelphrey, K. (2007). Anorexia nervosa and autism spectrum disorders: Guided investigation of social cognitive endophenotypes. *Psychological Bulletin, 133,* 976–1006.

CHAPTER 9

Psychopharmacological Treatment of Asperger Syndrome

Alexander Westphal
Dana Kober
Avery Voos
Fred R. Volkmar

This chapter discusses the pharmacological approaches used to treat individuals with Asperger syndrome (AS). As noted in other chapters, the features that define AS are a disabling impairment in social ability coupled with a pattern of restricted and repetitive behaviors, interests, or activities (American Psychiatric Association, 1994). There are currently no pharmacological treatments that directly address the social disability in AS, nor are such treatments yet available for any of the autism spectrum disorders (ASD). However, as research on both AS and the other ASD expands, and the physiological substrates that underlie social behavior are better understood, therapeutic targets have been identified. For example, preliminary support exists for a positive effect of oxytocin, a hormone that modulates affiliative behavior, on the retention of social information in subjects with ASD (Andari et al., 2010; Hollander et al., 2007). This type of symptom-specific pharmacological intervention is at a preliminary stage, and its development will depend on the coordinated efforts of research in the fields of pharmacology, genetics, neuroimaging, psychiatry, and psychology. As it stands, the evidence available to practitioners involved in the ongoing care of people with AS and ASD suggests that the most effective role for pharmacology currently is to address problematic symptom clusters associated with the disorder and other conditions that might, if appropriately treated, facilitate adjustment of the individuals with AS. Thus, pharmacology can serve as an adjunct to the behavioral interventions targeted at the core features of the disorder discussed elsewhere in this book.

A number of symptom clusters has been associated with AS, and the symptoms are appropriate targets for pharmacological interventions. In some cases symptom clusters may be both specific and pronounced enough to warrant another diagnosis, a so-called *comorbidity*. The concepts of both comorbidity and symptom clusters create challenges for psychiatric classification systems in general (Volkmar, 1997) and for AS in particular. The first edition of this volume cited significant issues relative to the comorbid diagnoses: namely, whether they are truly independent disorders or just one aspect of AS (Klin, Volkmar, & Sparrow, 2000). This type of problem occurs both in general medicine and in psychiatry, but is of particular relevance to childhood-onset disorders in which the presence of a major chronic condition may increase liability to other disorders (Volkmar, 1997). Historically, diagnosticians have erred toward ignoring secondary diagnoses to focus on the "primary" disorder, but by doing so, they risk "diagnostic overshadowing," overlooking treatable problems (Klin, 2003).

Another issue with comorbid diagnoses becomes very apparent when discussing repetitive behaviors, for example, which can be conceptualized as representing an artifact of the primary diagnosis, or, on the other hand, as comorbid obsessive–compulsive disorder (OCD). There are also more subtle but equally important examples: When a child with AS exhibits inattention in a school setting, does it represent a comorbid disorder of attention or rather an excessive focus on an inappropriate target that is more consistent with the core symptoms of AS? If an inappropriate focus were driving inattention, a standard treatment such as a stimulant might be expected to exacerbate the problem.

An emphasis on epidemiological studies is needed to clarify whether associations occur more frequently in individuals with AS than in the general population. At this point, such epidemiological data are limited; much of the data suggesting potential areas of comorbidity arise from case reports or case series. The applicability of such data is limited by the fact that only positive associations are likely to be reported.

One might argue that the symptom-focused approach would lead to more effective treatments, but sometimes the failure to appreciate the "big picture" leads to poor treatment planning and overmedication. On the other hand, "true" comorbidity may be helpful in highlighting areas for additional research. Thus, a symptom-cluster-based approach is not ideal. However, it is clear that psychopharmacological agents are regularly used in the population with AS, and what little research there is on the topic is based on ameliorating targeted symptoms.

We organize this chapter around the principle that the most appropriate targets for pharmacotherapy are currently the problematic symptom clusters that are associated with, but do not define, AS. Below, in the section titled "Medication Use Patterns," we discuss general trends in the pharmacological treatment of AS. A section titled "Symptom Clusters," in which the approach we have taken in this chapter is justified and explained, follows. The rest of the chapter is divided into sections based on each symptom cluster, discussing the evidence for various pharmacological agents, with a final section summarizing what is known, limitations of available research, and directions for the future.

Throughout this introduction we have discussed both AS and the more general category of ASD. AS was a diagnostic category in the DSM-IV-R that has been absorbed by the broader ASD category in the DSM-5 (American Psychiatric Association, 2013). However, most pharmacological approaches to AS rely heavily on what little is known about treatment of individuals with other ASD and, for the most part, on what is known about the treatment of individuals without ASD. These approaches reflect the paucity of research on pharmacological treatments specific to AS and the fact that research has not reliably isolated pharmacological targets specific to any individual ASD, let alone ASD in general. The general consensus among the research and clinical community, however, seems to be that some precision can be gained by applying what is known about treating ASD without co-occurring intellectual disability to the AS population. This approach blends well with the symptom-cluster approach, if we accept that certain symptom clusters are more or less likely to occur at different levels of intellectual ability. Thus, depression might be conceptualized as more characteristic of intact intellectual ability and aggression of intellectual disability. This approach, however, is by no means substantial and is still a controversial topic. We attempt to focus, whenever possible, on what is known about AS specifically and draw heavily on both what is known about the ASD in general and on what is known about the population with ASD and no intellectual disability.

MEDICATION USE PATTERNS

In the chapter on psychopharmacological treatment in the first edition of *Asperger Syndrome* (Martin, Patzer, & Volkmar, 2000), the authors presented the results of an initial survey undertaken at the Yale Child Study Center to describe medication use patterns (Martin, Scahill, Klin, & Volkmar, 1999). One of the purposes of this study was to document the rates and characteristics of psychotropic drug use among a representative sample of individuals with high-functioning ASD. Since the 2000 publication of

Asperger Syndrome, prescribing patterns have changed for a variety of reasons. In order to highlight this point, we present summary statistics for the subjects with AS evaluated at the Yale Child Study Center between 1999 and 2008 and compare them to some of the results described by Martin et al. (2000) (see Table 9.1). Our sample was made up of 45 males and 8 females, all with diagnoses of AS. The average Full Scale IQ score was 113, with a range of 81–146.

There was an overall decrease in the percentage of subjects receiving medications between the two time points. At the first time point, 6% of subjects was being treated with tricyclic antidepressants (TCAs). These were no longer used at the second time point, apparently replaced by the selective serotonin reuptake inhibitors (SSRIs), the use of which increased by 5% during the same period. The first-generation antipsychotics also disappeared, but without a concomitant increase in the use of second-generation antipsychotics. Although this finding may reflect a difference between the groups in that first-generation antipsychotics are more often used in treatment-refractory cases, it may also reflect a general shift in prescribing practice, both away from first-generation antipsychotics, in particular, and from antipsychotics in general.

In considering the observed changes, it should be noted that our follow-up study focuses only on subjects diagnosed with AS, in contrast to the broader high-functioning ASD sample employed in the prior study. Another source of bias may be that the data we present were collected during a period of massive increase in public knowledge about autism. As a result, cases of AS are more commonly identified, and families are more likely to seek specialized evaluations and care. Thus, any shift in medication prescribing patterns may reflect a dilution of the acuity level of the population seen at the previous time point. Finally, it is not clear that these data reflect general prescribing trends in the United States, because they were collected at the Yale Child Study Center, a tertiary care center with a specialty in ASD. The data may be skewed by the challenging cases, sometimes coming from all over the world, that are more often seen at tertiary care centers.

SYMPTOM CLUSTERS

In an early examination of psychiatric comorbidity in AS, Wing found that among 18 subjects, "four had an affective illness, four had become increasingly odd and withdrawn, probably with underlying depression, one had a psychosis with delusions and hallucinations that could not be classified, one had an episode of catatonic stupor, one had bizarre behavior and an unconfirmed diagnosis of schizophrenia, and two had bizarre behavior, but no psychiatric illness" (Wing, 1981, p. 118). The picture that emerges from Wing's work is of elevated affective and psychotic symptoms in AS in comparison to the general population. In a later study expanding this work,

TABLE 9.1. Changes in Prescribing Practices in Patients with Asperger Syndrome

Drug type	1999[a]		2010[b]	
	N	%	N	%
Any psychotropic (lifetime)	75	69	31	59
Any psychotropic (current)	60	55	25	47
One drug	28	26	11	20
Two drugs	25	23	9	17
Three drugs	5	5	5	9
Four drugs	2	2	1	2
Any antidepressant	35	32	17	31
SSRI	29	27	17	31
TCA	7	6	0	0
Stimulant	22	20	8	15
SNRI (atomoxetine)	—	—	2	4
Any neuroleptic	18	16	7	13
First-generation neuroleptic	5	5	0	0
Second-generation neuroleptic	14	13	7	13
Mood stabilizer	10	9	1	2
Anxiolytic	7	6	3	5
Antihypertensive	7	6	4	7

Note. SSRI, selective serotonin reuptake inhibitor; TCA, tricyclic antidepressant; SNRI, serotonin–norepinephrine reuptake inhibitor.
[a]$n = 109$; [b]$n = 53$.

Ghaziuddin used strict diagnostic criteria to define psychiatric comorbidity (Ghaziuddin, Weidmer-Mikhail, & Ghaziuddin, 1998). The majority (65%) of the 35 subjects were given a psychiatric diagnosis, most frequently attention-deficit/hyperactivity disorder (ADHD; $n = 10$) and depression ($n = 13$). There were also single cases of bipolar disorder, Tourette syndrome, OCD, and tic disorder in the cohort. In this sample, no subject had a psychotic disorder such as schizophrenia, a finding at odds with Wing's work.

Towbin (2003) described six symptoms clusters as a convenient way of talking about the pharmacological treatments for the ASD. The clusters he defined were aggression, anxiety, depression, hyperactivity–inattention, inflexibility and behavioral rigidity, and stereotypies and perseveration. This symptom-based organization complements and extends the strict diagnostic approach (e.g., that used by Ghaziuddin). For example, Towbin's "inflexibility and behavioral rigidity" might have been marked by Ghaziuddin as comorbid OCD. The previous edition of this book included discussion on "Target Symptoms, Clinical Heterogeneity, and Patterns of Comorbidity," identifying anxiety, aggression/irritability/self-injurious behaviors, mood disorders including depression, OCD, and ADHD as possible targets of pharmacological intervention.

Below we use a symptom-cluster approach, defining each cluster according to the first edition of this chapter and Towbin's work. In addition, we refer to a recent study on comorbidity in high-functioning ASD. In this study, comorbid psychopathology was assessed in 122 consecutively referred adults with ASD and normal intelligence, 67 of whom were diagnosed with AS. Lifetime psychiatric Axis I comorbidity was common, particularly mood, anxiety, and attention disorders, but also psychotic disorders (Hofvander et al., 2009).

INATTENTION AND HYPERACTIVITY

Individuals with ASD exhibit increased levels of hyperactivity, distractibility, and impulsivity compared to their typical counterparts (Volkmar, Paul, Klin, & Cohen, 2005). Seventy-five percent are estimated to have symptoms consistent with ADHD (Sturm, Fernell, & Gillberg, 2004). However, the revised edition of the fourth edition of the *Diagnostic and Statistical Manual of Mental Disorders* (DSM-IV-TR; American Psychiatric Association, 2000) precludes the diagnosis of ADHD if the symptoms occur during the course of an ASD. DSM-5 (American Psychiatric Association, 2013) has removed this restriction, hopefully supporting greater research on the overlap between the symptoms of ASD and ADHD. Irrespective of diagnostic convention, behaviors associated with ADHD have always been a significant concern while treating children with ASD. Among children with ADHD, autistic behaviors are also more common. In a study of 946 children with ADHD, Reierson and Todd (2008) found that 75% of females and 32% of males had clinically significant PDD-like behaviors. In fact, some researchers have argued that the convergence of ADHD and PDD behaviors is common enough to justify a unique diagnostic term (Gillberg, 1983).

Among the subgroup of individuals diagnosed with AS, difficulties with impulsivity, hyperactivity, and inattention are also common. In a study of 20 adults with AS, Tani, Lindberg, et al. (2006) found that almost 75% were above ADHD cutoff limits on a self-report measure of retrospective childhood behavior using the Wender–Utah Rating Scale. Studies using rigorous diagnostic criteria suggest that rates of ADHD among the population with AS are between 30 and 36%, and that inattention is more common than hyperactivity (Ghaziuddin et al., 1998; Hofvander et al., 2009). Schatz et al. raised the important question of whether inattention in AS is best conceived of as a comorbidity or as a consequence of the intrinsic character of AS (unusual use of language, odd socialization, obsessive thoughts, etc.), which, in turn, causes a secondary attention deficit (Schatz, Weimer, & Trauner, 2002). This distinction has significant implications for the pharmacological treatment of inattention in AS. As mentioned above, treatment decisions in the AS population often reflect what is known about treating the typical population. However, if inattention in a subject with AS reflects, for example, an inability to shift attention from a topic of focus rather than an inability to focus on any topic at all, the treatment implications would be significant, and we might, in fact, exacerbate an individual's inability to switch topic.

Consistent with the prevalence estimates of ADHD, almost 30% of the subjects in our survey were receiving treatment for attention or hyperactivity problems. Stimulants were the most commonly prescribed class of medication and accounted for 17% of all medications prescribed to patients with AS. Other agents were also prescribed, including alpha-2 adrenergics, atomoxetine, and bupropion. To date, stimulants are the most commonly used class of treatments for attention and hyperactivity problems in the population without ASD. This class, which includes methylphenidate and the amphetamine salts, is thought to affect levels of norepinephrine and dopamine in brain areas identified as fundamental to attention, motor planning, and impulse control (Solanto, 1998). The stimulants, in various forms, have been used for over 70 years to treat symptoms of ADHD. The short-term benefits of the stimulants, particularly methylphenidate, are well established in the treatment of ADHD in the typical population (Kavale, 1982). The long-term benefits are less clear. A 14-month study conducted by the Multimodal Treatment Study of ADHD (MTA) Cooperative Group demonstrated significant benefits of both methylphenidate (MPH) alone and combined with behavioral therapy in comparison to behavioral therapy alone and to "as usual" community care (MTA Cooperative Group, 1999). However, a long-term follow-up of the same cohort suggested that these benefits may be time limited, that the differences between the groups fade, and that all have worse behavioral outcomes than their non-ADHD counterparts (Molina et al., 2009). Furthermore, the MTA study also suggested concerns about growth suppression as a side effect of MPH (Swanson et al., 2007). Thus, within the typical population, stimulants appear to be very effective for immediate symptom relief, but these benefits may not carry into the long term and may suppress growth.

There are fewer data on the use of stimulants in the population with ASD. MPH is the only exception, as it has been the subject of three double-blind, placebo-controlled trials. These trials all found benefit from MPH (Handen, Johnson, & Lubetsky, 2000; Quintana et al., 1995; Research Units on Pediatric Psychopharmacology Autism Network, 2005a) in subjects with ASD and ADHD symptoms. The largest of these, conducted by the RUPP, was a multisite trial on 72 subjects. Results displayed a significant improvement in the ADHD target symptoms (Research Units on Pediatric Psychopharmacology Autism Network, 2005a), particularly hyperactivity and impulsivity (Posey et al., 2007). Despite these improvements, the magnitude of response to MPH was diminished in comparison to typical subjects.

Several other interesting findings emerged from this study. First, MPH was less effective for the treatment of inattention than for hyperactivity and impulsivity, a pattern that is not the case in typical subjects (Research Units on Pediatric Psychopharmacology Autism Network, 2005a). This finding raises the question of whether inattention may be qualitatively different in subjects with ASD than in typical subjects. Additionally, MPH was found to improve some social behaviors (Jahromi et al., 2009). Again, it is unclear whether this social improvement is mediated by a reduction in ADHD behaviors, or if it reflects a more fundamental change in sociability.

Stimulants other than MPH, although a mainstay of therapy in the typically developing population, are not well studied in subjects with PDD and ADHD symptoms. Early studies suggest that side effects of stimulants may outweigh the benefits (Campbell et al., 1972). However, this is definitely not an established finding, and further study of all stimulants is needed in the population with ASD. Although side effects are of concern in any patient treated with medication, specific concerns have been raised about whether stimulants may exacerbate preexisting rigid and stereotypic behaviors as well as tics in subjects with ASD (McDougle, 2004). These concerns reflect the fact that stimulants, at high doses, may induce new stereotypies in both animals and humans (Roffman & Raskin, 1997) and may lead to new compulsive behaviors in subjects with ADHD (Borcherding, Keysor, Rapoport, Elia, & Amass, 1990). In a study of 13 subjects with ASD five had an immediate worsening of stereotypies, tics, dysphoria, or hyperactivity (Di Martino, Melis, Cianchetti, & Zuddas, 2004). The RUPP MPH study, described above, found increased rates of adverse events, particularly a worsening of irritability but also "repetitive behaviors and thoughts," and suggested that adverse events in general occur more commonly than in typical subjects (Research Units on Pediatric Psychopharmacology Autism Network, 2005a).

Of the subjects with AS evaluated at the Yale Child Study Center between 1999 and 2008, 17% were being treated for attention and hyperactivity with stimulants, suggesting that stimulants are widely used in this population. But, other than a case report (Roy, Dillo, Bessling, Emrich, & Ohlmeier, 2009) and general discussion in review articles, the literature does not address this topic. This oversight surely reflects the fact that practitioners are comfortable applying what is known about stimulants in the general population to subjects with AS. However, results from the RUPP study suggest that providers should move with caution, as the therapeutic windows may be narrower than expected.

The alpha-2 antagonists, including clonidine and guanfacine, are a class of agents chiefly used to treat hypertension. They have also been used to treat inattention and hyperactivity for over 30 years and are thought to work by effects on the noradrenergic system that plays a role in the "modulation of higher cortical functions including attention, alertness, and vigilance" (Biederman & Spencer, 2000). A large trial of clonidine for the treatment of ADHD in typical children established modest effectiveness and good tolerability (Palumbo et al., 2008), corroborating a meta-analysis of 11 smaller trials (Connor, Fletcher, & Swanson, 1999). A randomized placebo-controlled trial indicated that guanfacine is also moderately effective for treating inattention in this population (Scahill et al., 2001). An extended-release formulation of guanfacine demonstrated modest efficacy in several trials (Biederman et al., 2008; Sallee et al., 2009), and was recently approved by the U.S. Food and Drug Administration (FDA) for the treatment of ADHD. In summary, the alpha-2 antagonists appear to be effective for the treatment of ADHD symptoms in typically developing children and are well tolerated, but may not be as effective as the stimulants.

Both clonidine and guanfacine have been studied in the ASD population. Several small trials using clonidine demonstrated improvements in hyperactivity and disruptive behaviors (Fankhauser, Karumanchi, German, Yates, & Karumanchi, 1992; Jaselskis, Cook, Fletcher, & Leventhal, 1992). However, adverse side effects were also common, including sedation, fatigue, and hypotension. Guanfacine has shown promise in two well-constructed trials and a retrospective review of a large sample treated with open-label guanfacine, although there is a consensus that further study is needed (Handen et al., 2000; Handen, Sahl, & Hardan, 2008; Scahill et al., 2006). To date, there are no reports on the extended formulation of guanfacine in the population with ASD.

Among the group of subjects seen at Yale Child Study Center, 7% were treated for ADHD symptoms with an alpha-2 adrenergic (listed in Table 9.1 as antihypertensive) such as clonidine or guanfacine. The rate of alpha-2 adrenergic use was similar between 1999 and 2008 (see Table 9.1) and they were the second most commonly prescribed class of agent used for treating ADHD symptoms in our sample. There is very little literature on the use of alpha-2 adrenergics in subjects with AS. In Posey's retrospective analysis, mentioned above, guanfacine was effective in 23.8% of subjects. When the results were examined on the basis of ASD diagnosis, subjects with PDD-NOS (39.3%) or AS (33.3%) showed a better response than subjects with AD (13%), possibly related to the fact that subjects without intellectual disability showed a better response than their disabled counterparts. Posey and colleagues concluded that "individuals with Asperger's disorder and PDD-NOS, and those persons without mental retardation, may respond better to [guanfacine] treatment and should be considered as covariates in any double-blind study" (Posey, Puntney, Sasher, Kem, & McDougle, 2004, p. 240). Although further research is needed, it is clear that practitioners treating individuals with AS for ADHD symptoms should closely consider the alpha-2 adrenergics, and that a trial examining extended-release guanfacine in those with AS or high-functioning autism (HFA) is warranted.

Although originally designed as an antidepressant, atomoxetine, a selective norepinephrine reuptake inhibitor, has been found to be more effective for the treatment of inattention and hyperactivity than for depression, and has FDA approval for the treatment of ADHD. Atomoxetine is thought to affect attention using a mechanism much like the TCAs, which are described below (Spencer & Biederman, 2002). Unlike the tricyclics, however, atomoxetine is not associated with cardiotoxic effects, and does not pose the same risks if taken in doses larger than prescribed. The effectiveness and tolerability of atomoxetine in the typical population are well documented (Adler, Spencer, Williams, Moore, & Michelson, 2008; Arnold et al., 2006; Michelson et al., 2001). Research has shown that in the population with ASD, atomoxetine is also effective. Posey demonstrated significant improvements in attention and reduction of hyperactivity in an 8-week open-label trial of children with high-functioning PDD (Posey, Erickson, et al., 2006). In a similar open-label trial in 12 children with PDD, Troost also demonstrated an effect, although five of the subjects withdrew from the trial because of adverse events, including sleep problems, irritability, fatigue, and gastrointestinal reactions (Troost et al., 2006). In a placebo-controlled crossover trial of atomoxetine in 16 children with PDD, Arnold demonstrated that atomoxetine has an effect on par with MPH, but as in Troost's study, gastrointestinal side effects were very common, as was fatigue. Four of the subjects also exhibited tachycardia, attributable to the drug. However, none of these side effects was significant enough for subjects to terminate the study (Arnold et al., 2006).

Atomoxetine was prescribed for two (4%) of the subjects with AS seen at the Yale Child Study Center. In the previous edition of this chapter, atomoxetine was not used at all, as it was not on the market at that point. The only evidence for atomoxetine in the population with AS comes from Posey, Erickson, et al.'s study (2006) of "high-functioning" ASD subjects (IQ 93.9 ± 18) cited above. Seven of Posey's 16 subjects had a diagnosis of AS. The other subjects were diagnosed with either autistic disorder or PDD-NOS. Although Posey did not compare results by diagnosis, five of the subjects (71%) with AS responded to the medication, in comparison to 86% ($n = 7$) of those with AD and 50% ($n = 2$) with PDD-NOS. In summary, atomoxetine has been on the market for a short time in comparison to the stimulants, but limited evidence suggests that it may be effective in subjects with AS. Although there are side effects frequently associated with atomoxetine, particularly gastrointestinal disturbances, there is no evidence to date suggesting that subjects with AS or ASD are more vulnerable to these than any other population.

Several types of antidepressant have proven effective in the treatment of ADHD. The antidepressant bupropion has been shown to be as effective as methylphenidate in typical subjects (Barrickman et al., 1995; Conners et al., 1996). No trials have been conducted in subjects with ASD, however. Given the fact that bupropion is a well-tolerated drug that addresses both ADHD symptoms and depression, perhaps the two most common comorbidities in AS, it is a natural candidate for further study in all of the ASD. TCAs are a class of drugs used primarily to treat depression and include

both clomipramine and desipramine. There are no studies directly addressing their utility for the treatment of ADHD symptoms in subjects with
AS, but both have shown benefits in treating ADHD in typical subjects
as well as those with PDD (Gordon, State, Nelson, Hamburger, & Rapoport, 1993; Remington, Sloman, Konstantareas, Parker, & Gow, 2001).
However, all TCAs have fallen from use. This is most likely a reflection of
a variety of factors, including the necessity that they be monitored using
electrocardiograms and plasma levels, the concern that they can be toxic in
high doses, and finally the increase in the number SSRIs available. At the
time that the survey described in the first edition of this chapter was completed, the TCAs accounted for 6% of the drugs prescribed. It is not clear
whether they were being used to treat ADHD or mood symptoms. They
had not been prescribed, however, in the treatment group seen at the Yale
Child Study Center during 1999–2008 (see Table 9.1), most likely reflecting
the general trend away from TCAs.

A variety of other drugs may address ADHD symptoms in subjects
with AS, but none has been evaluated in AS, and for various reasons these
agents are not recommended unless the options described earlier in this
chapter have failed. There is good evidence that several antipsychotic drugs,
including haloperidol (Anderson et al., 1989) and risperidone (Research
Units on Pediatric Psychopharmacology Autism Network, 2005b), can
reduce ADHD behaviors in subjects with ASD. However, they are also
associated with metabolic side effects. For the sole treatment of ADHD
symptoms, their risks appear to outweigh their benefit. Naltrexone, an opi-
ate antagonist, has been reasonably well studied in ASD but not specifically in AS. It appears to be well tolerated, but is only modestly effective in
reducing ADHD behaviors (Kolmen, Feldman, Handen, & Janosky, 1995;
Kolmen, Feldman, Handen, & Janosky, 1997). Modafinil, a recently introduced drug that promotes wakefulness, is also effective for the treatment
of ADHD in typical subjects (Greenhill et al., 2006; Kahbazi et al., 2009),
although to date, no trials have been conducted among subjects with any
ASD.

Hyperactivity, distractibility, and impulsivity commonly occur in people with the diagnosis of AS. Although there is evidence for several classes
of drug in the treatment of ADHD symptoms in subjects with ASD, there is
very little data on the treatment of these symptoms in AS specifically. Treatment recommendations depend heavily on the literature on ASD in general.
The strongest evidence exists for the stimulants, alpha-2 antagonists, and
atomoxetine, although all come with their associated side effects. As with
the other ASD, practitioners treating patients with AS for ADHD symptoms are urged to carefully consider several issues:

1. Do inattention and distractibility mark an alternative orientation of
   focus rather than a lack thereof? A feature of AS can be a tendency
   toward an intense focus on narrow topics. It is easy to imagine that

in a setting, such as a school, which demands constant shifts of attention, that an inability to shift focus could easily be understood as inattention. If this were the case, it would be no surprise that treatment for ADHD would exacerbate the problem.

2. Patients with AS may be more vulnerable to side effects than their typical counterparts. They are also less likely to be able to describe any side effect to their care team. Together these factors suggest that any medication trial should be conducted with more caution and more slowly than in typical subjects.

AFFECTIVE SYMPTOMS

The most commonly prescribed class of psychotropic medications in our sample was the antidepressants: 31% of our sample had been on an antidepressant at one time. This most likely reflects the prominent role that mood symptoms, and more specifically depressive symptoms, play in AS. On the other hand, antidepressants, particularly SSRIs, are also used to target anxiety and obsessive behavior.

Depression affects typically developing children with a prevalence of up to 8.3% (Shaffer et al., 1996). Depression also tends to be a common comorbidity in children and adolescents with an ASD, with estimates ranging from 4 to 38% (Lainhart, 1999). Children with autism or AS also demonstrate a higher rate of depression than their typically developing peers (Kim, Szatmari, Bryson, Streiner, & Wilson, 2000). A comparison of 68 preschool children with PDD to a random sample of 1,751 typically developing children found that 16.9% scored at least two standard deviations above the population mean on the measure of depression (Kim et al., 2000). Several studies have suggested even higher rates of depression once the impact of communication impairments on describing internal states is factored in (Stewart, Barnard, Pearson, Hasan, & O'Brien, 2006). Because of limited data on antidepressant use in the pediatric population, treatment has largely been influenced by data from adults. Current theories of depression are generally based on neurotransmitter receptor hypotheses in which a depletion of monoamine neurotransmitters causes an upregulation of postsynaptic neurotransmitters (Wagner & Ambrosini, 2001). Thus most of the newer-generation antidepressants aim to increase the levels of monoamines, norepinephrine, serotonin, or dopamine (Wagner & Ambrosini, 2001). A wide variety of antidepressants exist, although most recent controlled trials in typically developing children and adolescents have focused on the SSRIs and to a lesser degree on the TCAs.

The TCAs have continually failed to show a statistically significant superiority to placebo in children and adolescents (Puig-Antich et al., 1987; Wagner & Ambrosini, 2001), and in our sample had fallen out of use in the population with AS. In a meta-analysis of the pharmacotherapy of childhood depression, Wagner and Ambrosini (2001) found that, despite methodological differences across studies, the use of TCAs in the treatment of depression in children and adolescents produced negative findings. Because of the ineffectiveness of TCAs and their prevalent side effects, SSRIs have become first-line treatment for children and adolescents (Hazell, O'Connell, Heathcote, Robertson, & Henry, 1995). In a large multisite trial of 219 depressed youth (ages 8–17), Emslie, Mayes, and Hughes (2000) found fluoxetine, an SSRI, to be superior to placebo. By the completion of the study, subjects treated with fluoxetine had significantly better Clinical Global Impressions (CGI) scores and were more likely than subjects randomized to the placebo group to meet recovery criteria. A similar study of 275 adolescents (ages 12–18) with major depressive disorder compared paroxetine and imipramine to placebo (Wagner et al., 1998). Results showed that 63% of adolescents randomized to paroxetine were considered responders. Imipramine (with 50% responding) did not differ significantly from placebo (46%).

For the most part, the medications used for the treatment of depression in typically developing children are also used for children with autism. The SSRIs are the most widely used class of antidepressant in the typical population. There are several reasons that the SSRIs may have a particular role for the treatment of depression in ASD. Serotonin dysfunction has been widely documented in ASD (Cook & Leventhal, 1996; Cook et al., 1997), and abnormal levels of serotonin have been identified in individuals with ASD (Cook & Leventhal, 1996). Due to these findings, it has been hypothesized that the medications altering serotonin function might also alter depressive symptoms in youth with autism (Posey, Erickson, et al., 2006). SSRIs have also been successful in the treatment of behaviors associated with OCD, many of which are also common symptoms of ASD (Posey, Erickson, et al., 2006). Two agents in particular, fluvoxamine and fluoxetine, have been tested in children with ASD in a placebo-controlled study. Mixed results have been found for both agents, although they have proven effective in the areas of mood disturbance and repetitive phenomena (Posey, Erickson, Stigler, & McDougle, 2006). The SSRIs have been the most widely used in the treatment of depression in AS but with additional caution, as children and adolescents with AS may be particularly susceptible to side effects (Tantam, 2000).

In addition to unipolar depression, symptoms of affective instability, including irritability and lability, are a frequent trigger for clinical intervention in the population with ASD (Arnold et al., 2003). The diagnosis of bipolar disorder is often made when these behaviors are present. However, as with attention problems, determining whether the symptoms represent some core ASD feature, or a true comorbidity, is both challenging and vital to treatment. A variety of other behaviors may also be associated with irritability and labile moods in the population with ASDs, including aggression, elevated mood, and psychomotor agitation (Towbin, Pradell, Gorrindo, Pine, & Leibenluft, 2005). Interestingly, among the population with a primary diagnosis of mood disorder, rates of ASD behavior are much more common (Towbin et al., 2005). In a sample made up of 19 children with AS and 40 children with HFA, Kim et al. (2000) found higher rates of externalizing mood symptoms when the groups were combined and compared to the typical population, but similar rates when the groups were compared to each other. In a sample comprised of 67 adults with AS and 55 adults with other high-functioning ASD, Hofvander found that 8% had been diagnosed with bipolar disorder (Hofvander et al., 2009). Neither study reported the rates in the AS population alone, however.

Two main classes of drugs, the mood stabilizers and the antipsychotics, are used to treat affective instability in the typical population. The antipsychotics, or neuroleptics, are a class of drugs that blocks dopamine receptors, leading to various effects, including the reduction of psychosis and mood stabilization. The first generation of antipsychotics (e.g., haloperidol and chlorpromazine) were not used in the sample we examined, representing a significant shift from the use patterns reported in the first edition of this chapter. The second-generation antipsychotics (or atypicals, e.g., risperidone and aripiprazole), distinguished from the first generation, in part, by their effects on serotonin, were used in 13% of our sample. It is unlikely, however, that mood instability, including aggression, was the primary target in all of these cases.

Both classes of antipsychotics have been studied in ASD. In autism, haloperidol has been the most extensively studied of the first generation, and showed some promise for improving an array of behaviors, including lability and anger (Anderson et al., 1989). Unfortunately, extrapyramidal symptoms, particularly tardive and withdrawal dyskinesias, were found to be common side effects (Campbell et al., 1997). Haloperidol is thus only used in treatment-refractory situations. The other first-generation antipsychotics have not been studied as closely as haloperidol, also carry similar side effects, and are no longer commonly used. None of these drugs has been studied systematically in AS.

The second-generation antipsychotics have also shown some positive effects in ASD. As a class, they less commonly produce extrapyramidal symptoms, although most are still associated with adverse metabolic effects. Risperidone has been the most extensively studied of the second generation and has been approved for the treatment of disruptive behaviors in ASD. This approval was partly attributable to the RUPP study, a large, multisite trial that was conducted in three phases: an initial 8-week double-blind, placebo-controlled phase, followed by a 4-month open-label extension for the responders (and the opportunity for those randomized to placebo to get the active drug), and a placebo-controlled discontinuation (McCracken et al., 2002). The primary outcome was the Aberrant Behavior Checklist Irritability subscale along with a CGI scale. The trial found a significant reduction of disruptive behaviors, including aggression, with risperidone. Several other atypical antipsychotics, including olanzapine, have shown similar effects in a small double-blind, placebo-controlled trial (Hollander, Wasserman, et al., 2006).

The atypical antipsychotics have also been the subject of several studies in AS. In an open-label study of a group of children with AS or PDD-NOS, aripiprazole reduced severe irritability (Stigler et al., 2009). In another open-label study, olanzapine improved externalizing symptoms such as irritability and aggression, but also the so-called "negative symptoms" such as the affective flattening often associated with AS (Milin et al., 2006). Similarly, risperidone has also shown some promise as a treatment for negative symptoms (Rausch et al., 2005). Although negative symptoms can be associated with mood problems, particularly depression, they also may be more directly generated by the core social deficit in AS. Thus, these effects need to be explored carefully in order to determine whether they actually represent a shift in core sociability.

Very little research has been done on the use of mood stabilizers in ASD. There are several reasons to suggest that mood stabilizers may be worth further study. Firstly, most mood stabilizers are also anticonvulsants. Given the higher rates of epilepsy and mood instability in ASD, this class of drugs may be used to target several problems. The most well-studied mood stabilizer in ASD is valproate, which has been shown to address repetitive behaviors in a double-blind, placebo-controlled study (Hollander, Soorya, et al., 2006) and aggression, mood lability, and social relatedness in an open-label study (Hollander, Dolgoff-Kaspar, Cartwright, Rawitt, & Novotny, 2001). An open-label trial of lamotrigene showed similar effects in a group of children with seizure disorders and some ASD behaviors (Uvebrant & Bauziene, 1994), although these results were not sustained in a follow-up placebo-controlled trial in ASD (Belsito, Law, Kirk, Landa, & Zimmerman, 2001). Case reports describe the use of carbamazepine and lithium in ASD. A mood stabilizer was used in only one patient with AS from our sample, mirroring Hofvander's finding (Hofvander et al., 2009) that only 2% of a group with high-functioning ASD had ever been treated with these medications. The only evidence for the use of mood stabilizers in AS comes from case reports (Duggal, 2001; Frazier, Doyle, Chiu, & Coyle, 2002). However, given the positive effects of mood stabilizers described in ASD in general, they certainly deserve evaluation in AS.

REPETITIVE PATTERNS OF BEHAVIOR AND THOUGHT

One of the defining criteria of AS is "restricted, repetitive, and stereotyped patterns of behavior, interests, and activities" (American Psychiatric Association, 1994, p. 84), a constellation of behaviors that shares features with other psychiatric disorders, including Tourette syndrome (TS) and OCD.

TS, a childhood-onset neuropsychiatric disorder, is defined by the presence of vocal and motor tics and occurs at a higher rate in people with

ASD (Baron-Cohen, Scahill, Izaguirre, Hornsey, & Robertson, 1999; Kerbeshian & Burd, 1996; Realmuto & Main, 1982). Tics are defined as involuntary movements that are typically sudden, nonrhythmic, and nonchoreiform (Leckman et al., 1998; Swain, Scahill, Lombroso, King, & Leckman, 2007). A study of 447 children with ASD by Baron-Cohen et al. (1999) estimated that comorbid TS occurs in 6.5% of subjects with AS, whereas the international prevalence of TS is estimated to be 1% (Robertson, Eapen, & Cavanna, 2009). Hereditary associations have been implied through a variety of mechanisms, from co-associated deletion within the *NLGN4* gene (Lawson-Yuen, Saldivar, Sommer, & Picker, 2008) to increased expression of a lymphocyte antigen (Hollander et al., 1999). However, the stereotyped movements that define autism can be difficult to distinguish from tics, and may even share pathophysiology based in abnormalities in dopaminergic and glutamatergic systems (Graybiel, Canales, & Capper-Loup, 2000; King et al., 2001).

Although there are multiple studies linking ASD and TS, none addresses the specifics of treating TS in the context of an ASD. The first step in treatment is to educate the family about the waxing and waning nature of tics. Parents should keep detailed records of tic occurrences, both to aid in defining the temporal characteristics of the tics and to identify stressors that can worsen tics. A number of modalities is used to address tics, including pharmacological, procedural, and behavioral approaches. For a review of all treatments used for TS, Bloch (2008) or Swain et al. (2007) are recommended. Commonly used psychopharmacological treatment for tics includes dopamine receptor blockers (typical and atypical antipsychotics) as well as alpha-agonists (Swain et al., 2007). Haloperidol and pimozide remain the only FDA-approved medications for tic disorders (Silay & Jankovic, 2005). As in TS without ASD, the treatment of tics in ASD with medications depends on whether the movements impair academic and interpersonal functions.

OCD is defined by the presence of intrusive, recurrent thoughts or obsessions. OCD is also associated with compulsive behaviors often thematically linked to specific obsessions. To meet diagnostic criteria for OCD, the obsession or compulsion must take up a significant part of the person's day, interfering with adaptive function and undermining academic and social skills. It is unclear whether OCD is a true comorbidity of autism. Baron-Cohen (1989), for example, warned that repetitive behaviors in ASD are not necessarily an indication of OCD, raising the concern that the communication limitations of many children diagnosed with ASD may obscure whether compulsive behaviors are, in fact, rooted in obsessions. On the other hand, the obsessions and compulsions that occur with OCD are generally egodystonic, at odds with the idealized self-image a person may have. The circumscribed interests and rituals that accompany ASD, on the other hand, tend to be egosyntonic, in harmony with the subject's self-image.

McDougle et al. (1995) showed that subjects with ASD, many of whom had intellectual disability, were less likely to have thoughts in the aggressive, contamination, sexual, religious, symmetry, and somatic content categories compared to the OCD group (McDougle et al., 1995). Regarding behaviors, the patients with ASD were more likely to exhibit repetitive ordering, repetitive questioning, hoarding, touching, tapping or rubbing, and self-injurious behavior than patients with OCD. The OCD group showed more cleaning, checking, and counting behaviors. Ruta, Mugno, D'Arrigo, Vitiello, and Mazzone (2010) demonstrated that hoarding thoughts and behaviors as well as repeating and ordering behaviors occurred more frequently in AS, whereas contamination and aggressive obsessions and checking compulsions occurred more in OCD. Russell, Mataix-Cols, Anson, and Murphy (2005) compared obsessive and compulsive behaviors in adults with OCD and AS, finding somatic and repeating rituals more common in the OCD group. In this study, the OCD group also had higher symptom-severity ratings.

On the basis of the fact that collecting behaviors occur in typical development, particularly between ages 3 and 6 years, Jacob, Landeros-Weisenberger, and Leckman (2009) have proposed that these behaviors, sustained over time, may reflect developmental delay. Of note, children with ASD often collect unusual objects. A further argument for an OCD–ASD connection can be made on the basis that researchers have found that OCD occurs at higher frequencies among the relatives of people with ASD than in the typical population (Bolton, Pickles, Murphy, & Rutter, 1998; Micali, Chakrabarti, & Fombonne, 2004). Moreover, OCD is more common in parents of those children with ASD with high levels of repetitive behavior and stereotypies (Hollander, King, Delaney, Smith, & Silverman, 2003). Neurohormonal, neuroimaging, and genetics studies have been conducted to search for biological abnormalities common between OCD and ASD, with limited results (see Gross-Isseroff, Hermesh, & Weizman, 2001). Imaging studies have tended to demonstrate the differences between autism and OCD rather than the similarities. However, several regions of common dysfunction have been identified, specifically the cerebellum, cingulate gyri, and orbitofrontal cortex (Gross-Isseroff et al., 2001; Saxena, Brody, Schwartz, & Baxter, 1998). The genetic connection is supported by a genetic study linking treatment-resistant OCD with AS and ASD, but is by no means definitive (Ozaki et al., 2003). There were no studies at the time of publication on psychopharmacological treatments of OCD or repetitive behaviors in AS.

Although SSRIs have been effective for repetitive behavior in adults with ASD, the same has not been the case in pediatric populations (McDougle, Kresch, & Posey, 2000; McDougle et al., 1996; Posey, Erickson, et al., 2006). In an open-label study using sertraline for adults with ASD, those with AS showed less improvement than those with autistic disorder or PDD-NOS (McDougle et al., 1998). Two reviews of the use of SSRIs in ASD concluded that open-label and retrospective studies indicate some benefits, but that more randomized controlled trials are needed (Kolevzon, Mathewson, & Hollander, 2006; Posey, Erickson, et al., 2006). The STAART Psychopharmacology Network published a controlled trial of 149 children and adolescents with ASD randomized to placebo or citalopram (King et al., 2009). Results showed no significant reduction of repetitive behaviors on the Children's Yale–Brown Obsessive Compulsive Scales (modified for PDD) and on the CGI Improvement subscale.

There is some suggestion that children with ASD may be more likely to experience adverse effects to SSRIs, although one study of fluoxetine in children with autism showed no increase in adverse events in comparison to placebo (Hollander et al., 2005; McDougle et al., 1996). Other pharmacological interventions have fewer data. Divalproex sodium and its derivatives are the subjects of several case reports and a small study by Hollander, Dolgoff-Kaspar, et al. (2006) that included two subjects with AS. These studies indicate that divalproex sodium may be useful for the treatment of obsessive symptoms. Other studies and case reports have been done for the treatment of pediatric OCD, including the use of antipsychotics, but not specifically in an ASD population.

Several studies have demonstrated increased anxiety symptoms in people with AS and other ASD (Gillott, Furniss, & Walter, 2001; Hofvander et al., 2009; Kim et al., 2000; Kuusikko et al., 2008; Mattila et al., 2010; Russell et al., 2005; White, Oswald, Ollendick, & Scahill, 2009). Children with AS seem to experience more anxiety symptoms than children with autism or PDD-NOS (Weisbrot, Gadow, DeVincent, & Pomeroy, 2005). At least one study has found a positive correlation between IQ and social impairment and anxiety (Sukhodolsky et al., 2008). There are no psychopharmacological studies specifically targeting the treatment of anxiety in AS. There are several case reports of positive effects of SSRIs (Bhardwaj, Agarwal, & Sitholey, 2005; Ozbayrak, 1997) and aripiprazole (Staller, 2003). In a study of citalopram, six subjects with AS showed improvement on the CGI score for anxiety (Namerow, Thomas, Bostic, Prince, & Monuteaux, 2003). However, in this case, all subjects were simultaneously on other psychotropic medications. Most treatment studies for anxiety in AS populations focus on cognitive therapy (see Lang, Regester, Lauderdale, Ashbaugh, & Haring, 2010, for a review).

THOUGHT DISORDER

As described above, Wing (1981) found that psychosis can be associated with AS. Historically, this association led some researchers to argue that AS was at the intersection between schizophrenia and ASD (Wolff & McGuire, 1995). However, some data suggest no increase in the frequency of schizophrenia above that seen in the general population (Volkmar, Paul, et al., 2005; Ghaziuddin, 1992). More recently, Hofvander et al. (2009)

found that 15% of a sample of 67 adults with AS had been diagnosed with a psychotic disorder. In the first edition of this book Martin et al. (2000) raised the significant concern that the impulsive verbalization of thoughts might result in an erroneous presumption of a thought disorder and inappropriate attribution of schizophrenia. Even if a diagnosis of schizophrenia were not the end result, this "verbalization of thoughts" could take a variety of forms, including statements that sound paranoid, threatening, or delusional—factors that might trigger the use of antipsychotic agents. Furthermore, there is a phenomenological overlap between the negative symptoms of schizophrenia (affective flattening, social withdrawal) and the core features of AS. In a clinical setting it is easy to imagine a scenario in which antipsychotics are used to address schizophrenic-like behaviors in a subject with AS. However, it is not clear that antipsychotics treat either of these behaviors in the absence of a comorbid psychotic disorder, although there is some preliminary work suggesting that haloperidol (Anderson et al., 1989; Kolmen et al., 1995) and risperidone (Williams et al., 2006) improve sociability in subjects with ASD and that risperidone may alter the negative symptoms of AS (Rausch et al., 2005). It is unclear, however, whether these effects are mediated by a reduction in disruptive behaviors or represent an actual effect on the core social disability.

Although antipsychotics have not been studied in ASD for the treatment of psychosis, they have been fairly extensively studied for the treatment of aggressive behaviors (see mood section) and have FDA approval for this purpose. As in typical subjects, subjects with ASD are vulnerable to significant metabolic side effects. In the case of AS, it may be more difficult to modify dietary and exercise habits to offset these effects. At this point the only guidance that can be offered for the treatment of comorbid psychosis is to consider carefully whether what is being diagnosed as psychosis truly represents psychosis. With this caution in mind, we can only suggest proceeding conservatively and using guidelines drawn from the existing literature on psychosis in subjects without ASD.

SLEEP DISORDERS

The association between ASD and sleep abnormalities has been well established (Limoges, Mottron, Bolduc, Berthiaume, & Godbout, 2005) and may be related to abnormalities in serotonin (Horner, Sanford, Annis, Pack, & Morrison, 1997) and melatonin (Nir et al., 1995), both of which play an important role in sleep regulation. Sleep abnormalities have also been documented in AS, most frequently with sleep initiation (Allik, Larsson, & Smedje, 2006; Bruni et al., 2007), with the ultimate effect of advancing the phase of sleep–wake cycles. Some researchers have identified abnormal movements during sleep (Godbout, Bergeron, Limoges, Stip, & Mottron, 2000) in subjects with AS, although other groups have not found this and have argued for these sleep abnormalities as an "anxiety based phenomen[on]" (Tani et al., 2004; Tani et al., 2006).

A variety of pharmacological agents exists to treat sleep disorders in the typical population. One such agent that has received attention by autism researchers is the naturally occurring hormone melatonin, which plays a role in regulating the sleep–wake cycle. The use of melatonin as a pharmacological agent has been an area of focus because its naturally occurring counterpart has been shown to be abnormal in subjects with ASD (Melke et al., 2008; Nir et al., 1995). Melatonin has shown promise in the population with ASD. A randomized, placebo-controlled, double-blind crossover trial of melatonin for the treatment of sleep problems in 11 children with ASD found significant reductions in sleep latency and nighttime awakening and an increase in sleep duration (Garstang & Wallis, 2006). In an open clinical trial of 15 children between the ages of 6 and 17 years with AS, melatonin decreased sleep latency but did not change sleep duration. These changes were also associated with behavioral improvements (Paavonen, Nieminen-von Wendt, Vanhala, Aronen, & von Wendt, 2003). In both studies melatonin was well tolerated. Unfortunately, no trials of any other pharmacological agent used in the treatment of sleep disorders in AS exist.

SEIZURES

Seizures are more common in ASD than in the typical population. In a sample of 100 males with AS and an average age of 11 years old, Cederlund found that four also had a seizure disorder (Cederlund & Gillberg, 2004). Seizures are generally treated in AS as they would be in the typical population. There are, however, several factors that should be considered that may alter treatment. Many of the drugs used to treat seizure disorders are also used to treat mood lability or comorbid bipolar disorder. This should be factored in to minimize the number of pharmacological agents used. Seizure disorders may interfere with sleep, and conversely sleep disruptions can trigger seizures (Bazil, 2000). Given the sleep irregularities discussed in AS above, it is important to consider the role of sleep in any treatment of comorbid seizures.

FUTURE DIRECTIONS

Progress in the psychopharmacological treatment of ASD may be hampered by the fact that the diagnostic categories themselves are based on criteria generated by clinical impressions rather than biological markers. This may, in part, explain the heterogeneity of ASD and some of the variability in response to treatment. We are, however, at an exciting time in

autism research, where progress in a variety of fields is beginning to elucidate the anatomical and physiological substrates that underlie the complex phenomenology of ASD. Application of some of the recent advances in
neuroimaging and genetics to the psychopharmacology of ASD may allow
care providers to ultimately define the relationship between genes, brain
phenotype, and clinical presentation on an individual basis, making it possible to provide tailored, effective drug treatment.

REFERENCES

Adler, L. A., Spencer, T. J., Williams, D. W., Moore, R. J., & Michelson, D.
    (2008). Long-term, open-label safety and efficacy of atomoxetine in adults
    with ADHD: Final report of a 4-year study. *Journal of Attention Disorders,*
    12(3), 248–253.
Allik, H., Larsson, J. O., & Smedje, H. (2006). Sleep patterns of school-age chil-
    dren with Asperger syndrome or high-functioning autism. *Journal of Autism*
    and Developmental Disorders, 36(5), 585–595.
American Psychiatric Association. (1994). *Diagnostic and statistical manual of*
    mental disorders (4th ed.). Washington, DC: Author.
American Psychiatric Association. (2000). *Diagnostic and statistical manual of*
    mental disorders (4th ed., text rev.). Washington, DC: Author.
American Psychiatric Association. (2013). *Diagnostic and statistical manual of*
    mental disorders IV-TR. Arlington, VA: Author.
Andari, E., Duhamel, J. R., Zalla, T., Herbrecht, E., Leboyer, M., & Sirigu, A.
    (2010). Promoting social behavior with oxytocin in high-functioning autism
    spectrum disorders. *Proceedings of the National Academy of Sciences of the*
    United States of America, 107(9), 4389–4394.
Anderson, L. T., Campbell, M., Adams, P., Small, A. M., Perry, R., & Shell, J.
    (1989). The effects of haloperidol on discrimination learning and behavioral
    symptoms in autistic children. *Journal of Autism and Developmental Disor-*
    ders, 19(2), 227–239.
Arnold, L. E., Aman, M. G., Cook, A. M., Witwer, A. N., Hall, K. L., Thompson,
    S., et al. (2006). Atomoxetine for hyperactivity in autism spectrum disorders:
    Placebo-controlled crossover pilot trial. *Journal of the American Academy of*
    Child and Adolescent Psychiatry, 45(10), 1196–1205.
Arnold, L. E., Vitiello, B., McDougle, C., Scahill, L., Shah, B., Gonzalez, N. M.,
    et al. (2003). Parent-defined target symptoms respond to risperidone in RUPP
    autism study: Customer approach to clinical trials. *Journal of the American*
    Academy of Child and Adolescent Psychiatry, 42(12), 1443–1450.
Baron-Cohen, S. (1989). Do autistic children have obsessions and compulsions?
    British Journal Clinical Psychology, 28(Pt. 3), 193–200.
Baron-Cohen, S., Scahill, V. L., Izaguirre, J., Hornsey, H., & Robertson, M. M.
    (1999). The prevalence of Gilles de la Tourette syndrome in children and
    adolescents with autism: A large scale study. *Psychological Medicine, 29*(5),
    1151–1159.
Barrickman, L. L., Perry, P. J., Allen, A. J., Kuperman, S., Arndt, S. V., Herrmann,
    K. J., et al. (1995). Bupropion versus methylphenidate in the treatment of

attention-deficit hyperactivity disorder. *Journal of the American Academy of Child and Adolescent Psychiatry, 34*(5), 649–657.

Bazil, C. W. (2000). Sleep and epilepsy. *Current Opinion in Neurology, 13*(2), 171–175.

Bejerot, S., Nylander, L., & Lindstrom, E. (2001). Autistic traits in obsessive–compulsive disorder. *Nordic Journal of Psychiatry, 55*(3), 169–176.

Belsito, K. M., Law, P. A., Kirk, K. S., Landa, R. J., & Zimmerman, A. W. (2001). Lamotrigine therapy for autistic disorder: A randomized, double-blind, placebo-controlled trial. *Journal of Autism and Developmental Disorders, 31*(2), 175–181.

Bhardwaj, A., Agarwal, V., & Sitholey, P. (2005). Asperger's disorder with co-morbid separation anxiety disorder: A case report. *Journal of Autism and Developmental Disorders, 35*(1), 135–136.

Biederman, J., Melmed, R. D., Patel, A., McBurnett, K., Konow, J., Lyne, A., et al. (2008). A randomized, double-blind, placebo-controlled study of guanfacine extended release in children and adolescents with attention-deficit/hyperactivity disorder. *Pediatrics, 121*(1), e73–e84.

Biederman, J., & Spencer, T. J. (2000). Genetics of childhood disorders: XIX ADHD, Part 3: Is ADHD a noradrenergic disorder. AACAP, 39–10.

Bloch, M. H. (2008). Emerging treatments for Tourette's disorder. *Current Psychiatry Report, 10*(4), 323–330.

Bolton, P. F., Pickles, A., Murphy, M., & Rutter, M. (1998). Autism, affective and other psychiatric disorders: Patterns of familial aggregation. *Psychololgical Medicine, 28*(2), 385–395.

Borcherding, B. G., Keysor, C. S., Rapoport, J. L., Elia, J., & Amass, J. (1990). Motor/vocal tics and compulsive behaviors on stimulant drugs: Is there a common vulnerability? *Psychiatry Research, 33*(1), 83–94.

Bruni, O., Ferri, R., Vittori, E., Novelli, L., Vignati, M., Porfirio, M. C., et al. (2007). Sleep architecture and nREM alterations in children and adolescents with Asperger syndrome. *Sleep, 30*(11), 1577–1585.

Campbell, M., Armenteros, J. L., Malone, R. P., Adams, P. B., Eisenberg, Z. W., & Overall, J. E. (1997). Neuroleptic-related dyskinesias in autistic children: A prospective, longitudinal study. *Journal of the American Academy of Child and Adolescent Psychiatry, 36*(6), 835–843.

Campbell, M., Fish, B., David, R., Shapiro, T., Collins, P., & Koh, C. (1972). Response to triiodothyronine and dextroamphetamine: A study of preschool schizophrenic children. *Journal of Autism and Childhood Schizophrenia, 2*(4), 343–358.

Cath, D. C., Ran, N., Smit, J. H., van Balkom, A. J., & Comijs, H. C. (2008). Symptom overlap between autism spectrum disorder, generalized social anxiety disorder, and obsessive–compulsive disorder in adults: A preliminary case-controlled study. *Psychopathology, 41*(2), 101–110.

Cederlund, M., & Gillberg, C. (2004). One hundred males with Asperger syndrome: A clinical study of background and associated factors. *Developmental Medicine and Child Neurology, 46*(10), 652–660.

Conners, C. K., Casat, C. D., Gualtieri, C. T., Weller, E., Reader, M., Reiss, A., et al. (1996). Bupropion hydrochloride in attention deficit disorder with hyperactivity. *Journal of the American Academy of Child and Adolescent Psychiatry, 35*(10), 1314–1321.

Connor, D. F., Fletcher, K. E., & Swanson, J. M. (1999). A meta-analysis of clonidine for symptoms of attention-deficit hyperactivity disorder. *Journal of the American Academy of Child and Adolescent Psychiatry, 38*(12), 1551–1559.

Cook, E., Courchesne, R., Lord, C., Cox, N., Yan, S., Lincoln, A., et al. (1997). Evidence of linkage between the serotonin transporter and autistic disorder. *Molecular Psychiatry, 2*(3), 247–250.

Cook, E., & Leventhal, B. (1996). The serotonin system in autism. *Current Opinions in Pediatrics, 8*(4), 348–354.

Di Martino, A., Melis, G., Cianchetti, C., & Zuddas, A. (2004). Methylphenidate for pervasive developmental disorders: Safety and efficacy of acute single dose test and ongoing therapy: An open-pilot study. *Journal of Child and Adolescent Psychopharmacology, 14*(2), 207–218.

Duggal, H. S. (2001). Mood stabilizers in Asperger's syndrome. *Australian and New Zealand Journal of Psychiatry, 35*(3), 390–391.

Emslie, G. J., & Mayes, T. (2001). Mood disorders in children and adolescents: Psychopharmacological treatment. *Biological Psychiatry, 49*(12), 1082–1090.

Emslie, G. J., Mayes, T. L., & Hughes, C. W. (2000). Updates in the pharmacologic treatment of childhood depression. *Psychiatric Clinics of North America, 23*(4), 813–835.

Fankhauser, M. P., Karumanchi, V. C., German, M. L., Yates, A., & Karumanchi, S. D. (1992). A double-blind, placebo-controlled study of the efficacy of transdermal clonidine in autism. *Journal of Clinical Psychiatry, 53*(3), 77–82.

Frazier, J. A., Doyle, R., Chiu, S., & Coyle, J. T. (2002). Treating a child with Asperger's disorder and comorbid bipolar disorder. *American Journal of Psychiatry, 159*(1), 13–21.

Garstang, J., & Wallis, M. (2006). Randomized controlled trial of melatonin for children with autistic spectrum disorders and sleep problems. *Child: Care, Health and Development, 32*(5), 585–589.

Ghaziuddin, M., Ghaziuddin, N., & Greden, J. (2002). Depression in persons with autism: Implications for research and clinical care. *Journal of Autism and Developmental Disorders, 32*(4), 299–306.

Ghaziuddin, M., Weidmer-Mikhail, E., & Ghaziuddin, N. (1998). Comorbidity of Asperger syndrome: A preliminary report. *Journal of Intellectual Disability Research, 42*(Pt. 4), 279–283.

Gillberg, C. (1983). Perceptual, motor, and attentional deficits in Swedish primary school children: Some child psychiatric aspects. *Journal of Child Psychology and Psychiatry and Allied Disciplines, 24*(3), 377–403.

Gillott, A., Furniss, F., & Walter, A. (2001). Anxiety in high-functioning children with autism. *Autism, 5*(3), 277–286.

Godbout, R., Bergeron, C., Limoges, E., Stip, E., & Mottron, L. (2000). A laboratory study of sleep in Asperger's syndrome. *NeuroReport, 11*(1), 127–130.

Goodman, W. K., Price, L. H., Rasmussen, S. A., Mazure, C., Fleischmann, R. L., Hill, C. L., et al. (1989). The Yale–Brown Obsessive Compulsive Scale: I. Development, use, and reliability. *Archives of General Psychiatry, 46*(11), 1006–1011.

Gordon, C. T., State, R. C., Nelson, J. E., Hamburger, S. D., & Rapoport, J. L. (1993). A double-blind comparison of clomipramine, desipramine, and placebo in the treatment of autistic disorder. *Archives of General Psychiatry, 50*(6), 441–447.

Graybiel, A. M., Canales, J. J., & Capper-Loup, C. (2000). Levodopa-induced dyskinesias and dopamine-dependent stereotypies: A new hypothesis. *Trends in Neurosciences, 23*(10 Suppl.), S71–S77.

Greenhill, L. L., Biederman, J., Boellner, S. W., Rugino, T. A., Sangal, R. B., Earl, C. Q., et al. (2006). A randomized, double-blind, placebo-controlled study of modafinil film-coated tablets in children and adolescents with attention-deficit/hyperactivity disorder. *Journal of the American Academy of Child and Adolescent Psychiatry, 45*(5), 503–511.

Gross-Isseroff, R., Hermesh, H., & Weizman, A. (2001). Obsessive compulsive behaviour in autism: Towards an autistic–obsessive compulsive syndrome? *World Journal of Biological Psychiatry, 2*(4), 193–197.

Handen, B. L., Johnson, C. R., & Lubetsky, M. (2000). Efficacy of methylphenidate among children with autism and symptoms of attention-deficit hyperactivity disorder. *Journal of Autism and Developmental Disorders, 30*(3), 245–255.

Handen, B. L., Sahl, R., & Hardan, A. Y. (2008). Guanfacine in children with autism and/or intellectual disabilities. *Journal of Developmental and Behavioral Pediatrics, 29*(4), 303–308.

Hazell, P., O'Connell, D., Heathcote, D., Robertson, J., & Henry, D. (1995). Efficacy of tricyclic drugs in treating child and adolescent depression: A meta-analysis. *British Medical Journal, 310*(6984), 897–901.

Hofvander, B., Delorme, R., Chaste, P., Nyden, A., Wentz, E., Stahlberg, O., et al. (2009). Psychiatric and psychosocial problems in adults with normal-intelligence autism spectrum disorders. *BMC Psychiatry, 9*, 35.

Hollander, E., Bartz, J., Chaplin, W., Phillips, A., Sumner, J., Soorya, L., et al. (2007). Oxytocin increases retention of social cognition in autism. *Biological Psychiatry, 61*(4), 498–503.

Hollander, E., DelGiudice-Asch, G., Simon, L., Schmeidler, J., Cartwright, C., DeCaria, C. M., et al. (1999). B lymphocyte antigen D8/17 and repetitive behaviors in autism. *American Journal of Psychiatry, 156*(2), 317–320.

Hollander, E., Dolgoff-Kaspar, R., Cartwright, C., Rawitt, R., & Novotny, S. (2001). An open trial of divalproex sodium in autism spectrum disorders. *Journal of Clinical Psychiatry, 62*(7), 530–534.

Hollander, E., King, A., Delaney, K., Smith, C. J., & Silverman, J. M. (2003). Obsessive–compulsive behaviors in parents of multiplex autism families. *Psychiatry Research, 117*(1), 11–16.

Hollander, E., Phillips, A., Chaplin, W., Zagursky, K., Novotny, S., Wasserman, S., et al. (2005). A placebo controlled crossover trial of liquid fluoxetine on repetitive behaviors in childhood and adolescent autism. *Neuropsychopharmacology, 30*(3), 582–589.

Hollander, E., Soorya, L., Wasserman, S., Esposito, K., Chaplin, W., & Anagnostou, E. (2006). Divalproex sodium vs. placebo in the treatment of repetitive behaviours in autism spectrum disorder. *International Journal of Neuropsychopharmacology, 9*(2), 209–213.

Hollander, E., Wasserman, S., Swanson, E. N., Chaplin, W., Schapiro, M. L., Zagursky, K., et al. (2006). A double-blind placebo-controlled pilot study of olanzapine in childhood/adolescent pervasive developmental disorder. *Journal of Child and Adolescent Psychopharmacology, 16*(5), 541–548.

Horner, R. L., Sanford, L. D., Annis, D., Pack, A. I., & Morrison, A. R. (1997).

Serotonin at the laterodorsal tegmental nucleus suppresses rapid-eye-move-ment sleep in freely behaving rats. *Journal of Neuroscience, 17*(19), 7541–7552.

Jacob, S., Landeros-Weisenberger, A., & Leckman, J. F. (2009). Autism spectrum and obsessive–compulsive disorders: OC behaviors, phenotypes, and genetics. *Autism Research, 2*(6), 293–311.

Jahromi, L. B., Kasari, C. L., McCracken, J. T., Lee, L. S., Aman, M. G., McDou-gle, C. J., et al. (2009). Positive effects of methylphenidate on social communi-cation and self-regulation in children with pervasive developmental disorders and hyperactivity. *Journal of Autism and Developmental Disorders, 39*(3), 395–404.

Jaselskis, C. A., Cook, E. H., Jr., Fletcher, K. E., & Leventhal, B. L. (1992). Cloni-dine treatment of hyperactive and impulsive children with autistic disorder. *Journal of Clinical Psychopharmacology, 12*(5), 322–327.

Kahbazi, M., Ghoreishi, A., Rahiminejad, F., Mohammadi, M. R., Kamalipour, A., & Akhondzadeh, S. (2009). A randomized, double-blind, and placebo-controlled trial of modafinil in children and adolescents with attention deficit and hyperactivity disorder. *Psychiatry Research, 168*(3), 234–237.

Kavale, K. (1982). The efficacy of stimulant drug treatment for hyperactivity: A meta-analysis. *Journal of Learning Disabilities, 15*(5), 280–289.

Kerbeshian, J., & Burd, L. (1996). Case study: Comorbidity among Tourette's syn-drome, autistic disorder, and bipolar disorder. *Journal of the American Acad-emy of Child Adolescent Psychiatry, 35*(5), 681–685.

Kim, J. A., Szatmari, P., Bryson, S. E., Streiner, D. L., & Wilson, F. J. (2000). The prevalence of anxiety and mood problems among children with autism and Asperger syndrome. *Autism, 4*(2), 117–132.

King, B. H., Hollander, E., Sikich, L., McCracken, J. T., Scahill, L., Bregman, J. D., et al. (2009). Lack of efficacy of citalopram in children with autism spec-trum disorders and high levels of repetitive behavior: Citalopram ineffective in children with autism. *Archives of General Psychiatry, 66*(6), 583–590.

King, B. H., Wright, D. M., Handen, B. L., Sikich, L., Zimmerman, A. W., McMahon, W., et al. (2001). Double-blind, placebo-controlled study of aman-tadine hydrochloride in the treatment of children with autistic disorder. *Journal of the American Academy of Child and Adolescent Psychiatry, 40*(6), 658–665.

Klin, A., Volkmar, F. R., & Sparrow, S. S. (2000). *Asperger syndrome.* New York: Guilford Press.

Kolevzon, A., Mathewson, K. A., & Hollander, E. (2006). Selective serotonin reup-take inhibitors in autism: A review of efficacy and tolerability. *Journal of Clinical Psychiatry, 67*(3), 407–414.

Kolmen, B. K., Feldman, H. M., Handen, B. L., & Janosky, J. E. (1995). Naltrex-one in young autistic children: A double-blind, placebo-controlled crossover study. *Journal of the American Academy of Child and Adolescent Psychiatry, 34*(2), 223–231.

Kolmen, B. K., Feldman, H. M., Handen, B. L., & Janosky, J. E. (1997). Naltrex-one in young autistic children: Replication study and learning measures. *Jour-nal of the American Academy of Child and Adolescent Psychiatry, 36*(11), 1570–1578.

Kuusikko, S., Pollock-Wurman, R., Jussila, K., Carter, A. S., Mattila, M. L., Ebeling, H., et al. (2008). Social anxiety in high-functioning children and adolescents with autism and Asperger syndrome. *Journal of Autism and Developmental Disorders, 38*(9), 1697–1709.

Lainhart, J. (1999). Psychiatric problems in individuals with autism, their parents and siblings. *International Review of Psychiatry, 11*(4), 278–298.

Lang, R., Regester, A., Lauderdale, S., Ashbaugh, K., & Haring, A. (2010). Treatment of anxiety in autism spectrum disorders using cognitive behaviour therapy: A systematic review. *Developmental Neurorehabilitation, 13*(1), 53–63.

Lawson-Yuen, A., Saldivar, J. S., Sommer, S., & Picker, J. (2008). Familial deletion within *NLGN4* associated with autism and Tourette syndrome. *European Journal of Human Genetics, 16*(5), 614–618.

Leckman, J. F., Grice, D. E., Boardman, J., Zhang, H., Vitale, A., Bondi, C., et al. (1997). Symptoms of obsessive–compulsive disorder. *American Journal of Psychiatry, 154*(7), 911–917.

Leckman, J. F., Zhang, H., Vitale, A., Lahnin, F., Lynch, K., Bondi, C., et al. (1998). Course of tic severity in Tourette syndrome: The first two decades. *Pediatrics, 102*(1, Pt. 1), 14–19.

Limoges, E., Mottron, L., Bolduc, C., Berthiaume, C., & Godbout, R. (2005). Atypical sleep architecture and the autism phenotype. *Brain, 128*(Pt. 5), 1049–1061.

Martin, A., Patzer, D. K., & Volkmar, F. R. (2000) Psychopharmacological treatment. In A. Klin, F. R. Volkmar, & S. A. Sparrow (Eds.), *Asperger syndrome* (pp. 210–228). New York: Guilford Press.

Martin, A., Scahill, L., Klin, A., & Volkmar, F. R. (1999). Higher-functioning pervasive developmental disorders: Rates and patterns of psychotropic drug use. *Journal of the American Academy of Child and Adolescent Psychiatry, 38*(9), 923–931.

Mataix-Cols, D., Rauch, S. L., Manzo, P. A., Jenike, M. A., & Baer, L. (1999). Use of factor-analyzed symptom dimensions to predict outcome with serotonin reuptake inhibitors and placebo in the treatment of obsessive–compulsive disorder. *American Journal of Psychiatry, 156*(9), 1409–1416.

Mattila, M. L., Hurtig, T., Haapsamo, H., Jussila, K., Kuusikko-Gauffin, S., Kielinen, M., et al. (2010). Comorbid psychiatric disorders associated with Asperger syndrome/high-functioning autism: A community- and clinic-based study. *Journal of Autism and Developmental Disorders, 40*(9), 1080–1093.

McCracken, J. T., McGough, J., Shah, B., Cronin, P., Hong, D., Aman, M. G., et al. (2002). Risperidone in children with autism and serious behavioral problems. *New England Journal of Medicine, 347*(5), 314–321.

McDougle, C. J. (2004). Methylphenidate an effective treatment for ADHD? *Journal of Autism and Developmental Disorders, 34*(5), 593–594.

McDougle, C. J., Brodkin, E. S., Naylor, S. T., Carlson, D. C., Cohen, D. J., & Price, L. H. (1998). Sertraline in adults with pervasive developmental disorders: A prospective open-label investigation. *Journal of Clinical Psychopharmacology, 18*(1), 62–66.

McDougle, C. J., Kresch, L. E., Goodman, W. K., Naylor, S. T., Volkmar, F. R., Cohen, D. J., et al. (1995). A case-controlled study of repetitive thoughts and behavior in adults with autistic disorder and obsessive–compulsive disorder. *American Journal of Psychiatry, 152*(5), 772–777.

McDougle, C. J., Kresch, L. E., & Posey, D. J. (2000). Repetitive thoughts and behavior in pervasive developmental disorders: Treatment with serotonin reuptake inhibitors. *Journal of Autism and Developmental Disord, 30*(5), 427–435.

McDougle, C. J., Naylor, S. T., Cohen, D. J., Volkmar, F. R., Heninger, G. R., & Price, L. H. (1996). A double-blind, placebo-controlled study of fluvoxamine in adults with autistic disorder. *Archives of General Psychiatry, 53*(11), 1001–1008.

Melke, J., Goubran Botros, H., Chaste, P., Betancur, C., Nygren, G., Anckarsater, H., et al. (2008). Abnormal melatonin synthesis in autism spectrum disorders. *Molecular Psychiatry, 13*(1), 90–98.

Micali, N., Chakrabarti, S., & Fombonne, E. (2004). The broad autism phenotype: Findings from an epidemiological survey. *Autism, 8*(1), 21–37.

Michelson, D., Faries, D., Wernicke, J., Kelsey, D., Kendrick, K., Sallee, F. R., et al. (2001). Atomoxetine in the treatment of children and adolescents with attention-deficit/hyperactivity disorder: A randomized, placebo-controlled, dose–response study. *Pediatrics, 108*(5), E83.

Milin, R., Simeon, J. G., Batth, S., Thatte, S., Dare, G. J., & Walker, S. (2006). An open trial of olanzapine in children and adolescents with Asperger disorder. *Journal of Clinical Psychopharmacology, 26*(1), 90–92.

Molina, B. S., Hinshaw, S. P., Swanson, J. M., Arnold, L. E., Vitiello, B., Jensen, P. S., et al. (2009). The MTA at 8 years: Prospective follow-up of children treated for combined-type ADHD in a multisite study. *Journal of the American Academy of Child and Adolescent Psychiatry, 48*(5), 484–500.

MTA Cooperative Group. (1999). A 14-month randomized clinical trial of treatment strategies for attention-deficit/hyperactivity disorder. *Archives of General Psychiatry, 56*(12), 1073–1086.

Namerow, L. B., Thomas, P., Bostic, J. Q., Prince, J., & Monuteaux, M. C. (2003). Use of citalopram in pervasive developmental disorders. *Journal of Developmental and Behavioral Pediatrics, 24*(2), 104–108.

Nilsson, B. M., & Ekselius, L. (2009). Acute and maintenance electroconvulsive therapy for treatment of severely disabling obsessive–compulsive symptoms in a patient with Asperger syndrome. *Journal of ECT, 25*(3), 205–207.

Nir, I., Meir, D., Zilber, N., Knobler, H., Hadjez, J., & Lerner, Y. (1995). Brief report: Circadian melatonin, thyroid-stimulating hormone, prolactin, and cortisol levels in serum of young adults with autism. *Journal of Autism and Developmental Disorders, 25*(6), 641–654.

Ozaki, N., Goldman, D., Kaye, W. H., Plotnicov, K., Greenberg, B. D., Lappalainen, J., et al. (2003). Serotonin transporter missense mutation associated with a complex neuropsychiatric phenotype. *Molecular Psychiatry, 8*(11), 933–936.

Ozbayrak, K. R. (1997). Sertraline in PDD. *Journal of the American Academy of Child Adolescent Psychiatry, 36*(1), 7–8.

Paavonen, E. J., Nieminen-von Wendt, T., Vanhala, R., Aronen, E. T., & von Wendt, L. (2003). Effectiveness of melatonin in the treatment of sleep disturbances in children with Asperger disorder. *Journal of Child and Adolescent Psychopharmacology, 13*(1), 83–95.

Palumbo, D. R., Sallee, F. R., Pelham, W. E., Jr., Bukstein, O. G., Daviss, W. B., & McDermott, M. P. (2008). Clonidine for attention-deficit/hyperactivity disorder: I. Efficacy and tolerability outcomes. *Journal of the American Academy of Child and Adolescent Psychiatry, 47*(2), 180–188.

Posey, D. J., Aman, M. G., McCracken, J. T., Scahill, L., Tierney, E., Arnold, L. E., et al. (2007). Positive effects of methylphenidate on inattention and hyperactivity in pervasive developmental disorders: An analysis of secondary measures. *Biological Psychiatry, 61*(4), 538–544.

Posey, D., Erickson, C., Stigler, K., & McDougle, C. (2006). The use of selective serotonin reuptake inhibitors in autism and related disorders. *Journal of Child and Adolescent Psychopharmacology, 16*(1–2), 181–186.

Posey, D. J., Puntney, J. I., Sasher, T. M., Kem, D. L., & McDougle, C. J. (2004). Guanfacine treatment of hyperactivity and inattention in pervasive developmental disorders: A retrospective analysis of 80 cases. *Journal of Child and Adolescent Psychopharmacology, 14*(2), 233–241.

Posey, D. J., Wiegand, R. E., Wilkerson, J., Maynard, M., Stigler, K. A., & McDougle, C. J. (2006). Open-label atomoxetine for attention-deficit/hyperactivity disorder symptoms associated with high-functioning pervasive developmental disorders. *Journal of Child and Adolescent Psychopharmacology, 16*(5), 599–610.

Puig-Antich, J., Perel, J., Lupatkin, W., Chambers, W., Tabrizi, M., King, J., et al. (1987). Imipramine in prepubertal major depressive disorders. *Archives of General Psychiatry, 44*(1), 81–89.

Quintana, H., Birmaher, B., Stedge, D., Lennon, S., Freed, J., Bridge, J., et al. (1995). Use of methylphenidate in the treatment of children with autistic disorder. *Journal of Autism and Developmental Disorders, 25*(3), 283–294.

Rausch, J. L., Sirota, E. L., Londino, D. L., Johnson, M. E., Carr, B. M., Bhatia, R., et al. (2005). Open-label risperidone for Asperger's disorder: Negative symptom spectrum response. *Journal of Clinical Psychiatry, 66*(12), 1592–1597.

Realmuto, G. M., & Main, B. (1982). Coincidence of Tourette's disorder and infantile autism. *Journal of Autism and Developmental Disorders, 12*(4), 367–372.

Reiersen, A. M., & Todd, R. D. (2008). Co-occurrence of ADHD and autism spectrum disorders: Phenomenology and treatment. *Expert Review of Neurotherapeutics, 8*(4), 657–669.

Remington, G., Sloman, L., Konstantareas, M., Parker, K., & Gow, R. (2001). Clomipramine versus haloperidol in the treatment of autistic disorder: A double-blind, placebo-controlled, crossover study. *Journal of Clinical Psychopharmacology, 21*(4), 440–444.

Research Units on Pediatric Psychopharmacology Autism Network. (2005a). Randomized, controlled, crossover trial of methylphenidate in pervasive developmental disorders with hyperactivity. *Archives of General Psychiatry, 62*(11), 1266–1274.

Research Units on Pediatric Psychopharmacology Autism Network. (2005b). Risperidone treatment of autistic disorder: Longer-term benefits and blinded discontinuation after 6 months. *American Journal of Psychiatry, 162*(7), 1361–1369.

Robertson, M. M., Eapen, V., & Cavanna, A. E. (2009). The international prevalence, epidemiology, and clinical phenomenology of Tourette syndrome: A cross-cultural perspective. *Journal of Psychosomatic Research, 67*(6), 475–483.

Roffman, J. L., & Raskin, L. A. (1997). Stereotyped behavior: Effects of d-amphetamine and methylphenidate in the young rat. *Pharmacology, Biochemistry, and Behavior, 58*(4), 1095–1102.

Roy, M., Dillo, W., Bessling, S., Emrich, H. M., & Ohlmeier, M. D. (2009). Effective methylphenidate treatment of an adult Asperger's syndrome and a comorbid ADHD: A clinical investigation with fMRI. *Journal of Attention Disorders, 12*(4), 381–385.

Russell, A. J., Mataix-Cols, D., Anson, M., & Murphy, D. G. (2005). Obsessions and compulsions in Asperger syndrome and high-functioning autism. *Britsh Journal of Psychiatry, 186*, 525–528.

Ruta, L., Mugno, D., D'Arrigo, V. G., Vitiello, B., & Mazzone, L. (2010). Obsessive–compulsive traits in children and adolescents with Asperger syndrome. *European Child and Adolescent Psychiatry, 19*(1), 17–24.

Sallee, F. R., McGough, J., Wigal, T., Donahue, J., Lyne, A., Biederman, J., et al. (2009). Guanfacine extended release in children and adolescents with attention-deficit/hyperactivity disorder: A placebo-controlled trial. *Journal of the American Academy of Child and Adolescent Psychiatry, 48*(2), 155–165.

Saxena, S., Brody, A. L., Schwartz, J. M., & Baxter, L. R. (1998). Neuroimaging and frontal–subcortical circuitry in obsessive–compulsive disorder. *British Journal of Psychiatry*, (Suppl. 35), 26–37.

Scahill, L., Aman, M. G., McDougle, C. J., McCracken, J. T., Tierney, E., Dziura, J., et al. (2006). A prospective open trial of guanfacine in children with pervasive developmental disorders. *Journal of Child and Adolescent Psychopharmacology, 16*(5), 589–598.

Scahill, L., Chappell, P. B., Kim, Y. S., Schultz, R. T., Katsovich, L., Shepherd, E., et al. (2001). A placebo-controlled study of guanfacine in the treatment of children with tic disorders and attention deficit hyperactivity disorder. *American Journal of Psychiatry, 158*(7), 1067–1074.

Schatz, A. M., Weimer, A. K., & Trauner, D. A. (2002). Brief report: Attention differences in Asperger syndrome. *Journal of Autism and Developmental Disorders, 32*(4), 333–336.

Shaffer, D., Fisher, P., Dulcan, M., Davies, M., Piacentini, J., Schwab-Stone, M., et al. (1996). The NIMH Diagnostic Interview Schedule for Children—Version 2.3 (DISC-2.3): Description, acceptability, prevalence rates, and performance in the MECA study. *Journal of the American Academy of Child and Adolescent Psychiatry, 35*(7), 865–877.

Silay, Y. S., & Jankovic, J. (2005). Emerging drugs in Tourette syndrome. *Expert Opinion on Emerging Drugs, 10*(2), 365–80.

Solanto, M. V. (1998). Neuropsychopharmacological mechanisms of stimulant drug action in attention-deficit hyperactivity disorder: A review and integration. *Behavioural Brain Research, 94*(1), 127–152.

Spencer, T., & Biederman, J. (2002). Non-stimulant treatment for attention-deficit/hyperactivity disorder. *Journal of Attention Disorders, 6*(Suppl. 1), S109–S119.

Staller, J. A. (2003). Aripiprazole in an adult with Asperger disorder. *Annals of Pharmacotherapy, 37*(11), 1628–1631.

Stewart, M., Barnard, L., Pearson, J., Hasan, R., & O'Brien, G. (2006). Presentation of depression in autism and Asperger syndrome: A review. *Autism, 10*(1), 103–116.

Stigler, K. A., Diener, J. T., Kohn, A. E., Li, L., Erickson, C. A., Posey, D. J., et al. (2009). Aripiprazole in pervasive developmental disorder not otherwise specified and Asperger's disorder: A 14–week, prospective, open-label study. *Journal of Child and Adolescent Psychopharmacology, 19*(3), 265–274.

Sturm, H., Fernell, E., & Gillberg, C. (2004). Autism spectrum disorders in children with normal intellectual levels: Associated impairments and subgroups. *Developmental Medicine and Child Neurology, 46*(7), 444–447.

Sukhodolsky, D. G., Scahill, L., Gadow, K. D., Arnold, L. E., Aman, M. G., McDougle, C. J., et al. (2008). Parent-rated anxiety symptoms in children with pervasive developmental disorders: Frequency and association with core autism symptoms and cognitive functioning. *Journal of Abnormal Child Psychology, 36*(1), 117–128.

Swain, J. E., Scahill, L., Lombroso, P. J., King, R. A., & Leckman, J. F. (2007). Tourette syndrome and tic disorders: A decade of progress. *Journal of the American Academy of Child and Adolescent Psychiatry, 46*(8), 947–968.

Swanson, J. M., Elliott, G. R., Greenhill, L. L., Wigal, T., Arnold, L. E., Vitiello, B., et al. (2007). Effects of stimulant medication on growth rates across 3 years in the MTA follow-up. *Journal of the American Academy of Child and Adolescent Psychiatry, 46*(8), 1015–1027.

Tani, P., Lindberg, N., Appelberg, B., Nieminen-von Wendt, T., von Wendt, L., & Porkka-Heiskanen, T. (2006). Childhood inattention and hyperactivity symptoms self-reported by adults with Asperger syndrome. *Psychopathology, 39*(1), 49–54.

Tani, P., Lindberg, N., Nieminen-von Wendt, T., von Wendt, L., Virkkala, J., Appelberg, B., et al. (2004). Sleep in young adults with Asperger syndrome. *Neuropsychobiology, 50*(2), 147–152.

Tani, P., Tuisku, K., Lindberg, N., Virkkala, J., Nieminen-von Wendt, T., von Wendt, L., et al. (2006). Is Asperger syndrome associated with abnormal nocturnal motor phenomena? *Psychiatry and Clinical Neurosciences, 60*(4), 527–528.

Tantam, D. (2000). Psychological disorder in adolescents and adults with Asperger syndrome. *Autism, 4*(1), 47–62.

Towbin, K. E. (2003). Strategies for pharmacologic treatment of high functioning autism and Asperger syndrome. *Child and Adolescent Psychiatric Clinics of North America, 12*(1), 23–45.

Towbin, K. E., Pradella, A., Gorrindo, T., Pine, D. S., & Leibenluft, E. (2005). Autism spectrum traits in children with mood and anxiety disorders. *Journal of Child and Adolescent Psychopharmacology, 15*(3), 452–464.

Troost P. W., Steenhuis, M. P., Tuynman-Qua, H. G., Kalverdijk, L. J., Buitelaar, J. K., Minderaa, R. B., et al. (2006). Atomoxetine for attention-deficit/hyperactivity disorder symptoms in children with pervasive developmental disorders: a pilot study. *Journal of Child and Adolescent Psychopharmacology, 16*(5), 611–619.

Uvebrant, P., & Bauziene, R. (1994). Intractable epilepsy in children: The efficacy of lamotrigine treatment, including non-seizure-related benefits. *Neuropediatrics, 25*(6), 284–289.

Volkmar, F. R., Paul, R., Klin, A., & Cohen, D. (2005). *Handbook of autism and pervasive developmental disorders* (3rd ed.). Hoboken, NJ: Wiley.

Wagner, K., & Ambrosini, P. (2001). Childhood depression: pharmacological therapy/treatment (pharmacotherapy of childhood depression). *Journal of Clinical Child Psychology, 30*(1), 88–97.

Wagner, K. D., Birmaher, B., Carlson, G., et al. (1998). Safety of paroxetine and imipramine in the treatment of adolescent depression. Paper presented at the

New Clinical Drug Evaluation Unit Program (NCDEU) 38th annual meeting, Boca Raton, FL.

Weisbrot, D. M., Gadow, K. D., DeVincent, C. J., & Pomeroy, J. (2005). The presentation of anxiety in children with pervasive developmental disorders. *Journal of Child and Adolescent Psychopharmacology, 15*(3), 477–496.

White, S. W., Oswald, D., Ollendick, T., & Scahill, L. (2009). Anxiety in children and adolescents with autism spectrum disorders. *Clinical Psychology Review, 29*(3), 216–229.

Williams, S. K., Scahill, L., Vitiello, B., Aman, M. G., Arnold, L. E., McDougle, C. J., et al. (2006). Risperidone and adaptive behavior in children with autism. *Journal of the American Academy of Child and Adolescent Psychiatry, 45*(4), 431–439.

Wing, L. (1981). Asperger's syndrome: A clinical account. *Psychological Medicine, 11*(1), 115–129.

Wolff, S., & McGuire, R. J. (1995). Schizoid personality in girls: A follow-up study—what are the links with Asperger's syndrome? *Journal of Child Psychology and Psychiatry and Allied Disciplines, 36*(5), 793–817.

CHAPTER 10

Asperger Syndrome in Adolescence and Adulthood

Michael D. Powers
James W. Loomis

The continuing challenges facing individuals with Asperger syndrome (AS) as they negotiate the shift from later adolescence to adulthood are in many ways a continuation of those hurdles encountered previously, but they also represent a new set of considerations not likely experienced earlier in their lives. Sadly, whereas the literature on younger persons with this disability has expanded exponentially over the past 30 years, research on adults (and especially those in middle age and beyond) with this disability has not. In this chapter we outline issues of importance for those with AS who have reached later adolescence and are entering adulthood and those who are already adults. We recognize that this transitional process is not fixed; indeed, the process is more likely to be elongated as compared to those developing typically who are launched by their families into adulthood. However, as a necessary developmental task we appreciate that those with AS must eventually become more fully integrated into a productive, adult community—vocationally, socially, and with respect to independent living and often will require special supports to do so.

Earlier in this book, the various diagnostic and clinical characteristics and commensurate needs of younger individuals with AS have been thoroughly discussed. Therefore, we focus more specifically on the nature of these presentations in later adolescence and adulthood, and the needs of individuals as they confront a range of issues, including transitions, employment, continuing social-developmental tasks, independent living, maintaining family support while developing greater independence, and considerations for individual and group therapy as the need presents. We conclude with a discussion of the need for developing coordinated systems of care through adulthood and a discussion of future needs and directions for research. In our discussions we provide a heuristic for thinking about AS in adulthood that diverges from the sometimes too-frequent misunderstanding that those with this disability in adulthood are simply grown-up children. Indeed, whereas adult development provides a series of reasonably consistent developmental challenges for those who are typical, the very nature of the developmental *discontinuity* of AS in adulthood requires a thoughtful discussion of the points of parallel and divergent opportunity and need. As such, we describe needs, evidence-based solutions (where they exist), and opportunities for ongoing investigation with the stated understanding that we researchers and clinicians working with adults with AS have much to accomplish before we can articulate a clear set of practice parameters that will enable the full and comprehensive integration of those with this disability into society.

THE NATURE AND NEEDS OF OLDER ADOLESCENTS AND ADULTS WITH ASPERGER SYNDROME

By later adolescence many families have an understanding of the academic assets and challenges faced by their children with AS. Decisions about postsecondary opportunities may already have been explored, or vocational opportunities may already be in process. As we consider the overarching needs of this group beyond academics or the technical skills needed for gainful employment, generalization and expansion of a wide range of skills mastered in more circumscribed settings (e.g., the classroom) to the broader, more natural environments of the community and workplace take prominence. To that end, several domains of need should be considered.

Enhancing Social Functioning with Peers

The congregate nature of school provides an established potential peer group for students. Although we recognize that these peers may or may not always facilitate friendships, nonetheless there are increased opportunities simply by the presence of these peers and the mandates for skill teaching established through individualized education plans (IEPs) or other means in school programs. However, leaving school often means leaving a network of peers for the adolescent with AS. As well, given the difficulties transferring skills across settings and people typically experienced by these individuals, independently identifying and joining another peer network is a typical and very frustrating hurdle. The ongoing need for social learning, for friendship development, and for building and maintaining an active and supportive social network is therefore a critical one at this time. This area of need includes the task of first identifying appropriate individuals or groups of peers with whom to engage as well as knowing the proper etiquette for initiations and responses to affiliative overtures. Being able to discern those who might be interested in the person with AS but who would not be appropriate to engage with is also essential. Ongoing difficulties with social perspective taking (Klin, McPartland, & Volkmar, 2005) and a history of social isolation may make moving across the continuum of acquaintance to friendship even more challenging for some. The interest in more intimate (and socially demanding) interpersonal relationships can be especially confusing and devastating for some individuals with AS (Stokes & Kaur, 2005). Unfortunately, with less attention given to such issues during a person's educational program, this often is new territory whose terrain is made more difficult to traverse by the absence of any mandated service delivery system or option to address it.

As those with AS age, their developmental needs and social expectations sometimes can be at odds. Consider the middle-age man with AS who, because of his parents' failing health, is now thrust into the role of primary caregiver when, throughout his life living with his parents, he was cared *for* and therefore far less independent. Having developed neither adequate independent health care access skills nor the ability to separate from his parents as an adult child, this person may be ill-equipped emotionally, socially, and cognitively (i.e., with respect to critical judgment and thinking skills) to assume the role in which he now finds himself. Later in this chapter we discuss considerations relevant to establishing forms of family functioning that respect both the needs of maturing adults with AS and also the ongoing challenges faced by these individuals.

Enhancing the Impact of the Educational Curriculum in a Postsecondary Environment

The completion of an educational program (whether supported by an IEP or not) does not imply the end of social learning or the assumption that material mastered in school automatically will be transferred, generalized, or fluent in other settings. The emphasis on academic achievement for so many adolescents with AS—often to the relative exclusion of social achievement—presents certain challenges. Whereas the need for ongoing social teaching is clear throughout later adolescence and into adulthood, the parallel need to ensure that academic achievement is expanded, generalized, and applied in noneducational settings is no less important. Special emphasis must be placed on targeting functional academic skills and determining where, and how, to expand and integrate these. For example, a student who excelled in geography and history may find greater opportunities for advancement with postsecondary education, whereas an individual who is more interested in the details and functioning of police scanners and radio dispatching may enter the workforce successfully without additional formal education. What becomes important at this point in time is the process of assessment and placement considerations, as well as the actual skills available to the person with AS.

Often, a student can exit an educational setting at 18 or 21 years of age with a set of skills or instructional objectives mastered in the instruction setting but not in the natural environment. Although this state of affairs clearly would constitute poor practice (Eren & Bruckner, 2011; Doehring & Winterling, 2011; Powers, Palmieri, D'Eramo, & Powers, 2011), the situation is anything but rare. As such it is essential to ensure that mastery of academic, social, communication, and behavioral/coping skill objectives be recognized only when they have been demonstrated with fluency across multiple environments outside the classroom. While it is beyond the scope of this chapter to review these in detail (see Brown & Wolf, Chapter 11, this volume), a number of evidence-based strategies is available to accomplish this important task (Horner, Dunlap, & Koegel, 1988). Further, it is sometimes the case that a skill has been mastered and generalized across settings, but is not fluent in a functional environment (i.e., is not demonstrated *both* correctly *and* quickly wherever necessary). Direct instruction opportunities must be guided by the need to establish correct and socially valid responding in all settings and to ensure that such responding is flexible and fluent.

Enhancing Functioning in the Community

Ultimately, educational opportunities from preschool through the completion of secondary school are of diminished value if they do not prepare a person for life beyond the classroom. The special deficits inherent to AS, especially those related to problems with social cognition, magnify the potential problems and their impact on the short- and longer-term options of a person with this disability. It becomes critical, therefore, that targeted interventions to develop appropriate and effective *functional* social relationships with significant persons in the community be expanded. Teaching the skills to engage and participate with community merchants, municipal and public health personnel, neighbors, first responders, and others typically are not part of a comprehensive curriculum for those completing their secondary school career, but the failure to demonstrate competency with each of these community sectors can have far-reaching negative consequences.

Similarly, the adult with AS who pursues a more independent employment and residential experience is at risk for failure without well-established safety routines and decision-making strategies to apply in ambiguous safety situations (e.g., what to do when an odd smell in the kitchen is detected and how to decide whether to clean out the refrigerator, turn off the unlit gas burner, or leave the house and call the gas company). Predicting potential danger becomes an important skill to master as well, considering that all of us receive unexpected visitors to our homes, as well as phone solicitations for items, for credit cards, and other financial instruments, and unwanted requests for information. Although it may seem appealing (and simple) to provide a person with a list of rules about who or what should and shouldn't be discussed (e.g., you would never give out your Social Security number to an unknown phone solicitor, but you might give out the last four digits of it to a bank or credit card representative during a billing inquiry), not all situations and circumstances can be clearly predicted. Evaluating the person's understanding of the potential problems that may occur, and the correct responses to them, becomes an assessment task of importance. The development of necessary teaching plans for skill deficits and for expansion of skills that are emerging but not yet fluent becomes the overarching goal.

Enhancing Functioning in the Workplace

Information processing and executive functioning difficulties experienced by many individuals with AS have been described comprehensively elsewhere in this book. As the individual with AS enters the workplace, he or she may discover that the more forgiving family or school environment often has not adequately prepared him or her for the harsher expectations and realities of a job. To the extent that adequate adaptations, modifications, and accommodations are not developed, the employee with AS may continue to have difficulty with demands for rapid decision making, changes in supervision or supervisors, applying skills across job settings, and cross-training. Job placement and maintenance efforts must consider the need to develop these supports proactively and to familiarize both the employee with AS and supervisors and coworkers (as appropriate) with these supports.

The social-communication demands of the workplace may also be challenging. Expectations of working without excess talking, of asking for assistance only when needed, engaging in problem solving based on prior training before asking for help, and various other "soft skills" (e.g., proper dress and general appearance, maintaining proper hygiene, following breakroom etiquette, and allowing the supervisor to offer corrective feedback rather than the person with AS assuming that responsibility for him-or herself) all may be implicit—and unspoken. When discussing school-age individuals, the term "hidden social curriculum" (Myles, Trautman, & Schelvan, 2004) has been instructive, and with expansion this term is equally applicable to adults. It is important to consider that successful integration into the workplace is often as dependent upon the fluency demonstrated with soft skills as with the technical demands of the job.

Enhancing Awareness and Self-Monitoring of Personal Needs

Those with AS may have a history of circumscribed interests, aversion to particular sensory events (e.g., halogen lighting, high-pitched sound, smells, clothing textures), or defined "rules for engagement" with others that are well practiced but less functional beyond the confines of the family or school. These areas must be addressed explicitly in the process of selecting and integrating the person with AS into an adult community. Self-awareness and self-monitoring of reactions to unpredicted aversive sensory events; awareness of one's personal "rules" and the need to demonstrate more flexibility with others where these rules are concerned; and learning to "map" social, communication, and behavioral expectations and conventions onto specific events or tasks should be part of a supportive curriculum when transitioning an adolescent with AS into adulthood, but through all of life's other transitions as well. This usually will require direct instruction initially, with fading of supportive mentoring as skill proficiency is demonstrated by the person with AS.

DEVELOPMENTAL CONSIDERATIONS ACROSS THE LIFESPAN

Just as we understand that adults with AS are not simply larger versions of themselves as children, so too do we appreciate that the various phases of adulthood and adult life impact those with AS as they do all of us. Unfortunately, continuing difficulties with social thinking and "mindblindness" (Baron-Cohen, 1995) often prevent the person with AS from benefiting more fully from the social learning opportunities afforded typical peers. The result often is a struggle with predictable developmental tasks for which the person is either poorly prepared, bewildered by, or both. Understanding and predicting these potential dilemmas permits proactive planning, ultimately enhancing both quality of life and the options available to the person with AS. A brief discussion of important developmental considerations confronted by those with AS follows.

One of the critical tasks of later adolescence and early adulthood is *separating from one's family of origin* and establishing oneself as a separate yet related entity. This task requires expanding beyond the social and decision-making orbit of one's parents and shifting one's attention to, and seeking social guidance from, peers, other adults, and one's own prior experience. While this is difficult for many nondisabled young adults, it is especially hard for many with AS. Close bonds—sometimes excessively so—may have developed over the years by necessity between parents and their child with AS, and these can be difficult to disentangle. Although few would argue that independence is a good thing for someone with AS, many parents still have reservations (often justified) about the ability of their now-adult child to safely and competently negotiate life's challenges.

Helping families and the individual with AS set reasonable, well-defined goals toward more independent functioning outside of school is an important transitional objective.

Creating or expanding social networks is a related developmental task of young adulthood. As we rely less on parents for guidance and decision making, we seek the counsel of friends to provide that guidance and help us address problems. Unfortunately, those with AS may have had difficulty establishing and maintaining friendships historically, and now have few resources to correct this problem when it is most needed. Peer relationships in AS often initially are driven by common (sometimes circumscribed) interests, with affiliative interests (e.g., "I want to spend time with my friend because she makes me feel happy") often a secondary consideration. As a result, the basic strategies for initiating peer interactions and developing ongoing relationships may be unavailable to individuals with AS or, worse yet, under poor functional control. For example, consider the individual who expects that initiating and maintaining one-sided conversation on a particular topic is a way to show his interest in someone else. Or, the person who believes that "honesty is a must" and makes blunt, sometimes unflattering remarks (albeit true, according to her) to a potential friend. In such cases, few would doubt the eagerness to make friends, but the less competent strategies used in the process are unsuccessful. It is sad reality that for many with AS, the absence of a learned social repertoire has devastating consequences, but the person with AS may be among the last to realize this. Recognizing this potential problem early in the life of a child with AS and providing effective social instruction to address these needs is the most obvious solution. But for those without benefit of good prior instruction, continuing awareness and instruction can make the difference between a life with others and a life alone.

Young adults eventually *enter the workforce*. The trajectory of this transition may be sooner, with some forgoing postsecondary education, or later for someone with AS who advances through undergraduate and graduate degrees, only to ultimately confront the same social realities (and confusions) that existed for him or her when much younger. In either case, as we discuss later in this chapter, the issues of "hard" and "soft" skill competencies, underemployment, and difficult economic realities for the chosen skill set of the person with AS must be anticipated and addressed with effective instruction.

Balancing work, personal interests, and leisure can be a challenging triad for the most competent among us, but is a particular problem for many with AS. Organizational challenges secondary to executive functioning deficits make the task of prioritizing, planning, and executing activities more difficult. Preferences for more sedentary activities, or those revolving around circumscribed interests, may contribute to a restricted repertoire of choices. Long-standing social deficits may contribute to continuing isolation, despite the desire of the person with AS to broaden social contacts. As well, when there is an imbalance in the triad (as when the personal/social dimension is more poorly realized and the leisure dimension consists of sedentary and solitary activities), work may become all-consuming. Helping an individual with AS achieve a realistic balance requires not only support but competencies in each of the three domains of this triad. Establishing skill sets, activities, and coping strategies for each helps to ensure better functioning as well as balance.

Young adults without developmental disabilities typically are expected to *assume responsibility for their own health and personal care*, even when chronic conditions (e.g., diabetes) are present. For some with AS, however, long-standing family or parental patterns of caretaking may undermine this process of taking responsibility. For others, poor judgment and organizational skills, poor working memory, or other factors well known to the family may have made it unrealistic for the person with AS to take a primary, responsible role. When we consider that most individuals with AS will likely outlive their parents, and that society is increasingly mobile with adult siblings often more likely to move away than remain living in the family hometown, it becomes imperative to address the development of more independent personal care, health care, and health maintenance skills in adults with AS. Learning to monitor medications, status of physical conditions requiring careful scrutiny (e.g., type 1 diabetes), personal appearance and hygiene, and diet are worthwhile skill targets for the person with AS. Ideally, this process would have begun in later adolescence or earlier as part of an IEP and individual transition plan (ITP), but if functional personal care and health maintenance and promotion skills are not demonstrated and generalized, these must become objectives that are developed and taught during early adulthood.

Perhaps one of the developmental tasks most challenging and fraught with potential for disaster is the *independent management of personal finances* by many with AS. While in childhood money management is somewhat more circumscribed and agenda-driven (we save for what you want, say, trading cards or the newest Matchbox car), in adulthood we must learn to save for what we need and those things that we really cannot do without. An example of the former might be the need for a fire extinguisher that can be kept in the kitchen of a newly rented apartment, and in the latter case, money must be saved to pay the monthly heating bill. These contingencies of daily life all require planning, prioritizing, and critical judgments (e.g., this month I have enough to pay either half my outstanding credit card bill, or my entire heating bill—which is more important?) that may be very difficult to recognize. That we can anticipate these needs and determine the degree of full or relative independence that is possible for the young adult with AS is the first step, to be followed by development of comprehensive teaching plans to ensure mastery and generalization.

The primary developmental tasks of middle adulthood involve maintaining those skills developed earlier, but also adjusting to change. For example, employment transitions, transitions in family status or constellation, and the impact of changes in personal or health status on social, community, and work initiatives all can be challenging. Hopefully, those social and friendship relationships that developed earlier in adulthood will continue to be available, but there is no guarantee of this. *Working to maintain friendships* and to develop new ones is an ongoing process for all successful adults, and although it is no less important for those with AS, it typically requires a greater effort, flexibility, and persistence as well as enhanced social understanding and perspective taking. For example, consider the person with AS whose friendship with a neurotypical person revolved around a common interest in railroading. Whereas this may have been a very successful relationship in the past, the marriage and addition of children to the family of the typical peer will obviously alter the relationship in terms of available time and priority setting for hobbies. To the extent that the person with AS is unable to adjust flexibly to these changes, the relationship may be at risk or lost. Recognizing the potential for risk associated with change and working to develop the necessary skills to neutralize this risk becomes a very important task to address during middle adulthood.

Many individuals with AS become employed and enjoy advancement opportunities in the workplace because of their skills. Others fall victim to layoffs, job contraction, corporate takeovers, and other exigencies of business life. *Coping with the planned and unpredictable changes of the workplace* becomes a set of skills to be mastered and also a focus of instruction as the need arises. It is not uncommon that with advancement often comes new technical *and* social responsibilities. Consider the well-respected mechanical engineer who is promoted into a managerial position, only to be confronted by the social and personnel management skill demands for which he is poorly equipped by virtue of his AS. Without an understanding senior administrative manager, the engineer's failure to demonstrate the "soft" skills needed to manage a team of others may influence perceptions of the technical expertise already present, and may negatively affect job stability. We have worked with individuals who were highly successful in a technical area in the military who, upon retirement from the service, were unable to transfer their competencies into a less-structured and less-hierarchical work environment. In many ways this type of dilemma can be predicted and resolved proactively if we understand the challenges AS places on an individual.

For those with AS who become involved in close and intimate relationships in their adult life, *the ability to maintain a healthy intimacy* that is anchored by common expectations and mutual understanding is no less important than for those without AS. However, inflexibility, entrenchment into circumscribed interests, "mindblindness" (Baron-Cohen, 1995), and a more agenda-driven egocentric interpersonal style can prevent the necessary personal change and adjustment that is often brought on by more advancing age. As it is for all of us who wish to maintain and strengthen our relationship with a significant other as we grow older, learning the skills that underlie flexibility and applying them effectively become important developmental tasks of middle (and later) adulthood.

With later adulthood comes the inevitable need to regroup, reconsider, and restructure. Advancing health concerns; loss of parents, siblings, or supportive friends through death or disability; job loss or retirement; and decreased physical stamina (and sometimes interest) in those things that motivated one's younger self all increase the risk factors for poor adjustment to this phase of life. Therefore, the need to *maintain activities that promote social and physical health* becomes a prominent priority at this time. Considering that very little research has been done on the impact of chronic physical illness, treatment compliance, and treatment outcome on older individuals with ASD (Gerhardt, 2009; Tantam, 2003), we must be especially mindful of the effects of the social-cognitive implications of AS in the context of advancing age and the social isolation that may become the default position of those with AS facing difficult life changes and challenges.

ISSUES AND DILEMMAS IN THE DIAGNOSIS AND DIFFERENTIAL DIAGNOSIS OF ASPERGER SYNDROME IN LATER ADOLESCENCE AND ADULTHOOD

The diagnostic and differential diagnostic considerations in AS have been well described earlier in this book (see Volkmar et al., Chapter 1, and Campbell et al., Chapter 2, this volume) and we refer the reader to that work as a foundation for the following discussion of distinctions in both clinical and practical implications of AS for those in later adolescence and adulthood. In a pragmatic sense, the question is this: *What do we make of the person with AS whose disability is becoming invisible by virtue of expanding social and adaptive competencies?* The developmental psychopathology of AS does not follow an identical course in all individuals accurately diagnosed earlier in life. Indeed, enough variation occurs so as to prompt some clinicians to posit that distinctions between AS and autism without intellectual disability are difficult to make, supporting a conceptualization of multiple pathways to the same virtual end point. The decision of the framers of the newly revised edition of the *Diagnostic and Statistical Manual of Mental Disorders* (DSM-5; American Psychiatric Association, 2013) to remove AS from the official diagnostic nomenclature and subsume it under the broader term ASD is one such example. Although we do not find that the research supports the homogenizing of AS (see Volkmar et al., Chapter 1, this volume, for discussion), we certainly appreciate that many with AS improve in very important ways and may be far less noticeable in the natural environment where, by dint of life's opportunities and choices made, they are doing well.

Later adolescents and adults present for evaluation and diagnosis for reasons often different than those of toddlers or younger children. For those in their late teen years and beyond, the functional implications of the diagnosis predominate. Diagnosis is a pathway to service access and treatment. Considering that many adults diagnosed with AS are also diagnosed with another psychiatric condition (Ghaziuddin, Wieder-Mikhail, & Ghaziuddin, 1998; Volkmar, Lord, Klin, Schultz, & Cook, 2007), accurate representation of needs and assets consistent with a proper diagnosis can lead to crucial services. The Connecticut Pilot Project, described at the end of this chapter, clearly articulates these concerns and the solutions that may be needed and then made available. For others, first diagnosis in adulthood is precipitated by a crisis or a more serious problem or need. For example, one of us (J. W. L.) has been involved in clarifying the diagnosis of individuals with AS who are part of the criminal justice system, so that the nature, motivation, and implications of their alleged offenses can be better understood and addressed by the courts. In such cases, the criminal offense precipitated the crisis that, in turn, led to proper identification and treatment.

Accurate diagnosis in later life often requires some degree of flexible thinking on the part of the clinician. Obviously, an earlier, accurate diagnosis of ASD provides a better starting point for understanding the social and pragmatic language deficits currently observed and their relation to "what was" in the past for the person. We do not always have access to such information, however. In this latter case, the clinician is faced with obtaining a detailed developmental history and a review of records (if these are even available). This process is often complicated by the absence of credible reporters. Parents may have died, older or younger siblings may recollect through their own prism of time, and the individual with AS may remember some benchmark facts that are of personal interest (where he or she lived and which exits on the highway to take to get there), but not the more nuanced details of social disability, pragmatic communication problems, or circumscribed interests. To support this process it becomes very important to survey comprehensively rituals, interests, preoccupations, and "obsessions" of the past and their relationship to present clinical features or observed behavior.

Consideration must also be given to the literality of language use; to the understanding and use of humor, idioms, metaphors, and other elements of figural speech; and to learned as opposed to more formulaic and patterned conventions of conversation. Social inefficiencies, egocentrism and social isolation, deficits of social reasoning and cognitive inflexibility, and the adaptive use of coping strategies should be surveyed. Finally, when coping failures or behavioral excesses and deficits are prominent, it is essential for the clinician to understand and describe those events functionally for the person suspected of AS, within the context of violations or breakdowns in routine, structure, predictability, order, and personal control.

Often, the true dilemma is this: In the face of credible historical data supporting a diagnosis of AS, but in the presence of adequate social and adaptive functioning that may well be highly supported by natural contingencies, how do we conceptualize the diagnostic process? The person may appear to be very competent but only within the confines of a well-organized supportive structure, and lack the ability to generalize those successful strategies to another similar but nonidentical situation as the need arises. Given the short-lived presence of AS in the diagnostic nomenclature, we do not have longitudinal studies on the developmental trajectories of those identified in early or middle childhood as they enter midlife. Under such circumstances it may be advisable to be cautious about underrepresenting the important needs that may have been present earlier, but have become subtler in the present, and to regard gains as fragile and in need of careful monitoring for fluency, generalization, and maintenance.

To address this dilemma it is often helpful to consider the parameters of the expanding social competencies and continuing social deficits we see in adults with AS. In adulthood, we may find many assets that have been learned through direct instruction or through a more natural accumulation of experiences. More competent social behavior for initiating and maintaining interactions, coping with unexpected change or frustrating conditions, and better self-regulation strategies are not uncommon. Conversation skills may have improved as well through instruction and practice. The ability to initiate, maintain, and shift conversation topics often becomes less problematic than in the person's earlier years. Finally, academic or vocational competence may be more evident due to the natural (or planned) selection of pursuits that have a "goodness of fit" with the interests and abilities of the person with AS. For example, we once worked with a young man of considerable ability who had a special affinity for numerical relationships and mathematical computations. His most successful job experiences were with a major rental car company where his responsibility was contract review of the franchise owners' past weeks' work. In this capacity, he quickly became a very valuable member of the company workforce because he could easily exceed (sometimes doubled and tripled) the industry standard for contracts reviewed in a day, and he identified errors that saved tens of thousands of dollars over the course of a year. In this environment, his symptoms of AS were perceived more as eccentricities than debilitating elements and, while still sometimes problematic, they were much less of an impediment than for other positions he held subsequently after the company was sold to a competitor and his job was eliminated. In later jobs, this man found work as a night clerk in hotels, where he came into more public contact and needed to exercise critical thinking skills that required him to interpret the hotel's rules flexibly late at night, when supervision was not immediately available to him (as when he left a line of potential hotel patrons waiting because the hotel computer server went down, and he could not enter credit card information into the computer as required by the hotel front desk policy).

AS brings with it continuing social deficits that are lifelong, even as personal choice making, job selection, and ongoing learning continue to mitigate the severity of these deficits for many. Literality and concrete thinking continue to be present (Tantam, 2003), as do problems with social perspective taking and theory-of-mind (ToM) considerations (Pennington & Ozonoff, 1996). Executive functions may have improved with intervention and positive learning experiences, but poorer capacity in this important area is still evident in most adults with AS (Klin et al., 2005). Behavioral rigidity is not at all uncommon, particularly with the need to comply with rules. Indeed, many social errors are the result of a person with AS making an accurate assessment of a relevant social rule to be applied, but failing to recognize that flexibility in the application of the rule is necessary for this situation. Finally, continuing difficulty with speech, prosody, and the metalinguistics of communication are evident (Shriberg et al., 2001). More nuanced understanding of adult humor, and knowing in whose company it should be offered (and where it should not), is an obvious example. Integrating and interpreting accurately a speaker's tone of voice, facial expression, words, body language, and proximity to a conversation partner are other common difficulties for even some of the most intellectually capable persons with AS.

ADOLESCENTS AND ADULTS WITH ASPERGER SYNDROME AND COMORBID PSYCHIATRIC CONDITIONS: CONSIDERATIONS OF BEHAVIORAL SEQUELAE

AS is not a prophylaxis against other concurrent and often debilitating psychiatric disorders. As well, someone with AS should not be automatically assumed to be affected by major depression, anxiety disorder, or obsessive–compulsive disorder (OCD), even as certain aspects of his or her adult clinical profile may appear to suggest this. Westphal, Kober, Voos, and Volkmar (Chapter 9, this volume) discuss the issue of comorbidity in detail, highlighting the differential diagnostic features of the more common issues that confront those with AS. Here we raise considerations about behavioral profiles that may be observed, but to the less well-initiated observer, may be less indicative of psychiatric problems than of poor coping strategies applied to problems in living.

As noted earlier, adolescents and adults with AS continue to (1) have difficulty extracting meaningful rules from social situations; (2) demonstrate significant problems with social perspective taking and with organizing information from many sources into coherent, cohesive constructs; and (3) may continue to be distressed or avoidant of situations that predict unexpected sensory stimuli, social ambiguity, or social challenge. These tendencies can lead to behavior that may be misinterpreted by others, to misunderstanding of the experience and behavior of the person with AS, and to misdiagnosis of comorbid conditions. For example, inefficiencies in the modulation and regulation of sensory stimuli by those with ASD have been discussed in the literature (Baranek, Wakeford, & David, 2008; Volkmar et al., 2007). Sensory-seeking or avoidant behavior can sometimes be misinterpreted because it may mimic other, less uncommon behavioral responses seen in adults. We once worked with a young man with AS who became fixated on touching black stockings worn by females and succeeded in creating a great deal of trouble for himself on his college campus. Functional assessment of this behavior revealed that he was motivated by automatic reinforcement, that is, the sensory features (in this case, texture) of the stockings rather than any sexual or social considerations. The situation was compounded by the fact that, consistent with his earlier school instruction about being polite and asking permission of others, this man would politely ask young women if he could touch their stockings. Finally, the selection of black stockings was contextual; at the time of his enrollment in college many fashionable young women were wearing black stockings. (At an earlier age our young man had been very interested in the texture of polyester clothing.) Unfortunately, his behavior was initially labeled as predatory sexual behavior by campus authorities.

Unexpected or unpredictable violations in routine or structure or violation of a rule from an authority source (e.g., a policy and procedure manual at one's place of employment) can sometimes cause behavioral agitation, excessive verbal expressions of distress, and requests or demands that the situation return to "normal" or that the violator be reprimanded. The more black-and-white demand for "fairness" sometimes comes into play here. One of our older adolescent clients with AS was very adept at both computers and videography, and also with reminding others of the need for strict adherence to the rules of conduct for students and staff at his academic high school. A careful observer of possible transgressions around him, he noticed that an assistant principal at his school regularly stood outside the school gym to smoke between certain class periods. He confronted the administrator but was rebuffed. Unfortunately, his next strategy led to him being suspended and referred for psychiatric evaluation. He proceeded to videotape the assistant principal and then uploaded the video to the school's community website with his own editorial about the violation of school policy. When confronted with his behavior, and the referral for psychiatric evaluation for "willful misconduct and possible conduct disorder," the young man argued that he was simply following school rules and trying to enforce those rules that would lead to better health for the school community.

We know of similar situations involving rule violation without redress that have led to behavioral agitation and expressed concerns about possible generalized anxiety disorder in other clients. Fortunately, a more thorough assessment of behavioral function and precursor events can often clarify the situation, and also lead to the development of more effective intervention strategies that might include developing alternative coping strategies, response and check-in communication systems to verify (or refute) the relative importance of the problem, and teaching self-monitoring and self-management of life circumstances that elicit agitated behavior.

The pattern of circumscribed interests observed in those with AS is sometimes confused with OCD. Circumscribed interests typically have a function and often become multifunctional in AS. Consider the adolescent who is passionately interested in World War II fighting aircraft and characteristically collects information on air battles over Europe, specific aircraft in those battles, the names and history of the air commanders involved, and the number of casualties suffered. While he will willingly share this information with anyone who seems interested (and with too many who are not), he continues to amass facts primarily for his own purposes rather than to impress others or to make friends. As this young man matures into adulthood, he locates a cohort of other adults who share a similar interest, but who are also amazed by his encyclopedic knowledge. Their high regard supports the development of social relationships among this group, and expanding his knowledge now takes on a social-access function. For us a key distinction here between a circumscribed interest and a more serious psychiatric condition is the motivating value of the behavior itself. In AS the motivation (*drive*, if you will) to collect information about a circumscribed interest is positively reinforcing. A person seeks to acquire information on his or her narrow interest because it brings reinforcing events (facts and knowledge to catalogue, or social regard because of his or her knowledge). In other conditions, such as OCD, the motivation to complete the behavior is the relief experienced by completion. This is a negatively reinforcing contingency, whereby the anxiety and excessive arousal of an aversive event are reduced by the performance of a behavior. Granted, the behavior is still more likely to occur in the future (that is the nature of reinforcement whether it is positive or negative). But the long-term motivation and behavioral sequelae of elation or release from acute distress is an operative element in conceptualizing and accurately treating an individual with these behavioral features.

In considering these examples, our intent is not to minimize the higher prevalence of comorbid psychiatric problems in adults with AS, but rather to highlight the importance of considering those neurocognitive features of AS that may influence client behavior, and potentially influence our understanding of that behavior out of context. Indeed, many persons with AS will experience a behavioral crisis that becomes better described as a psychiatric disorder over time and requires appropriate and effective intervention strategies that combine cognitive-behavioral and psychopharmacological elements. Recognizing, however, that the overt behavior and behavioral patterns of someone with AS may well be due to the fact that the disorder itself makes certain challenges in life that much more distressing and debilitating, and that these are often better conceptualized for treatment purposes as "problems in living" requiring the teaching of better adaptive and coping skills, is the primary intent in this discussion.

TRANSITIONS AND CHANGE

Few would argue that change is hard, and even more so for many individuals with AS. Transitions are a natural process throughout adolescence and adulthood, however, and the ability to negotiate them must be an area for specific intervention and supported for more independent social, vocational, and community realities to come to fruition for the individual with a social learning disability such as AS. In this section, we discuss the concept of transition as a process, the need to understand and assess readiness for change, and several questions of critical importance that must be considered in the process of a person with AS transitioning across the lifespan.

Transition as a Process

As a general rule, *predicted* transitions are more successful transitions. They are also dynamic and dependent on the interrelationship between environmental demands; the degree to which change in the transition is predictable, the degree to which the demands inherent in change are part of the repertoire of the individual with AS; the availability of internal and external coping systems and supports; and the specific social, communication, and cognitive strengths and challenges of the person with AS.

Consideration of transition as a process implies that it can be planned, and this planning is an essential element for success. Several components that support successful transitions can be described. Initially, it is important to have a thorough understanding of the social and communication processing assets and weaknesses of the person with AS. The individual who has a great deal of difficulty understanding the relationship between single activities or components of a task and the more holistic gestalt of the completed task may not be successful unless this linkage is made clear as part of the transition training and implementation process. For example, it is often helpful to provide an example of a completed product, task, or activity prior to expecting participation in order to "set the stage" for more successful participation. Mentoring and job coaching can facilitate this component. Those with AS who have more compromised visual–motor or visual–spatial skills may require specific accommodations and modifications to transition tasks in order to complete them more successfully, whereby motor demands are minimized or otherwise supported and reduced in their complexity.

An assessment of the ecology of the sending and receiving environment is also important. To the extent that the individual with AS has been successful in his or her current setting, those elements of that setting that are most responsible for success should be explicated. They will form the basis for understanding transition planning as a generalization gradient, where common (and transferrable) elements of the sending environment are brought into the receiving environment. For example, if an adult in a work environment is successful, in part, because the rules for job performance are clearly stated *and posted* for all to see, and if adherence to those stated rules leads to functional rewards (e.g., better ratings on job performance evaluations), then the element of stating and posting expectations may be considered a critical one to transfer to the new environment as part of the transition process.

New environments are differently, and sometimes less, defined than old environments for the person with AS, and this simple consideration underscores the importance of making the new setting "known" before transitioning there. By conducting an *ecological assessment* of the next, receiving environment, and then teaching to the new demands and expectations, the individual with AS enters a more predictable experience with greater established competencies. We have found it helpful to those facilitating transitions to request that they identify the social, communication, deportment, and physical setting expectations of the receiving environment as part of the pretransition planning process. This information then becomes a curriculum of target skills for assessment, and if necessary also for instruction, so that the person with AS is prepared for the demands of that new setting and is equipped with the behavioral repertoire necessary for success there. For example, some community activities for women that emphasize health promotion (e.g., Curves) have a structure and expectations for mutual support, encouragement, and confidentiality that may be very different from a physical education class in high school or college. To the extent that a woman with AS is aware of the expectations before participating in the new environment and equipped with an appropriate behavioral repertoire and effective strategies to resolve confusion (e.g., she attends initially with a mentor, community peer, or a female sibling for coaching as needed), her transition to this more independent community setting will be facilitated. The ecological assessment is the means of identifying skills and behavior critical to a successful transition. For the transition to the new setting to remain successful, however, those skills identified in the ecological assessment must be taught and mastered.

There is a robust, well-defined, evidence-based treatment literature for developing skills in persons with ASD (see Reichow, Doerhing, Cicchetti & Volkmar, 2011, for a comprehensive review). Broadly defined, these involve the use of teaching strategies derived from principles of learning described as *applied behavior analysis* and incorporate the use of reinforcement, shaping, prompting, and fading, among many others, to establish and generalize new behavioral repertoires. Although it is well beyond the scope of this chapter to review these in any detail, we later make reference to cognitive-behavioral treatment strategies for purposes of individual therapy, as necessary, and more structural behavioral family therapy strategies for working with families of adults with AS. Suffice it to say that the emphasis on precise, defined intervention that is objectively evaluated, with clear procedures for data-driven decision making is a hallmark of effective treatment for those with AS, including for developing requisite skills needed for successful transitions.

Transitions require the flexible and fluent use of adequate coping strategies by the person with AS. Given the more rigid, rule-governed, egocentric, and agenda-driven tendencies of many individuals with AS, the need for flexibility and fluency often creates a problem. There are two competing needs for resolution in such circumstances: (1) Prior learning must be utilized as it is well established and previously successful; and (2) prior learning must be stretched, modified, and sometimes altered considerably to meet the needs of the new transitional situation. This problem is one of stimulus-and-response generalization, whereby certain behaviors are under the more limited control of particular conditions (e.g., the presence of a certain type of written plan for action) and are not fluently used in novel, nontraining environments. A number of important and effective strategies can be used to facilitate generalization, including systematically introducing variability and novelty into the learning experience ("training loosely"), using material or stimuli in training that are common to the natural (and next) environment, teaching with multiple exemplars (e.g., teaching an employee to respond successfully to multiple forms of positive and corrective performance feedback), and providing functional mediators to support the transition of learned repertoires from familiar to novel settings. For example, an individual with AS who has learned time management and task priority skills through applications on an iPhone in one work environment would do well to continue to use that resource, with perhaps modified applications as the needs of the new job demands, in the new setting because it represents a well-understood memory and organizational guide. Horner, Dunlap, and Koegel (1988) provide a thorough review of these and other strategies.

We have also found it useful to accept that all transitions cannot be planned or predicted, and we have taught the use of more omnibus transition coping strategies. For example, teaching the coping strategy of "asking a coworker or supervisor" when a situation presents as ambiguous may be useful. Of course, it is rarely sufficient to simply tell someone to do this; as a skill to be taught the learning contingencies must be defined and practiced. For those persons with AS accustomed to using Social Stories™ (Gray, 1998), we have create an "Oops" Social Story that prescribes what to do when the proper response is unclear (as well as highlighting the possible perceptions of others to the situation, and the potential positive responses of others to better coping). In many respects, the important point is that the prior successful learning and behavioral repertoire of the person with AS should be utilized in developing skills necessary for a successful transition.

A final point about transition is that many individuals beyond the person with AS are part of the transition planning and implementation process. Those in the sending environment who have developed special knowledge and skills with the individual with AS must share that information with those in the receiving environment. Those in the receiving environment must have thorough knowledge of their own setting, and the demands and expectations in that setting, in order to adequately plan. A comprehensive and transparent process of sharing this information with individuals in both settings, the person with AS, parents or other stakeholders, and others as appropriate is an important element of the transition planning, implementation, and evaluation process to be maintained.

Understanding and Evaluating Readiness for Change

In any transition, motivation to change is a key consideration. With sufficient motivation (whether intrinsic or extrinsic) success is more likely; without it, resistance and sabotage are typical. In considering transitions and change for the adolescent and adult with AS, we must first determine whether there are sufficient motivators to effect and maintain the change, and whether the new setting will provide sufficient inherent motivation to stabilize new behavioral repertoires needed for growth and development. Powers and Handleman (1984) and Powers and Bruey (1988) have described a rubric for assessing and understanding readiness for change in persons with ASD and other developmental disabilities, adapted from earlier work on organizational change by Maher and Bennett (1984). A brief description follows.

Change requires not only readiness or motivation but also *resources* and the willingness to commit those resources to bring about the transition successfully. Resources include personnel with necessary skills, training, and experience; available funds to pay for necessary training and activities that may be part of the transition; and physical space for training or implementation of the transition. Philosophical constraints may need to be assessed. Parents or others working with the individual with AS may have differing views about the value, appropriateness, or benefit of a proposed transition. These concerns need to be clarified and resolved before the transition process is initiated because disagreement can promote inconsistency of expectation and of intervention, confusing the person with AS and ultimately derailing the transition itself. A related construct relates to the held *values* of the person with AS and parents as well as other important people. Behavioral expectations during and after a transition is accomplished, allowable tolerances for resistance or regression, and congruence with normative values of the individual, his or her family, and the new setting all will contribute to stability or instability. In the former case the person with AS has a consistent and established support system available to carry out specific tasks of the transition. In the latter case, however, expectations of incomplete progress based on family or staff perceptions of lack of competence on the part of the individual with AS may generate a self-fulfilling prophecy and ultimate failure. Knowing about these issues prior to beginning the transition helps focus priorities, hopefully allowing resolution of the differences to occur before moving ahead.

Circumstances of the sending and receiving environments provide the context for change and help to predict success or failure. Characteristics of the family system, transitional life events occurring within the family itself, instability in the receiving environment's staffing resources, and other related considerations can be evaluated for their ability to support or interfere with the transition process. For example, consider the parents who have kept the middle-age person with AS in the family home and have not supported more independent, community-based living opportunities for their son or daughter. A life crisis in the family, such as the death of the primary caretaking parent, may unbalance the parental system so substantially that living at home no longer is a viable option. However, without a developed repertoire of community access and safety skills, and with the ambivalent messages that may be proffered by the surviving parent, the person with AS is at a fragile state of compromise and will need more objective and dispassionate guidance to weather the crisis and negotiate the transition successfully.

The *timing* of a transition is based upon a multiplicity of factors, including the readiness and preparation of the individual, the preparedness of the receiving setting, and the congruence of expectations, learning objectives, and values of all involved. Although it is often said that "timing is everything," in the case of transitions for individuals who experience great difficulty with change, this truism has even greater credence. *Resistance* is a natural by-product of poor transition planning and premature implementation. As with most psychotherapeutic and psychoeducational interventions, resistance is to be expected and must be managed proactively and reactively. The only true crime would be a failure to predict and respond productively to resistance to change, as this would imply a less-than-comprehensive initial assessment of the needs of the person with AS, his or her current environment, and the new setting in which the transition will occur.

The concept of *obligation* has also been referred to as perception of a need for change and to the extent of personal distress experienced by an individual as a result of maintaining the status quo for a person with AS (Powers & Franks, 1988). Lower perceptions of obligation to promote a change through transition to more independent or adaptive learning opportunities may ultimately inhibit efforts of family and community members in supporting the transition in the face of difficulty.

Finally, an understanding of expected yield or outcome must be facilitated prior to embarking on a planned transition. *Yield* refers to the anticipated benefit of the proposed change, and whether the effort required to promote and execute the change would be worth the proposed outcome. For success to occur, the anticipated yield must exceed the effort. This is evident in simple terms if we consider parental support of a transition to teaching independent transportation skills to a person with AS. The ultimate savings in parental time and energy may seem obvious, and we would expect a parent to support such a transitional activity on a number of levels. But what about broader parent concerns for their "child's" failure to exercise good judgment in traffic or with a detour, to maintain their vehicle in safe working order, or to recognize socially and physically dangerous situations (e.g., picking up hitchhikers or allowing a new friend to drive the car while intoxicated)? These concerns raise the perception of yield beyond a more straightforward equation of the effort expended and the savings of future efforts achieved, to a broader systems level that incorporates skill repertoires of the person with AS, perceptions of those repertoires by significant others, and the environment of support that may (or may not) be accessible in an unanticipated crisis. Knowing these issues and concerns in advance permits more thoughtful planning for the transition, far beyond developing a set of steps to achieve the outcome.

Change and Growth in the Face of Developmental Discontinuity

For many years one of us (M. D. P.) worked with an adult man with AS who had lived alone with his mother for his entire life. Over the course of the years of our work together, his mother aged and became more infirm and debilitated by chronic illness, ultimately requiring him to assume more of the role of caretaker than the one being cared for. As there was a significant learning history both for him and his mother regarding who made important decisions (not the man with AS), some of his mother's insistent decisions regarding her own health care ultimately led to her demise. For this family the man's social disability was a predictor of overall less competent behavior (even though he possessed two graduate degrees!), and he had learned to perform less competently. More to the point, however, although he was an adult of some competence, he was still the less able child in the eyes of his family.

AS is at once a social disability and also a disorder of developmental discontinuity. This discontinuity creates certain inherent problems as the individual with AS matures through adolescence into adulthood and to later adulthood. The nature of therapeutic and other supportive relationships must adjust to the realities inherent in attaining the age of majority. Although it is certainly the case that some with AS will require, or request, a conservatorship to help manage their affairs, many neither seek nor need one. Regardless of the formality of such assistance, it is important to define the nature of need of the individual with AS entering and progressing through adulthood and differentiate those situations that require caregiving, caretaking, advice and support, or simply support. In short, the task becomes one of balancing the best interests of the person with AS in the age of majority. There is no simple equation for achieving this balance, and decisions will likely be made based upon some of the considerations noted above, such as readiness for change, history of success with more independent habilitation opportunities, and the overall profile of strengths and deficits of the individual him- or herself. That these various elements should be considered is a given, however.

UNDERSTANDING AND ADDRESSING EMPLOYMENT CHALLENGES

One of the most daunting challenges for adults with AS is finding and keeping employment that allows them to be financially self-sufficient and to derive satisfaction from work. Although there have been recent gains, outcome studies paint a bleak picture, with only up to 50% of adults with AS being employed and many studies showing less than 20% having jobs (e.g., Howlin, 2003, 2005; Tantam, 1991). The situation is more negative when we consider how many of these jobs are part-time (and consequently without benefits) and how many are entry-level positions paying minimum wage. Furthermore, individuals with AS are often the most vulnerable to layoffs or downsizing during hard times. And although there is little research addressing the issue of attitudes toward one's job, relatively high percentages of these employed individuals report great frustration and low levels of job satisfaction (e.g., Fast, 2004).

The employment picture cannot be explained simply by the impact of AS in reducing marketable work skills, motivation to work, or school success. In fact, workers with AS can be extremely dependable with excellent attendance records, high levels of consistency, thoroughness in job performance, strong attention to detail, and high intelligence (e.g., Attwood, 2007; Hawkins, 2004). Unfortunately, the social, communication, and executive functioning challenges that are central to AS can have a strongly negative impact on finding and maintaining employment.

A number of issues relevant to the individual with AS can complicate employment and job retention. For example, many jobs are found through social networks and for individuals with AS, this may be particularly true (e.g., Howling & Goode, 1998). Having contacts and knowing a large number of people who know other people can open the door to a job interview or tip the balance in one's favor when a hiring decision is made. Networking is a powerful strategy in finding employment. However, individuals with the social challenges of AS often have few friends and acquaintances, let alone networks of contacts.

The ability to create a positive first impression and to effectively interview with prospective employers is essential to attaining competitive employment. The hygiene and grooming deficits often seen with AS can make a negative impact on interviewers (e.g., Hawkins, 2004). Effective interviewing requires perspective taking (what is the interviewer looking for?), strong conversation skills (not interrupting, staying on topic rather than focusing on preferred topics), reading nonverbal cues ("Is the interviewer pleased with what I am saying?") and good listening skills—all areas of challenge for most individuals with AS. Additionally, negative attitudes in the general population about disability, autism, or just being "different" can cause employers to reject applicants with AS who present any manifest features of atypicality, such as unusual prosody, motor mannerisms, or inconsistent eye contact.

For those who secure employment, having AS can bring a number of challenges that make success on the job more difficult. The first and most basic of these is the physical work environment, which of course varies greatly depending on the type of job. Sensory-processing issues can make workplace noises, smells, or temperature unbearable (e.g., Hawkins, 2004; Howlin, 2003; Hurlbutt & Chalmers, 2004; Powers, 2002; Standifer, 2009). Work sites with a high level of activity by people or equipment can be overstimulating, and complex floor plans can make it difficult for individuals with AS to navigate and find their way around.

The level of structure in the environment is another key variable in this regard. Settings where there are well-established work task routines and schedules that do not vary provide a better fit for individuals with AS who struggle with change or transitions. Clear and unchanging expectations and rules to follow make it much easier for workers with AS to succeed, especially when this information is provided in a visual format (e.g., Hawkins, 2004; Hume, Loftin, & Lantz, 2009). Readily available and easy-to-find people or resources to provide needed information and direction (e.g., a supervisor, company manual, or visual charts and checklists) are another aspect of structure that can be very helpful. Many employment settings have more flexible and changing rules and duties, necessitated by the nature of the work or by the style of the supervisor. Jobs in these environments can confuse and overwhelm individuals with AS, and may lead to a deterioration in their work performance.

The most central aspect of employment success is the individual's ability to perform the actual duties of the job. Individuals with AS present a wide of range of skill profiles and thus fit different jobs to varying degrees. It is important to match basic job demands with the neuropsychological profile of the individual (e.g., Attwood, 2007; Hawkins, 2004; Standifer, 2009). Someone with visual–motor challenges and slow processing speed would not do well in a position on a fast-moving assembly line, or someone with short-term memory and auditory processing deficits would not do well in a role that involves taking complex orders from consumers. Conversely, an individual with strong visual analysis and visual–motor competencies and a preference for organization and structure would thrive with inventory control and sorting duties.

In this regard, there are three particularly important areas of skill that impact most individuals with AS (e.g., Attwood, 20007; Hawkins, 2004; Hurlbutt & Chalmers, 2004). *Communication challenges* can cause a bad fit with jobs that require exchanging information with people, such as teaching, customer service, running a cash register, or sales. In some of these situations, the job may entail using a script or structured body of information in a rote manner (e.g., telemarketing, phone-based customer service) and in these cases, job fit may be very good. Second, *social difficulties* with perspective taking, reading nonverbal cues, identifying and following social conventions (i.e., the "hidden curriculum"; Myles et al., 2004), and interpersonal problem solving make jobs in teaching, counseling, and human services a struggle for individuals with AS. Finally, *executive functioning skills* that involve being able to initiate a process or sequence of steps, move from one duty to another, set priorities, multitask, and organize bodies of information are essential to a number of management, professional, and research jobs. This area of skills is generally a relative weakness for individuals with AS and so impacts job success in a number of fields.

Of course, individuals with AS have found job and career success in many fields of endeavor (e.g., Attwood, 2007). Some authors offer a list of AS-friendly jobs in which the chance of a good fit is better (e.g., Grandin & Duffy, 2004; Hawkins, 2004). We are not suggesting that there is a list of jobs that should be considered for people with AS and a list of jobs that no individual with AS can manage. Rather, job placement and successful employment are processes involving (1) understanding the skill profile of the individual and (2) helping him or her explore areas that fit his or her interests and skills so as to make a good, long-term fit. Pursuing employment in areas that are not compatible will only lead to frustration and less employment.

Social demands within the work environment constitute another important set of challenges to employment success (e.g., Fast, 2004; Grandin & Duffy, 2004; Hawkins, 2004). Virtually all jobs require interaction with a supervisor and coworkers, and some require frequent and complex interactions among team members. The social challenges associated with AS can impede employment success even in situations where the individual performs extremely well with his or her job duties. If the worker does not interact in a way that is satisfying and functional for the supervisor, he or she is vulnerable to receiving poor evaluations, being passed over for promotions, and even being laid off. When social behaviors frustrate or alienate coworkers, it can set up social rejection and scapegoating by the work group as well as contribute to negative work evaluations.

There is a key set of social skills in any job environment that can be difficult for individuals with AS. With regard to the relationship with the supervisor, it is important to understand his or her intentions and needs so as to perform the job in a way that fits the team and is congruent with the expectations of the supervisor. This level of understanding requires a certain level of perspective taking, nonverbal communication, knowledge of the conventions around interacting with managers (e.g., how to address them, what you can and cannot talk about with them), and social problem solving. Individuals with AS are often seen to struggle with this area and to inadvertently alienate or frustrate their supervisors with repetitive questions, excessive talk about preferred topics, correcting the supervisor/insisting that they know the best way to do a job, hypersensitivity to feedback or criticism, or unintentional disrespect (e.g., laughing at the supervisor's mistakes, pointing out problems in front of the supervisor).

It is also important to fit in with the peer group of workers. Although it may be hard for individuals with AS to form close friendships with coworkers, it is important that they fit in and not alienate others. Basic skills such as going and receiving greetings, engaging in small talk, and following the rules of etiquette, as well as more difficult social skills such as sharing tools, compromising, and resolving conflicts, are important to being a good employee/team member and to not creating friction with others. Individuals who stand out because of poor social conduct are more vulnerable to teasing/bullying/scapegoating as well as to negative feedback from the supervisor (e.g., Shtayermman, 2007).

Behavioral challenges can also impede job success (Powers et al., 2011). Employers have little tolerance for any type of aggressive behavior (physical or verbal) and even high-performing employees will be severely disciplined or fired for this type of conduct. Similarly, emotional outbursts, tantrum-like episodes, or excessive arguing will jeopardize employment. Consequently, building strong self-regulation and behavioral control is essential to maintaining competitive employment for individuals with AS (e.g., Howlin, 2003).

Behavioral tendencies toward rigidity can also get in the way of employment success. Supervisors prefer workers who can respond to fluid conditions and follow changing instructions, rather than insist on a certain way of performing a task. A common example of this potential problem area involves perfectionistic employees with AS creating work outputs that meet an excessively high standard even when it takes long periods of time to complete. In many work situations, rapid completion that may not be "perfect" is what is required, and so taking the care and time to meet a higher standard becomes counterproductive (e.g., Hawkins, 2004).

In considering all of these challenges, the issue of disclosure and the extent to which the presence of a disability is evident plays a key role (e.g., Grandin & Duffy, 2004; Hawkins, 2004). When the AS is disclosed to management, the supervisor can be informed and trained with regard to the best ways to support and facilitate the work performance of the affected employee (e.g., Nesbitt, 2000). When social and communication challenges and atypical behaviors are evident to coworkers, they may demonstrate greater rejection or understanding. However, when the AS manifests in subtle ways, the individual may be misjudged as aloof, uncaring, or rejecting of others, and this misperception may lead to negative responses from others.

Assessment and Treatment Considerations for Employees with Asperger Syndrome

In recent years, there have been significant increases in vocational success for individuals with AS with some programs reporting high frequencies of success (e.g., Howlin, Alcock, & Burkin, 2005; Keel, Mesibov, & Woods, 1997; Hawkins, 2004). Several strategies have been found to be effective in addressing the problems of finding employment and work perfomance:

- Improving the fit between the job duties and the individual's skill profile.
- Disclosing the disability at the time of application for all but the highest functioning individuals with AS.
- Coordinating efforts with public and private agencies to utilize all available resources and access to disability-friendly employers.
- Working directly with employers, selling them on the strengths of employees with AS (e.g., reliability, consistency), and collaborating with them to develop positions that support the needs of the company and fit workers with AS.
- Extending periods of job coaching to allow full mastery of essential skills.
- Utilizing teaching methods that work with individuals with AS (e.g., high levels of repetition, using visual cues, chunking tasks).
- Teaching key social skills and hidden-curriculum aspects of the job.
- Using volunteer positions to develop basic vocational competencies and prepare for later paid employment.
- Teaching and rehearsing interview skills.
- Coaching grooming and hygiene skills.
- Searching when possible for positions that build on focal interests in order to maximize work motivation and satisfaction.

Although not exhaustive, this list provides a good starting point for initial assessment and placement activities, and will also facilitate ongoing evaluation of client progress when problems surface and troubleshooting is necessary.

DEVELOPING SOCIAL COMPETENCIES IN ADULTS WITH ASPERGER SYNDROME ACROSS THE LIFESPAN

Studies of social outcomes for adults with AS also reveal widespread challenges, with low incidences of friendships, dating relationships, and marriages. Although estimates vary and many of the investigations include individuals with ASD other than AS, as a whole, research consistently cites estimates of fewer than half of individuals having friendships (e.g., Howlin,

2003) and less than 25% being married (e.g., Howlin, 2003, 2005). Additionally, there are indications that relationships are generally less intimate, less strong, and less valued (e.g., Baron-Cohen & Wheelright, 2003). When considering the range of social and communication difficulties confronting individuals with AS, these outcomes are not surprising and point to the importance of social skills training and generalization throughout the lifespan (e.g., Baker, 2005; Bellini, 2006).

The primary social challenge for most adults with AS is to maintain their motivation to participate in social activities. For youngsters growing up with AS, social interactions are hard work and frequently frustrating. Developing their verbal and nonverbal communication skills, learning perspective taking, mastering the hidden curriculum, and figuring out social problem solving require a considerable effort. Furthermore, individuals with AS may encounter high levels of teasing, bullying, and rejection. As a result, when entering the adult world, where one is not forced into the highly social school environment, many individuals with AS choose to withdraw and engage in solitary pursuits such as playing videogames, using the Internet, or watching movies and television. In many cases, when parents or others provide financial support and daily room and board, the bulk of the individual's time is spent in these self-soothing pursuits, often related to focal interests.

The social challenges seen with adults with AS start with difficulties accessing social opportunities. They may not know where and when to find peers with whom they can share activities. In social situations, they often struggle with initiation and approach skills (e.g., Klin et al., 2005). They may demonstrate atypical behaviors that cause them to stand out and not fit in and may unintentionally alienate others because of poor conversation skills, repetitive questions, inappropriate comments, or violations of interpersonal boundaries (e.g., Attwood, 2007; Klin et al., 2005). Without necessarily intending to, they violate social conventions and appear to be out of step with what is going on around them. Their rigid adherence to rules and the truth can lead them to be overly pedantic, to point out misinformation, or to try to correct misbehavior that is within the social norms (e.g., Attwood, 2007).

As adults, individuals with AS continue to be vulnerable to being taken advantage of by others in social situations (e.g., Allen et al., 2007; Shtayerman, 2007). They often stand out as "different" and so present themselves as a target to predators. They are often willing to give things away or to engage in inappropriate behavior out of their wish to have friends or be part of a social group. They may not be aware that they are being financially exploited, that their rights are being disrespected, that they are being set up to commit inappropriate acts, or that they are being ridiculed by others.

For those individuals who master the hidden curriculum and develop reasonably good conversational skills, the challenge may not be only with social participation, but with going beyond forming acquaintances to building real friendships and dating relationships. Many individuals in this group experience intense frustration and sadness as they see relationships forming around them, but they cannot successfully build or experience this level of intimacy and interpersonal relatedness. They may desperately wish to have a girlfriend/boyfriend or even a spouse, but they cannot manage the intimacy and emotional sharing that accompany this type of bond (e.g., Attwood, 2007; Baron-Cohen & Wheelright, 2003). This is not to say that satisfying dating and marital relationships are not possible. In some cases, partners can build a relationship that works for them, even with the social challenges of AS. Often, when the spouse of an individual with AS understands the diagnosis, it allows him or her to understand what to expect from the partner and how to best respond to him or her (e.g., Attwood, 2007; Holliday Willey, 2001).

Sexuality plays a central role in the formation of dating and marital relationships, and it is another challenging component of social functioning with AS. Although there has not been a large body of research in this area, there are indications that individuals with AS experience sexual development and interests similar to the population at large and engage in masturbation as well as sexual exploration with partners at close to expected levels (e.g., Henault, 2006). However, the difficulties with perspective taking, self-concept, and behavioral rigidities can lead to inappropriate behaviors and challenges to marital sexual relations (Stokes & Kaur, 2005; Ray, Marks, & Bray-Garretson, 2004). Individuals with AS may also experience their gender identity and sexual orientation in unique ways (e.g., Galucci, Hackerman, & Schmidt, 2005; Ray et al., 2004). For example, seeking out gender reassignment without sufficient understanding and insight as to the consequences of this action, or experiencing arousal toward cartoon characters, animals, or objects.

For many, it is difficult to integrate sexuality into their relationships with potential partners because of the social processing challenges or the lack of available partners. The other person may be seen as a source of sexual pleasure without the context of romance, pursuit and response, or committed love. This narrow view leads the individual with AS to violate the rules and expectations of courtship. Because the social challenges of dating are so difficult, some adults with AS may direct their sexual interests toward pornography, obsessive sexualized interests or activities, or interactions with people on the internet or over the telephone (e.g., Haskins & Silva, 2006; Henault, 2006). These variations provide a higher level of structure and reduce demands for nonverbal communication, emotional sharing, and intimacy. In this context, women with AS may be particularly at risk, having multiple partners without attendant intimate or affectionate relationships (Henault, 2006).

The social challenges of AS can also lead to problems with the legal system. When approached by police or other authorities, communication challenges and rigid coping responses can make it difficult for individuals with AS to respond in the expected and appropriate manner (e.g., Deb-baudt, 2001). Officers may misinterpret their conduct as disrespectful, deceitful, or even dangerous, leading to situations in which people are unnecessarily arrested. Similar difficulties may then play out in the court-room, with judges and attorneys misunderstanding the individual and his or her disability. Recent efforts to educate first responders, attorneys, and judges have yielded some progress in this regard.

There are times when behavior without criminal intent results in the arrest of individuals with AS (e.g., Allen et al., 2007; Haskins & Silva, 2006). Sexual curiosity and drive (along with a lack of appropriate chan-nels for sexual expression and interaction) can lead individuals with AS to explore websites with child pornography without understanding the criminal and predatory context. They can be drawn into online sexualized communication with underage children and adolescents without perceiv-ing how old the person really is. Furthermore, social challenges leave indi-viduals with AS vulnerable to charges of inappropriately touching others or stalking when they are attracted or develop a crush on a person, but do not know how to appropriately initiate social contact.

The rigidity and lack of social judgment associated with AS also put individuals in legal jeopardy in situations where they respond to perceived injustices or unfairness with threats or violence. Although they may not have the means to carry out the threat, individuals with AS may not under-stand the social ramifications of their behavior and how the target of the threat and legal authorities will respond to it. Of course, individuals with dysregulation challenges that result in episodes of aggressive behavior are also at risk for arrest and criminal charges. The aggressive conduct that was managed, or even tolerated, in school and at home when the individual was a minor is viewed differently in adult settings and can lead to incar-ceration rather than school suspension or a loss of privileges.

Establishing Social Competency

The key to social success for individuals with AS is to start early and emphasize social skill development throughout the years of childhood and adolescence. There is a growing literature on interventions for youngsters with AS (e.g., Baker, 2003; Bellini, 2006; Dunn, 2006). Focusing on these competencies so essential to functional independence is particularly impor-tant during the high school years (see below). Building a foundation of skills in social initiation, conversation, perspective taking, reading social context, understanding the hidden curriculum, and social problem solving is essential to success as an adult. However, although teaching the skills is important, it is just as important to provide social opportunities in which people can practice and generalize these skills. Without appropriately structured social opportunities, the skills are not maintained and social motivation is lost.

Whereas these efforts during childhood and adolescence are vital to building a foundation of social competence, it is just as important to realize that social development continues into the adult years. During the young-adult period, it is helpful to continue the efforts at training and generalizing social skills. It is usually more difficult to access resources in this regard and to form a team such as is found during the school years. But, drawing from state programs, clinicians (e.g., psychologists, MFT therapists, social workers, counselors, speech therapists, behavior analysts), clinical agencies, as well as family and community resources (e.g., religious groups, clubs, recreational leagues), the process of building social competence continues.

The ultimate goal of these interventions is to provide the highest level of social skills so that the individual can access and enjoy as much social participation, friendships, and dating relationships as he or she chooses. It is important to add here that even for those who do not want a lot of social involvement, the social competencies remain crucial because they are central to functional independence. To function on your own in the community, the individual must be able to interact effectively with service personnel, merchants, workers in recreational settings, neighbors, and first responders.

INDEPENDENT LIVING

The concept of independent living actually falls along a continuum from full independence to needing around-the-clock care and supervision, with key components of independence including taking care of hygiene and health care, keeping oneself safe, managing money, establishing one's own residence, and getting around in the community. Individuals with AS struggle in these areas, with investigations showing a majority living with parents or in care settings and requiring help with adaptive skills (e.g., Howlin, 2003; Klin et al., 2005; Shea & Mesibov, 2005). There is a wide range of outcomes in this context, with some fully independent and self-supporting individuals with AS as well as many requiring high levels of care and support. This picture reflects, in part, the preference of many families to have adult children with AS live with them, under their care. This allows the parents to support and protect the individual in the way that they feel is most appropriate, but in time ultimately leads to situations when the parents are no longer able to care for the adult and other family members or community institutions must intervene.

Independence presents a range of challenges to individuals with AS. Hygiene and self-care may be impeded by problems with sequencing and following through with the steps of a task, and sensory-processing issues can make bathing, shaving, or brushing teeth quite aversive. The choice and care of clothing is another area of challenge. The lack of social perception, self-monitoring, and perspective taking can leave individuals with AS unaware and uncaring about how they appear or if they have an odor. As they go through adolescence and need to take more responsibility for their health, executive functioning deficits, limited social referencing, and poor self-monitoring can make it hard for them to follow through with health prevention activities, to know who to turn to for health care when something is wrong, and how to communicate what is wrong. Parents often have to manage the access to health care into adulthood, and adults with AS may require support from a health care advocate throughout their lives.

Independence also means keeping oneself safe from a range of dangers in the social and physical environments. Individuals with AS may struggle with mastering the basics of safety that come seemingly automatically to typical youngsters, including how to interact safely with sharp knives and hot ovens, how to lock up homes and cars, walk or drive in traffic, or respond to house fires, power outages, and dangerous weather events. They are vulnerable to being taken advantage of by predatory and antisocial people as well as by aggressive salesmen and abusive neighbors. In this age, there is a new set of hazards associated with the Internet and telecommunications, with safety rules about giving out information and interacting with people online. People with AS can be particularly vulnerable to making missteps in this area. Keeping safe also means knowing how to notify and interact with first responders and, as noted above, this can be difficult for individuals with AS.

Managing one's financial resources is another key component to functional independence. Problems with executive functioning, social judgment, and mathematical computation can impact skills in this area, from safely carrying money and counting change when making a purchase, to being able to comparison shop and get what is needed at the best possible price. A number of higher-order competencies requiring judgment, reasoning, and planning are difficult with AS and include budgeting, managing checking/savings accounts, and investing financial assets. Knowing where to get help and whom to trust with these processes can be daunting for individuals with AS. Long-term management of personal wealth can be further complicated by the need to establish a special needs trust or other arrangements to use assets while also qualifying for public health insurance and other programs.

Housing is a particular challenge for individuals with AS; recent surveys find that only about a third of adults with AS are living in their own residence (e.g., Howlin, 2003). Multiple factors contribute to this picture. Being financially self-sufficient is a major obstacle, as is having the ability to maintain and manage a residence (e.g., knowing what to do when the power goes out, cutting the grass, fixing broken appliances, cleaning house). Safety considerations, as noted above, also play a part in these challenges. To live in one's own place of residence one must know what to do when a stranger comes to the door, how to lock the home and make it secure, how to practice fire safety, and much more. A number of skills related to diet also must be considered, such as cooking and grocery shopping. These too can be difficult for individuals with AS. The possibility of accessing a residence that will work for adults with AS is also impeded by a lack of available housing that is affordably priced, in safe neighborhoods, accessible to public transportation, and near a shopping district (Resnick, 2009).

A final aspect of independent living concerns accessing the community. Many individuals with AS are not able to safely drive a car, an important restriction in many geographical areas. Being able to use mass transit requires a set of skills (e.g., knowing the routes and schedules, how to pay, managing transfers, where to sit, and how to act during transit) that are often difficult for adults with AS, but can be taught and mastered with practice. Being able to walk long distances or ride a bicycle also helps in this regard, if the person knows the area and is able to navigate his or her way around.

Community access also includes knowing how to find recreational facilities (e.g., restaurants, bowling alleys, community centers), gain admission and arrange payment, and master the social conventions associated with the various settings. In today's world, it also requires competence with communication technology such as phones, computers, and the Internet. The communication, cognitive, behavioral, and social challenges associated with AS can undermine the individual's ability to master these skills and ultimately participate in the community.

Strategies to Build Independence

Building independence for adults with AS requires careful assessment of each individual's skills and adapting effective teaching strategies to help him or her develop as many needed competencies as possible (e.g., Baker, 2005). For many, cognitive, behavioral, or social challenges will reduce the extent to which they can be independent, and so the goal becomes to find ways to provide needed supports while allowing for as much autonomy as possible. In other cases, their motivation may be limited, and copious support provided by their family puts them in a position where they do not need to be independent, and so long-term dependence results.

For those individuals who are motivated to become more independent or for those whose family/support system is pushing for more independence, the process becomes one of identifying needed skills, applying effective ways to teach the skills, and providing opportunities to practice and generalize their skills. This process entails establishing enough support that the individual can be successful in the situation and then systematically fading or removing the supports to build greater independence. Ideally, this process starts in early childhood and continues past the age of majority or when typical peers are leaving home and becoming independent. For most individuals, great steps forward toward independence occur during their 20s and 30s.

Key strategies to this process include starting in childhood and then building the focus on transition in early adolescence, assessing the competence of the individual and prioritizing the skills that are most needed to allow functional competence. This focus usually means deemphasizing academic objectives and putting more efforts into building social skills, adaptive daily living skills, and community-based competencies. There is a group of functional skills related to communication, social interaction, and problem solving that are central to success across the domains—independent living, vocational success, community participation, and forming friendships. These need to be emphasized.

As noted earlier in this chapter, the importance of generalization cannot be overstated (Hume et al., 2009). Generalizing presents a critical learning challenge for individuals with AS and will obstruct independence if skills are not applied across different settings: at home, at work, and in the community. Generalization can be addressed by using coaching in the actual environment, be it in the workplace or a community setting.

Prompt dependency is another learning challenge that must be taken into consideration (e.g., Hume et al., 2009). Individuals with AS will often master skills but then only demonstrate them with a cue from teachers or others. Throughout the school years, we noted earlier that it is essential that instructors aggressively address this area by fading prompts and supports as they are no longer needed and to reinforce truly independent performance of learned skills. When working with adults with AS, coaches and teachers need to monitor the amount of verbal prompting they provide and utilize visual/gestural tools as a way to fully fade the supports being used by individuals.

Perhaps the greatest obstacle to building independence in adults is motivation. If the individual is overwhelmed by a lifetime of frustration, rejection, and perceived failure, taking a supportive, engaging approach with him or her is important. In these cases, one must proceed slowly and ensure successful experiences by limiting the degree of challenge, providing a lot of praise and acceptance, and building enjoyment into all activities. The key is to help the individual realize that being independent gives him or her more control, a greater feeling of mastery, and access to a wider range of desired activities.

Alternately, for individuals who are in a situation where there are receiving everything they need from their family (i.e., room and board, access to entertainment and recreation), with few demands being placed on them, the objective becomes to make them uncomfortable by requiring greater independence in order to have access to preferred activities. Taking on the challenges of independence can be hard work and very anxiety provoking. If you are receiving everything you need, then it is understandable that you would not be motivated to learn new skills or try new experiences.

Finally, facilitating independence also requires community advocacy to help build acceptance for individuals with AS (and other disabilities) and open doors to social, recreational, housing, and vocational opportunities. Helping the public understand individuals with AS can lead to greater acceptance and less intolerance in the community, while reducing scapegoating or negative treatment. It can help to establish more affordable housing that fits the needs of individuals with AS, transit systems that are accessible to people with AS, and jobs that can be successfully performed by individuals with AS.

FAMILY CONSIDERATIONS

We all dream about our children's future lives, about whether they will be happily and gainfully employed, sustain committed relationships, and contribute to their community in meaningful and fulfilling ways. For parents of a child with AS these dreams are often accompanied by anxieties about whether any or all of these hopes could be meaningfully achieved. As importantly, many parents worry about what will become of their sons and daughters if they cannot meet these goals. While the diversity of presentation in AS makes it impossible to say with certainty what any one person can or cannot reasonably achieve, we should always consider those (sibling's) issues that parents (or siblings) will likely confront as they seek to optimize their child's future. In this section we discuss the issues families face, the developmental gains needed to launch the person with AS into adulthood, and the relationships and dilemmas of confronting this disability in the age of majority.

Parents who have guided their child with AS successfully for 18 or 21 years typically have much to celebrate, though often with a sense of fatigue. In the best scenario, the sense of shared accomplishment and recognition of new opportunities for their child's continuing growth and development attenuates the fatigue while leaving parental motivation intact. In its worst form, however, parents have experienced the trauma of burnout and have altered their expectations for their child's future, feeling more bitterness than accomplishment, and looking more pessimistically toward the future. Several issues consistently arise for families experiencing either end of this continuum, as well as for those in between. We discuss these briefly here.

Whether families are close partners or distant participants in their child's care, later adolescence and young adulthood bring with them a shift in case management, planning, and intervention from the family to external agencies, including community service providers, social service agencies, state departments of vocational rehabilitation, etc. For the family accustomed to an active role in decision making, this shift can be concerning and even traumatic. For the disengaged family, it can lead to relief (and sometimes further disengagement) or to abrogation of parental responsibilities. Thankfully, the responses of many families fall in between these poles. The critical consideration in this instance is to effect a balance between participation—at whatever level the family and child find functional—and independence. A second important consideration, however, is finding the right people and services in those external agencies and learning both to work with them and to advocate within them. This latter point requires a clear and objective understanding of the needs of the person with AS, as well as diplomacy and transparency on the part of everyone engaged in the process. Many parents have become accustomed to working on a daily or weekly basis with their child's school team to address needs and advance opportunities. Transferring some of that control and decreasing one's participation can be difficult at times. Other families participated less frequently and may be unable to reengage with providers to their now-adult child. Both types of families benefit from an active process of interaction that focuses on shared goal setting and participation on the part of the person with AS, his or her family, and the providers.

The attainment of legal majority brings with it certain rights and responsibilities. Although it is true that many with AS continue to rely on the judgment and wisdom of others in planning for their community, vocational, medical, and financial needs, in a legal sense there is a presumption of greater independence unless determined otherwise. As a result, there is the presumption of increased participation by the person with AS in personal decision making across a number of domains. Hopefully, this evolving independence has been considered—and taught—over a long period of time. In such a case, the leap is not a great one. However, when the person with AS achieves a majority age and there is no compelling rationale for assigned guardianship or conservatorship, personal choices and decisions may be at odds with the prevailing opinion of parents and school or agency staff. The best "cure" for such a scenario, obviously, is an ongoing collaborative and transparent working relationship whereby the student with AS is taught to recognize options and make good decisions (and to explicitly recognize and avoid bad ones), and to do so in a collaborative manner with trusted friends, family, and caregivers. This complex process comes neither automatically nor with fluency to those with AS, however. Problem solving and decision making must be identified as pivotal skills and taught from an early age. Attempting to begin this instruction as the adolescent nears the end of his or her minority status or transitions out of school and into adulthood is nearly always fraught with problems.

Launching a child into the world can be daunting for anyone, but especially so for parents who perceive (correctly or incorrectly) that their child is less equipped socially or emotionally to do so. When coupled with a long history of guidance and interdependence, "letting go" can be a hard thing to do for families unless viewed in a planful, gradual, and transparent manner. In the final analysis, persons with AS need to separate from their families in a healthy way, shedding the role of the child of parents, becoming instead the adult child of parents. (We write this approaching a major family holiday with personal recognition of just how hard this is to do for those with neurotypical conditions!) This healthy separation promotes the emotional development of the individual with AS as an entity in his or her own right, and not as an adult person who must forever rely on the guidance and opinions of others to proceed to the next decision.

TASKS THAT FACILITATE A SMOOTH LAUNCH INTO ADULTHOOD

As families prepare to launch their adolescent or young adult into adulthood, we have found it useful to emphasize several developmental tasks. These have been discussed elsewhere in detail (Powers & Bruey, 1988; Powers, 2002) and are summarized below.

Supporting Empowerment of the Person with Asperger Syndrome and His or Her Family

The tasks of early childhood include empowering parents to understand, teach, and advocate for their child. With emerging adulthood, however, comes the need to redefine that role to incorporate the person with AS into the role of self-advocate. Empowerment is a direct benefit of equality in the client–parent–professional partnership. Family members and professionals working with them must work to develop services and responses to special client needs that enhance the status and dignity of the individual with AS as well as his or her family.

Supporting a Healthy Response to the Diagnosis

Although the age of first diagnosis of AS varies widely, once established it is important to place this information in its proper context both for the family and for the individuals themselves. An accurate diagnosis is useful for understanding signs and symptoms and for highlighting certain potential future symptoms that may become problematic, such as an anxiety disorder (White, Ollendick, Scahill, Oswald, & Albano, 2009) or right-hemisphere learning challenges (Klin, Volkmar, Sparrow, Cicchetti, & Rourke, 1995). The diagnosis is also a heuristic, a kind of shorthand for understanding information-processing assets and weaknesses that help to differentiate the range of needs that may be common to, or discrepant from, those with other ASD. When a diagnosis of AS becomes a justification for attention to certain social needs that may be less evident to the uninitiated observer, it promotes better advocacy to address those needs. When it becomes an excuse used to restrict learning opportunities, it fails on all counts. The individual with AS and the family sometimes walk a fine line in supporting independence without creating unwitting dependence, but the solution to the problem lies partly in creating an objective understanding of how the symptoms of AS affect a particular person and his or her family, and partly in moving intervention efforts forward in a steady, progressive manner to achieve a criterion of ultimate functioning that is relevant to the person with AS. This process requires knowledge, objectivity, and transparency.

Supporting Service Access and Coordination

Just as each change in a family's life cycle brings with it new needs and opportunities for the person with AS (see Harris, 1982, 1983, and Harris & Powers, 1984, for a thoughtful discussion of the family life cycle in ASD), the shift into adulthood brings with it the need to identify or create services without benefit of post-21 years of age entitlement programs. School-age children with AS have a basic mechanism for accessing a wide range of needed services through their educational programs and the mandates of the Individuals with Disabilities Education Act (IDEA). No such mandate exists for those who have left the educational system, and locating services of any kind, much less those that understand and respect the needs of someone with AS, can be daunting. The importance of service access, service utilization, and service coordination cannot be overemphasized. Given the important problems with executive functions experienced by many with AS, however, locating and coordinating such services can itself be a significant problem. For these tasks it is often helpful to have a community mentor, coach, or support person who helps to keep priorities organized and emphasized. Such a person can make the difference between a successful employment and community living experience and one that is a failure. Both of us have worked with an individual, now 50 years of age, who is advanced educationally (holding two master's degrees) but who has had a consistent history of underemployment due to his social deficits. The addition of a community mentor/coach to his support team has helped him make significant improvements with his employment stability and to his quality of life outside of work by both preparing him for expectations in new environments and by preparing the new employment setting for his needs and highlighting his assets. Although many parents continue to serve this function by default, the goal of greater independence as an adult may be better served by shifting this task away from parents and onto the individual with AS and appropriate support persons.

Supporting Structural Balance within the Family System

The needs of a person with AS can place excessive demands on both individual family members and also on the various subsystems within the family. For example, one parent may historically have assumed primary responsibility for all aspects of service access and intervention planning, or a particular sibling may have been expected to function as a surrogate parent through his or her time in the family household (Harris, 1983). Although it is not possible to speak of an "ideal family" as it pertains to

AS, it would seem important that certain family structures be supported. These include the maintenance of role boundaries between parental and sibling subsystems, and the maintenance of a balanced relationship within the marital system.

With the evolving adulthood of the person with AS, structural balance may be challenged by the advancing age of parents or the mobility of siblings and lack of frequent contact with them. One of us (M. D. P.) has worked for many years with a middle-age man who earlier in his life relied on his widowed mother for nearly all important decisions (a role she relished, to be fair), but with her advancing age and significant health concerns, this man has now experienced something of a role reversal. He is now required to manage the household, respond to his mother's increasingly frequent health emergencies, and attempt to maintain a job to support the family. Not surprisingly, he has developed more acute symptoms of stress and anxiety. Only by providing additional organizational support and care for his mother has this situation improved. Because there is a dearth of research on those with ASD who are aging into middle and later adulthood, we are often left with the incomplete solution of doing the best we can, but without clear guidelines for practice or care. As the bubble of newly identified young children with ASD moves through adolescence and adulthood into middle and old age over the next 30+ years, we continue to ignore these issues at our peril.

Supporting Functional Forms of Family Organization

Irrespective of its source, added stress can lead to the establishment of dysfunctional forms of behavior in the nuclear and extended family of a person with AS. Family members, friends, and community service providers should be aware of several potential forms of family dysfunction and be prepared to address them. These include:

• Cross-generational coalitions, whereby members of different subsystems work against a common good for the person with AS, by joining forces to advance a particular position of another member. For example, a father and the grandparents of the person with AS advance the position that the individual with AS is simply being lazy at work, or failing to work hard enough on the job, as a way of explaining the serial employment terminations of the person with AS.

• Conflict between the parents on issues unrelated to AS may lead to disagreement or inconsistency in the treatment sought or offered to the person with AS. This dynamic may infiltrate into conversations with community supports, employers, and others in a position to advance the opportunities of the individual with AS, only to reduce those opportunities.

• Sibling subsystem dysfunction may occur because of role diffusion (the evolution of a "parentified child" in the sibling group, as noted earlier), whereby one sibling assumes the role of first among equals with the person with AS, effectively shutting out other family members who are important stakeholders. Or, following many long years of subjugation to the needs of the sibling with AS as primary, siblings may have disengaged from the family, effectively leaving aging parents and others to serve as primary stakeholders in the care of their brother or sister with AS.

Supporting the Development and Maintenance of Social Networks

Insularity and isolation are not uncommon in families of a person with a developmental disability. Although the availability of social media and networking sites has opened the world of information and mutual support to many parents and individuals with AS alike, few would disagree that a social life comprised of interactions with a computer screen would lead to more adaptive personal, social, and vocational functioning in the longer term. The emerging adult with AS needs to establish and maintain social networks that are fulfilling and that expand opportunities for social advancement in the community. Later in this chapter, we discuss these networks and relationships in greater detail. All are particularly important, but also socially risky.

With AS we often have the opportunity to evolve social opportunities through areas of expertise or interest. These interests can be the opening to a relationship or activity network, but sustaining a relationship requires a more complex set of coping strategies, flexibility of thinking and action, and motivation. These efforts necessarily *cannot* begin as adolescence nears an end, but must be incorporated into the earliest phases of instruction. Embedded instruction in natural environments, ensuring mastery and generalization of social coping skills, and providing early instruction and practice in social perspective taking all will support later competencies. The goal is to prevent the development of insularity as a lifestyle choice, and to position the person with AS, and his or her stakeholders, in such a way that new opportunities to expand socially can build upon older, successful ones.

ADULTHOOD AT THE CROSSROADS: WHERE INDEPENDENCE, COMPETENCY, AND INTERDEPENDENCE MEET

For most individuals with AS who enter adulthood, uncertainty is common. Where transition planning, postsecondary learning, and community supports have been maximized, some will move forward into a job or career, but often with more challenges and impediments to full participation than their nondisabled peers. However, as noted later in this chapter, the percentage of those who do manage to live independently and who maintain typical adult activities and relationships is relatively small. Many parents, siblings, and extended family members find themselves in some role of guidance or oversight, if not responsibility, for an individual with AS in early adulthood. The issue of conservatorship is sometimes raised, in the service of determining whether an individual with AS will be able to make decisions about health, finances, and daily events and needs in a way that will support greater independence and prevent risk or exposure to harm. Estate planning and the question of creating a special needs trust may come up (although hopefully, it has been resolved much earlier). Allocation of parental estates and the competency of an adult sibling with AS to make sound long-term decisions when faced with a sudden financial windfall can stress even the most caring and cohesive of families. Recognizing that the age of majority occurs for most people regardless of a diagnosis of AS, it appears wise to assess needs and intervene proactively when a child is young, then adjust expectations up or down in the face of experience and demonstrated competencies. For the person with AS who has considerable cognitive and academic prowess, the need for teachers and even sometimes parents to anticipate such issues appears foreign. But whereas the "hard" or technical skill is often a precondition of getting a job interview, it is the "soft," interpersonal skills that win the interview and hold the job. Instruction in these skills from an early age certainly appears prudent if we are to maximize success for those with AS.

THERAPEUTIC INTERVENTIONS WITH OLDER ADOLESCENTS AND ADULTS WITH ASPERGER SYNDROME

Individuals with AS, like any other person who may be experiencing problems in living or adaptive coping, sometimes benefit from therapeutic supports of a more formal nature. These experiences can be delivered in individual, group, or family formats depending on the needs and resources of the person and significant others. In nearly all cases, however, the conduct of the intervention must specifically address the information-processing strengths and weaknesses of the person with AS, and work explicitly toward problem resolution with subsequent insight to follow, rather than emphasizing deeper insight initially that then leads to problem understanding and resolution. In this section we discuss three formats: individual treatment, group-based interventions, and behavioral family therapy. Given the scope of this chapter our focus is necessarily more descriptive than comprehensive in nature, but important elements of each approach are addressed.

Throughout this discussion, several themes are evident, often present as a dynamic tension during intervention. These include (1) knowing the difference between caregiving and caretaking; (2) balancing the well-informed best interest of the individual with AS in relation to the new rights as an adult who, in many circumstances, is the legal holder of privilege; (3) dealing with significant problems with social judgment even as other cognitive and academic abilities surpass the normative peer group;

and (4) addressing that age-old question: Do children ever grow up in the eyes of their parents?

Individual Treatment

Given the learning and information-processing assets and weaknesses of those with AS, there is a clear need for individual therapy or counseling to be problem-focused, structured, and to define explicitly the relationship between treatment goals and their component steps. Further, the context of treatment and the need to plan and program explicitly for generalization become prominent considerations. Finally, because of lack of social insight, the tendency toward more literal black-and-white thinking, and problems with the accurate perception and regulation of emotions are common among those with AS, explicit work on social perspective taking, social coping skills development, and the fluent demonstration of those skills in nontherapeutic settings all are critical treatment objectives. Traditional insight-oriented, reflective models of therapy have enjoyed less success than more objective cognitive-behavioral models. A brief introduction to the use of cognitive-behavioral models of therapy with those with AS follows.

Cognitive-behavioral therapy (CBT) has been identified as an evidence-based procedure for children and adults with a wide range of difficulties, including anxiety disorders (Ollendick, King, & Chorpita, 2006), OCD (Piacentini & Langley, 2004), conduct disorders (Kendall, Reber, McLeer, Epps, & Ronan, 1990), and tic disorders (Woods, 2001). An expanding body of research has also demonstrated the utility of this approach to treat individuals with ASD (White et al., 2009; Wood et al., 2009; Lehmkuhl, Storch, Bodfish, & Geftken, 2008). With children and adolescents who do not have developmental disabilities, there are numerous well-designed assessment and treatment approaches available (see Kazdin, 2004, for a comprehensive review). Indeed, CBT is mandated in residency training in child and adolescent psychiatry in the United States (Albano, 2005). The particular features of ASD make these treatment strategies broadly viable, but they do require modification to address the individual needs of the client and the presenting problem. Given the relatively small but well-done research literature available currently, it is most reasonable to describe CBT with individuals with AS as a very promising approach, warranting use and ongoing research.

CBT is based upon the premise that a person's *interpretation* of events, in combination with the event itself, influences behavior and psychological distress. It follows, then, that it is important to modify not only overt behaviors, but also cognitions about the event itself as one component of changing thoughts and behavior associated with the distress caused by the event. As a treatment modality, CBT is firmly grounded in learning theory and experimental psychology, and places a significant emphasis on the empirical validation of treatment effects and ongoing data-driven decision

making throughout treatment, as well as on the generalization and maintenance of treatment effects.

There are several components to treatment based upon CBT, including (1) active client participation with treatment strategy implementation;
(2) homework for the client to complete on an ongoing basis; (3) rigorous
outcome evaluation of intervention strategies and subsequent modification
of treatment procedures if the intervention is not successful; (4) a focus on
symptom presentation as it affects daily functioning; (5) an emphasis on
short-term treatment that allows for opportunities to practice new strategies in natural environments while incorporating these new behaviors into
a more consistent response repertoire; and (6) active efforts at training for
generalization, maintenance, and relapse prevention (Friedman, Thase, &
Wright, 2003).

Several authors have incorporated these basic components into a modified treatment format that addresses the neurocognitive assets and deficits of AS, including problems with empathy and social perspective taking,
cognitive distortions, and dysfunctional beliefs (Attwood, 2004; Chalfant,
Rapee, & Carroll, 2007; Sze & Wood, 2007; White et al., 2009). Some have
been oriented to more single-component, individual intervention activities (e.g., Attwood, 2004), whereas others have adopted a multicomponent
integrated treatment approach incorporating individual treatment, parent
education, and group practice (e.g., White et al., 2009). In all cases, treatment has emphasized the importance of providing affective education (to
facilitate understanding of emotions and emotional regulation), cognitive
restructuring (to identify and confront dysfunctional beliefs and replace
them with more accurate and functional thoughts and actions), guided
practice opportunities (to promote generalization and maintenance), and
the incorporation of relevant stakeholders (parents, teachers) into different
phases of treatment implementation. Attwood (2004) has elaborated on a
particular rubric termed the *emotional toolbox* as a means of conceptualizing and understanding the needs and compensatory assets to be used with
people with AS during CBT efforts. This rubric stresses the importance of
using tools (and icons representing them) as a means of helping individuals with AS to recall and resolve difficult situations. Physical tools represent activities that serve to release energy, whereas relaxation tools support
arousal reduction and self-calming. Social tools address social misperceptions through mediation by others who can provide more accurate and more
adaptive social responses to challenging situations. Thinking tools aim to
use logic to address misunderstandings and misinterpretations, and special-
interest tools recognize the function of many circumscribed interests (e.g.,
arousal and stress reduction) and seek to incorporate the individual's special interest into a more adaptive format that engenders social engagement.

White and her colleagues (2009) have examined the effects of a more
broad-based intervention approach in treating anxiety and phobias in adolescents with AS. Their manualized, time-limited approach incorporated

the elements contained in Atwood's rubric but more specifically included evidence-based practices for the treatment of childhood anxiety disorders and social deficits associated with AS concurrently. Their results indicated greater success with treatment of anxiety than in developing sustained and generalized social repertoires. Although promising, these findings are preliminary and highlight the critical need for additional research into this important area.

The emerging research literature on the use of CBT in treating those with AS enjoys the advantage of utilizing well-established treatment parameters for particular comorbid conditions (e.g., generalized anxiety disorder) with a concurrent robust research literature on the social, affective, and neuropsychological challenges faced by those with AS. Incorporating these two research foundations into evidence-based clinical practice is the opportunity and challenge ahead, but one that shows every promise of being achieved.

Group Interventions

Group-based interventions are a valuable tool for helping adults with AS (e.g., Baker, 2003; Bellini, 2006; Hillier, Fish, Cloppert, & Beversdorf, 2007). The group format creates a forum for teaching skills, practicing interpersonal behaviors with other group members, and even forming real friendships. The group brings a cost-effective delivery of instruction and intervention with the opportunity for direct interactions with, and feedback from, other group members.

Groups can be conducted in a wide range of ways. Some are more highly structured and psychoeducational, whereas others may be more free-flowing and process-oriented. Individuals with AS are usually best served in more structured groups that have a clear instructional approach. They do best in groups that maintain a predictable, consistent format, with communication adapted to their level, and few demands for emotional processing and perspective taking (areas of challenge for them).

There are two general types of groups. Some are led by a trained provider (e.g., psychologist, social worker, speech therapist, counselor) who provides instruction and facilitates practice through exercises and structured activities. These groups usually follow a curriculum drawn from published resources (e.g., Baker, 2003; Bellini, 2006; Garcia Winner, 2000) yet tailored to the group. Others are activity groups without a structured approach to learning and a stronger emphasis on enjoyable interaction and participation in activities. Some of these groups may be led by individuals with AS who share their unique expertise with the group. With both types of groups, it is essential to create an environment that works for these individuals, with communication they can follow, instruction they can apply, fellow members they trust and like, and activities that are enjoyable.

The group sessions should be challenging and instructive, but they must also provide an accessible social environment for the participants. The complexity and pacing of communication should not be too challenging. The level of social demands (e.g., related to perspective taking, hidden-curriculum rules) should not overwhelm group members. There should be a mood of acceptance and warmth, with a good use of humor. To support the motivation of group members, enjoyment and having fun need to be one of the group objectives. The experience of attending group should be associated with a positive context (i.e., building skills, making friends, having fun) rather than negative connotations of having problems, not being liked, or not fitting in. Most of all, the group room must be a safe place where members are free from teasing or antagonism, and where they can be vulnerable and truly talk about their experiences without fear of being denigrated or judged. Any teasing or unsupportive conduct should be addressed immediately so that members know that the group is indeed a safe place. Care should be taken when encountering the use of sarcasm and more pointed types of humor to ensure the protection of members' feelings.

The size of the group may vary from two or three members to large groups. It is important to design the group so that there is enough time for all the members to accomplish the group objectives. For a group that lasts an hour, it is difficult to provide enough practice and speaking opportunities for more than five or six members. With a larger group, members can withdraw and remain passive bystanders rather than active learners. There are advantages and drawbacks to any size group. In smaller groups, more intensive coaching and practice are possible. But larger groups are needed to allow members to role-play many social situations or help members to experience a range of interactions in the room.

When forming groups, it is important to find members that share similar social skills objectives. This commonality makes it easier to address most group members with instruction and activities. A group with members who present widely varying functional levels and objectives allows only some of the participants to be reached at any one time and the others get bored or feel overwhelmed. Some variation in this regard can be advantageous as some group members emerge as leaders and teachers. But too wide a gap in the needs of group members and participants question why they are in the room with the others.

The dynamics of the group will vary depending on whether both genders are present. With men and women, there is the opportunity to practice interactions with the opposite sex and to get direct feedback across gender. However, in groups with only one gender, there is greater opportunity to comfortably discuss issues related to sexuality in detail. In many cases, there are many more referrals of men, and so a group may contain just a woman or two. In such situations, it is very important to set clear rules about what can be discussed, ensure a respectful attitude among group members, and check in with the female participants to see if they are comfortable.

Groups may also include individuals with other ASD diagnoses, or even individuals with anxiety and communication disorders. This combination usually works well if the social skills objectives are consistent and the level of functioning similar. However, it is important to exclude individuals who act out in negative ways toward peers. Their inclusion would undermine the safety of the group, and much time and effort that should be directed at teaching social skills would be spent on setting limits and repairing negative interactions.

Groups utilize a wide range of formats and activities. Still, there are four components that should always be included to varying degrees. First, conversation skills are of prime importance to social and communication success. Although they may be challenging to work on, they need to take a high priority during group sessions. Some form of structured discussion or conversational practice is essential. Depending on the skill level of the group, this could mean unstructured group conversation, discussion with the facilitator guiding turn taking and rules, conversational exercises working with partners or in triads, or discussions with scripting support.

Second, teaching objectives should be addressed through didactic presentations and exercises. Building from social skills curricula and guided by the skill needs presented by group members, there should be instruction addressing topics, specific skills (e.g., topic maintenance, modulating voice volume, using gestures), or challenging situations (e.g., phone invitations, making social bids in the work setting, holiday practices). This instruction should utilize strategies known to be effective with individuals with AS (e.g., repetition, chunking, visuals) and should be followed by practice exercises involving role playing, rehearsal, and/or video feedback.

As noted above, it is essential to include enjoyment and fun as objectives for the group to promote motivation. In this light, there should be regular inclusion of games or other enjoyable activities. Games should be chosen to encourage members to use and practice social skills while having fun. Games such as charades or Pictionary, which require communication and perspective taking, are very effective toward this end. Games where the focus is on game-based strategy and analysis, such as chess or Scrabble, provide less social practice and should be avoided.

Finally, the group should always include strategies that promote the generalization of skills from the group setting to the outside world. The easiest way to do this is through homework assignments (e.g., to make an invitation, sit with someone at lunch, attend a club meeting). In some situations, more ambitious efforts may include working with family members and community providers to identify generalization opportunities and structure situations to allow application of group-learned skills in the community. For example, a young man attending college was doing well in classes but avoiding all social contacts with peers. In the group, he was working on learning how to engage in small talk. We were able to collaborate with the college's Disability Services Office and arrange for a peer mentor in one of the young man's classes to approach him and elicit conversation.

Family Therapy

Individuals with AS exist within the context of many environments, including the school, community, and vocational settings. None, however, is more important than their family. Whereas parent training and education have been long considered an essential component to the treatment of those with AS, the needs of, and treatment for, the family as a system have not been well represented in the literature.

In many regards, family needs can be best conceptualized structurally, with specific attention to the various systems and subsystems that typically exist (for a more comprehensive description, see Harris, 1983 and Haley, 1976). For example, the parental (or marital) subsystem is traditionally invested with certain roles and functions, including care and protection, guidance to the children, imparting social norms and expectations, providing appropriate models for behavior, and demonstrating effective and appropriate coping skills and conflict resolution strategies. The sibling subsystem is invested with the task of nurturing one another, providing hierarchical guidance (e.g., older children provide models for younger siblings), and providing a cohesive unit to balance the group itself in light of the structural demands of the parents (e.g., as when one sibling advocates for another to the parents). Intergenerational subsystems may be present as well, including grandparents, aunts and uncles, older cousins, etc. In addition, subsystems can become more fluid and dynamic, as when family structure changes through divorce or death and stepparents or stepbrothers and -sisters enter the family. Each subsystem can exert functional or dysfunctional control over the person with AS, and can contribute to success or failure of a well-designed intervention plan.

There is no ideal family structure, although certain forms of family organization can better support adaptive functioning. Structural balance between and within subsystems is important. For example, an overbearing, authoritarian spouse can diminish the role of the other parent in both the marital subsystem and also with the children. Similarly, a sibling who takes on inordinate parental responsibilities, effectively becoming a "parentified child," can disrupt the relationship among the sibling group, but also within the parental subsystem. A child with ASD in the family can increase the likelihood of system and subsystem imbalance and possible dysfunction in some vulnerable families, but does not necessarily do so (Harris & Powers, 1984). It is important for the clinician working with the family of an adolescent or young adult with AS to recognize this potential impact, assess for it as appropriate, and consider these factors when planning, implementing, and evaluating treatment efforts.

The position in the life cycle of the family of an individual with AS can also be considered. Different phases of the life cycle of a family are typically associated with different developmental tasks and challenges. For example, as a child with ASD reaches adolescence, many parents report fatigue and discouragement associated with a less-than-expected pace of progress, ongoing difficulties with school programs, or disruptive behavior that may become more prominent. As well, families sometimes become more acutely aware of the discrepancies between their child with AS and those of friends or family who do not have AS. The child with AS who continues to be socially isolated and preoccupied with a circumscribed interest stands in stark contrast to children of friends and neighbors who are dating, attending social functions, and broadening their interests in a more developmentally anticipated manner.

With the transition into adulthood, parents not only see the distinctions more acutely, but are more likely to confront "ultimate" questions. These include worries about their own mortality, who will advocate and care for their son or daughter with AS if they are no longer able to do so, financial security for their child, and employment and living arrangements that may or may not be available. These concerns can contribute to a renewed sense of urgency for some families, prompting energized advocacy and planning. For others, however, these worries can be overwhelming and lead to disengagement. It is incumbent upon the clinician working with families to appreciate not only the needs of the individual with AS, but the abilities and needs of the family of that child in selecting socially valid treatment goals, intervention strategies, and outcomes. Harris and Powers (1984) and Powers and Bruey (1988) discuss these considerations in greater detail.

HIGH SCHOOL PROGRAMMING
TO SUPPORT SUCCESS IN ADULTHOOD

Over recent years, educational systems have improved their ability to understand AS, recognize it in students, and provide appropriate programs. One area of particular challenge in this regard is the schools' approach to the transition to adulthood (Baker, 2005). Although emphasis is placed on helping students with AS succeed in the high school environment—that is, achieve academic objectives and minimize disruptive behaviors—schools often overlook preparing the student for life after high school, be it at college, in vocational training, or on a job. Academic goals, even those that might not relate to post-high school activities, are addressed and supports are given through the resource room or a paraprofessional; success is measured by the student's successful completion of the academic program of study. At the same time, the student's ability to become independent, function in the community, survive in a college dorm, or succeed in a job is overlooked.

AS carries with it developmental challenges related to a number of functions that are essential to adult independence. These include executive functions (e.g., initiating a series of steps to solve a problem, organizing information, making and following a plan), social skills (e.g., forming friendships, negotiating with people in the community, establishing relations with a supervisor and coworkers), and self-care abilities (e.g., maintaining hygiene, managing health care). Neurotypical students develop most of these skills (more or less) on their own through the normal developmental process and grow into independent adults without the need for explicit school-based interventions. However, the presence of AS means that without specific skill teaching and generalization, the capacity for independence will be restricted. Consequently, an appropriate educational program needs to teach these skills (social, adaptive, vocational) to prepare students with AS for independent living and community participation (e.g., Connecticut Interagency Transition Task Force, 2004).

A valuable tool in these endeavors is a person-centered planning process using a "futures planning" format that brings together all the people who know the individual well (including the person with AS, as well as family, friends, providers, and school team) to inventory his or her strengths, weaknesses, and aspirations for the future. Participants then consider short- and long-term goals and plan steps to reach them. With the wide range of strengths and weaknesses found with AS, the path to independence can follow many different routes, depending on the person. This type of meeting helps to create an individualized plan going forward that incorporates the person's profile of strengths as well as his or her aspirations.

Considering this type of plan, the school team must look beyond academics to identify those skills that are needed for success in the adult, postsecondary environment. It may mean changing priorities and passing over higher-level academic classes to allow more time for social and adaptive skill training. Or it may lead to adding time to the high school program and taking additional years to complete it.

The high school curriculum should address the challenges discussed above. Social skills should take on an increased focus with groups addressing the skills involved in reciprocal conversation, social bids, friendship formation, and social conventions. Adaptive skills should be taught as needed, including hygiene/grooming, domestic skills (e.g., cooking, cleaning), home maintenance, time management, money skills, and safety practices. And in both of these areas, teachers must include generalization strategies to ensure that the skills will be used in the actual settings. Generalization requires actual community-based experiences with shopping, participating in recreational activities, and using utilities. Care should be taken to assess, on an ongoing basis, the degree to which the student needs prompts or supports to demonstrate these skills, and efforts should be made to fade prompts and build truly autonomous skills.

Vocational programming is another essential component to the high school program. Even for those students who have the skills and motivation to go to college (see Brown & Wolf, Chapter 11, this volume), basic vocational skills may be lacking and later lead to problems with getting and holding a job, even after receiving a college or graduate degree. Vocational programming should start with assessments of interests and skills to help guide the process of choosing a vocational direction. Following this assessment, students with AS benefit from direct experiences with jobs and work settings, with instruction in basic vocational skills provided in the setting by a job coach. These skills include communicating with a supervisor and coworkers, asking for help, dressing and grooming appropriately, following directions, and problem solving. Although short-term internships or "job shadows" are a good first step, students with AS often require longer time periods and opportunities to practice operations in order to learn and master the skills they need. Consequently, extended work placements and internships are often recommended.

High school programming will vary widely depending on the needs of the individual. For some college-bound students with minimal levels of challenge related to the AS, there may just be the need to assess these key functional skills and provide minimal facilitation and teaching. For others with severe challenges, the adaptive, social, and vocational aspects become the primary components to the program. In any case, the school team should graduate the student with AS with the best possible range of skills in these areas and the ability to use these skills independently in the actual settings where they are needed.

DEVELOPING COORDINATED SYSTEMS OF CARE TO SUPPORT INDIVIDUALS

One particular challenge for people working to help adults with AS is the difficulty of coordinating care among a disparate group of providers, family members, and community supporters. When the individual is in the school system, there is usually a team approach with school personnel working together, meeting and communicating with the family and community providers. This team approach is much harder to enact (but still worth the effort) after graduation from high school because the resources and organizational structure of the school are absent.

As the numbers of adults with AS increases, a new type of approach is emerging in various parts of the country, addressing this challenge through the establishment of a coordinated care program. By drawing together the resources and providers under the umbrella of a single agency, it is possible to better coordinate care, monitor progress, identify challenges, and make the most efficient use of resources. Some of these programs are residential, with adults living in apartments with supports and provided with classes, job internships, and college placement (Gerhardt, 2009). This type of model offers an intensive approach with around-the-clock support as needed, yet brings with it high costs and generalization challenges as the individual transitions back to the community.

There are also community-based programs designed around a coordinated care model emerging in a number of states. One example is the Pilot Program for Individuals with Autism Spectrum Disorders in Connecticut. The pilot program started providing services in September of 2006 and now serves approximately 50 clients with AS and other ASD in two counties. The program's model emphasizes client-centered planning and community-based services. Participants and their families meet with program staff to identify objectives and plan the range of services that are needed. Core services include case management, community-based life skills coaching, community mentoring, job development/coaching (through the Connecticut Bureau of Rehabilitation Services), and social skills training. Clinical services, including occupational therapy and speech therapy, are also provided as needed.

Among other areas, clients work on skills related to self-care (e.g., hygiene, diet/weight, exercise), domestic skills (e.g., cooking, cleaning, organizing materials), college skills (e.g., multitasking, talking in class), vocational skills (e.g., communicating with supervisor, following directions), social skills (e.g., friendship formation, perspective taking), communication (e.g., reciprocal conversation, nonverbal communication), and community-based skills (e.g., riding mass transit, shopping). Instruction is provided in the community, on the job site, and in the home by life skills coaches, utilizing instructional strategies effective with individuals with ASD. The amount of instruction varies, depending on the client's needs and motivation, and could be as little as an hour or 2 per week, to 15–20 hours per week.

Community mentors help clients gain comfort in leaving the home setting and joining the community and social activities while generalizing the skills that they are learning. Most of the participants attend weekly social skills groups addressing the key social skills with which they are struggling. The structure of the program provides a case manager who coordinates the range of services and regular meetings among coaches, mentors, social skills group facilitators, and the program staff.

Initial assessment of the program shows some promising results with more participants working and experiencing greater job satisfaction, increases in ratings of independent behavior, family-reported progress on individual goals, and cost-effective delivery of services (Robison, Reed, Shugrue, Kleppinger, & Gruman, 2008).

FUTURE DIRECTIONS

There is much that we know about the needs of those with AS as they transition through adolescence into adulthood, but there is much more that is less well understood. For example, we have some, but unfortunately not many, studies of how those with AS fare later in adulthood. We assume (correctly or incorrectly) that earlier intervention efforts to teach various communication, social, adaptive, and coping skills generalize and are maintained in ever-expanding novel family, social, and vocational environments. Research on the development and maintenance of self-advocacy skills in adults is sparse. Given the finding that the majority of those with a diagnosis of AS are likely to be underemployed as adults, we have few outcome studies of the effect of intervention to address this issue and reverse the trend. Are those with AS who are identified before ages 18–21 more likely to experience better long-term outcomes than those identified later in adulthood? We have only anecdotal reports to rely on, surely not the stuff of good science. Concerning AS and aging, we know little about intervention success in promoting long-term health and health maintenance, management of chronic health problems (e.g., diabetes or cardiovascular disease) by those with AS, or strategies to support those with AS in accessing health care providers for routine or critical care needs. Finally, with the general population of all citizens living longer, we know virtually nothing about how to help those with AS support *their* aging or infirm parents toward the end of their lives. This responsibility is arising more frequently for those without a developmental disability. Will the cognitively and vocationally capable middle-age person with AS fare as well with this situation as his or her neurotypical peers? While we hope so, we also recognize that there are inherent social-processing deficits in AS that may preclude the most successful outcomes.

The lack of research available today to answer these questions is less troubling to us than the opportunity before us. AS has a long past, but a short history. Considering that we have come to better understand the needs and abilities of those with the condition only in the past 30 years, we know quite a lot. The knowledge we have acquired, however, is the impetus for developing an even better understanding of strategies that will help us develop better educational programs, postsecondary learning opportunities, vocational experiences, and better participation in the warp and weft of family and community life. That is both the challenge and the opportunity. Given the remarkable talents and abilities of those with AS, we would do well to embrace the task of expanding with enthusiasm.

REFERENCES

Albano, A. (2005). Cognitive-behavioral psychology for children and adolescents. In B. Saddock & V. Sadock (Eds.), *Comprehensive Textbook of Psychiatry,* (8th ed., Vol. 2, pp. 3332–3342). Philadelphia: Lippincott Williams & Wilkins.

Allen, D., Evans, C., Hider, A., Hawkins, S., Peckett, H., & Morgan, H. (2007). Offending behavior in adults with Asperger syndrome. *Journal of Autism and Developmental Disorders, 38,* 748–758.

American Psychiatric Association. (2013). *Diagnostic and statistical manual of mental disorders* (5th ed.). Arlington, VA: Author.

Attwood, T. (2004). Cognitive behaviour therapy for children and adults with Asperger's syndrome. *Behaviour Change, 21*(3), 147–161.

Attwood, T. (2007). *The complete guide to Asperger's syndrome.* London: Jessica Kingsley.

Baker, J. E. (2003). *Social skills training for children and adolescents with Asperger syndrome and social-communication problems.* Shawnee Mission, KS: Autism Asperger Publishing Company.

Baker, J. E. (2005). *Preparing for life: The complete guide for transitioning to adulthood for those with autism and Asperger's syndrome.* Arlington, TX: Future Horizons.

Baranek, G. T., Wakeford, L., & David, F. (2008). Understanding, assessing, and treating sensory–motor issues. In K. Chawarsksa, A. Klin, & F. Volkmar (Eds.), *Autism spectrum disorders in infants and toddlers* (pp. 104–140). New York: Guilford.

Baron-Cohen, S. (1995). *Mindblindness: An essay on autism and theory of mind.* Cambridge, MA: MIT Press.

Baron-Cohen, S., & Wheelright, S. (2003). The friendship questionnaire: An investigation of adults with Asperger syndrome or high-functioning autism and normal sex differences. *Journal of Autism and Developmental Disorders, 33*(5), 509–517.

Bellini, S. (2006). *Building social relationships: A systematic approach to teaching social interaction skills to children and adolescents with autism spectrum disorders and other social difficulties.* Shawnee Mission, KS: Autism Asperger Publishing Company.

Chalfant, A., Rapee, R., & Carroll, L. (2007). Treating anxiety disorders in children with high-functioning autism spectrum disorders: A controlled trial. *Journal of Autism and Developmental Disorders, 37*, 1842–1857.

Chorpita, B. F. (2007). *Modular cognitive-behavioral therapy for childhood anxiety disorders.* New York: Guilford Press.

Connecticut Interagency Transition Task Force. (2004). *Connecticut's transition training manual and resource directory.* Hartford: Connecticut Department of Education.

Debbaudt, D. (2001). *Autism, advocates, and law enforcement professionals: Recognizing and reducing risk situations for people with autism spectrum disorders.* London: Jessica Kingsley.

Doehring, P., & Winterling, V. (2011). The implementation of evidence-based practices in public schools. In B. Reichow, P. Doehring, D. V. Cicchetti, & F. R. Volkmar (Eds.), *Evidence-based practices and treatments for children with autism* (pp. 343–363). New York: Springer.

Dunn, M. A. (2006). *S.O.S. social skills in our schools: A social skills program for children including pervasive developmental disorders, high functioning autism and Asperger syndrome, and their typical peers.* Shawnee Mission, KS: Autism Asperger Publishing Company.

Eren, R. B., & Bruckner, P. O. (2011). Practicing evidence-based practices. In B. Reichow, P. Doehring, D. V. Cicchetti, & F. R. Volkmar (Eds.). *Evidence-based practices and treatments for children with autism* (pp. 309–326). New York: Springer.

Fast, Y. (2004). *Employment for individuals with Asperger syndrome or non-verbal learning disability: Stories and strategies.* London: Jessica Kingsley.

Friedman, E. S., Thase, M. E., & Wright J. H. (2003). *Cognitive and behavioral therapies.* New York: Wiley.

Galucci, G., Hackerman, F., & Schmidt, C. W. (2005). Gender identity disorder in an adult male with Asperger's syndrome. *Sexuality and Disability, 23*(1), 35–40.

Garcia Winner, M. (2000). *Inside out: What makes a person with cognitive deficits tick?* San Jose, CA: Author.

Gaus, V. L. (2007). *Cognitive-behavioral therapy for adult Asperger syndrome.* New York: Guilford Press.

Gerhardt, P. F. (2009). *The current state of services for adults with autism.* New York: New York Center for Autism.

Ghaziuddin, M., Wieder-Mikhail, W., & Ghaziuddin, N. (1988). Comorbidity of Asperger syndrome: A preliminary report. *Journal of Intellectual Disability Research, 42,* 279–283.

Grandin, T., & Duffy, K. (2004). *Developing talents: Careers for individuals with Asperger syndrome and high functioning autism.* Shawnee Mission, KS: Autism Asperger Publishing Company.

Gray, C. (1988). Social Stories and comic strip conversations with students with Asperger syndrome and high-functioning autism. In E. Schopler, G. B. Mesibov, & L. J. Kunce (Eds.), *Asperger syndrome or high-functioning autism?* (pp. 167–198). New York: Plenum Press.

Haley, J. (1976). *Problem-solving therapy.* San Francisco: Jossey-Bass.

Hare, D. J., & Paine, C. (1977). Developing cognitive behavioural treatments for people with Asperger's syndrome. *Clinical Psychology Forum, 110,* 5–8.

Harris, S. L. (1982). A family systems approach to behavioral training with parents of autistic children. *Child and Family Behavior Therapy, 4,* 21–35.

Harris, S. L. (1983). *Families of the developmentally disabled.* Elmsford, NY: Pergamon Press.

Harris, S. L., & Powers, M. D. (1984). Behavior therapists look at the impact of an autistic child on the family system. In E. Schopler & G. Mesibov (Eds.), *The effects of autism on the family* (pp. 207–274). New York: Plenum Press.

Haskins, B. G., & Silva, J. A. (2006). Asperger's disorder and criminal behavior: Forensic–psychiatric considerations. *Journal of the American Academy of Psychiatry and the Law, 34,* 374–384.

Hawkins, G. (2004). *How to find work that works for people with Asperger syndrome.* London: Jessica Kingsley.

Henault, I. (2006). *Asperger's syndrome and sexuality: From adolescence through adulthood.* London: Jessica Kingsley.

Hillier, A., Fish, T., Cloppert, P., & Beversdorf, D. Q. (2007). Outcomes of a social and vocational skills support group for adolescents and young adults on the autism spectrum. *Focus on Autism and Other Developmental Disabilities, 22*(2), 107–115.

Holliday Willey, L. (2001). *Asperger syndrome in the family: Redefining normal.* London: Jessica Kingsley.

Horner, R. H., Dunlap, G., & Koegel, R. L. (1988). *Generalization and maintenance: Life-style changes in applied settings.* Baltimore: Brookes.

Howlin, P. (2003). Longer term educational and employment outcomes. In M. Prior

(Ed.), *Learning and behavior problems in Asperger syndrome* (pp. 269–293). New York: Guilford Press.

Howlin, P. (2005). Outcomes in autism spectrum disorders. In F. R. Volkmar, R. Paul, A. Klin, & D. Cohen (Eds.), *Handbook of autism and pervasive developmental disorders* (pp. 201–220). Hoboken, NJ: Wiley.

Howlin, P., Alcock, J., & Burkin, C. (2005). An eight-year follow-up of a specialist supported employment service for high ability adults with autism or Asperger syndrome. *Autism, 9*(5), 533–549.

Howlin, P., & Goode, S. (1998). Outcome in adult life for individuals with autism. In F. R. Volkmar (Ed.), *Autism and developmental disorders* (pp. 209–241). New York: Cambridge University Press.

Hume, K., Loftin, R., & Lantz, J. (2009). Increasing independence in autism spectrum disorders: A review of three focused interventions. *Journal of Autism and Developmental Disorders, 39,* 1329–1338.

Hurlbutt, K., & Chalmers, L. (2004). Employment and adults with Asperger's syndrome. *Focus on Autism and Other Developmental Disabilities, 19*(4), 215–222.

Kazdin, A. E. (2004). Cognitive-behavior modification. In J. M. Weiner & M. K. Dulcan (Eds.), *Textbook of child and adolescent psychiatry* (pp. 985–1006). Arlington, VA: American Psychiatric Association.

Keel, J. H., Mesibov, G., & Woods, A. V. (1997). TEACCH: Supported employment program. *Journal of Autism and Developmental Disorders, 27,* 3–10.

Kendall, P. C., Reber, M., McLeer, S., Epps, J., & Ronan, K. R. (1990). Cognitive behavioral treatment of conduct disordered children. *Cognitive Therapy and Research, 14,* 279–297.

Klin, A., McPartland, J., & Volkmar, F. (2005). Asperger syndrome. In F. R. Volkmar, R. Paul, A. Klin, & D. Cohen (Eds.), *Handbook of autism and pervasive developmental disorders* (pp. 88–125). Hoboken, NJ: Wiley.

Klin, A., Volkmar, F. R., Sparrow, S. S., Cicchetti, D. V., & Rourke, B. P. (1995). Validity and neuropsychological characteristics of Asperger syndrome. *Journal of Child Psychology and Psychiatry, 36*(7), 1127–1140.

Lehmkuhl, H. D., Storch, E. A., Bodfish, J. W., & Geftken, G. R. (2008). Brief report: Exposure and response prevention for obsessive compulsive disorder in a 12-year-old with autism. *Journal of Autism and Developmental Disorders, 38,* 977–981.

Maher, C. A., & Bennett, R. E. (1984). *Program planning and evaluation.* Englewood Cliffs, NJ: Prentice Hall.

Myles, B. S., Trautman, M. L., & Schelvan, R. L. (2004). *The hidden curriculum: Practical solutions for understanding unstated rules in social situations.* Shawnee Mission, KS: Autism Asperger Publishing Company.

Nesbitt, S. (2000). Why and why not?: Factors influencing employment for individuals with Asperger syndrome. *Autism, 4*(4), 357–369.

Ollendick, T. H., King, N. J., & Chorpita, B. F. (2006). Empirically supported treatments for children and adolescents. In P. C. Kendall (Ed.), *Child and adolescent therapy: Cognitive-behavioral procedures* (3rd ed., pp. 492–520). New York: Guilford Press.

Pennington, B. F., & Ozonoff, S. (1996). Executive functions and developmental psychopathology. *Journal of Child Psychology and Psychiatry Annual Research Review, 37,* 51–87.

Piacentini, J., & Langley, A. (2004). Cognitive behavior therapy for children with obsessive compulsive disorder. *In Session: Journal of Clinical Psychology, 60,* 1181–1194.

Powers, M. D. (2002). *Asperger syndrome and your child: A parent's guide.* New York: HarperCollins.

Powers, M. D., & Bruey, C. (1988). Treating the family system. In M. D. Powers (Ed.), *Expanding systems of service delivery for persons with developmental disabilities* (pp. 17–41). Baltimore: Brookes.

Powers, M. D., & Franks, C. M. (1988). Behavior therapy and the educative process. In J. Witt, S. Elliott, & F. Gresham (Eds.), *The handbook of behavior therapy in education* (pp. 3–36). New York: Plenum Press.

Powers, M. D., & Handleman, J. S. (1984). *Behavioral assessment of severe developmental disabilities.* Rockville, MD: Aspen.

Powers, M. D., Palmieri, M. J., D'Eramo, K. S., & Powers, K. M. (2011). Evidence-based treatment of behavioral excesses and deficits in individuals with autism spectrum disorders. In B. Reichow, P. Doehring, D. Cicchetti, & F. R. Volkmar (Eds.), *Evidence-based practices and treatmernts for children with autism* (pp. 55–92). New York: Springer.

Ray, F., Marks, C., & Bray-Garretson, H. (2004). Challenges to treating adolescents with Asperger's syndrome who are sexually abusive. *Sexual Addiction and Compulsivity, 11,* 265–285.

Reaven, J., & Hepburn, S. (2003). Cognitive-behavioral treatment of obsessive-compulsive disorder in a young child with Asperger syndrome. *Autism, 7,* 145–164.

Reichow, B., Doehring, P., Cicchetti, D. V., & Volkmar, F. R. (Eds.). (2011). *Evidence-based practices and treatments for children with autism.* New York: Springer.

Resnick, D. D. (2009). *Opening doors: A discussion of residential options for adults living with autism and related disorders.* Phoenix, AZ: Southwest Autism Research and Resource Center.

Robison, J., Reed, I., Shugrue, N., Kleppinger, A., & Gruman, C. (2008). *An evaluation of the Autism Pilot Program of the Division of Autism Services of the Department of Developmental Services.* Hartford: State of Connecticut.

Shea, V., & Mesibov, G. (2005). Adolescents and adults with autism. In F. R. Volkmar, R. Paul, A. Klin, & D. Cohen (Eds.), *Handbook of autism and pervasive developmental disorders* (pp. 288–311). Hoboken, NJ: Wiley.

Shriberg, L., Paul, R., McSweeney, J., Klin, A., Cohen, D., & Volkmar, F. (2001). Speech and prosody characteristics of adolescents and adults with high functioning autism and Asperger syndrome. *Journal of Speech, Language, and Hearing Research, 44,* 1097–1115.

Shtayermman, O. (2007). Peer victimization in adolescents and young adults diagnosed with Asperger's syndrome: A link to depressive symptomatology, anxiety symptomatology, and suicidal ideation. *Issues in Comprehensive Pediatric Nursing, 30,* 87–107.

Standifer, S. (2009). *Adult autism and employment: A guide for vocational rehabilitation professionals.* Columbia: University of Missouri School of Health Professions.

Stokes, M. A., & Kaur, A. (2005). High-functioning autism and sexuality: A parental perspective. *Autism, 9*(3), 266–289.

Sze, K. M., & Wood, J. J. (2007). Cognitive behavioral treatment of comorbid anxiety disorders and social difficulties in children with high-functioning autism: A case report. *Journal of Contemporary Psychotherapy, 37,* 133–143.

Tantam, D. (1991). Asperger's syndrome in adulthood. In U. Frith (Ed.), *Autism and Asperger syndrome* (pp. 147–183). Cambridge, UK: Cambridge University Press.

Tantam, D. (2003). The challenge of adolescents and adults with Asperger syndrome. *Child and Adolescent Psychiatric Clinics of North America, 12,* 143–163.

Volkmar, F. R., Lord, C., Klin, A., Schultz, R., & Cook, E. H. (2007). Autism and pervasive developmental disorders. In A. Martin & F. R. Volkmar (Eds.), *Lewis's child and adolescent psychiatry* (4th ed., pp. 384–400). Philadelphia: Lippincott, Williams & Wilkins.

White, S. W., Ollendick, T., Scahill, L., Oswald, D., & Albano, A. (2009). Preliminary efficacy of a cognitive-behavioral treatment program for anxious youth with autism spectrum disorders. *Journal of Autism and Developmental Disorders, 39,* 1652–1662.

Wood, J. J., Drahota, A., Sze, K., Har, K., Chiu, A., & Langer, D. A. (2009). Cognitive behavioral therapy for anxiety in children with autism spectrum disorders: A randomized, controlled trial. *Journal of Child Psychology and Psychiatry, 50*(3), 224–234.

Woods, D. W. (2001). Habit reversal treatment manual for tic disorders. In D. W. Woods & R. G. Miltenberger (Eds.), *Tic disorders, trichotillomania, and other repetitive behavior disorders: Behavioral approaches to analysis and treatment* (pp. 97–131). Norwell, MA, Kluwer Academic.

CHAPTER 11

Transition to Higher Education for Students with Autism Spectrum Disorder

Jane Thierfeld Brown
Lorraine Wolf

Asperger syndrome (AS) is a genetic neurodevelopmental disorder at the mildest end of the autism spectrum (Asperger, 1991; American Psychiatric Association, 1994). It carries the best prognosis for independent function in adulthood, as many individuals complete high school and college and go on to successful careers. Recent coverage in the popular press and national talk shows has highlighted the upsurge in the diagnosis of autism and related disorders, often harbingered at an "epidemic" level. Although the cause(s) remain unclear, there is no doubt that school districts are facing an increase in the numbers of students in this population. This increase has prompted many parents, schools, and medical and allied health professionals to deliver enhanced supports for youngsters with autism, enabling many to successfully navigate high school. Consequently, colleges and universities nationwide are also seeing a marked increase in the numbers of students who carry autism spectrum diagnoses, such as AS, and are often unsure of the best way to respond to their needs (Wolf & Thierfeld Brown, 2004).

Students with AS may be very advanced in terms of intelligence and academic ability. Yet these intellectually brilliant students struggle in the realm of higher education. Despite intellectual and academic gifts, persons with AS suffer from a marked inability to decipher the minds of others, to integrate many streams of incoming information, and to navigate an increasingly complex social world. Students may be rigid and perfectionistic, and resist changing to meet the demands of their environment. Often students with AS are naïve and can be easily victimized by others. As college students, they are challenged by deficits in social and interpersonal skills, organization, and self-advocacy. Yet these are the very skills that are essential for success in college and beyond (Wolf & Thierfeld Brown, 2007).

LIFE AFTER HIGH SCHOOL: THE TRANSITION PROCESS

For many families, impending graduation is cause for celebration and the beginning of the separation process for young adults to leave home. Families of children with autism spectrum disorders (ASD) have a very different road to travel in terms of planning and separation. Often that road is fraught with confusion, questions, and very few resources. It takes enormous effort, determination, and skill on the part of the student and the family to negotiate adolescence and the special education system to reach the college transition stage. To better understand the transition process and work together with families to make the best possible move, it is important for professionals working with prospective college students with ASD to understand the process that these families have undergone. It is important as well for postsecondary providers to understand the landscape of raising a child with disabilities so that they may be better prepared to assist with this key life phase.

WHERE HAVE FAMILIES BEEN?

The diagnostic process for an ASD is often complicated, fraught with misdiagnosis and misunderstanding. Many students are assigned multiple diagnoses prior to ASD. Often students have been diagnosed with an anxiety disorder (social anxiety or obsessive–compulsive disorder [OCD] most commonly; see Tantam, 2000), speech–language impairment, attention-deficit or attention-deficit/hyperactivity disorder (ADHD) (Ehlers et al., 1997), a nonverbal learning disorder (Klin et al., 1991), or a mood disorder (Tantam, 2000), to name but a few (see Gillberg & Billsted, 2000). Some families have pursued nonscientific assessments and treatments, including dietary or vitamin treatments. This multitude of diagnoses has kept families searching for treatment options and medical/psychological advice. Having secured a diagnosis, the parents must come to grips with the reality of an autistic disorder and all that it implies, often with little or no support in dealing with the long-term impact of the disability. Families often must find their own way in a maze of jargon and therapists, hoping to discover an optimal path for their child. Many families never truly accept the diagnosis and bring that anger and frustration to the college transition process for their child. Yet one of the best indicators of college success for a student with a disability is that the student understands and accepts his or her own disability. Clearly this cannot happen in the setting of parents who continue to fight the diagnosis.

Families and caregivers enter a confusing minefield of treatment options, but must also learn to secure necessary services for their child (medical, disability, educational). Many families have been frustrated with their school system, which could not more aptly assist their son or daughter. Students with ASD are often extremely bright and the academics have gone well for the most part. There are times that certain subjects have posed a particular challenge to the student with ASD. The larger concern in K–12 has been the social issues. A team has followed the student's progress and provided services that have assisted in social functioning in the K–12 setting. That team no longer exists in higher education.

Parents have learned to act as the main advocate and CEO of their child's education to this point. As mentioned above, this has often been a contentious relationship. Relinquishing that role and teaching the son or daughter with ASD to manage his or her life and education with proper assistance is a frightening proposition. It is imperative that parents, caregivers, physicians, and special education teams recognize that this teaching must begin early, certainly before the student's senior year and often in the face of strong resistance on the part of the student. Often parents do not see their child with ASD as ready to practice taking on these roles at age 14 or 15. However, the early teen years are the appropriate time to begin learning independence skills with parental guidance. Teens with ASD will need additional time to master the multiple skills necessary for living independently and succeeding in higher education. Because ASD is a developmental disability, we must assume that students are behind their typically developing peers.

WHERE ARE FAMILIES GOING?

Roles are changing for everyone in the family as the young person goes to college. Parents may have difficulty separating from their child with ASD in more ways than just the physical move from home. Entrusting a college student with the ability to make decisions that affect their education is difficult for parents of the most typical children, especially when the financial costs are so high. At $20,000 per semester at some private liberal arts schools, do parents really feel comfortable trusting that their students will understand the school's core requirements and will know which courses to take? Are they willing to risk the student's needing an extra semester of college? How does this translate to the student with ASD? Will the student call the advisor to make and keep appointments? Will the student understand the preregistration process well enough and ask questions in order to obtain the courses he or she needs? This is a tremendous task requiring adequate executive function and assumption of responsibility, two areas in which we know our students with ASD have trouble.

The student and his or her parents must grapple with the reality that the student now has certain legal rights and responsibilities. The student must become the CEO and learn to be his or her own self-advocate. For parents who have been accustomed to taking charge, with some degree of support from school districts, aides, therapists, and other caregivers, this transfer of power is enormous. Yet the student must assume this role as a function of the new legal framework in which he or she must learn to operate. The university considers that students over the age of majority are adults and expects that they behave as such. Accordingly, students now have rights to privacy (which often can exclude parental involvement) as well as the responsibility to comply with certain polices, procedures, and codes of conduct (academic and behavioral) that now govern many aspects of their experience.

As families move forward to higher education, different laws shift the focus from entitlement and remediation to protection from discrimination and equal access. Increasingly, students must be able to self-identify as a person with a disability and demonstrate that they are they qualified as a member of a protected group. Adult students must now take charge of their own education and their disability, which comes as a shock to many highly (sometimes overly) involved families who now find their function limited by the policies of the university. Families discover that documentation guidelines and the review processes for eligibility are more stringent, as the diagnosis alone is no longer the only criteria for services. Students may face, for the first time, a rejection for accommodations and services. This may be the case particularly when symptoms and impairment are relatively mild. Even when approved, families discover that services and accommodations are usually more limited than what they enjoyed in high school. For example, aides and social coaches are no longer typically provided by colleges and universities for qualified undergraduates (we return to this point later).

TYPICAL COLLEGE DEVELOPMENT

One of the most difficult aspects for professionals working with young adults with ASD to keep in mind is the developmental nature of the syndrome. Students may be intellectually superior; however, developmentally the same students may be significantly delayed. Thus the problem for families and professionals is to find an appropriate college or educational institution that will match students' intelligence and learning needs to their significant delays in other areas. As college-age students become more autonomous and independent, they typically develop skills that include exploring areas of individual competency, managing their emotions, developing more mature relationships, establishing their identity (including motivation and personal choice), and developing internal goals and a sense of purposes. These advances culminate in an adult identity, with a personal sense of integrity and system of values (adapted from Barkley, 1997; also see Wolf, 2001).

Few studies have examined milestones of adult development in persons with ASD. Yet we can understand how most of these areas would be extremely challenging for the student with ASD. In order to assist the student, time should be spent in the high school (and preferably middle school) years on developing some of these milestones. In higher education, it has been helpful to have assistance from a social skills group or a counselor. This individual provides resources and assists with the social and developmental delays experienced by the college student with ASD.

THE DIFFERENCE BETWEEN HIGH SCHOOL AND COLLEGE

In order to transition successfully, students must recognize the key differences between college and high school. Many are ill-prepared for the enormity of this leap. High school students are accustomed to 5 to 6 hours of class per day with 1–2 hours of homework. Quizzes are frequent and, most often, the tests are not cumulative. Teachers usually have 20–25 students in a class and form personal relationships with every student. Teaching content typically comes from textbooks, which can be reviewed to reinforce in-class learning. Most high schools are housed in one or two buildings with all classes taking place in that building. This is most certainly not the typical college scenario, however.

In stark contrast, when students move to higher education, they usually take four or five courses, plus labs and discussions. Classes may meet three to four times per week, with class lengths as much as 3 hours. Optimally, students will study 2 hours per day for each hour they spend in class (this estimate may be double for students with disabilities). Each class usually has two or three cumulative exams per semester. Classes are often taught through lecture, discussion, and seminar, not directly from the textbook. The books for classes now are resources, with lecture, independent primary source readings, and research reports as the main learning tools. Syllabi contain an entire semester's worth of readings, exams, and other course requirements. Often for the first time, good note taking becomes particularly important. Class size can be anywhere from 10 students for a seminar class to 400 for a survey course. Most often, students will have a combination of small and large classes in multiple buildings, depending on the size of the campus.

Cognitive and Academic Skills

Beginning college students with or without disabilities do require new and advanced skills that have not been drilled in high school. Little direct instruction in classroom preparation, deportment, and study strategies occurs in most high schools for typical students, let alone those with ASD. Yet many students will require additional instruction in how to prepare for, and interact in, the classroom. All students must be able to self-advocate with faculty, administration, and peers. This is an essential skill in order to survive and succeed in college. Excellent study habits are also crucial, along with advanced test-taking skills and strategies. Students must understand how to prepare in advance for class and figure out what to do to learn necessary material. They must understand that professors may deduct points for lateness or sloppiness, and that no one will call to remind them when their project is due. Thus executive function deficits are at issue as organization, time management, and classroom social rules become more important. Students need to understand the classroom culture and learn new ways to interact with faculty and peers. Some conventions, such as staying seated, not interrupting, or not raising one's hand may be particularly difficult for students with ASD to comply with. They must be able to negotiate successfully with professors and administrators. (See WNY Collegiate Consortium of Disability Advocates, Technology for Transition Project at the State University of New York at Buffalo; also see *www.ccdanet.org/ecp_index.html* for a list of major skills needed by beginning college students.)

College professors expect that students are mature thinkers and possess excellent reasoning skills. Thus such attributes as flexibility, categorical thinking, the ability to use logic and sequence, abstraction, inference, and insight are essential to success in a college. For example, it is no longer acceptable for students to use encyclopedias or web pages such as Wikipedia as primary reference sources. Students are now learning to think for themselves and to integrate multiple sources of information form lectures, readings, and independent thought to construct new ideas. Neuropsychologists refer to the term *executive function* when discussing some of these concepts. We return to this concept below.

THE LEGAL FRAMEWORK

The Individuals with Disabilities Education Act, Section 504 of the Rehabilitation Act of 1973, and the Americans with Disabilities Act

Families are typically unprepared for the fact that having achieved high school graduation, students with ASD now leave the familiar territory covered by the Individuals with Disabilities Education Act (IDEA) and enter the higher education realm of Section 504 of the Rehabilitation Act of 1973 and the Americans with Disabilities Act (ADA) of 1990 (see Macurdy &

Geetter, 2008, for a review). The differences are important for planning when a student should graduate from high school and what services are needed or possible once attending college. In our experience, failing to understand the legal framework of higher education is the source of most strife between the college student with a disability, his or her family, the evaluator, members of the professional team, and the college or University disability service providers. Physicians and other professionals can play a key role in educating the family before the fact.

There are many key differences between the special education laws (IDEA) and the disability statutes that protect college students with disabilities. We summarize some of these below.

Fundamentals of the Individuals with Disabilities Education Act

The IDEA (*http://idea.ed.gov*) is an education act that provides federal financial assistance to state and local education agencies to guarantee special education and related services to eligible children with disabilities. In general, the IDEA ensures that educational programs in public schools (K–12) provide "specifically designed instruction at no cost to the parents, to meet the unique needs of the child with a disability." Under the IDEA, children with disabilities are guaranteed a free and appropriate education in the least restrictive environment with an individualized program designed to meet their educational needs. One of the goals of the program is to remediate the student to a success level.

Eligibility

Under IDEA, students may become eligible for special education, accommodations, and related services by virtue of having been diagnosed with one of several prescribed medical or psychological conditions (ASD diagnoses are on this list). The school district is responsible for identifying and assessing children at risk for developing school-related difficulties, those with documented medical or other diagnoses, or those suspected of having disabilities (although this is changing with the recent reauthorization of IDEA; see *www.nichcy.org/reauth/index.html*). It is unclear how this will affect children with ASD. The criteria that mandate diagnosis and service can vary state by state and district to district. However, services are typically dependent on a combination of diagnosis and educational need. Parental involvement is mandatory, and parents must be notified of the school's plan or intent to evaluate their child.

The Individualized Education Plan

Once a student has been determined to have a disability, an individualized education plan (IEP) is developed by the special education team, which outlines the nature, timing, and setting for all services and accommodations for which the student is found entitled. The definition of disability under the IDEA is tied to eligibility for special education. This qualification also mandates review and reassessment by a multidisciplinary team at regular periods during the educational career of the child.

Parents must participate in the IEP process, and they have the right to bring an advocate to the team meeting if they wish. Parents can either sign the IEP if they approve of the plan or contest the plan. They may also call for another review of the student and the plan, should they disagree with any of the findings. For example, if the parents disagree with the diagnosis or feel that the proposed class setting is too restrictive, or if they feel that another school, district, or even private school would be more appropriate for their child, they can refuse the plan and call for a hearing. Parents have the right to ask for an independent evaluation outside of the school district, and they can ask the district to cover the costs of such evaluations (see Disability Rights and Education Defense Fund, *www.dredf.org*, for more information; also see Wrightslaw at *www.wrightslaw.com*).

Transition Planning

The child and the IEP goals must be reevaluated by the team at regular intervals to assess progress, continued eligibility, and to revise the plan if necessary. Most importantly for the college-bound student, the IDEA coverage extends only until high school graduation or age 21, whichever comes first (although this may vary in some states and for some conditions). The IEP language contains mandatory transition planning for all exiting students, including those who are college bound. Importantly, families and professionals must understand that the transition plan does not require students to be retested, which is often a source of confusion when students are asked for current documentation of disability when they arrive at college.

The 504 Plan

The 504 plan is a device used in many school districts to provide limited assistance to students who would not be eligible for special education services but Need/want accommodations. This includes students with ADHD and "other health-impaired" students whose diagnoses and needs do not fit the traditional special education definitions. Often this 504 status is used as the means by which exam accommodations (such as extra time or computers) can be provided to students. Parents are often led to believe that this accommodation will carry over to college, since colleges are mandated under Section 504. However, this is a misunderstanding on the part of evaluators and high schools that should not be communicated to the family, as they may lose the chance to mandate the district to conduct exit testing.

Section 504 of the Rehabilitation Act of 1973

Section 504 (*www.hhs.gov/ocr/504.pdf*) is a civil rights law that prohibits discrimination on the basis of disability in programs and activities, public and private, which receive federal financial assistance. Section 504a states that "no otherwise qualified individual with a disability in the United States, as defined in section 7(20), shall, solely by reason of her or his disability, be excluded from the participation in, be denied the benefits of, or be subjected to discrimination under any program or activity receiving Federal financial assistance or under any program or activity conducted by any Executive agency or by the United States Postal Service."

The Americans with Disabilities Act

Section 504 is paralleled in the ADA of 1990 (see *www.ada.gov*), a federal civil rights statute that also prohibits discrimination solely on the basis of disability. The ADA extends Section 504 to protect against discrimination for reasons related to disabilities in employment, education, public facilities (e.g., mandates for wheelchair ramps), and accommodations (see *www.ada.gov*). It applies to public and private entities that receive federal funds and thus covers accommodations in most colleges and universities.

Titles II and III of the ADA prohibit discrimination on the basis of disability in employment, government, public accommodations, commercial facilities, transportation, and telecommunications. It includes access to building and facilities, employment practices, self-evaluations, and grievances. The ADA also contains the language that guides the definition of disability for the purposes of accommodation and sets guidelines for who is eligible. It sets forth the obligations of the institution and the individual. These guidelines and the statutory language are vague enough to be open to interpretation—hence the frequent redefinition of the criteria by the courts (Macurdy & Geetter, 2008).

THE LAW IN HIGHER EDUCATION

Section 504 and the ADA both protect individuals with disabilities from discrimination. There is no funding associated with either. Both laws guide how institutions of higher education provide accommodations and services to level the playing field for students with disabilities. Students at this level must meet program requirements and be otherwise qualified to participate in the program in which they are enrolled. Accommodations are made without altering essential curriculum. Therefore, students must now fit the program, with accommodations that are determined by an outside agent (i.e., not the family) to be reasonable and appropriate. Often parents want to continue the special education entitlements into the college setting. Not only does the law not cover this, but the practice is counterproductive for the student who needs to develop independence and self-advocacy skills. (Further details regarding the differences between these laws can be found at *www.ccdanet.org/differenceschart.html*; also see *www.hhs.gov/ocr/504*.)

When young people with ASD transition to college under ADA and Section 504, the landscape changes dramatically. No longer is the school charged with identifying or assessing students to remediate their weaknesses. Rather, these laws are civil rights statutes that aim to protect persons with disabilities from discrimination in the workplace and in the educational environment. In brief, the formal definition of disability is "a physical or mental impairment that substantially limits one or more major life activities" that renders the individual "unable to perform a major life activity, or significantly restricted as to the condition, manner, or duration under which a major life activity can be performed, in comparison to the average person" (Section 504; ADA 1990; ADAAA, 2008).

This distinction is one of the cruxes of successful transition, as the student and the family must come to understand that the university no longer considers them to have a disability simply because they have been diagnosed with an ASD. Indeed, we often explain to frustrated parents and providers that having a diagnosis is not equivalent to being disabled within the meaning of the law. Thus, counterintuitive as most families find it, having a diagnosis of ASD does not equal having a disability in the absence of demonstration of significant functional limitation. This is sometimes an issue with higher-functioning students who do not actually qualify for accommodations when they enter college.

The core of ADA and Section 504 is self-disclosure of disability. Although students are not obligated to disclose their disability, if they are asking for accommodations or services, they must self-identify to the appropriate agency on campus (usually the disability services office) and explain their disability and the functional limitations (note that this must be done by the student, not the parents). Having disclosed their disability and provided documentation, their disability eligibility and the merits of their accommodation request are reviewed separately. In practical terms, this means that each accommodation is rereviewed without consideration of what was previously provided in high school.

Another distinction that is difficult for many families to understand is that students requesting accommodations in college must show that they are "otherwise qualified" to attend classes and complete required work (i.e., the academic standards of the university are enforced) and be able maintain appropriate behavioral standards (i.e., the university conduct codes are enforced). A final benchmark of being otherwise qualified is that students are expected to be able to advocate for themselves with the minimal level of assistance.

Documentation

Appropriate and current documentation validates services based on current level of function in an academic setting. The high school IEPs or 504 plans are insufficient documentation of a disability for the purposes of accommodations in college. Clear and specific evidence in the documentation that the disorder substantially limits one or more major life activities in an academic setting (usually learning) is very important in order to access services.

Students with ASD often arrive at this diagnosis only after multiple assessments. Therefore, it is not unusual for students to present the results of occupational therapy, speech and language, optometric, neurological, educational, psychological, neuropsychological, and/or psychiatric evaluations dating back to early childhood. Different assessment reports may have come to different conclusions, including diagnoses thought to be related to the autism spectrum (Williams, 1996). Most commonly, one or two of the above are presented (although all may be useful, especially comorbid psychiatric diagnoses such as ADHD, OCD, or depression). There is no gold standard for acceptable documentation, and formal guidelines have not yet been adopted for this disorder in the same fashion as for attention or learning disorders (see Educational Testing Services, *www.ets.org/disability* for examples of formal documentation guidelines for those conditions). Rather, most disability service offices deal with whatever documentation is available and reasonably current. Recall that the transition IEP no longer mandates testing, so families and professionals must determine together whether the student will require an update of documentation and plan for how that will be accomplished. In most cases, the disability services staff is happy to discuss this issue with prospective families.

We prefer that documentation of ASD be in the form of a current, comprehensive neuropsychological evaluation that is tailored toward elucidating areas of functional impairment. Students with AS are typically quite bright and do not evidence "classic" learning disabilities. Thus testing must go beyond the standard psychoeducational assessment to pinpoint specific areas of weakness that may require accommodation. For example, the need for a note taker or clarification of exam answers may not be clear without additional testing that targets oral listening skills, working memory, or written language organization. Additional documentation by a psychiatrist is often useful to better understand a student's reactions to stress, mitigating measures in terms of anxiety reduction, depression, and so forth. Accordingly, we have developed guidelines for ASD that are being considered by the major testing agencies.

It is imperative that families and professionals understand that provision of documentation of the current condition is only the first step in establishing eligibility for reasonable and appropriate accommodations. Recall that a diagnosis does not necessarily equate with disability, and that the disability services officer will make a determination that a student is a qualified student with a disability. In the same fashion, a disability does not guarantee a particular accommodation. Accommodations are determined by the disability services professional and not by a team as they were in high school. Accommodations are individually determined based on the functional limitations of the particular disability. Just because a student requests, for example, to have his or her exams scribed does not mean that this accommodation will be provided. The disability officer may determine, among a range of effective accommodations, which one will be provided (we discuss this area further below). Finally, families and providers must understand that individual accommodations do not guarantee success, and that equal access under the law means that some students will succeed and some will fail.

University Rights and Responsibilities

Under Section 504/ADA, a college or university must provide the qualified student with a disability with equal access to all educational programs, services, facilities, and activities. The university must also provide reasonable accommodations, academic adjustments, and/or auxiliary aids and services to eligible persons with disabilities. The university or college is also responsible for maintaining student confidentiality as far as the disability is concerned, and must establish and maintain written policies and procedures (including procedures for filing grievances).

In addition to the university's responsibilities, the educational institutions also hold rights. Universities have the right to maintain academic standards, integrity and freedom, and to determine the fundamental requirements of their individual courses and programs. Fundamental requirements are essential aspects of a course or program that do not need to be altered or modified for a student with a disability. One example might be a math or foreign language requirement in a liberal arts course of study. Once this fundamental requirement has been established (following the legal guidelines for such determination, *Wynne v. Tufts University School of Medicine*, 1991; also see Macurdy & Geetter, 2008), the college or university would not need to waive or modify the requirement as an accommodation for a student with a disability, even if the student had demonstrated that he or she would benefit from such an adjustment. Universities also have the right to maintain and enforce conduct codes without regard to a student's disability as a mitigating factor (unlike public schools, which often cannot discipline unless the disability is taken into account).

With regard to accommodations, the university may determine what is reasonable and appropriate and select among effective alternatives. This means that despite the student's request for a note taker, the university may determine that another alternative would be reasonable and appropriate (such as audiotaping lectures). Finally, the university may deny unreasonable or inappropriate accommodation requests. An accommodation request is considered unreasonable when the accommodation would confer an unfair advantage on the student receiving the adjustment; pose an undue burden on the agency being asked to provide the accommodation; compromise the academic integrity of academic standards of a course, degree, or program; or fundamentally alter the nature of a course, examination, or program of study (see *Southeastern Community College v. Davis*, 1979, where the Supreme Court determined that colleges and universities are not required to make changes to program standards that can be demonstrated to be fundamental or essential to the program of study; also see Macurdy & Geetter, 2008).

Student Rights and Responsibilities

Under the law, students with disabilities have the right to equal access to all university programs and activities, including equal access to all educational activities. Other rights that the universities must recognize include the right to receive effective, appropriate, and reasonable accommodations. This is often the first point of intersection between the student and the university, as the student and/or family contact the university to arrange accommodations for tests or in residence halls. Unlike high school, students must engage in an interactive process with the disability services office in requesting and monitoring their accommodations.

Of course, along with student rights come the student responsibilities. Students are ultimately responsible for self-disclosing their disability to the designated entity on campus. Failure to do so means that the university is not obligated to recognize the student as having a disability or to offer the legal protection which that affords. Self-disclosure also includes providing documentation of disability in compliance with campus policy. The student is responsible for requesting his or her own accommodations and monitoring their effectiveness. Finally, the student must follow established policies and procedures for disabilities accommodations and must meet required academic and behavioral standards (i.e., be otherwise qualified).

In addition, if a student is attending a residential college, he or she takes on extra responsibilities, such as independence in the living environment (laundry, food prep, cleaning, roommate issues, etc.). All students must learn effective time management and organization strategies in their personal (as well as academic) lives, as they manage their free time and impose structure on themselves in the absence of their parents. They must learn to navigate their individual campuses, driving or using mass transportation if needed. Students must learn to assess when they need help or when they are sick, and know what to do or whom to call in such instances. Often they must learn money management and budgeting for the first time. They must establish friendships and negotiate and advocate for themselves without parental involvement.

In making the decision as to whether a student is ready to live away from home, families and professionals must take into account the big issues (e.g., friendship skills, maturity, and compliance with basic rules) but should also try to envision their student engaging in many of the smaller aspects of student life. Would the student be able to purchase his or her textbooks at the bookstore and exchange them should he or she drop a course? Would he or she be able to use student health services, or could the student do so with simple help from a parent on the phone? Would the student know to call home or require assistance in order to keep in touch? For a large campus, could the student figure out the bus or shuttle system? On small campuses, could the student find his or her way around from class to class? If the answer to these scenarios is negative, the student and family may be best considering a commuter campus while the student lives at home and develops better self-care skills. Professionals working with the student and family should assist in considering whether the student is truly able to leave home and function independently. In our experience, more students with ASD leave college because of residential or behavioral problems rather than academic issues, largely due to not being adequately prepared to fend for themselves.

Social and Independent Living Skills

Academics are only part of the total college experience. Consistent with the developmental goals of adulthood reviewed above, students must also develop independent living skills as they move away from home. Beginning students learn to interact appropriately with a wide range of people on campus, including professors, administrators, staff, and peers. They learn to interact as adults rather than adolescents, including navigating areas such as dating, sexuality, and parties (e.g., dealing with peer pressures around alcohol and drugs). They are called on to behave according to student conduct codes, which provide strict guidelines for campus behavior in class and in residences, and are rarely forgiving based on a student's status as a person with a disability. Students who are found in violation of student behavioral standards are subject to judicial review and sanction and are not protected because they are disabled. Importantly, unlike secondary school, there will not be widespread knowledge that a particular student is disabled by AS, nor will faculty and staff routinely be notified of the student's diagnosis, learning preferences, habits, and so forth. Indeed, faculty may provide accommodations in the absence of knowing the student's disability, because the disability services offices is prohibited by law from disclosing diagnostic information without students' explicit permission to do so. Similarly, residence hall staff may not know about a student's AS or sensory difficulties until and unless this information is provided to them by the student and his or her family. Families often believe that the information on the medical forms that they complete prior to enrollment will be distilled and transmitted to all persons working with or encountering their son or daughter on campus. This is categorically not the case, and families must understand that the student will need to set the boundaries in terms of what will and will not be disclosed and to whom.

CAMPUS LIFE FOR STUDENTS AND FAMILIES

Who's Who on Campus

Parents of typical children dream of college from the time their children are in diapers. However, families affected by ASD may defer or modify this dream. In doing so, they may distance themselves from the knowledge of what college life is all about. Yet it is imperative that everyone in the system understand the mechanics of higher education if a successful family partnership is to be fostered for the transitioning college student.

Particular attention must be paid to orienting the student to the size and culture of the chosen college. These factors (size and culture) can also be important considerations in the college search for a young person with an ASD. How is the campus navigated? How complicated is the transportation system? How far apart are the buildings and how far from the residence halls? Students with visual-perceptual and spatial difficulties may struggle with multiple bus routes or difficult driving directions and require some additional training to manage such a campus.

Both the student and the family are now exposed to unfamiliar people, places, and terminology. Who is the bursar? What does the registrar handle? Since the university expects students to handle their affairs as adults, again we pay particular attention to briefing the family about who the important stakeholders are on campus. Students with ASD are well advised to familiarize themselves with the divisions of their particular campus. To the extent that they can commit to memory the hierarchy, they may avoid some predictable pitfalls (e.g., not calling a dean by his or her first name unless invited to do so).

Campuses are typically divided into academic, student affairs, and business wings, all reporting to the Office of the President. The academic wing is comprised of the provost as the chief academic officer, assisted by academic deans who typically manage smaller schools within a large university. These deans manage academic affairs, academic standards, faculty, grants, budgets, and other academic issues in their individual schools. Department chairs do the same for their individual departments, managing the classroom and academic issues encountered by their professors (typically ranked as full, associate, assistant, instructor, fellow, and teaching assistant). Faculty advisors may be professors or student affairs professionals who work within academic affairs to provide varying levels of student support and counseling. Finally, the division of academic affairs is assisted by a host of clerical, support, and research staff.

The business wing of the university is usually comprised of the Office of the Registrar, which handles such details as full-time or part-time registration, tuition and fees levels, and leaves of absence. Business Affairs and the Office of the Bursar (or student accounts) are responsible for finances and may also encompass financial assistance and scholarships. Enrollment and retention, admissions, development, and alumni affairs are also typical offices within the business division of most universities and colleges, each with its own hierarchy of directors, managers, and support personnel.

Students and their families should become very familiar with the various offices within Student Affairs. This division typically falls under the direction of the Dean of Students, and may include such offices as disability services, judicial affairs, counseling and wellness, housing and residence life, dining services, tutoring services, and career services. Students need to understand that this dean can be very helpful to them and that the offices directly under the Dean of Students are critical supports as well. For example, there is a body of residential support staff that can assist students with roommate conflicts, social activities, and handling meltdowns; however, the staff must be notified directly by the family and the student, or by disability services but only with permission. However, students with ASD may also interact with this office regarding violations of student conduct codes or difficulties in the residence halls.

Conduct Codes

Every institution of higher education has a code of conduct by which all students must abide. General behavior such as, "students shall not disrupt the educational environment," are standard at every college and university in some form. Many other standards are unique to each institution and are not required to be accommodated for students with disabilities. These may include academic impropriety (plagiarism, cheating), classroom behaviors (creating a hostile atmosphere or one that interferes with the academic mission of the professor and the university), campus behavior (hate speech, stalking, intimidation), and behavior in the residence halls (drugs and alcohol). Depending on the disciplinary structure in place at the college or university, infractions of the conduct code may be reported to the dean, to the Office of Judicial Affairs, or to the campus or city police. Any of these offices has the right to sanction the student for conduct code violations. Sanctions can be harsh and can include arrest for criminal behavior, removal from housing, or suspension or expulsion depending on the nature of the violation. (We discuss judicial affairs later in this chapter.) Students and their families need to understand explicitly that there is no protection from conduct code violations contained within the language of either ADA or Section 504.

Disability Services

On most campuses, the Office of Disability Services (variably named) is the authorizing body for students with disabilities. In other words, students must first be cleared through this office in order to be recognized as students with disabilities for the purposes of services and accommodations. Numerous lawsuits have turned on whether the student had properly self-identified to the appropriate body on campus. Failure to do so jeopardizes students' legal rights under the ADA and Section 504.

All campuses in the United States are required to have a designated agent on campus that is responsible for students with disabilities. Smaller colleges may have a professor, counselor, or dean under whom these duties fall. Such persons may not be particularly expert in different disability types, and may have available only the basics of disability compliance. Larger colleges and universities typically have free-standing offices that are professionally staffed by disability experts. These offices are typically housed within Student Affairs (under the Dean of Students) or within a department of Counseling and Mental Health.

This administrative structure fosters good relationships between disability experts and student residence life, dining, career services, tutoring services, and judicial affairs. Because the needs of students with ASD are so far reaching, such partnerships become very valuable. Alternately, the mental health and crisis needs of students with ASD may be addressed when disability services (DSS) is housed within the counseling department. Some additional coordination may be required between counseling services, disability services, and the other offices within student affairs.

Although smaller colleges with one designated disability contact may be an excellent choice for the student with ASD, comprehensive understanding of the particulars of theses disorders may require more specialized knowledge and skills. Larger colleges and universities may have support staff with expertise in working with students with psychiatric disabilities, learning disabilities, or attention disorders who may also have experience with ASD.

Many families and professionals view DSS as a barrier to accommodations and services, and indeed the more stringent processes of higher education may give that impression. However, DSS can serve as the main resource for qualified students with ASD on campuses. DSS providers can authorize accommodations in class, negotiate special housing requests, and work with students to understand their rights and responsibilities. In a broader role, this office can also educate faculty, administration, and staff about students with ASD and mediate any misunderstandings. DSS may act as the "point person" for crisis management, a source of professional information and referrals, and as a "safe space" for the student.

DSS offices are typically staffed with professional disability experts who may work with students with physical and medical, sensory, learning, cognitive, psychiatric, and other disabilities. Whereas few DSS providers would consider themselves expert in working with ASDs, over the past five years, more providers have sought special training in this area. A small but growing number of colleges and universities are even developing specialized ASD support programs (some, with very large price tags). We caution all students with ASD, their families, and their professional support staff to inquire specifically whether the disability staff is experienced with ASD students. Regardless of the experience of the DSS office with ASD, the student, the family, and the health providers must be prepared to inquire, educate (when necessary), and fully disclose to the providers responsible for the student.

In most cases, DSS will not disclose for the student, and indeed is strictly prohibited by law from doing so. As well, most offices will not negotiate accommodations or adjustments for students but will work with students so that they develop self-advocacy skills independently. Understanding that many students with ASD lack the social acumen to be good self-advocates, disability providers may find themselves working more intensively with these students so that they can achieve the highest level of self-determination possible. In our experience, partnering with the family in the early stage of the transition process is important in communicating to the student the necessity of his or her developing these negotiating skills.

By providing necessary information to the DSS staff, in terms of all relevant documentation (especially psychiatric), information about personal habits, soothing strategies, response to stress, changes in family dynamics, etc., the family enters a partnership that is often new to the DSS provider as well. Recall that we emphasized above that students are expected to become their own CEOs. This is certainly the case; however, it is often the case that some more communication between the student, DSS, and the parents is useful in making the transition to higher education.

ASPERGER SYNDROME IN COLLEGE: SOME BASICS

In 2001, when we began to present to the disability service community (Wolf, Thierfeld Brown, & Bork, 2001), the diagnosis of AS was largely unfamiliar to disability providers. The recent prevalence estimate of 1:88 by the Centers for Disease Control and Prevention (2012) predicts that this increase will continue. We suspect that the increase in numbers reflects (in part) the inclusion of more individuals at the boundaries of autism who would not have been previously diagnosed. It is these young people with milder symptoms who may well be our incoming population of college students in the future.

The reasons for this increase are unknown, but campuses are working to develop improved programming to support this very able yet challenging population of young people. Students with AS are not like other groups of students with disabilities. They experience pervasive difficulties in all aspects of the higher educational experience, including social as well as cognitive and academic domains. Accommodating students whose disabilities may very likely affect social and regulatory capacities is a particular challenge for service providers who are not accustomed to reaching out into many areas of student life.

The social disability of college students with AS include development of self-awareness and sense of self, as well as core social skills such as social perception, reading social cures, and social language. The social skills deficits become particularly problematic when students are required to negotiate with faculty, staff, and administrators as they try to arrange accommodations or register for classes. Other classroom interactions such as forming study groups or working on group projects require particular attention, as students may be prone to being victimized in a group setting (if indeed they are willing to enter into it at all; we return to this topic below). Obvious difficulties are also seen in residence halls where managing roommate conflicts (never easy for any student) can quickly become a full-blown AS meltdown.

The cognitive disability in AS has been explored in many excellent sources (Minshew, 2001; Russell, 1997; Wetherby & Prizant, 2000; Schopler, Mesibov, & Kunce, 1998). We distill this information very briefly here. Due to widespread integrative and regulatory deficits, students with AS have difficulty grasping the bigger picture of assignments, tests, and reading. They may struggle with understating what the professor actually wants or expects from an assignment. Interpreting graphical information and managing science or math requirements may be problematic, especially if a neuropsychological pattern consistent with a nonverbal learning disorder is present (Klin, Volkmar, Sparrow, Cicchetti, & Rourke, 1997). Other students may have no difficulty in those areas at all. The organization of writing is typically problematic, as managing long-range projects requires time management and planning skills along with an ability to maintain momentum.

Thus we see that the "big problems" may arise due to overall faulty integration and synthesis mechanisms. Students tend to miss the big picture; they miss the forest for the trees. Students may become quite anxious and rigid in the face of this widespread confusion. As well as a core feature of the diagnosis, rigidity serves the additional function of helping individuals cope with the anxiety aroused by novel situations and change (Rosenn, 1999). Planning, shifting, prioritizing, and other aspects of executive and regulatory control may be affected (Happé, Booth, Charlton, & Hughes, 2006; Hill, 2004; Joseph, McGrath, & Tager-Flusberg, 2005; also see Wolf & Thierfeld Brown, 2007, for review). Finally, deficits in the social arena that impede these students' efficacy as social agents who are able to take the perspective of another (theory of mind; Baron-Cohen, 1999) may be problematic in a university environment.

Executive Functioning and Self-Regulation in College

The term *executive function* is typically used to describe a set of behaviors often attributed to systems in the frontal and subcortical regions of the brain (see Wolf & Kaplan, 2008, and Wolf & Wasserstein, 2001, for reviews). Tasks often associated with the executive system include self-reflection, inhibition, planning, flexibility, and delay of gratification (Stuss, 2007; also see Wolf & Kaplan, 2008, for review). Executive function abilities permit the individual to adopt a more mature, forward-thinking stance and disengage from immediate concerns and rewards (Wolf & Wasserstein, 2001, for review).

In addition to the familiar cognitive processes of the executive system is a parallel system that regulates affect, motivation, and social–emotional functioning (Stuss, 2007; also see Wolf & Kaplan, 2008, for review). The combination of executive and motivational deficits results in a dysregulated college student. This student appears to be unable to organize work or plan ahead, does not sustain and regulate his or her level of energy and effort, and has difficulty completing and following through with tasks. Furthermore, he or she is typically rigid and inflexible, and has difficulty using feedback from others to alter his or her approach to tasks. Core organizational tasks such as managing and structuring time, materials, and space may be seriously compromised (Wolf, 2001; also Wolf & Thierfeld Brown, 2007). This student may also struggle to set personal goals and remain motivated, especially in the face new or difficult tasks (Wolf & Kaplan, 2008). Obviously, such a student will struggle in the university setting, where demands for organization, follow through, motivation, and flexibility are critical for success.

Students with ASD who also have executive deficits can suffer in the academic environment. In our experience, traditional accommodations (e.g., extra time for exams) designed to mitigate the academic effects of other disabilities are often not effective with these students. Deficits in the ability to organize and shift among concepts, behaviors, ideas, and goals can be debilitating in college students, as so much of academic life requires good planning (Wolf & Kaplan, 2008; Wolf, 2001).

Academic Accommodations

The ADA states that

> institutions must make modifications to academic requirements as necessary to ensure that such requirements do not discriminate against students with disabilities, or have the effect of excluding students solely on the basis of disability. An institution may not impose rules or restrictions that have the effect of limiting participation of students with disabilities in educational programs or activities." (ADA)

This means that students with disabilities have the right to receive accommodations to mitigate the impact of their disability on their academic performance as part of "leveling the playing field" viz a viz students without disabilities.

Students with AS often need academic support in subjects in which they are not strong. For example, a student who is strong in math and science but weak in English and humanities may require extended time for tests in the weaker areas but no accommodations in the strong subjects. Extended time, a private room for exams, assistance with organization and time management, and time to discuss questions privately with a professor are all common accommodations for students with AS. Examples of accommodations that would not be provided in most higher education settings include personal aides for academics or housing, social coaches, disability-specific content tutoring, and one-to-one assistance for out-of-class work (homework). However, some schools offer specialized programs in which these services are offered for a fee.

We believe that the best practice for developing accommodation plans for students with ASD includes ensuring that (1) the disability service professional understands the cognitive, linguistic, and behavioral deficits of the diagnosis and (2) comprehensive information is provided to that professional concerning how well the individual student functions in each of these domains. Some accommodation planning will be relatively straightforward (e.g., allowing extra time on computers), whereas other aspects may require more creativity and collaboration between the student and various offices or faculty (e.g., renegotiating the means by which a student demonstrates that he or she has mastered the fundamental requirements of a course).

Academic Problem Areas

Students with AS often have trouble in predictable areas. Some of these areas include the following.

Writing

Students with AS may struggle with essay questions on exams. Others encounter difficulty with term papers, as the long-range planning and organizing are challenging. Still others may have difficulty writing creatively or synthetically, and prefer to write lengthy, factual treatises that do not contain much insight or synthesis of ideas. Assignments that emphasize taking another's perspective or analyzing the personal motivation of characters, typical of many freshman literature courses, may be particularly problematic as the student does not possess the ability to put themselves in someone else's shoes. Many students with AS require intervention to teach them better organizational skills for writing projects. In some cases, students may require special accommodations to allow them to demonstrate their course mastery in an alternate manner.

Group Work

College students typically have many opportunities to work in groups on projects, for presentations, and in lab courses where they are assigned a lab group. Students with AS have the potential to become overwhelmed by the interpersonal aspects of these classes, and may require some intervention to help them navigate the demands of the situation. They may be bullied or taken advantage of, and rarely possess the interpersonal acumen to avoid, resist, or rebuff this treatment.

Executive Issues

Many students with AS struggle with time management issues that impedes their ability, for example, to reduce a syllabus into a semester game plan. They easily become overwhelmed and frustrated, or insist that they do not need to use organizational strategies to stay on top of their work. Indeed, the sheer intellectual gifts of many students with AS has enabled them to manage remarkably well, but at an inordinate cost. Many cannot surmount the demands of an academic calendar that requires them to be able to multitask, study for several exams in a short period of time, or have several long-range projects on the table at the same time. Others struggle with task initiation and motivation maintenance, and require external assistance to "keep their eye on the prize." Others struggle with the multitasking demands inherent in a full course load.

Exams

Taking exams is often not problematic for students with AS, in that they are good at memorizing large amounts of information and regurgitating them on demand. Some students with nonverbal learning disability profiles may have difficulty with scantron-type format exams. Others may not fully read test instructions or listen for any additional instructions in the exam room. Essay format exams, again, may be problematic due to the demand for organized, concise writing. Distraction and sensory issues in an exam setting must be closely monitored, as rectifying these issues may make the difference between good and abysmal exam performance.

Classroom Behaviors

It is not uncommon for professors to call disability services regarding the classroom behavior of a student with AS who does not appreciate the rules of comportment. Students need to understand that interruptions and speaking out of turn, correcting the instructor, walking out of the classroom, or eating and drinking in class are not permitted. Some students require sensory integration materials, such as squeeze balls, to remain focused in the classroom. Sensitivity to ambient conditions such as lighting, temperature, noise, or smells can be easily accommodated simply by moving a class or an exam for the student with ASD. Such interventions should be explained to the professor in a manner such that he or she understands that the student is not being disrespectful. The reactions of other students to the student with AS may need to be monitored and the student helped to understand the impact of his or her behaviors on peers.

Judicial Affairs

Conduct codes, as mentioned earlier in the chapter, are strictly applied. Academic conduct codes involve issues such as cheating and plagiarism. Students with AS may not commit these conduct breaches on purpose, but may participate in behavior that is prohibited by not understanding the consequences of their actions. For example, a student with AS may be so excited that someone has asked for his or her help with a science lab that he or she may not realize that part of the exercise was to work independently. Though the other student initiated the assistance, the student with AS would be seen as participating in the cheating. Another example might be the student who is accused of plagiarism because of an essay that reproduces the original text—thanks to the student's prodigious memory. In this case, the student would need to be counseled to check and double-check his or her wording and references to assure that such instances do not occur.

Behavior within the college community is also governed by codes. Students who do not understand social rules can be at a particular disadvantage. Stalking and harassment are two large problems that students with AS experience on campus. For example, a student's awkward social approach may be misconstrued as unwanted advances, even as harassment or stalking, toward a student of the opposite sex, especially should the recipient make a judicial report. Often the student with AS does not understand what he or she has done, but again, disability does not excuse conduct code violations. Some behaviors (e.g., stalking) can be "translated" for personnel in judicial affairs so that they understand the context. In short, it is very important that students understands the rules and the consequences for breaking them.

Disability is not an excuse for breach of conduct code. Students with AS are often somewhat rule-bound and appreciate having clear expectations about what they can and can't do. Accordingly, they usually benefit from working with someone on campus as well as at home to understand the rules of academic conduct prior to matriculating on campus. These rules can even take the form of a "manual" that clearly lays out the expectations and the consequences for a student should he or she violate any conduct or behavior codes.

Residential Issues

The most difficult aspect of higher education for students with AS is the residential piece. Many students want to live on campus, or their parents want them to, in order to "fully experience college." For many students, however, this aspect of their educational experience is overwhelming. The idea of living with a roommate, sharing a bathroom with a wide range of people, dealing with noise, partying, drugs, and sex is more than many students with AS can handle. The level of flexibility and executive functioning required to succeed in the residence halls and in the classroom is often not present in our students with AS. The stress and sensory issues involved often make the residence halls an unwelcoming place to live for students on the spectrum. For more information on residence life for students with AS, see Wolf, Thierfeld Brown, and Bork (2001).

Residence halls have many levels of professionals and students working on site. Students, usually known as resident assistants or RAs, live on each floor and are the first layer of information and support for the student. Of course, we believe that RAs should know about the student(s) with AS on their floor, but recall that there is no automatic disclosure of the AS condition to these critical staff members. The family and the student with AS optimally should consult with the DSS office to make a plan for informing residence hall staff about a student's issues in a manner that will not embarrass or cause undue discomfort for the student. RAs can assist the student in their transition, with roommate issues, and in handling any teasing or bullying that take place. Conduct codes can also work to the student's benefit to reduce bullying, etc.

Stress Management

In our experience on college campuses, we have found that students with AS who are very affected by stress and anxiety need ongoing counseling support from the outset of their college career. Students who become depressed or overanxious should be treated quickly and aggressively with therapy and often with medication. We have found that students who try to recoup from severe depression or anxiety usually do not catch up academically (or socially) and lose the semester. Often the students go deeper into depression or experience the increased anxiety if they attempt to continue in school and stay on campus. It is crucial to know what can precipitate a student's crisis, how his or her stress manifests, and what behaviors to look for. This information should be communicated to the campus disability services and mental health or counseling center staff in order to obtain the best services possible. Calming methods for the student and the medications the student is taking are also crucial information to communicate.

In April 2007 a student at Virginia Tech University went on a shooting rampage killing 33 people. The student had been hospitalized for mental illness and a family member said that when the shooter was young, they thought he was autistic. This national attention to mental health issues on college campuses changed the reactions and expectations of many in higher education regarding students who exhibit odd or unacceptable behavior. Professionals understand that students on the spectrum are not typically dangerous and do not usually display aggressive behavior. However, when an incident as dramatic as the events at Virginia Tech occurs and images from the massacre are all over the air waves, we must do even more to educate our colleagues, the campus community and other professionals about students on the autism spectrum.

CONCLUDING THOUGHTS

Students with AS can and do succeed in college. Families, professionals, and the student must choose carefully, selecting a school that is a good fit for the student and has appropriate services. This choice cannot be taken lightly; it is the single most important factor in the success of the educational experience for students with AS.

To foster a good transition, students and their families must be prepared for the changes in the roles of the household. A good transition to higher education depends on careful planning and excellent communication. Families and professionals working with college-bound students with AS should be familiar with the culture of their selected campus, and be familiar with the important people who will be involved in the student's education. They should be counseled to become involved when needed, but not at the expense of teaching the student important self-advocacy skills. Students must be prepared to assume their new legal status as adults with disabilities (and their families, to adjust to the huge change that includes self-advocacy, disability awareness, and compliance with campus policy (including compliance with academic and conduct codes).

The ultimate goal for everyone in the system is for the student with AS to function independently and successfully in school, at work, and in life. Though many supports and services may appear to be the goal, discovering that the student can learn to succeed with fewer services and less intervention is the pathway to ultimate success.

ACKNOWLEDGMENTS

Portions of this chapter are adapted from *Students with Asperger Syndrome: A Guide for College Personnel* by G. R. Bork, J. Thierfeld Brown, and L. Wolf (2009) and *The Parent's Guide to College for Students on the Autism Spectrum* by J. Thierfeld Brown, L. E. Wolf, L. King, and G. R. K. Bork (2012). Adapted with permission from AAPC Publishing.

REFERENCES

Americans with Disabilities Act of 1990. *www.ada.gov.*

American Psychiatric Association. (1994). *Diagnostic and statistical manual of mental disorders* (4th ed.). Washington, DC: Author.

Asperger, H. (1991). Autistic psychopathy in childhood. In U. Frith (Ed.), *Autism and Asperger syndrome* (pp. 37–92). Cambridge, UK: Cambridge University Press.

Barkley, R. A. (1997). Behavioral inhibition, sustained attention, and executive functions: Constructing a unified theory of ADHD. *Psychological Bulletin, 121,* 65–94.

Baron-Cohen, S. (1999). *Mindblindness: An essay on autism and theory of mind.* Cambridge, MA: MIT Press.

Centers for Disease Control and Prevention. (2007). Prevalence of autism spectrum disorders—autism and developmental disabilities monitoring network, 14 sites, United States 2002. *www.cdc.gov.*

Disability Rights and Education Defense Fund. *http://www.dredf.org.*

Educational Testing Service, Guidelines for Documenting Learning Disabilities in Adults. *www.ets.org/disabilty.*

Gillberg, C., & Billstedt, E. (2000). Autism and Asperger syndrome: Coexistence with other clinical disorders. *Acta Psychiatrica Scandinavica, 102*(5), 321–330.

Happé, F., Booth, R., Charlton, R., & Hughes, C. (2006). Executive function deficits in autism spectrum disorders and attention deficit/hyperactivity disorder: Examining profiles across domains and ages. *Brain and Cognition, 61,* 25–39.

Hill, E. L. (2004). Executive function in autism. *Trends in Cognitive Science, 8,* 26–32.

Individuals with Disabilities Education Act. *http://idea.ed.gov.*

Joseph, R. M., McGrath, L. M., & Tager-Flusberg, H. (2005). Executive dysfunction and its relation to language ability in verbal school-age children with autism. *Developmental Neuropsychology, 27,* 361–378.

Klin, A., Volkmar, F. R., Sparrow, S. S., Cicchetti, D. V., & Rourke, B. P. (1997). Validity and neuropsychological characterization of Asperger syndrome: Convergence with nonverbal learning disabilities syndrome. In M. E. Hertzig & E. A. Farber (Eds.), *Annual progress in child psychiatry and child development* (pp. 241–259). New York: Brunner/Mazel.

Macurdy, A., & Geetter, E. (2008). Legal issues for adults with learning disabilities in higher education and employment. In L. E. Wolf, H. E. Schreiber, & J. Wasserstein (Eds.), *Current issues in adult learning disorders* (pp. 415–432). New York: Psychology Press.

Minshew, N. J. (2001). The core deficit in autism and autism spectrum disorders. *Journal of Developmental and Learning Disorders, 5,* 107–118.

National Dissemination Center for Children with Disabilities. *www.nichcy.org/reauth/index.html.*

Piven, J., Palmer, P., Jacobi, D., Childress, D., & Arndt, S. (1997). Broader autism phenotype: Evidence from a family history study of multiple-incidence autism families. *American Journal of Psychiatry, 154,* 185–190.

Rosenn, D. W. (1999). What is Asperger's disorder? *Harvard Mental Health Letter, 16,* 4–8.

Russell, J. (Ed.). (1997). *Autism as an executive disorder.* New York: Oxford University Press.

Schopler, E., Mesibov, G. B., & Kunce, L. J. (Eds.). (1998). *Asperger syndrome or high functioning autism?* New York: Plenum Press.

Section 504 of the Rehabilitation Act of 1973. *www.hhs.gov/ocr/504.pdf.*

Southeastern Community College v. Davis, 442 U.S. 397, 423 (1979).

Stuss, D. R. (2007). New approaches to prefrontal lobe testing. In J. L. Cummings & B. L. Miller (Eds.), *The human frontal lobes: Functions and disorders* (pp. 292–305). New York: Guilford Press.

Tantam, D. (2000). Psychological disorder in adolescents and adults with Asperger syndrome. *Autism, 4,* 47–62.

Wetherby, A. M., & Prizant, B. M. (Eds.). (2000). *Autism spectrum disorders: A transactional developmental approach.* Baltimore: Brookes.

Williams, D. (1996). *Autism: An inside-out approach: An innovative look at the "mechanics" of "autism" and its developmental "cousins."* London: Jessica Kingsley.

WNY Collegiate Consortium of Disability Advocates, Technology for Transition Project at the State University of New York at Buffalo. *www.ccdanet.org/ecp_index.html.*

Wolf, L. E. (2001). College students with ADHD and other hidden disabilities. *Annals of the New York Academy of Sciences, 931,* 385–395.

Wolf, L. E., & Kaplan, E. (2008). Executive functioning and self-regulation in young adults: Implications for neurodevelopmental learning disorders. In L. E. Wolf, H. E. Schreiber, & J. Wasserstein (Eds.), *Adult learning disorders: Contemporary issues* (pp. 219–244). New York: Psychology Press.

Wolf, L. E., & Thierfeld Brown, J. (2005a, April 20). *College transition for students with Asperger disorder.* Invited full-day presentation, Asperger Syndrome Education Network, Short Hills, NJ.

Wolf, L. E., & Thierfeld Brown, J. (2005b, August 4). *Managing executive dysfunction in attention disorders and Asperger syndrome.* Paper presented at the annual conference of the Association of Higher Education and Disabilities, Milwaukee, WI.

Wolf, L. E., & Thierfeld Brown, J. (2007). *Strategic education for university students with Asperger syndrome: A model demonstration project.* Manuscript submitted for publication.

Wolf, L. E., Thierfeld Brown, J., & Bork, R. (2001, July 12–15). *Asperger's syndrome in college students.* Paper presented at the meeting of the Association for Higher Education and Disability, Portland, OR.

Wolf, L. E., & Wasserstein, J. (2001). Adult ADHD: Concluding thoughts. *Annals of the New York Academy of Sciences, 931,* 396–408.

Wrightslaw. *www.wrightslaw.com.*

Wynne v. Tufts Univ. School of Medicine, 932 F.2d 19, 26 (1st Cir. 1991).

CHAPTER 12

Asperger Syndrome and Forensic Issues

Marc Woodbury-Smith

Since the publication of Wing's paper in 1981, a small yet significant body of literature has emerged describing people who have Asperger syndrome (AS), and who have engaged in problematic behavior (Woodbury-Smith et al., 2005 and references therein). Crucially, as will become apparent later in this chapter, the significance of this literature does not lie in the strength of the association, if indeed there is one, because it is clear that such problematic behaviors are not a common occurrence. Instead, it is important to understand the factors that might be associated with such behaviors, and perhaps more importantly, how the criminal justice system and other statutory authorities might appropriately respond.

The need to identify such individuals as a means by which they may be more effectively rehabilitated, rather than "punished," was raised as early as 1992 in the United Kingdom, in the Reed Report, *Services for Mentally Disordered Offenders* (Department of Health, 2002). Sadly, 20 years later, little is still understood about offending among people with AS, and people with AS who engage in more serious offending may find themselves in maximum-secure psychiatric hospitals for prolonged periods of time, and those who engage in more minor offending may find themselves increasingly socially excluded.

This chapter critically reviews the literature concerned with problematic behaviours among people with AS, examines factors that may increase propensity to such behaviors, and considers management options using exemplification. Throughout, I refer to AS for simplification, but problematic behaviors may also be seen among those described as having "high-functioning autism," although, in contrast, such behaviors may be less likely among those who are intellectually impaired. Moreover, although the term "problematic behaviors" implies a range of transgressions, from relatively minor infringements of conventional rules to more serious behaviors impacting on the well-being of others, this chapter is concerned with the more serious behaviors that may lead to contact with the criminal justice system. As will become apparent, such behaviors may not be criminally driven, per se, among people with AS but more often than not result from social naïveté and misunderstanding.

Although the focus of this chapter is people with AS who engage in serious behaviors, it is important to emphasize that such behaviors are rare. This point is particularly important to recognize as the media has been guilty on a number of occasions, both in the United Kingdom and the United States, of misrepresenting AS, which may ultimately have an impact on the public perception of people with AS.

EVIDENCE OF PROBLEMATIC BEHAVIORS: HISTORICAL CONTEXT

When Asperger described a group of boys with core deficits in social interaction and communication and with inflexible patterns of behavior, he additionally commented on other aspects of their behavior. For example, Fritz V. "never got on with other children [and] quickly became aggressive and lashed out with anything he could get hold of (once a hammer) regardless of the danger to others" (Asperger, 1944, as cited in Frith, 1991, p. 40). Another patient, Harro L., was referred by his school because of his "savage tendency to fight" (p. 57); Asperger commented that "little things drove him to senseless fury, whereupon he attacked other children" (p. 57). Similar conduct disordered behaviours were seen in Asperger's other patients. Asperger believed that such "autistic acts of malice" (to use his terminology) reflected a limited ability of these individuals to reflect upon how much they hurt others, a reference to their poorly developed empathy.

A review of the clinical records of cases seen by Asperger in his clinic in Vienna during the 1960s and 1970s (Hippler & Klicpera, 2003 identified more detailed information about the behaviors. Of the 46 children whose files were available for examination, seven (15%) had been admitted to the ward because their behavior was no longer acceptable at school and exclusion was imminent. Asperger described the occurrence of "autistic malice" in seven patients (15%). These children were described as showing intentional acts of malice, "with malicious pleasure and apparent pride in what they had done. Some of the children were said to experiment on others, that is, they seemed to do things on purpose to see how others reacted or to provoke a certain reaction" (Hippler & Klicpera, 2003, p. 294).

Wing, too (Wing, 1981), described a propensity for violent behavior among a few of the individuals in her case series, noting that "a small minority have a history of rather bizarre antisocial acts, perhaps because of their lack of empathy" (p. 116). This was true of four of the individuals she described. One child, for example, with a particular interest in chemistry, injured a colleague during the course of a "scientific" experiment. Wing also commented more specifically on how a lack of social understanding could lead to contact with the criminal justice system. For example, "he has no idea of how to indicate his interest and attract a partner in a socially acceptable fashion. If he has a strong sex drive, he may approach or touch or kiss a stranger, or someone much older or younger than himself and as a consequence find himself in trouble with the police" (Wing, 1981, p. 116).

Since Wing's seminal paper, interest in AS as a diagnostic entity has ballooned, reflected in the exponential rise in published articles concerned with delineating its clinical characteristics, its relationship to autism, and its biological underpinning. Paralleling this proliferation has been a steady flow of case reports describing people purported to have AS who have engaged in serious offending behaviors (Chesterman & Rutter, 1993; Mawson, Grounds, & Tantam, 1985; Baron-Cohen, 1988; Chen et al., 2003; Murrie, Warren, Kristiansson, & Dietz, 2002; Everall & Lecouter, 1990; Kohn, Fahum, Ratzoni, & Apter, 1998; Silva, Ferrari, & Leong, 2002; Palermo, 2004). In addition to these single-case studies and small-case series, noteworthy too are the cases described as "schizoid disorder of childhood" by Wolff (2000) and with "lifelong eccentricity" by Tantam (1988a, 1988b). Wolff identified a group of children who shared the core impairment of social isolation and followed their progress into adulthood, and Tantam studied a group of young adults who had been referred to his clinic with a lifelong history of social isolation and eccentricity. In both groups phenomenological similarities to AS were observed, and in both a small minority had engaged in problematic behaviors in adulthood.

In isolation, the case study literature is not particularly compelling for several reasons. For example, many ascribe retrospective diagnoses to detained individuals. This is particularly apparent in the claim that the serial murderer Jeffrey Dahmer may have had AS (Silva et al., 2002). Problematically, this and other similar retrospective analyses have not carried out detailed developmental histories, being based instead on patchy background information accumulated from different, sometimes "second-hand" sources; in the case of Dahmer, considering the bizarre nature of his offense, it is perhaps unsurprising that his childhood was characterized by an unusual social and emotional development. It is important not to equate his developmental abnormalities with the specific impairments seen in autism spectrum disorders (ASD).

Moreover, due to publication bias evidence of a positive association is more likely to be reported, therefore inflating any apparent association. In a similar fashion, only those cases involving more severe behaviors are described in the literature. As such, they provide little information concerning the pattern and prevalence of less severe problematic behaviors among people with AS more generally.

PREVALENCE OF PROBLEMATIC BEHAVIORS AMONG PEOPLE WITH AS

Whereas the case studies and case series provide no clues to the prevalence of problematic behaviors in AS, other researchers have attempted to more explicitly examine the prevalence of such behaviors. Focusing on violent behavior, Ghaziuddin and his colleagues reviewed 132 cases described in the literature (excluding those of Wolff and Tantam) and identified only a small number recorded to have been violent, indicative of a prevalence of offending in the community that is probably much lower than among their general population counterparts (Ghaziuddin, Tsai, & Ghaziuddin, 1991). This finding is consistent with the assertion made by Howlin (2004) that people with AS have a strong sense of right from wrong and therefore will probably offend much less than others (Howlin, 2004). This point notwithstanding, the nature of the study means that the small number is likely to be an underestimate of the exact figure, particularly as the large case series of Tantam and Wolff were specifically excluded. In fact, if all these reports are included in the type of analysis conducted by Ghazziudin, the prevalence of offending in AS would be 20% (46 out of 224) instead of the 2.27% reported.

Woodbury-Smith and colleagues (Woodbury-Smith, Clare, Holland, & Kearns, 2006) similarly attempted to examine rates of problematic behaviors in the community using a self-report questionnaire about offending administered during a face-to-face interview ($n = 25$) and compared with a community comparison group ($n = 25$). Although a recognized valid and robust measure of crime, it has not been used in such samples previously. This limitation notwithstanding, and the fact that the study sample sizes were small, the study did demonstrate that the AS group was significantly less likely than the general population peers to report having engaged in many of the problematic behaviors recorded (e.g., theft or behaviors related to illicit substance use), and was more likely to have engaged in other behaviors (e.g., criminal damage), albeit nonsignificantly so.

Wolff also specifically examined prevalence of offending in her schizoid children by following up with both the boys and girls into adulthood to determine the outcome (Wolff, Townshend, McGuire, & Weeks, 1991). In considering the schizoid boys, there was no evidence of any raised prevalence of delinquency, measured by self-report methodology, compared to a psychiatric control group. However, the self-report results of the schizoid girls indicated that they had rates of delinquency similar to the boys and higher than the control girls.

Wolff also approached the Scottish Criminal Records Office to undertake a search of official convictions for the 109 schizoid boys, 32 schizoid girls, and the matched psychiatric controls. Compared to the population "norms" of 22% for men and 5% for women, 32% of the schizoid men and 34.5% of the schizoid women had convictions. When compared with the control sample, recruited from a psychiatric clinic, the rates for schizoid men were comparable (34.5% of control men with a conviction), whereas the rates for schizoid women were still significantly higher (15.5% of control women with a conviction). Of note is that there was no difference in the nature of offenses between the schizoid and control groups, and none had committed a particularly violent offense. However, 3 years after this survey was undertaken, one of the schizoidal men "had entered the home of a housewife by posing as a priest, attacked her with a poker, and sexually assaulted her" (Wolff, 2000, p. 293).

By way of investigating the numbers of people with AS in high-secure psychiatric hospitals and comparing such figures with reasonable estimates of community prevalence (Scragg & Shah, 1994; Hare, Gould, Mills, & Wing, 1999), two such studies both found a higher prevalence of AS in such establishments. The first (Scragg & Shah, 1994) examined the prevalence of AS, as diagnosed according to the criteria developed by Gillberg & Gillberg (1989), and found four definite cases and four possible cases among the population of Broadmoor Special Hospital (a maximum secure psychiatric hospital in England) representing a prevalence rate of 2.4%, and contrasting with the general population prevalence of AS using the same diagnostic criteria of 7.1/10,000. The second study examined the prevalence in the same way in all three maximum secure psychiatric hospitals in England and found similar rates (Hare et al., 1999).

These results seem to suggest that since people with AS are overrepresented, they are at an increased risk of engaging in problematic behaviors, and more specifically, violent behaviors. This conclusion is perhaps premature, as the findings may simply be a reflection of sentencing policy and practice; for example, people with AS who have engaged in more serious offending may end up detained in such places rather than in prisons. There is certainly evidence that before the 1980s some individuals were incorrectly diagnosed as having schizophrenia and directed to such hospitals for this reason. The other possible reason for an apparently inflated prevalence is that being more "treatment resistant" than their peers with mental illness, those with AS may end up detained for longer, and the accumulation of such individuals would thereby inflate the prevalence figure in these institutions. Interestingly, the rates of *conviction* of people with AS (in a Danish sample) were found to be similar to those of people without AS, and the conviction rate of people with atypical autism was lower than that of the comparison group (Mouridsen, Rich, Isager, & Nedergaard, 2007).

In summary, it seems reasonable to conclude that a small number of people with AS may engage in serious offending, as evidenced by the case studies and high-secure hospital studies, although it is not clear whether this finding represents a prevalence of violent offending that is higher or lower than general population counterparts. In the community the evidence seems to suggest that the prevalence of offending is lower than in the general population, but that the offenses may occur as a direct result of the AS/response to having AS, as exemplified in the study of Woodbury-Smith and colleagues (2006). It is therefore important to consider whether anything in the phenotype increases propensity to problematic behavior—a factor that would greatly inform better management.

TYPES OF PROBLEMATIC BEHAVIORS OBSERVED

Considering these case studies together, a range of offenses is represented, including for example assaults on others (Mawson et al., 1985), fire setting (Everall & Lecouteur, 1990), sexual offending (Kohn et al., 1998), and theft (Chen et al., 2003). Among the individuals described by Tantam (1988a, 1988b), 14 of 64 were known to have committed offenses punishable by imprisonment, including criminal damage (4), assault (3), arson (3), indecent exposure (3), and attempted rape (1). Similarly, in the studies of Woodbury-Smith et al. (2005, 2006, 2010) described later in this chapter, a range of offenses is seen, including theft, criminal damage, violence toward others, and sexual offenses. It has been suggested that fire setting is more common among offenders with AS than the non AS-offending population (Mouridsen et al., 2007; Siponmaa, Kristiansson, Jonson, Nyden, & Gillberg, 2001; Hare et al., 1999). Moreover, although some studies indicate that people with AS commit sexual offenses (Hare et al., 1999; Murphy, 2003), others suggest that the rates of sexual offending (Hare et al., 1999) and child sex offenses (Elvish, 2005) are lower in offenders with ASD.

In conclusion, a range of problematic behaviors has been described, with no specific observable pattern. As becomes apparent later, however, relatively minor transgressions that occur as a direct result of social misunderstanding or as a result of the pursuit of circumscribed interests are perhaps those that are seen most frequently in clinical practice.

REASONS FOR THE PROBLEMATIC BEHAVIORS

On the whole, people with AS or ASD are law-abiding citizens and have been described as having a strong sense of right from wrong. They may also adhere rigidly to rules and reprimand others during the course of a perceived wrongdoing (and in the process, may inadvertently end up as the perceived wrongdoer). People with AS may also not have the "opportunities" for crime. For example, it is rare for someone with AS to be part of a gang unless his or her social difficulties have made the person vulnerable to being "enticed" into this culture.

However, a number of factors might lead some people with AS to come into contact with the criminal justice system. These factors include those related to the clinical phenotype, such as the pursuit of a circumscribed interest or as a result of social naïveté, and those related to the "neuropsychological phenotype," such as impaired theory of mind or impairment of executive functioning. In addition, other factors such as adjustment to the disorder (i.e., being different) or vulnerability to manipulation by dominant others might be important. Comorbidity may also be of etiological significance. Wing (1997) has also suggested a number of other factors that might be associated with offending among people with AS, including isolation and the belief that others are hostile, perhaps as a result of previous unhappy experiences, such as being bullied at school. Many other more general criminological risk factors may also be relevant, including specific learning difficulties and disorders of attention and motor control. These various factors, discussed in more detail below, are summarized in Table 12.1.

SOCIAL-COMMUNICATIVE IMPAIRMENTS AND OFFENDING

The impairment of reciprocal social interaction skills is the sine qua non of AS and other ASD. (The characteristics of the social impairment are described elsewhere in this volume; see also Klin, McPartland, & Volkmar, 2005). More often than not, people with AS wish to seek relationships

TABLE 12.1. Possible Factors Associated with Offending by People with ASD

- As a result of social-communicative impairments
  Social naïveté, social misunderstanding
  Isolation
  Reaction to being bullied
  Resentment
  Adjustment to diagnosis

- As a result of rigidity and circumscribed interests
  Pursuit of a circumscribed interest

- Neuropsychological factors
  Impairment of theory of mind
  Impairment of emotional processing
  Impairment of executive functioning

- Comorbid mental health problem (e.g., depression, anxiety disorder, obsessive–compulsive disorder [OCD])

- Childhood correlates
  Learning difficulties
  Disorders of attention/motor control

with others but may be clumsy in their approach. This clumsiness may be particularly apparent in the individual who wishes for an intimate relationship but does not know how to make the first move. Some may follow a person, perhaps trying to "pluck up the courage" to talk to him or her, only later to find themselves arrested for harassment/stalking. One young man with AS recalled how he used to phone girls in his class, but not knowing what to say would remain speechless. One girl's father eventually called the police, and the boy received a formal caution. Others may attempt to make contact, but do so inappropriately. For example, one young man with AS, age 21, decided to go to a nightclub to "find a girlfriend." Not knowing how to approach others but observing intimate behavior between people, he decided to introduce himself by inappropriately touching a young girl and was arrested and charged with indecent assault. Another young man indecently exposed himself over a period of many years, because, according to him, it was the only way he could get girls to pay him attention.

Some published case studies have also described people with AS seeking social relationships in an inappropriate way. For example, in the paper of Haskins and Silva (2006) two cases are described in which the adults with AS have come into contact with the criminal justice system as a result of inappropriate sexualized behavior, in one case involving touching adolescent girls and the other, soliciting male strangers for sexual intercourse. Similarly, Barry-Walsh and Mullen (2004) described one individual with AS who became fixated on professionals who had been involved in his care, phoning them, writing to them, and ultimately being charged with stalking.

The social impairment might also be involved in nonsexualized offending behaviors. For example, people with AS are often critically aware of their differences from their peers, and as they reach early adulthood, and opportunities such as relationships, family, and employment do not come as easy, might experience a feeling of jealousy.

People with AS may also be vulnerable to being "dragged into" crime. For example, their strong wish for friendships may make them particularly vulnerable to agree to do something they would not normally consider doing if the "reward" of "friendship" is on offer. This vulnerability may be compounded by their social naïveté, whereby they are unaware that what they are doing is wrong or that their actions may have a negative impact on their "victim."

RIGIDITY, CIRCUMSCRIBED INTERESTS, AND OFFENDING

A person's circumscribed interests may also lead to contact with the criminal justice system. For example, an 18-year-old man with AS, whose interest was in electronics, had the habit, from a young age, of taking electronic equipment apart. He stole large quantities of electronic equipment for the purpose of disassembling it and figuring out "how it worked," and was convicted of theft. Similarly, the published case studies also describe people with AS who have come into contact with the criminal justice system as a result of their interests. Chen et al. (2003) describe theft in the context of a circumscribed interest, and Chesterman and Rutter (1993) described a young male with AS who was arrested following a series of burglaries of underwear from other people's houses. The case clearly describes an offense occurring in the context of a special interest, but it was also clear that he was more likely to commit an offense if his need to adhere to routine was not appreciated.

Woodbury-Smith et al. (2010) also examined the pattern of circum-scribed interests among 21 offenders with ASD. In the absence of an estab-lished structured method whereby information regarding circumscribed interests can be collected, the researchers constructed a questionnaire to allow relevant details regarding interests to be collected, including its nature and time spent engaged in it. This information was collected during a face-to-face interview. It was hypothesized that there would be a greater prevalence of interests rated as "violent" among offenders with ASD, and that for some a direct relationship between their interest and their offense could be demonstrated. Strikingly, only four of the 21 could be considered to have interests rated as violent compared to none of the 23 nonoffenders with ASD. However, their categorization as violent was debatable, with two having an interest in collecting World War II memorabilia, one an interest in weapons, and the fourth an interest in fires.

Conversely, and more importantly, however, an association between their interest and their offense could be argued in four cases. For example, one had an interest in an aspect of complimentary medicine. He displayed a deep knowledge and understanding of healing and would talk at great length about it. He also practiced healing on people with whom he came into contact. During the course of such "healing" on an 8-year-old girl, an allegation was made and he was subsequently convicted of indecent assault. Another young female claimed a long-standing interest in fires and, in par-ticular, used to enjoy the arrival of the firefighters. She had a history of set-ting fires but was adamant that her primary aim was to watch the arrival and subsequent activity of the emergency services. She believed that she did not place anyone in immediate danger because she carefully planned her fires to avoid this possible outcome.

Paradoxically, people with ASD may end up in difficult situations as a result of their strong adherence to rules. For example, they might inappro-priately reprimand a person for a real or perceived wrongdoing.

NEUROPSYCHOLOGICAL IMPAIRMENTS AND OFFENDING

AS is also defined according to a specific pattern of neuropsychological strengths and vulnerabilities, as discussed elsewhere in this volume (see

Tsatsanis, Chapter 3, this volume). A number of these vulnerabilities might theoretically be associated with offending, including impairments in mentalizing, executive function, and processing others' emotions. Indeed, such factors have been investigated in other groups, such as those with antisocial personality disorder (ASPD) and those with psychopathy. Briefly, there is a body of literature indicating that executive function impairments may be associated with offending among people with ASPD (Dolan & Park, 2002), and individuals with psychopathy show impairment in the recognition of fear and sadness (Blair et al., 2004). Both psychopathy and ASPD are strongly associated with offending behavior (Fazel & Danesh, 2002). In contrast, the literature does not support an association between impairment in theory of mind (ToM) and offending in such groups (Blair et al., 1996).

Two studies have systematically investigated whether the core neuropsychological impairments seen among people with AS are in any way associated with offending. The first (Murphy, 2003) examined cognitive characteristics of patients with AS ($n = 13$) in one maximum secure psychiatric hospital in comparison with detained patients with schizophrenia ($n = 13$) and personality disorder ($n = 13$). On a measure of executive function all three groups performed similarly.

In another cross-sectional case–control study (Woodbury-Smith et al., 2005), the neuropsychological and clinical characteristics of adults with ASD who had offended ($n = 21$) were compared with a matched community sample ($n = 23$) and a comparison group of adults without an ASD ($n = 23$). In this study only individuals functioning intellectually in the normal range and who met the DSM-IV diagnostic criteria for either AS or high-functioning autism (HFA) were included. The researchers were interested in determining whether impairments in ToM, emotion recognition, or executive function were associated with offending. After controlling for the confounding effect of IQ, impairment for the recognition of fear was associated with offending. In contrast, ToM and executive function were not associated. Indeed, as a group the "ASD offenders" demonstrated a superior performance on both ToM and executive function compared to their nonoffending counterparts with ASD, and unlike them, their performance on both of these did not significantly differ from the general population control group.

It is interesting to consider these findings in light of the research that has demonstrated a similar pattern of neuropsychological strengths and vulnerabilities among people described as having psychopathy. This similarity led Woodbury-Smith et al. (2005) to propose that people with AS who offend may be characterized by risk factors for both disorders. Although the clinical descriptions of the disorders are quite different, as discussed above, there are similarities in the neuropsychological characteristics of psychopathy and the offenders with ASD, and impairments of interpersonal behavior are central to both. Furthermore, the same regions of the brain, the amygdala and regions of the frontal cortices (Brower & Price, 2001), are implicated. Similar conclusions were reached by Rogers, Viding, Blair, Frith, and Happé (2006), who measured psychopathic traits among 28 boys with AS who also had aggressive behavior. Psychopathic traits were recorded among their sample, but were not correlated with the degree of severity of their autistic behavior, and were not related to the neuropsychological vulnerabilities. This finding supports the possibility of a double hit, rather than the offending being related to autism per se.

Other studies, however, have contradicted this conclusion. Murphy (2007) found that none of the patients with AS in a maximum secure psychiatric hospital received a diagnosis of psychopathy. Interestingly, comparison of the scores in the different domains of the Psychopathy Checklist—Revised (PCL-R) suggested that patients with AS frequently received higher scores in the affective facet (including features such as lack of remorse or guilt, a shallow affect, lack of empathy, and a failure to accept responsibility for ones actions), and lower scores on the other components when compared to a control group of patients without AS. The mean PCL-R score in the patients with AS was comparable to other patients.

In contrast, Siponmaa et al. (2001) found that the total PCL-R scores, as well as the Factor 2 (unemotionality) and Factor 3 (behavioral dyscontrol) scores, were significantly correlated with HFA traits. The interpersonal Factor 1 of the PCL-R showed none of these correlations, leading the authors to conclude that Factor 1 scores may capture features that are specific to psychopathy, distinguishing core psychopathy from other diagnostic definitions. These findings clearly need further investigation before any firm conclusions can be drawn.

COMORBIDITY

Among children and adults with ASD, so-called *comorbidity* (i.e., meeting the diagnosis for another mental disorder) is relatively common. In particular, studies have pointed toward high rates of depression and anxiety, whereas the rate of schizophrenia is relatively low. As a number of mental disorders are known to be associated with an increased risk of offending, it might be argued theoretically that such comorbidity accounts for offending by people with AS. For example, Palermo (2004) described problematic behaviors occurring during manic and depressive illnesses in individuals with AS, and therefore not as a direct consequence of the core autistic phenotype.

Although no studies have specifically examined whether comorbidity is associated with offending in larger samples of people with ASD, it has become clear from the longitudinal studies of delinquent development that childhood developmental traits, such as those of hyperactivity, impulsivity, and inattention, are associated with later criminal behavior (Babinski,

Hartsough, & Lambert, 1999; Farrington, Loeber, Yin, & Anderson, 2002; Loeber & Farrington, 2000). It is no surprise, therefore, that attention-deficit/hyperactivity disorder (ADHD), in which inattention, hyperactivity, and impulsivity form the core diagnostic features, has been found to be associated with vulnerability to criminal behavior (Farrington, 1990; Soderstrom, Sjodin, Carlstedt, & Forsman, 2004). At least part of this vulnerability is due the strong comorbidity between ADHD and conduct disorder (Manuzza, Klein, Konig, & Giampino, 1989), the childhood precursor of adult ASPD. However, an independent effect for ADHD remains even when conduct disorder is controlled for (Babinski et al., 1999). As there is an increased rate of ADHD among people with AS, this, too, may be a contributing factor, but the possibility has not been formally examined.

THE CONCEPT OF MALICE

Asperger (1944) first used the term "malice" to describe some of the problematic behaviors he observed among the young boys seen in his clinic. Tantam (1999) later described a series of people who have engaged in apparently purposefully hurtful behavior toward others and described such behaviors as "autistic acts of malice." For example, a young man is described who "[phoned] his favourite aunt to say that her husband had been killed in a road accident. . . . The report was a complete fabrication as became apparent an hour later when his uncle arrived home from work." Tantam, in attempting to understand such acts of seeming malice, hypothesized that some people with AS, rather than being motivated by evil intent—which such acts of malice might imply—instead are motivated by a sense of powerlessness that they attempt to circumvent by marshaling their power to shock or disrupt. At the same time, while attempting to shock, it is also likely that such behavior is the consequence of a lack of understanding the emotional impact of the "joke" on the other person. People with AS are also described as having a somewhat concrete sense of humor, which might also explain why they would find such a statement funny.

MANAGEMENT ISSUES

General Considerations

For individuals with ASD who come into contact with the criminal justice system, it is important to recognize the potential impact of their disorder on their fitness to be interviewed, as well as their fitness to plead and their criminal responsibility (Royal College of Psychiatrists, 2006).

From the outset, people with AS may be vulnerable during the police interview. For example, they may not fully appreciate (or understand the implications of) their right to remain silent, or they may be particularly vulnerable to suggestibility. Legislation in the United States, United Kingdom, and other countries has been developed to ensure that such vulnerable people are identified and offered appropriate support. In the United Kingdom, the Police and Criminal Evidence Act of 1994 identified the "Appropriate Adult" as a person who is not directly involved in the interviewing of a vulnerable witness, but who is present to ensure that the person understands what is going on and is interviewed fairly. In the United States, the Americans with Disabilities Act states that reasonable accommodation should be made to allow people with disabilities to participate in many activities including court proceedings.

People with AS may be more suggestible in criminal proceedings for a number of reasons. For example, they may have a heightened state of anxiety in the unfamiliar surroundings of the police station or courtroom. They may not fully understand the questions asked and may be more likely to simply wish to please the questioner. It has been shown that accuracy and amount of recall can be improved by open and free questions (e.g., "Describe him [her]"), whereas closed questions (e.g., "Describe his shirt") result in more complete but less accurate information. Extremely closed questions that are leading (e.g., "Was he wearing a red shirt?"), are more likely to result in a "yeah" response. The Gudjonnson Suggestibility Scale (GSS; Gudjonnson, 1984) is now widely used both in research circles and in clinical services and the criminal justice system to decide on a person's acquiescence to closed and leading questions. It has been shown to have good reliability and validity for men and women across the spectrum of intellectual ability. It measures two aspects of suggestibility: first, the tendency to give in to leading questions, and second, the tendency to shift responses under conditions of interrogative pressure.

The courtroom itself may also be a daunting experience that may raise the level of anxiety. Among people who are intellectually impaired, measures to address this factor have included the allowance of videotaped interview evidence, video/radio live link, pretrial preparation, friend-in-court assistance, the removal of wigs and gowns by barristers/lawyers/attorneys (in the United Kingdom), and the use of screens and other measures. Consideration should be given to whether similar measures might be appropriate for a defendant/witness with AS. What is also sometimes observed both during the police interview and during court proceedings, is that people with AS may not appreciate the required formality of such proceedings. Alternatively, they may come across as emotionally detached and thereby give the opinion that they do not care about the victim, when, in fact, the "detachment" is simply their AS. Regarding fitness to plead, some have argued that the broad capacity required by U.S. courts would be difficult to establish in many cases of AS (Barry-Walsh & Mullen, 2004), although in my view, most people with AS are able to follow the proceedings in court and effectively instruct a lawyer.

In relation to *mens rea*—that is, the ability to form criminal intent—it might be argued that some people with AS may have an inadequate understanding of the consequences to be morally (or criminally) responsible for their offending (Barry-Walsh & Mullen, 2004; Schwartz-Watts, 2005). In most cases, however, people with AS will not deny their actions and will be fully cognizant of the fact that what they were doing was at least legally wrong, even if they fail to understand their behavior from the victim's point of view (and therefore fully understand their transgression from a moral standpoint). For example, one 18-year-old boy with AS involved in the brutal torture of one of his peers described recognizing at the time that if he got caught he would be in serious trouble, but at the same time he was unaware of exactly what his victim was going through.

Clearly, it is vital for professionals working in the criminal justice system to be aware of AS and its presentation. It is also important for clinicians who have expertise in AS to be involved from an early stage in any criminal proceedings. In order to facilitate this involvement, court diversion schemes were set up in the United Kingdom in response to Home Office circulars 66/90 and 12/95, which encouraged health, social care, and criminal justice agencies to work together to provide services for people with mental health problems (including those with ASD) who have offended. However, even with this safeguard, one of the difficulties faced when people with AS are involved in criminal proceedings is that there has been little research to inform the development of policy to meet the rehabilitative needs of such individuals.

As a result, where a community order is suggested, there may not be any specialist rehabilitation to reduce risk of further offending. Conversely, for those who have committed more serious offending, a failure to understand and address the risk factors may result in incarceration for many years. Although there are services for children and adolescents with AS that may be able to address their rehabilitation needs, including residential placements, this is less true for adults. As a consequence, they may end up in generic services for mentally disordered offenders or prisons where there is a lack of expertise with individuals who have AS.

In all but the most severe of cases, prison sentences are not appropriate. Despite being an environment that is characterized by structure, routine, and little requirement to conform to rules of social interaction, there are no therapeutic programs suitable for people with AS, or, indeed, developmental disabilities more generally. The environment encourages social withdrawal, removes individuals from their established routines and predictable environment, and perhaps most importantly, people with any form of disability are vulnerable to bullying, abuse, and exploitation by more dominant and antisocial types. These factors notwithstanding, for those individuals who do commit serious crimes, prison may be the only option, and a diagnosis of AS should not preclude their participation in those therapeutic programs that are on offer, such as the Sex Offender Treatment Programme (SOTP) or the Enhanced Thinking Skills (ETS) program. What should be recognized, however, is that participation of individuals with AS in group work, particularly work that involves role play, may cause anxiety, and that their ability to self-reflect may be limited and require additional work, perhaps on a one-to-one basis with a suitably trained therapist.

Offending and the Social Impairment

As described above, offending by people with AS is likely to have occurred as a result of a variety of factors, and for some, these factors may include their social impairment. Arguably, therefore, among such individuals, reducing their risk of reoffending will involve work to reduce the impact of their social impairment on their everyday interactions. This can be achieved in several different ways. For example, social skills training is now widely used among children with ASD, and groups for adults are being established. Such groups often consist of a small number of people with ASD who meet at an agreed location for an agreed length of time, along with a suitably trained facilitator. Issues such as how to cope in different situations are discussed, facilitated by the development of "social scripts" to achieve more flexible and successful communication with others. In this way individuals with AS learn rules of interaction and ways to avoid committing faux pas.

Alternatively, strategies to "teach" empathy skills may be appropriate. These include, for example, attempting to teach an understanding of others' feelings through individual or group treatments, as has been carried out with sexual offenders (Pithers, 1999). Role playing as a means to develop perspective-taking skills form a central part of many such groups, but may be particularly difficult for people with ASD.

Alternatively, teaching empathy in a more "concrete" way may be helpful. At a more basic level, a software package has been developed, using lessons, quizzes, and games, to help develop individuals' understanding of emotions (University of Cambridge, 2002). This approach was found to significantly improve the ability of adults with AS to recognize a variety of complex emotions and mental states over a period of 10–15 weeks (Golan, Baron-Cohen, & Hill, 2006). Research by Klin, Jones, Schultz, and Cohen (2002) suggests that the impairments in social and emotional understanding are evident very early in life, implying that a developmental approach to promoting empathy is likely to be helpful. This is also consistent with the potential for an attachment-based perspective in the treatment and management of people with severe and long-standing difficulties.

Offending in the Context of Circumscribed Interests

Particular challenges are faced when people with AS offend in the context of their circumscribed interest. Most people's circumscribed interests are not inherently problematic in a criminal sense, and, as such, might not require any specific interventions. It is important to recognize that, in the best-case scenario, interests may have a positive impact on self-esteem, may facilitate the establishment of relationships, provide a topic of conversation, and may lead to employment in some cases. Careful consideration therefore needs to be given to this area before attempts are made to modify or minimize the focus of a person's interest.

This point notwithstanding, as is evident from the literature reviewed above and in my clinical experience, some circumscribed interests are problematic, either inherently or because during their pursuit, a legal transgression is made. In these circumstances it may be appropriate to intervene. Some circumstances may require that the interest be stopped completely, although in most cases it may be possible to "mold" the interest into one that is more acceptable, one that is pursued with less intensity, or one that is pursued only in certain places or at certain times of the day (e.g., an interest in fire fighting could be shaped into volunteering at a local fire station).

It is also important to be clear whether the behavior of concern is best conceptualized as a circumscribed interest or whether it is phenomenologically "obsessive" in nature and a manifestation of OCD. Obsessions are common among higher-functioning people with ASD (Russell, Mataix-Cols, Anson, & Murphy, 2005; McDougle et al., 1995), and making the distinction in everyday clinical practice can be difficult. As a general rule, as a result of their fundamentally rewarding and interesting nature, circumscribed interests are associated with a positive affect and have a positive impact on self-esteem, whereas obsessions are experienced as intrusive and distressing and can be associated with dysphoria and anxiety.

It is important to make this distinction because treatment will be dictated by diagnosis. Specific treatments, such as medication and cognitive-behavioral therapy (CBT), are known to help reduce OCD symptoms in the general population of adults and children, although the efficacy of such interventions is poorly established among people with ASD.

Conversely, there is very little known about the most useful techniques to modify a person's circumscribed interest. Here, CBT may also be beneficial in reducing preoccupation with violent and sexual themes (Barry-Walsh & Mullen, 2004). A behavioral approach, introducing reward and punishment contingencies, might be more useful to "mold" a circumscribed interest toward something more acceptable. A supportive behavioral approach may also help teach the individual about the inappropriateness of the behavior and through a mutual understanding, a set of "rules" could be drawn up regarding times and places where pursuit of the interest is acceptable.

Employment and Offending

In terms of more general therapeutic provision, facilitating employment is likely to have several beneficial effects. First, employment provides a means whereby an individual can make positive social relationships, as well as giving the opportunity to develop social-communicative skills. Secondly, it also provides structure for much of the day. For those individuals with circumscribed interests, employment will reduce the amount of time spent engaging in an interest, and may even provide legitimate avenues for their pursuit. Finally, employment provides financial gain and, along with its other positive benefits, will improve self-esteem.

Alternatively, recognizing that employment opportunities are not always easy to identify, there are other social activities that may be beneficial. For example, social skills groups have been developed to provide a forum to focus on the development of social-communicative skills through role play and discussion of difficult everyday situations (these are discussed in detail elsewhere in this volume). In a similar way to employment, such groups also allow a wider network of social relationships to be developed. Considering circumscribed interests specifically, these groups may provide the opportunity to share an interest with others or learn from others ways of shaping an interest either by reducing its nature, intensity, or avenues for pursuit. In a similar way, other social activities, such as joining a gym, can be useful. Table 12.2 summarizes strategies and approaches to dealing with forensic issues in the AS population.

CONCLUDING REMARKS

There is now little doubt that a small number of people with ASD will come into contact with the criminal justice system as a result of criminal behavior. It remains unclear exactly what factors contribute to this risk, but it is likely to be multifactorial. Importantly, core clinical and neuropsychological

---

TABLE 12.2. Summary of Management Strategies for the Forensic ASD Population

General strategies
- Availability of appropriate adult during interrogation.
- Involvement of health professional with expertise in ASD early in criminal justice process.
- Diversion from criminal justice system to mental health services/specialist ASD provision.

Provision of Employment

Social impairment
- Provision of social support
- Social skills training
- Empathy training

Circumscribed interests/obsessive behavior
- CBT
- Behavioral strategies
- Medication

---

impairments may contribute. Experts in the field of ASD have a crucial role to play in facilitating the rehabilitation of such individuals and protecting them from further social exclusion. There is now an urgent need for more research to help facilitate an understanding of this risk and to inform the development of management strategies and ultimately inform policy.

ACKNOWLEDGMENTS

I would like to thank the Wellcome Trust and Department of Health (UK) for their support in funding my project concerning criminal behavior among people with AS. I would also like to acknowledge the support of colleagues at Cambridge University and Yale Child Study Center.

REFERENCES

Asperger, H. (1944). Die "autistichen Psychopathen" im Kindersalter. *Archiv für psychiatrie und Nervenkrankheiten, 117,* 76–136.

Babinski, L. M., Hartsough, C. S., & Lambert, N. M. (1999). Childhood conduct problems, hyperactivity–impulsivity, and inattention as predictors of adult criminal activity. *Journal of Child Psychology and Psychiatry, 40*(3), 347–355.

Baron-Cohen, S. (1988). An assessment of violence in a young man with Asperger's syndrome. *Journal of Child Psychology and Psychiatry, 29*(3), 351–360.

Barry-Walsh, J. B., & Mullen, P. E. (2004). Forensic aspects of Asperger's syndrome. *Journal of Forensic Psychiatry and Psychology, 15*(1), 96–107.

Blair, J., Sellers, C., Strickland, I., Clark, F., Williams, A., Smith, M., et al. (1996). Theory of mind in the psychopath. *Journal of Forensic Psychiatry, 7*(1), 15–25.

Blair, R., Mitchell, D., Peschardt, K., Colledge, E., Leonard, R., Shine, J., et al. (2004). Reduced sensitivity to others' fearful expressions in psychopathic individuals. *Personality and Individual Difference, 37,* 1111–1122.

Brower, M., & Price, B. (2001). Neuropsychiatry of frontal lobe dysfunction in violent and criminal behavior: A critical review. *Journal of Neurology, Neurosurgery, and Psychiatry, 71,* 720–726.

Chen, P. S., Chen, S. J., Yang, Y. K., Yeh, T. L., Chen, C. C., & Lo, H. Y. (2003). Asperger's disorder: A case report of repeated stealing and the collecting behaviours of an adolescent patient. *Acta Psychiatrica Scandinavica, 107*(1), 73–75; discussion 75–76.

Chesterman, P., & Rutter, S. C. (1993). Case report: Asperger's syndrome and sexual offending. *Journal of Forensic Psychiatry, 4*(3), 555–562.

Department of Health (2002). *Review of health and social services for mentally disordered offenders and others requiring similar services.* Final summary report. London, UK: HMSO, 1992.

Dolan, M., & Park, I. (2002). The neuropsychology of antisocial personality disorder. *Psychological Medicine, 32*(3), 417–427.

Elvish, J. (2005). *The exploration of autistic spectrum disorder characteristics in individuals within a secure service for people with learning disabilities.* Unpublished doctoral dissertation.

Everall, I. P., & Lecouter, A. (1990). Firesetting in an adolescent boy with Asperger's syndrome. *British Journal of Psychiatry, 157,* 284–287.

Farrington, D. P. (1990). Implications of criminal career research for the prevention of offending. *Journal of Adolescence, 13,* 93–113.

Farrington, D. P., Loeber, R., Yin, Y. M., & Anderson, S. J. (2002). Are within-individual causes of delinquency the same as between-individual causes? *Criminal Behaviour and Mental Health, 12,* 53–68.

Fazel, S., & Danesh, J. (2002). Serious mental disorder in 23,000 prisoners: A systematic review of 62 surveys. *Lancet, 359,* 545–550.

Frith, U. (Ed.). (1991). Asperger and his syndrome. *Autism and Asperger syndrome.* Cambridge, UK: Cambridge University Press.

Ghaziuddin, M., Tsai, L. Y., & Ghaziuddin, N. (1991). Brief report: Violence in Asperger syndrome: A critique. *Journal of Autism and Developmental Disorders, 21*(3), 349–354.

Gillberg, C., & Gillberg, C. (1989). Asperger syndrome—some epidemiological considerations: A research note. *Journal of Child Psychology and Psychiatry, 30,* 631–638.

Golan, O., Baron-Cohen, S., & Hill, J. (2006). The Cambridge Mindreading (CAM) Face–Voice Battery: Testing complex emotion recognition in adults with and without Asperger syndrome. *Journal of Autism and Developmental Disorders, 36*(2), 169–183.

Gudjonsson, G. H. (1984). A new scale of interrogative suggestibility. *Personality and Individual Differences, 5*(3), 303–314.

Hare, D. J., Gould, J., Mills, R., & Wing, L. (1999). *A preliminary study of individuals with autistic spectrum disorders in three special hospitals in England.* London: National Autistic Society.

Haskins, B. G., & Silva, J. A. (2006). Asperger's disorder and criminal behavior: Forensic–psychiatric considerations. *Journal of the American Academy of Psychiatry and the Law, 34*(3), 374–384.

Hippler, K., & Klicpera, C. (2003). A retrospective analysis of the clinical case records of "autistic psychopaths" diagnosed by Hans Asperger and his team at the University Children's Hospital, Vienna. *Philosophical Transactions of the Royal Society of London Series B: Biological Sciences, 358*(1430), 291–301.

Howlin, P. (2004). *Autism and Asperger syndrome: Preparing for adulthood* (2nd ed.). London: Routledge.

Klin, A., Jones, W., Schultz, R., Volkmar, F., & Cohen, D. (2002). Visual fixation patterns during viewing of naturalistic social situations as predictors of social competence in individuals with autism. *Archives of General Psychiatry, 59*(9), 809–816.

Klin, A., McPartland, J., & Volkmar, F. R. (2005). Asperger syndrome. In F. R. Volkmar, A. Klin, R. Paul, & D. J. Cohen (Eds.), *Handbook of autism and pervasive developmental disorders* (3rd ed., pp. 88–125). Hoboken, NJ: Wiley.

Kohn, Y., Fahum, T., Ratzoni, G., & Apter, A. (1998). Aggression and sexual offence in Asperger's syndrome. *Israeli Journal of Psychiatry and Related Sciences, 35*(4), 293–299.

Loeber, R., & Farrington, D. P. (2000). Young children who commit crime:

Epidemiology, developmental origins, risk factors, early interventions, and policy implications. *Development and Psychopathology, 12*(4), 737–762.

Manuzza, S., Klein, R., Konig, P., & Giampino, T. (1989). Hyperactive boys almost grown up: IV. Criminality and its relationship to psychiatric status. *Archives of General Psychiatry, 46,* 1073–1079.

Mawson, D., Grounds, A., & Tantam, D. (1985). Violence and Asperger's syndrome: A case study. *British Journal of Psychiatry, 147,* 566–569.

McDougle, C. J., Kresch, L. E., Goodman, W. K., Naylor, S. T., Volkmar, F. R., Cohen, D. J., et al. (1995). A case-controlled study of repetitive thoughts and behavior in adults with autistic disorder and obsessive–compulsive disorder. *American Journal of Psychiatry, 152*(5), 772–777.

Mouridsen, S. E., Rich, B., Isager, T., & Nedergaard, N. J. (2008). Pervasive developmental disorders and criminal behaviour: A case–control study. *International Journal of Offender Therapy and Comparative Criminology, 52*(2), 196–205.

Murphy, D. G. (2003). Admission and cognitive details of male patients diagnosed with Asperger's syndrome detained in special hospital: Comparison with a schizophrenia and personality disorder sample. *Journal of Forensic Psychiatry and Psychology, 14*(3), 506–524.

Murphy, D. G. (2007). Hare Psychopathy Checklist Revised profiles of male patients with Asperger's syndrome detained in high security psychiatric care. *Journal of Forensic Psychiatry and Psychology, 18*(1), 20–26.

Murrie, D. C., Warren, J. I., Kristiansson, M., & Dietz, P. E. (2002). Asperger's syndrome in forensic settings. *International Journal of Forensic Mental Health, 1*(1), 59–70.

Palermo, M. T. (2004). Pervasive developmental disorders, psychiatric comorbidities, and the law. *International Journal of Offender Therapy and Comparative Criminology, 48*(1), 40–48.

Pithers, W. (1999). Empathy: Definitions, enhancement, and relevance to the treatment of the sexual abuser. *Journal of Interpersonal Violence, 14,* 257–284.

Rogers, J. S. C., Viding, E., Blair, R. J. R., Frith, U., & Happé, F. (2006). Autism spectrum disorder and psychopathy: Shared cognitive underpinnings or double-hit? *Psychological Medicine, 36,* 1789–1798.

Royal College of Psychiatrists. (2006). *Psychiatric services for adolescents and adults with Asperger syndrome and other autistic-spectrum disorders* (No. CR 136). London: Author.

Russell, A. J., Mataix-Cols, D., Anson, M., & Murphy, D. G. (2005). Obsessions and compulsions in Asperger syndrome and high-functioning autism. *British Journal of Psychiatry, 186,* 525–528.

Schwartz-Watts, D. M. (2005). Asperger's disorder and murder. *Journal of the American Academy of Psychiatry and the Law, 33*(3), 390–393.

Scragg, P., & Shah, A. (1994). Prevalence of Asperger's syndrome in a secure hospital. *British Journal of Psychiatry, 165*(5), 679–682.

Silva, J. A., Ferrari, M. M., & Leong, G. B. (2002). The case of Jeffrey Dahmer: Sexual serial homicide from a neuropsychiatric developmental perspective. *Journal of Forensic Sciences, 47*(6), 1347–1359.

Siponmaa, L., Kristiansson, M., Jonson, C., Nyden, A., & Gillberg, C. (2001). Juvenile and young adult mentally disordered offenders: The role of child neuropsychiatric disorders. *Journal of the American Academy of Psychiatry and the Law, 29*(4), 420–426.

Soderstrom, H., Sjodin, A.-K., Carlstedt, A., & Forsman, A. (2004). Adult psychopathic personality with childhood-onset hyperactivity and conduct disorder: A central problem constellation in forensic psychiatry. *Psychiatry Research, 121*(3), 271–280.

Tantam, D. (1988a). Lifelong eccentricity and social isolation: I. Psychiatric, social, and forensic aspects. *British Journal of Psychiatry, 153*, 777–782.

Tantam, D. (1988b). Lifelong eccentricity and social isolation: II. Asperger's syndrome or schizoid personality disorder? *British Journal of Psychiatry, 153*, 783–791.

Tantam, D. (1999). *Malice and Asperger syndrome.* Paper presented at Autism99 International Online Conference. Available at *www.autismuk.com/?page_id=262.*

University of Cambridge. (2002). Mind Reading: The Interactive Guide to Emotions (Version 1.0). Cambridge, UK: Human Emotions.

Wing, L. (1981). Asperger's syndrome: A clinical account. *Psychological Medicine, 11*(1), 115–129.

Wing, L. (1997). Asperger's syndrome: Management requires diagnosis. *Journal of Forensic Psychiatry, 8*(2), 253–257.

Wolff, S. (2000). Schizoid personality in childhood and Asperger syndrome. In A. Klin & F. R. Volkmar (Eds.), *Asperger syndrome* (pp. 278–305). New York: Guilford Press.

Wolff, S., Townshend, R., McGuire, R. J., & Weeks, D. J. (1991). "Schizoid" personality in childhood and adult life: II. Adult adjustment and the continuity with schizotypal personality disorder. *British Journal of Psychiatry, 159*, 620–629, 634–625.

Woodbury-Smith, M., Clare, I. C., Holland, A., & Kearns, A. (2006). High functioning autistic spectrum disorders, offending and other law-breaking: Findings from a community sample. *Journal of Forensic Psychiatry and Psychology, 17*(1), 108–120.

Woodbury-Smith, M., Clare, I. C., Holland, A., Kearns, A., Staufenberg, E., & Watson, P. (2005). A case–control study of offenders with high functioning autistic spectrum disorders. *Journal of Forensic Psychiatry and Psychology, 16*(4), 747–763.

Woodbury-Smith, M., Clare, I. C., Holland, A. J., Watson, P., Bambrick, M., Kearns, A., et al. (2010). Circumscribed interests and "offenders" with autism spectrum disorders: A case–control study. *Journal of Forensic Psychology, 21*(3), 366–377.

CHAPTER 13

Social Brain Function and Its Development

New Insights into Autism Spectrum Disorders

Kevin A. Pelphrey
Brent C. Vander Wyk
Sarah Shultz
Caitlin M. Hudac

Asperger syndrome (AS) is one of a group of neurodevelopmental disorders collectively known as autism spectrum disorders (ASD). ASD include autistic disorder, AS, pervasive developmental disorder not otherwise specified (PDD-NOS), Rett disorder, and childhood disintegrative disorder. As an ASD, AS features significant deficits in the capacity to engage in normal reciprocal social interactions. Ritualized patterns of interests and repetitive behaviors co-occur with these social deficits. AS differs from other ASD in its relative preservation of linguistic and cognitive development; also commonly present is a significant degree of motor clumsiness (McPartland & Klin, 2006; Wing, 1981).

FUNCTIONAL NEUROIMAGING AS A TOOL FOR UNDERSTANDING AUTISM SPECTRUM DISORDERS

Extensive efforts are currently underway to examine the pathogenesis of ASD at multiple levels of the developing person: from the genes, to the brain, to behavior and cognition and beyond the person to the broader social context. Whereas approaches involving research on genes, the brain, and behavior have typically operated in parallel with little cross-fertilization, scientists are now undertaking the challenge of bridging these levels of analysis to understand the key developmental transactions that give rise to ASD. As a technique, functional magnetic resonance imaging (fMRI) is well suited for such multiple-levels-of-analysis efforts. fMRI can provide critical links between discoveries concerning genetic and molecular pathophysiological mechanisms and the core behavioral deficits in social engagement that are identified as uniquely characterizing ASD. In particular, fMRI can provide powerful endophenotypes to facilitate the search for genetic mechanisms and to provide a neural systems level context for their interpretation.

Originally described in the psychiatric literature by Gottesman and Shields (1972, 1973), *endophenotypes* are characteristics (behavioral, physiological, neuropsychological, etc.) reflecting genetic liability for disease that exist midstream between genotype and clinical phenotype and are often measurable in both affected and unaffected individuals (Gottesman & Gould, 2003). Such endophenotypes are thought to reflect more elementary phenomena (or the more basic components of a complex phenotype), and thus are more closely related to the underlying pathophysiology than downstream clinical syndromes that are often conceptualized as a synthesis of a number of such endophenotypes. Genetic factors contributing to endophenotypes are therefore generally considered to be easier to identify because of the increased proportion of the variance explained at a given genetic locus versus that explained by the traditional clinical end point.

Longitudinal studies of the neural circuitry supporting key aspects of social information processing in young children with and without autism, as well as prospective studies of infants at increased risk for being identified with autism by virtue of their status as a sibling of a child with an ASD, are likely to generate fundamental insights into the underlying components of the full syndrome of ASD, particularly via the contribution of genetically meaningful endophenotypes. The structural MRI findings of Schumann and colleagues (2004) provide a glimpse of this promise. They measured the volumes of the amygdala, the hippocampus, and the cerebrum in cross-sectional samples of 7- to 18.5-year-old male children and adolescents. There were four groups of individuals: (1) those with autism and mental retardation, (2) those with autism but without mental retardation, (3) those with AS, and (4) age-matched, typically developing comparison individuals. Overall, they found no group differences in total cerebral volume. Children ages 7.5–12.5 years with an ASD (autism with or without mental retardation or AS) had larger right and left amygdala volumes than did the typically developing children. However, there were no group differences in amygdala volumes among the adolescents (12.75–18.5 years of age). The developmental pattern was such that the amygdala, in typically developing children, increased substantially in volume from 7.5 to 18.5 years of age. In contrast, the amygdala in children with an ASD was initially larger, but failed to exhibit the age-related increase observed in typically developing children. Strikingly, these cross-sectional findings suggest an abnormal developmental pattern specific to the amygdala in individuals with an ASD. This pattern of development could serve as a key endophenotype in a research agenda focused on identifying the developmental transactions that give rise to ASD.

Figure 13.1 outlines the ways in which developmental trajectories of brain function in key social brain regions might serve as endophenotypes for the study of ASD. At the top of Figure 13.1 is a reaction surface, which is modeled after Gottesman and Gould's (2003) discussion of endophenotypes in schizophrenia, and is intended to represent the liability for developing the observable phenotype with regard to key behaviors that define ASD (i.e., deficits in social reciprocity and engagement, language abilities, the presence of restricted and repetitive behaviors). The surface is generated via the transactions, occurring across developmental time among genetic,

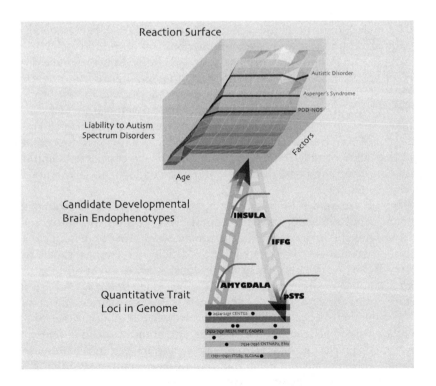

FIGURE 13.1. Developmental trajectories of brain function in key social brain regions as endophenotypes for the study of ASD. lFFG, lateral fusiform gyrus; pSTS, posterior superior temporal sulcus.

brain, environmental, and epigenetic factors. Levels, which are admittedly somewhat arbitrary, demark autistic disorder, AS, and PDD-NOS. The bottom panel identifies some of the gene regions where linkage findings have been observed repeatedly in the field of autism. Then, in the panel immediately above the genetic findings, we have illustrated several, now replicated findings regarding the social brain and its development in individuals with autism. It is important to emphasize here that although function in each of the featured brain regions has been identified as differentiating individuals with and without ASD, the developmental trajectories of function in these brain regions over time are predicted to be the better correlate of ASD. Above the level of the social brain systems and their development, embedded in the reaction surface, are developmental trajectories in key social behaviors, which are also known to be disrupted in ASD.

Note that the lines connecting brain and behavior are bidirectional, as are the lines connecting the brain and the genes. This bidirectionality emphasizes the hypothesis that over time, as social development is disrupted, this disruption in turn restricts the experiences of the individual, thereby further deflecting social brain development off its normative course. Some progress has been made toward identifying the brain systems and brain developmental processes that characterize ASD. Few studies have attempted to link these findings to the development of specific social behaviors of interest. Almost no work has addressed linkages between the development of specific social brain systems and potential genetic mechanisms. We believe that these steps are crucial for moving the field forward toward an accounting of how so many different genetic mechanisms, and a smaller number of molecular pathophysiological mechanisms, might give rise to consistently abnormal social brain development. Finally, it is important to note that none of the sections of this figure can be considered definitive; many genes and candidate developmental brain endophenotypes remain to be discovered.

In the remainder of this chapter, we present recent neuroimaging, computational modeling, and behavioral evidence from our program of research into the impairments in the functioning of neuroanatomical systems that are thought to be related to ASD deficits in reciprocal social interaction. We recognize that these disruptions in brain function may arise from a number of different genetic and molecular etiologies and are also further transformed across development by the experiences and activity of the individual in the world (Kandel, 1998). We argue that the reciprocal relationship between brain disruption and atypical social development drives homogeneity in the syndrome's presentation even in the presence of enormous phenotypic and genotypic heterogeneity. Our contention is that despite the etiological heterogeneity and despite such high phenotypic variability, it is the case that the various factors contributing to the now well-characterized triad of impairments in autism exert their effect through a circumscribed set of neural structures and their interconnections that both give rise to, and are shaped by, social development. That is, it is possible that the simplest and potentially most powerful marker of autism will be found at the level of brain systems and their development (i.e., the dynamic interactions among genes, brain, and behavior over time), rather than solely at the genetic, neural, or behavioral levels.

DIFFERENTIATING ASPERGER SYNDROME FROM OTHER AUTISM SPECTRUM DISORDERS

To date, there is relatively little neuroimaging research directed at defining what differentiates AS from other ASD at the level of brain phenotype. Indeed, the preponderance of evidence seems to point toward more similarities than differences. Thus, in this chapter, we discuss evidence from studies of ASD more broadly as opposed to distinguishing between AS and other ASD. However, a few recent structural neuroimaging studies have demonstrated important differences and are reviewed here.

McAlonan and colleagues (2008) identified distinct patterns of gray matter abnormality in high-functioning autism (HFA) versus AS. Children with autism had significantly smaller gray matter volumes in subcortical, posterior cingulate, and precuneus regions than did the group of individuals with AS. This same group of researchers also examined white matter development in these two groups (McAlonan et al., 2009). White matter volumes around the basal ganglia were higher in the group of children with HFA than in those with AS and higher in both ASD groups than in the comparison children. Lotspeich et al. (2004) reported that cerebral gray matter volume was enlarged in both HFA and low-functioning autism compared with controls. Cerebral gray matter volume in individuals with AS was intermediate between individuals with HFA and typically developing children.

A PRIMER ON THE SOCIAL BRAIN

Social perception is the initial stage of evaluating the intentions and psychological dispositions of others using their gaze direction, body movements, hand gestures, facial expressions, and other biological motion cues (Allison, Puce, & McCarthy, 2000). We use the term *biological motion* to refer to the visual perception of a biological entity engaged in a recognizable activity, including walking and making eye, mouth, and arm movements. Neuroscientists became keenly interested in social perception when it was discovered that neurons within the temporal cortex and amygdala of monkeys were sensitive to and selective for social objects (e.g., faces and hands) and complex social stimuli (actions in a social context and direction of gaze) (Brothers & Ring, 1993; Brothers, Ring, & Kling, 1990;

Desimone, 1991; Desimone, Albright, Gross, & Bruce, 1984; Perrett, Rolls, & Caan, 1979, 1982; Perrett et al., 1984, 1985; Rolls, 1981, 1995). On the basis of these findings, the field began to think seriously about the possibility of a network of brain regions dedicated to processing social information. The label "social brain" was coined by Leslie Brothers (1990) and defined as the network of neuroanatomical structures that enable us to recognize other individuals and to evaluate their mental states (e.g., intentions, dispositions, desires, and beliefs). The key idea is that human beings, in response to the unique computational demands of their highly social environments, have evolved cognitive mechanisms and an associated, dedicated neural system supporting such abilities as recognizing other agents and their actions, individuating others, perceiving the emotional states of others, analyzing the intentions and dispositions of others, sharing attention with one another, and representing another person's perceptions and beliefs.

In a model of the social brain, Brothers (1990) emphasized the contributions of the superior temporal sulcus (STS), amygdala, orbital frontal cortex (OFC), and fusiform gyrus (FFG). In humans, the STS region, particularly the posterior STS in the right hemisphere, analyzes biological motion cues, including eye, hand, and other body movements, to interpret and predict the actions and intentions of others (e.g., Bonda, Petrides, Ostry, & Evans, 1996; Pelphrey, Morris, Michelich, Allison, & McCarthy, 2005). The FFG, located in the ventral occipitotemporal cortex, contains a region termed the *fusiform face area* (FFA), which has been implicated in face detection (identifying a face as a face) and face recognition (identifying one's friend vs. a stranger) (e.g., Kanwisher, McDermott, & Chun, 1997; Puce, Allison, Asgari, Gore, & McCarthy, 1996). These two processes may well occur at different points in time within the FFA, with face detection preceding face recognition. The OFC has been implicated in social reinforcement and reward processes more broadly (e.g., Rolls, 2000, 2009). Finally, the amygdala, a complex structure that is highly interconnected with cortical and other subcortical brain structures, has been implicated in helping to recognize the emotional states of others through analysis of facial expressions (e.g., Morris et al., 1996), as well as in multiple aspects of the experience and regulation of emotion (e.g., Davis & Whalen, 2001; Klüver & Bucy, 1997; LeDoux, 2000).

To understand social brain functions, we must be as attentive to the interconnections of neuroanatomical structures as we are to their individual contributions. Currently, in humans, much is known about the roles played by the individual brain regions, but very little is known about the ways in which they are interconnected, and thus even less is known about how they interact functionally. However, we can take some initial guidance from the monkey brain. Here, it is known that the STS region has reciprocal connections to the amygdala (Amaral, Price, Pitkanen, & Carmichael, 1992). The amygdala, in turn, is connected to the OFC (Amaral et al., 1992), and the STS is also connected with the OFC (Barbas, 1988). The

OFC is connected to prefrontal cortex (Pandya & Yererian, 1996), which is connected to motor cortex and the basal ganglia, thus completing what Allison and colleagues (2000) described as a pathway from social perception to social action.

In the following sections, we present evidence from our laboratory implicating the STS region as a key player in the set of neural structures giving rise to ASD. However, we want to state clearly here that we view each of the components of the social brain (those mentioned here and others) and their interconnections as important players in ASD. We emphasize the posterior STS simply because it has, to date, been a key focus in our research program, and because it can serve as a good example of how work in this area might make progress toward identifying the brain mechanisms involved in core deficits within ASD.

THE FUNCTIONAL ROLE OF THE SUPERIOR TEMPORAL SULCUS REGION AND ITS DISRUPTION IN AUTISM SPECTRUM DISORDERS

Recognizing Agents and Actions

In an initial fMRI study of typically developing adults, we compared the response from the posterior STS to four different types of motion conveyed via animated virtual reality characters (Pelphrey, Mitchell, McKeown, Goldstein, Allison, et al., 2003). Participants viewed walking, a biological motion conveyed by a robot or a human. They also viewed a nonmeaningful but complex nonbiological motion in the form of a disjointed mechanical figure, and a complex, meaningful, and nameable nonbiological motion involving the movements of a grandfather clock. We reasoned that a region selectively responsive to biological motion should respond strongly to both the man and the robot walking, but not respond to the mechanical figure or the grandfather clock.

We found strong and equivalent activity in the right-hemisphere posterior STS region to the human and robot walking and very little activity to the moving clock and the mechanical figure. This pattern of results was very different from that observed in the nearby motion-responsive visual area called MT (Zeki, Watson, Lueck, Friston, Kennard, et al., 1991), which responded robustly to all four of our stimulus conditions. We concluded that the posterior STS responds selectively to biological motion. This finding led us to begin to view the posterior STS as one component of the neural system supporting social perception, via the identification and representation of observed human actions as compared to the movements of other objects.

Analyzing Intentions

Having established a basic role for the posterior STS region in social perception, we went on to examine whether this region simply serves as a biological motion detector or if it is involved more broadly in aspects of social perception through the evaluation of the intentions and dispositions that are conveyed by biological motions. For example, we asked if this region might be involved in representing another person's intentions with respect to the objects in his or her visual field (Vander Wyk, Hudac, Carter, Sobel, & Pelphrey, 2009). This understanding of intention would involve integrating actions with the social and physical context, and the STS may show regional sensitivity to environmental or cognitive sources of information that enrich this context. An especially salient component of social context is the perceived emotions of other individuals, particularly when a perceived emotion indicates another person's like or dislike of an object or event. We examined whether the posterior STS exhibits differences in activity that are dependent on the previous emotional context related to understanding another's preferences, which would inform the viewer about that person's underlying intentions. This experiment used a paradigm, adapted from a study of young children by Phillips, Wellman, and Spelke (2002), in which the participants observed an actress on video express positive or negative regard toward one of two cups. She then reached for and picked up that same object or the other one. Viewing the actress's emotional expression allowed the participant to attribute an intention to her: Positive expressions toward an object warranted the attribution of the intent to pick up the object, whereas negative expressions warranted the opposite attribution. The subsequent reaching gesture was then interpreted as being either congruent or incongruent with the intention.

Our results indicated that the right posterior STS exhibited significantly more activity for the incongruent trials than for the congruent trials. This finding indicated that the activity of the right posterior STS to a given biological motion is sensitive to prior emotional context. Specifically, the posterior STS showed a greater response when participants viewed a reach that was incongruent with a prior emotional expression (i.e., when the actress reached for the object not targeted by a prior positive expression, or when she reached for the object targeted by a prior negative expression) than when they viewed a reach congruent with the actress's expression. In both cases in which positive and negative emotions set up these expectations about the actress's future behaviors toward an object, the response in the posterior STS was greater upon viewing unanticipated actions.

This finding lends support to our proposal that the posterior STS region plays a role both in representing biological motion and in performing an analysis of the intentions and dispositions conveyed by that biological motion. This view of the functional role of the posterior STS is further bolstered by additional findings regarding a role for the posterior STS in analyzing the intentions and dispositions of others as conveyed by biological motion (e.g., Brass, Schmitt, Spengler, & Gergely, 2007; Castelli, Happé, Frith, & Frith, 2000; Pelphrey, Singerman, Allison, & McCarthy, 2003; Saxe, Xiao, Kovacs, Perrett, & Kanwisher, 2004).

Failing to Analyze Intentions: Superior Temporal Sulcus Dysfunction in Autism

A large body of research demonstrates that individuals with autism exhibit early-appearing deficits in using gaze information to understand the intentions and mental states of others, as well as to coordinate joint attention (Baron-Cohen et al., 1999; Baron-Cohen, Wheelwright, Hill, Raste, & Plumb, 2001; Dawson, Meltzoff, Osterling, Rinaldi, & Brown, 1998; Frith & Frith, 1999; Leekam, Hunnisett, & Moore, 1998; Leekam, López, & Moore, 2000; Loveland & Landry, 1986; Mundy, Sigman, Ungerer, & Sherman, 1986). This failure to understand the mentalistic significance of eye gaze and the focus of another person's attention motivated a recent study of posterior STS function in individuals with autism.

Adolescent and young-adult participants with and without HFA viewed actions that were either congruent or incongruent with expectations formed during the viewing of positive or negative emotional content. This experiment made use of the identical reach-to-cups paradigm as did our prior study of typical adults (Vander Wyk et al., 2009). To recap, participants were instructed to attentively watch videos in which an actress was seated in front of a red cup and a green cup. At the start of a trial, the actress shifted her head and gaze to show preference to a cup by either smiling (positive regard) or frowning (negative regard), followed by a return to a neutral expression and eye contact with the camera. She maintained this pose while reaching toward, lifting, and setting down either cup to end the trial. Thus, given the initial preference and whether the actress chose to reach toward and pick up the ignored or attended cup, four conditions were created: (1) a positive–congruent condition wherein the actress expressed a positive emotion toward an object and then reached for that object; (2) a positive–incongruent condition, in which the actress reached for the ignored object; (3) a negative–congruent condition wherein the actress expressed a negative emotion and reach to the ignored object; and (4) a negative–incongruent condition, in which the actress expressed a negative emotion toward an object, but then reached to that object.

Based on our prior work, we hypothesized that the right posterior STS would not differentiate incongruent and congruent actions in autism (Pelphrey, Morris, Michelich, Allison, & McCarthy, et al., 2005). The new sample of typically developing participants demonstrated a strong effect of congruency (incongruent > congruent) within the right posterior STS. This area of activation nicely overlaps with the previously published reference region, clearly replicating our prior findings (Vander Wyk et al., 2009). In sharp contrast, individuals with autism failed to exhibit incongruent > congruent activation in the posterior STS region. Participants with autism responded with significant activation to the two stimulus categories; however, the activation levels did not differ as a function of congruency.

Consistent with our findings, other neuroimaging studies have revealed dysfunction of the STS in autism during tasks involving eye movement perception (Pelphrey et al., 2005), the attribution of intentions to moving geometric figures (Castelli, Frith, Happé, & Frith, 2002), and human speech perception (Boddaert et al., 2003; Gervais et al., 2004). Bilateral hypoperfusion of temporal lobe areas at rest has been observed in children with autism (Ohnishi et al., 2000; Zilbovicius, Boddaert, Belin, Poline, Remy, et al., 2000). A positron emission tomography (PET) study of speech perception reported abnormal laterality of responses and hypoactivation of the left superior temporal gyrus (Boddaert et al., 2003), and an fMRI study observed abnormal responses in the STS to human voices (Gervais et al., 2004). Finally, a study comparing cortical sulcal maps in individuals with and without autism found anterior and superior displacements of the STS (Levitt et al., 2003), and Boddaert and colleagues (2004) reported abnormal STS volumes in ASD.

A COMPUTATIONAL MODEL OF SOCIAL PERCEPTION DYSFUNCTION IN AUTISM

Our studies have demonstrated that a region of the right posterior STS exhibits increased activity in typically developing individuals when they view an action that is unexpected or incongruent given the environmental or social context (Pelphrey, Morris, & McCarthy, 2004; Pelphrey, Singerman, et al., 2003; Pelphrey, Viola, & McCarthy, 2004; Vander Wyk et al., 2009). In contrast, individuals with autism do not exhibit this increase in activity (Pelphrey, Morris, & McCarthy, 2005). Here we present a simple connectionist network to help flesh out a mechanistic understanding of these neuroimaging findings. Central to this model is the assumption that the cognitive function of this region includes the *anticipation* of future actions.

To accurately anticipate a reach, the brain regions involved need to integrate both the observations of the present limb configuration and other sources of information to the extent that they enable anticipation. In our reaching-to-cups experiment, typically developing individuals integrate three sources of information to successfully anticipate a reach: the location of objects that are potential targets of a reach, the current position of the arm to be used to carry out the reach, and the meaning of the expression made to an object. In the congruent condition, the emotional information, together with the spatial location of the cups, would warrant the activation of representations anticipating a reach to one of the targets.

An unsuccessful anticipation would be disadvantageous, and the system cannot continue to activate representations that are no longer veridical. Thus, the system needs to continually monitor the state of the world, adjusting the anticipatory representations in light of new or incongruent information as it becomes available. In the congruent case, the observed reach unfolds largely in accord with the anticipated reach, so anticipatory representations would require little revision. However, in the incongruent conditions, the reach unfolds differently than anticipated, necessitating a relatively greater revision in the anticipated body motion representations. The differential blood oxygen level dependent (BOLD) signal associated with the incongruent and congruent conditions may reflect this revisionist processes.

Individuals with an ASD may not utilize all potential sources of information available in the environment, especially sources of social information, to the same extent as typically developing individuals. In our fMRI experiment described above, they may have failed to make use of the emotional expression and, in failing to do so, had no basis on which to anticipate different subsequent motions. Thus, any reach subsequent to the expression would have been no more or less congruent than any other. We sought to evaluate this proposal by building a connectionist model that is a necessary simplification, but captures the essential details of the phenomena.

Connectionist models have a number of properties that make them an attractive option for use with neuroimaging data. A network is made up of a number of simple neuron-like units that change activation over time based on their input. These units are arranged in layers that (similar to cortical regions) collectively encode and process some aspect relevant to the task. Thus, a measure of the activation of the units within a layer can be thought of as somewhat analogous to the BOLD signal from a cortical region.

In the current model, the task is to use immediately available information to activate a representation of the full trajectory of a reach, including an anticipation of components of the reach yet to be carried out. The architecture of the model is depicted schematically in the left panel of Figure 13.2. In the typically developing model, the network takes in information from several input layers, including (1) information about the emotion expression, (2) information about the trajectory of the reach up to a given moment in time, and (3) information about the position of objects. Input units pass activation along weighted connections to a set of hidden units that are, in turn, connected to an output layer. The output layer sends recurrent projections back to the hidden layer. The ASD model differs from the typically developing model in only one respect: Information propagated from the emotional input to the hidden units was degraded by different levels of noise. As noise increases, the network becomes less able to use the emotion expression information as a cue to anticipate one kind of reach or another

Figure 13.2 (left panel) also provides an example of the inputs and targets for a specific exemplar. At both the input and output layers, reaches are represented by a set of activated units on a topographically organized 5 × 5 lattice. On the input side, active units encode the trajectory of the reach, always initiated from the upper left unit in the grid, up to the present moment. At each time step, an additional unit in the trajectory is activated.

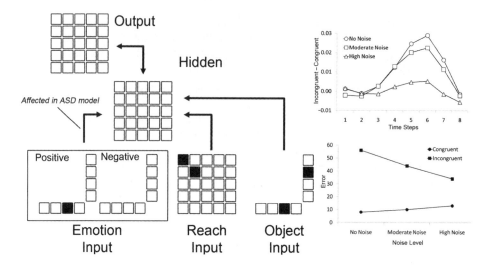

FIGURE 13.2. A connectionist model of posterior superior temporal sulcus function in individuals with and without autism.

Thus, the input representation of the reach gradually unfolds in time. At the output side, targets are set for the full trajectory of the reach. Figure 13.2 depicts the second time step of a reach toward the third unit from the left in the bottom row of the grid. The locations of the objects and the location toward which an emotion was directed have a similar (but reduced) topographic organization. The location of an object is represented as an active unit that corresponded to a location along the bottom or right side of the grid (eight possible locations). Emotions are similarly represented, with valence (positive and negative) encoded by separate pools of units. Figure 13.2 depicts a positive expression toward a location represented by the third unit from the left in the bottom row. There is an object at that location and a second object in the second row.

The hypothesized deficits in utilizing emotional information to inform processing of movements could arise from functional problems within (1) regions that represent and process the meaning or import of emotional expressions, (2) regions that process body motions, or (3) the connections between these sets of regions. Since our imaging data are largely equivocal on this issue, we modeled deficits in the processing of the emotional expression by injecting noise into those model components involved in representing this information. Critically, this noise obscures the information conveyed in the emotion expression, making the model less able to use it, while allowing us to remain relatively agnostic about the source of this obfuscation.

Both the typically developing and ASD models were implemented as continuous recurrent networks. During training, examples were presented over five time steps (as the input reach unfolded), which were individualized into four *ticks*, for simulation purposes. For testing, three additional time steps were added before and after an example, during which no input was given to the model, but activation was allowed to continue to flow around the network. This was done to assess the activation dynamics over a larger quantity of time. Hidden and output units integrated their input over time and their output was computed based on the sigmoid function. For each example, units were initialized in a quiescent state (initial input = –2.95, initial output = 0.0). Inputs were clamped to 0.0 or 1.0. Network weights were initialized to small random values and the network was trained for 500 sweeps through the training set. Weights were adjusted using back-propagation-through-time (learning rate = 0.01) with momentum (momentum = 0.9). Training consisted of all possible congruent examples where a reach could be anticipated by a concurrent emotional expression. Additionally, all possible neutral reaches were trained. These consisted of reaches in which no expression was active and a target was optionally presented. Testing was performed on the aforementioned congruent reaches as well as a set of incongruent reaches on which the network was not trained, which consisted of a reach that was not consistent with concurrent emotional expression.

In the ASD models, emotion input was degraded by adding or subtracting a random quantity from the unit output values, then normalizing the activation within both pools of emotional units (positive and negative), each to a total activation of 1.0. Thus, total input to the network from each of these pools is equivalent to the typically developing model. For the typically developing model, no noise was injected. To model differences in severity, two levels of noise injection were tested. For a moderate level of noise a value of ±0.2 was added or subtracted, and for a high level of noise a value of ±0.8 was injected.

After training, all networks successfully learned to generate predictions of reaches in the reach output layer. The top right panel of Figure 13.2 depicts the total error *per* training epoch on the three versions of the network. Both versions of the ASD model, one with high and one with moderate noise levels, did learn to represent future actions, though not as well as the typically developing model, with no injected noise. The result in the average reach output unit activation per example showed a clear differentiation between congruent and incongruent reaches for the typically developing model (Figure 13.2, middle right panel). However, this differentiation was attenuated proportional to level of impairment (i.e., amount of injected noise). Thus, the moderately impaired network exhibited a smaller differentiation. The highly impaired network showed little to no differentiation in activity. Interestingly, although the error in predicting congruent reaches increased with the level of impairment, the error corresponding to incongruent reaches, although always higher than the congruent reaches, *decreased* with impairment. This result is depicted in the lower right panel of Figure 13.2.

Our models were trained to predict simulated reaches given information about the current position of an arm, the location of potential targets, and congruent emotional expressions toward those targets. Because these cues are informative of a future reach, the typically developing network, where the emotion expression was undegraded by noise, learns to utilize them to rapidly activate a predicted reach ahead of observing the actual reach. These predictions could be used by other, unmodeled components of a social perception system to anticipate future actions and guide one's own actions. However, when these cues turn out to be misinformative, as in the case of an incongruent emotional expression, the predicted reach based on the emotional cue is different from that predicted by the unfolding reach that the network observes. For some period of time, the pattern of activation that reaches the output layer reflects both these predictions; hence, the increased activity to incongruent reaches relative to congruent ones in the typically developing network. It is possible that this increased activity may serve an adaptive purpose, cueing the system that something "unexpected" has occurred and thus demanding a reorienting of attention. In the case of the ASD models, where the emotional input is degraded by noise, the model has less of a basis for predicting a future reach from that cue. Because they less strongly activate patterns corresponding to a predicted reach, they also show less differentiation in their activity when the emotional cues are misinforming. These patterns of activation are consistent with patterns of BOLD signal within the posterior STS observed in our fMRI study of individuals with and without autism, described above, and are consistent with those reported elsewhere (e.g., Vander Wyk et al., 2009).

The network is also broadly consistent with behavioral reports of biological motion processing in autism, which show varying levels of impairments relative to typically developing individuals. Interestingly, whereas the ASD models reported here are less good at predicting congruent reaches than the typically developing network, they are also less negatively impacted by incongruent expressions. Thus, the most impaired model is the best at predicting incongruent reaches. This effect simply reflects the lack of activation of a competing predicted reach. We might expect that competition between representations in typically developing individuals to have behaviorally measurable consequences, such as slower reaction times to incongruent reaches. The lack of such competition in the ASD model suggests that they would be less subject to these consequences, but that remains to be tested in future work.

In interpreting the results of these models, however, it is important to bear in mind that they are grossly simplified. The observation of action often takes place in dynamic and interactive social contexts that require representations more elaborate than those modeled here. Indeed, in some ways, the model could be considered a "best case scenario" in which, despite a continuous failure to successfully link emotional expressions to subsequent actions, and despite a diminished ability to anticipate observed actions, the input to the ASD model remains identical to that of the typically developing one. In the real world, where the input a person receives is, in part, structured by the person him- or herself, successes or failures likely provide a cumulative effect. Early successes in anticipating others' actions, especially those anticipations that lead to goal achievement and rewards, are likely to motivate increased attention to other people, whereas failures may reduce a child's attending to others, which would lead to relatively impoverished social input, and so on. Success at this simple task may provide motivation or the foundation for the development of more sophisticated representations and processes for predicting others, which extend out further in time and are broader in their applicability, such as action schemas and "theories of mind." Under this view, high-level social cognition may be the natural result of developmental processes that begin with the simple anticipation of body motions, and normal social development depends on the ability to perceive others as things that are *able to be predicted*.

The ability to predict depends on the functioning of several brain regions. The regions critical to this particular set of models are the posterior STS and the extended limbic network that evaluates emotional valence (e.g., the amygdala and interconnected regions of the prefrontal cortex) and possibly links it to objects or locations in space. Here, we happened to implement impairment to this system as noise injected in the emotional input layer. However, we also ran a simulation that directly lesioned connections between these layers, and we obtained highly similar results. If we take the noise manipulation as denoting a failure to properly activate the extended limbic system in response to emotional stimuli, and we take the lesioning manipulation to denote a deficiency in long-range connectivity, we have two dysfunctions (with presumably different etiologies) that have the same outcome because they affect the function of the same brain region.

USING EMOTION TO INFORM DECISION MAKING

Our fMRI studies and computational modeling efforts have pointed to failures in the use of information regarding the emotional states of other individuals to inform the analysis and understanding of their actions. This failure to use affective cues is reminiscent of Leo Kanner's (1944) first description of 11 children with "infantile autism" as lacking the necessary skills for normal social functioning and a particular impairment in emotional interactions. A critical component highlighted by Kanner's original description that has yet to be explored sufficiently is the area of experience and expression of emotion in people with autism. It is possible that the development of emotions in individuals with ASD is as delayed and incomplete as many other social abilities. Their emotional responses to, and associations with, objects, people, and situations could also be quite atypical relative to typically developing peers.

We conducted a study to explore the experience of emotion in individuals with autism and their use of emotional experiences to inform their own decision-making processes. In this study, adolescents and adults with and without HFA (n = 12 and 10, respectively; matched at the group level on IQ, age, and gender) performed an affective decision-making task: a computerized version of the Iowa Gambling Task (Bechara, Damasio, Tranel, & Anderson, 1998). The individuals with HFA met appropriate criteria using the Autism Diagnostic Observation Schedule (ADOS; Lord et al., 2000) and the Autism Diagnostic Interview—Revised (ADI-R, Lord, Rutter, & Le Couteur, 1994).

Participants received $2,000 in play money and were encouraged to pick a card, one at a time, from any one of four decks of cards. Every card had a monetary reward amount on it; however, some cards also had a financial penalty. Two of the decks had larger gains but also larger losses, leading to a net financial loss. The other two decks had smaller gains on each trial, but much smaller penalties, causing a larger net gain over the trials. Participants were told that some decks are more advantageous than others and that they may choose one card at a time from any of the decks with the goal to win as much money as possible. The reward or loss was printed on the chosen card, and their current total was shown at all times. The task lasted 100 trials, but participants were not informed of the length as a means to avoid risk-taking behavior toward the end. This task measures a person's ability to use his or her emotional reaction to the bad decks to inform good decision making. Prior work has shown that healthy people quickly learn which decks are "good" and which are "bad." In contrast, individuals with damage to the ventral medial prefrontal cortex/OFC do not learn to discriminate between good and bad decks.

As illustrated in Figure 13.3, we examined sets of 10 trials across the Iowa Gambling Task and measured performance for each set as the proportion of advantageous to disadvantageous deck choices. We then examined how that ratio changes across sets of trials to determine whether or not there was a trend toward improvement (i.e., learning) and how this pattern differed as a function of group membership. As can be seen, typically developing adolescents and adults (dark gray) started out by choosing the disadvantageous decks because of the larger rewards, but that after the first 30–40 trials, they consistently chose the advantageous decks. In contrast, adolescents and adults with autism (light gray) continued to choose the disadvantageous cards and did not exhibit significant learning over the 100 trials. This study suggests that individuals with HFA fail to integrate their current implicit emotional reactions to the disadvantageous decks into their future decision-making processes. Alternatively, they do not experience the same kind of implicit emotional responses to the disadvantageous

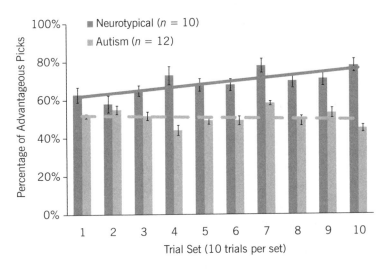

FIGURE 13.3. Results from a study of Iowa Gambling Task performance in individuals with and without autism.

decks. Our behavioral data, combined with our neuroimaging and computational model results, suggest that a failure to integrate emotional signals, both internally and externally generated, into ongoing cognitive processing might represent an important distinguishing feature of the neuropsychology of autism.

TAKING A DEVELOPMENTAL PERSPECTIVE ON SOCIAL BRAIN DYSFUNCTION IN AUTISM SPECTRUM DISORDERS

The work reviewed in this chapter indicates that specific brain regions in typically developing young adults are highly specialized for processing socially relevant stimuli. A fundamental question is how these regions become specialized for social information processing across development. Answers to this question will shed light not only on the development of social cognition and the social brain, but will also serve to constrain distinct, but not mutually exclusive, interpretations of findings of social brain dysfunction in autism. One interpretation is that very early disruptions in the social brain may drive the common deficits in social perception that are characteristic of ASD. Alternatively, social brain abnormalities in ASD may emerge as a consequence of the failure to follow the course of normative social development, causing increasing divergence in the processes impacting brain development (Jones & Klin, 2009).

Determining how the specialization of specific social brain regions emerges as a result of development will require longitudinal studies of infants in the first 2 years of life—the most significant and rapid period of neural and behavioral growth—and methodological approaches that allow for the consideration and measurement of the impact of genes and experience (and their interaction) on the developing brain.

At present, our knowledge of early typical and atypical development of social brain structures such as the posterior STS remains limited, in part due to technological and practical limitations. Imaging data are difficult to acquire for infants and young children who lack the ability to remain still while awake. Despite these limitations, studies have begun to elucidate the emergence of the specialization of brain regions for detecting agents, understanding emotions, and evaluating intentions.

Agents and Their Actions

Carter and Pelphrey (2006) investigated the development of social brain regions involved in the perception of biological motion in 7- to 10-year-old typically developing children using fMRI. As in adults (Pelphrey et al., 2003), BOLD activity in the posterior STS of school-age children clearly differentiated biological from nonbiological motion. However, a significant positive correlation was found between the magnitude of differentiation between biological and nonbiological motion in the right posterior STS and age. A recent functional near-infrared spectroscopy study examined whether 5-month-old infants show a differential hemodynamic response over the posterior temporal lobe (a region encompassing the posterior STS) in response to dynamic biological motion stimuli (an actress moving her hands, eyes, and mouth) compared with dynamic nonbiological motion (moving machinery; Lloyd-Fox, Blasi, Volein, Everdell, Elwell, & Johnson, 2009). Significant hemodynamic changes were observed in response to the dynamic biological motion stimuli in both left and right posterior sensors. Additionally, more activation was observed in response to biological, compared with nonbiological, motion, suggesting that in 5-month-old infants there are already areas of the temporal lobe, located roughly in an area corresponding to the adult posterior STS, dedicated to the perception of biological motion. Together these studies suggest early specialization of a cortical network for the perception of biological motion, which becomes increasingly fine-tuned throughout development.

Understanding Emotions

Behavioral studies have demonstrated that in the first day of life, newborns are able to discriminate facial expressions, preferring to look at happy, compared with neutral or fearful, emotional expressions (Farroni, Menon, Rigato, & Johnson, 2007). Discrimination of facial expressions becomes more fine-tuned throughout development (Kestenbaum & Nelson, 1990; Ludemann, 1991), and by 12 months of age typically developing infants can use others' positive and negative emotional expressions to regulate their own emotions and guide their behavior in ambiguous situations (Baldwin, & Moses, 1996; Sorce, Emde, Campos, & Klinnert, 1985; Carver & Vaccaro, 2007). Less is understood about the neural processes that occur while an infant is processing emotional expressions. Several studies have reported a shift in attention and neural resources to the processing of happy versus fearful faces between 5 and 7 months of age (Peltola, Leppänen, Mäki, & Hietanen, 2009; Nelson & de Haan, 1996). Peltola and colleagues (2009) demonstrated that although 5-month-olds attend equally to happy and fearful faces, an attentional bias for fearful faces emerges at 7 months of age. In addition, negative central mid-latency event-related potential (ERP) amplitudes were more negative in response to fearful faces in 7-month-olds, but not in 5-month-olds. In adults, enhanced neural response to fearful facial expressions is modulated by the amygdala (Morris et al., 1998; Vuilleumier & Pourtois, 2007; Leppänen & Kauppinen, 2007). Further research is needed to address whether the second half of the first year of life may be a critical period in the development of a brain network, including the amygdala, underlying processing of fearful faces (Leppänen & Nelson, 2009; Peltola et al., 2009).

Reading Intentions

Mosconi, Mack, McCarthy, and Pelphrey (2005) used fMRI to examine the neural circuitry underlying eye-gaze processing and intention understanding in 7- to 10-year-old typically developing children. Children viewed an animated actor who shifted her eyes toward a target object (a congruent gaze shift) or toward empty space (an incongruent gaze shift). Consistent with prior adult studies, the posterior STS was sensitive to the intentions underlying the actor's eye movements, suggesting that by 7 years of age the neural circuitry underlying the detection of intentions through eye-gaze shifts may already be specialized for this particular social perception task. A similar study, using the same paradigm, was conducted in both adults and 9-month-old infants using ERP measurements (Senju, Johnson, & Csibra, 2006). In adults, incongruent gaze shifts elicited larger amplitudes at occipitotemporal sites (N330). A similar posterior component (N290) was observed in infants in response to incongruent gaze shifts. An additional frontal component (N200), showing higher amplitude in response to congruent gaze shifts, was observed in infants but not in adults. Although these results suggest that infants and adults recruit a similar cortical network to encode intentions of others, the more widespread activation in infants may imply less specialization early in development.

Overall, the developmental patterns reported in these early studies indicate activation of social brain regions that becomes more fine-tuned throughout development. However, much work needs to be done to advance our understanding of the emerging functional specialization of the posterior STS, amygdala, and other areas of the social brain network. First, although infant studies demonstrate neural activity in response to social stimuli, such as biological motion versus mechanical motion, the exact degree of specialization of this response remains unclear. Second, although we have some understanding of brain development at the level of specific cortical regions (e.g., the posterior STS), few infant studies have examined how networks of brain regions become specialized for supporting social perception (Johnson, Grossman, & Cohen Kadosh, 2009). Similarly, few studies have directly examined how development of particular social abilities, such as perception of eye-gaze direction and the ability to discriminate facial expressions, may provide a foundation for higher-level forms of social cognition, such as reasoning about the intentions of others. Finally, few studies have addressed the disruption of neural systems for social perception in ASD. Because ASD are typically diagnosed after the second year of life, data on infants with ASD younger than 2 years of age are rare. However, research programs investigating infants at a high genetic risk for ASD may provide the opportunity for longitudinal studies of the development of cortical circuitry supporting social perception—an important step for understanding the time course and nature of the derailment of social mechanisms in ASD. For example, do disruptions in the processing of emotion in ASD arise from a failure to attend to socially relevant signals, or from a failure to understand the referential nature of emotional expressions? Do these early disruptions lead to cascading effects on other areas of social perception, such as reasoning about intentions? Do disruptions in brain mechanisms supporting these abilities give rise to the observed behavioral impairments, or do they result from abnormal experience with the social world early in life? Answers to these questions will have important implications for developing optimal treatments for ASD.

Scientists seeking to understand ASD face an important paradox: On the one hand, we clearly see enormous phenotypic and genetic heterogeneity. On the other hand, it is important to recognize that there is a great deal of homogeneity in ASD (Jones & Klin, 2009). Specifically, although diverse with regard to the severity of the core deficits and the underlying genetic etiology (Abrahams & Geschwind, 2008), ASD share the common feature of dysfunctional reciprocal social interaction. An understanding of the mechanisms generating this homogeneity might offer a way forward toward a clearer understanding of ASD (Jones & Klin, 2009).

REFERENCES

Abrahams, B. S., & Geschwind, D. H. (2008). Advances in autism genetics: On the threshold of a new neurobiology. *Nature Reviews Genetics, 9*(5), 341–355.
Allison, T., Puce, A., & McCarthy, G. (2000). Social perception from visual cues: Role of the STS region. *Trends in Cognitive Sciences, 4,* 267–278.

Amaral, D. G., Price, J. L., Pitkanen, A., & Carmichael, S. T. (1992). Anatomical organization of the primate amygdaloid complex. In J. P., Aggleton (Ed.), *The amygdala: Neurobiological aspects of emotion, memory, and mental dysfunction* (pp. 1–66). New York: Wiley-Liss.

Baldwin, D. A., & Moses, L. J. (1996). The ontogeny of social information gathering. *Child Development, 67,* 1915–1939.

Barbas, H. (1988). Anatomic organization of basoventral and mediodorsal visual recipient prefrontal regions in the rhesus monkey. *Journal of Comparative Neurology, 276,* 313–342.

Baron-Cohen, S., Ring, H. A., Wheelright, S., Bullmore, E. T., Brammer, M. J., Simmons, A., et al. (1999). Social intelligence in the normal and autistic brain: An fMRI study. *European Journal of Neuroscience, 11,* 1891–1898.

Baron-Cohen, S., Wheelwright, S., Hill, J., Raste, Y., & Plumb, I. (2001). The reading the mind in the eyes test revised version: A study with normal adults, and adults with Asperger syndrome or high-functioning autism. *Journal of Child Psychology and Psychiatry, 42,* 241–251.

Bechara, A., Damasio, H., Tranel, D., & Anderson, S. W. (1998). Dissociation of working memory from decision making within the human prefrontal cortex. *Journal of Neuroscience, 18,* 428–437.

Berument, S. K., Rutter, M., Lord, C., Pickles, A., & Bailey, A. (1999). Autism screening questionnaire: diagnostic validity. *British Journal of Psychiatry, 175,* 444–451.

Boddaert, N., Belin, P., Chabane, N., Poline, J. B., Barthélémy, C., Mouren-Simeoni, M. C., Brunelle, F., et al. (2003). Perception of complex sounds: Abnormal pattern of cortical activation in autism. *American Journal of Psychiatry, 160,* 2057–2060.

Boddaert, N., Chabane, N., Gervais, H., Good, C. D., Bourgeois, M., Plumet, M. H., et al. (2004). Superior temporal sulcus anatomical abnormalities in childhood autism: A voxel-based morphometry MRI study. *NeuroImage, 23*(1), 364–369.

Bonda, E., Petrides, M., Ostry, D., & Evans, A. (1996). Specific involvement of human parietal systems and the amygdala in the perception of biological motion. *Journal of Neuroscience, 16,* 3737–3744.

Brass, M., Schmitt, R. M., Spengler, S., & Gergely, G. (2007). Investigating action understanding: Inferential processes versus action simulation. *Current Biology, 17,* 2117–2121.

Brothers, L. (1990). The neural basis of primate social communication. *Motivation and Emotion, 14,* 81–91.

Brothers, L., & Ring, B. (1993). Mesial temporal neurons in the macaque monkey with responses selective for aspects of social stimuli. *Behavioural Brain Research, 57,* 53–61.

Brothers, L., Ring, B., & Kling, A. (1990). Response of neurons in the macaque amygdala to complex social stimuli. *Behavioural Brain Research, 41,* 199–213.

Carter, E. J., & Pelphrey, K. A. (2006). School-aged children exhibit domain-specific responses to biological motion. *Social Neuroscience, 1,* 396–411.

Carver, L. J., & Vaccaro, B. G. (2007). 12–month-old infants allocate increased neural resources to stimuli associated with negative adult emotion. *Developmental Psychology, 43*(1), 54–69.

Castelli, F., Frith, C., Happé, F., & Frith, U. (2002). Autism, Asperger syndrome and brain mechanisms for the attribution of mental states to animated shapes. *Brain, 125,* 1839–1849.

Castelli, F., Happé, F., Frith, U., & Frith, C. (2000). Movement and mind: A functional imaging study of perception and interpretation of complex intentional movement patterns. *NeuroImage, 12,* 314–325.

Davis, M., & Whalen, P. J. (2001). The amygdala: Vigilance and emotion. *Molecular Psychiatry, 6,* 13–34.

Dawson, G., Meltzoff, A. N., Osterling, J., Rinaldi, J., & Brown, E. (1998). Children with autism fail to orient to naturally occurring social stimuli. *Journal of Autism and Developmental Disorders, 28*(6), 479–485.

Desimone, R. (1991). Face-selective cells in the temporal cortex of monkeys: Special issue—face perception. *Journal of Cognitive Neuroscience, 3,* 1–8.

Desimone, R., Albright, T. D., Gross, C. G., & Bruce, C. (1984). Stimulus-selective properties of inferior temporal neurons in the macaque. *Journal of Neuroscience, 4,* 2051–2062.

Farroni, T., Menon, E., Rigato, S., & Johnson, M. H. (2007). The perception of facial expressions in newborns. *European Journal of Developmental Psychology, 4*(1), 2–13.

Frith, C. D., & Frith, U. (1999). Interacting minds: A biological basis. *Science, 286*(5445), 1692–1705.

Gervais, H., Belin, P., Boddaert, N., Leboyer, M., Coez, A., Sfaello, I., et al. (2004). Abnormal cortical voice processing in autism. *Nature Neuroscience, 7*(8), 801–802.

Gottesman, I. I., & Gould, T. D. (2003). The endophenotype concept in psychiatry: Etymology and strategic intentions. *American Journal of Psychiatry, 160*(4), 636–645.

Gottesman, I. I., & Shields, J. (1972). *Schizophrenia and genetics: A twin study vantage point.* New York: Academic Press.

Gottesman, I. I., & Shields, J. (1973). Genetic theorizing and schizophrenia. *British Journal of Psychiatry, 122,* 15–30.

Johnson, M. H. (2001). Functional brain development in humans. *Nature Reviews Neuroscience, 2,* 475–483

Johnson, M. H. (2005). Subcortical face processing. *Nature Reviews Neuroscience, 6,* 766–774.

Johnson, M. H., Grossman, T., & Cohen Kadosh, K. (2009). Mapping functional brain development: Building a social brain through interactive specialization. *Developmental Psychology, 45*(1), 151–159.

Johnson, M. H., Halit, H., Grice, S. J., & Karmiloff-Smith, A. (2002). Neuroimaging of typical and atypical development: A perspective from multiple levels of analysis. *Development and Psychopathology, 14,* 521–536.

Jones, W., & Klin, A. (2009). Heterogeneity and homogeneity across the autism spectrum: The role of development. *Journal of the American Academy of Child and Adolescent Psychiatry, 48*(5), 471–473.

Kandel, E. R. (1998). A new intellectual framework for psychiatry. *American Journal of Psychiatry, 155,* 457–469.

Kanner, L. (1944). Early infantile autism. *Journal of Pediatrics, 25*(3), 211–217.

Kanwisher, N., McDermott, J., & Chun, M. M. (1997). The fusiform face area: A module in human extrastriate cortex specialized for face perception. *Journal of Neuroscience, 17,* 4302–4311.

Kestenbaum, R., & Nelson, C. A. (1990). The recognition and categorization of upright and inverted emotional expressions by 7–month-old infants. *Infant Behavior and Development, 13,* 497–511.

Klüver, H., & Bucy, P. C. (1997). Preliminary analysis of functions of the temporal lobes in monkeys. *Journal of Neuropsychiatry and Clinical Neuroscience, 9,* 606–620.

Klin, A., Lin, D. J., Gorrindo, P., Ramsay, G., & Jones, W. (2009). Two-year-olds with autism orient to non-social contingencies rather than biological motion. *Nature, 459*(7244), 257–261.

LeDoux, J. E. (2000). Emotion circuits in the brain. *Annual Review of Neuroscience, 23,* 155–184.

Leekam, S. R., Hunnisett, E., & Moore, C. (1998). Targets and cues: Gaze-following in children with autism. *Journal of Child Psychology and Psychiatry, 39*(7), 951–962.

Leekam, S. R., López, B., & Moore, C. (2000). Attention and joint attention in preschool children with autism. *Developmental Psychology, 36*(2), 261–273.

Leppänen, J. M., Kauppinen, P., Pelota, M. J., & Hietanen, J. K. (2007). Differential electrocortical responses to increasing intensities of fearful and happy emotional expressions. *Brain Research, 1166,* 103–109.

Leppänen, J. M., & Nelson, C. A. (2009). Tuning the developing brain to social signals of emotion. *Nature Reviews Neuroscience, 10,* 37–47.

Levitt, J. G., Blanton, R. E., Smalley, S., Thompson, P. M., Guthrie, D., McCracken, J. T., et al. (2003) Cortical sulcal maps in autism. *Cerebral Cortex, 13*(7), 728–735.

Lloyd-Fox, S., Blasi, A., Volein, A., Everdell, N., Elwell, C. E., & Johnson, M. H. (2009). *Social perception in infancy: A near infrared spectroscopy study. Child Development, 80*(4), 986–999.

Lord, C., Risi, S., Lambrecht, L., Cook, E., Jr., Leventhal, B., DiLavore, P., et al. (2000). The Autism Diagnostic Observation Schedule—Generic: A standard measure of social and communication deficits associated with the spectrum of autism. *Journal of Autism and Developmental Disorders, 30*(3), 205–223.

Lord, C., Rutter, M., & Le Couteur, A. (1994). Autism Diagnostic Interview—Revised: A revised version of a diagnostic interview for caregivers of individuals with possible pervasive developmental disorders. *Journal of Autism and Developmental Disorders, 24*(5), 659–685.

Lotspeich, L. J., Kwon, H., Schumann, C. M., Fryer, S. L., Goodlin-Jones, B. L., Buonocore, M. H., et al. (2004). Investigation of neuroanatomical differences between autism and Asperger syndrome. *Archives of General Psychiatry, 61*(3), 291–298.

Loveland, K. A., & Landry, S. H. (1986). Joint attention and language in autism and developmental language delay. *Journal of Autism and Developmental Disorders,16*(3), 335–349.

Ludemann, P. M. (1991). Generalized discrimination of positive facial expressions by 7– to 10–month-old infants. *Child Development, 62,* 55–67.

McAlonan, G. M., Cheung, C., Cheung, V., Wong, N., Suckling, J., & Chua, S.

E. (2009). Differential effects on white-matter systems in high-functioning autism and Asperger's syndrome. *Psychological Medicine, 39,* 1885–1893.

McAlonan, G. M., Suckling, J., Wong, N., Cheung, V., Lienenkaemper, N., Cheun, C., et al. (2008). Distinct patterns of grey matter abnormality in high-functioning autism and Asperger's syndrome. *Journal of Child Psychology and Psychiatry, 49,* 1287–1295.

McPartland, J., & Klin, A. (2006). Asperger's syndrome. *Adolescent Medicine Clinics, 17,* 771–788.

Morris, J. S., Frith, C. D., Perrett, D. I., Rowland, D., Young, A. W., Calder, A. J., et al. (1996). A differential neural response in the human amygdala to fearful and happy facial expressions. *Nature, 383,* 812–815.

Morris, J. S., Friston, K. J., Buchel, C., Frith, C. D., Young, A. W., Calder, A. J., et al. (1998). A neuromodulatory role for the human amygdala in processing emotional facial expressions. *Brain, 121,* 47–57.

Mosconi, M. W., Mack, P. B., McCarthy, G., & Pelphrey, K. A. (2005). Taking an "intentional stance" on eye-gaze shifts: A functional neuroimaging study of social perception in children. *NeuroImage, 27,* 247–252.

Mundy, P., Sigman, M., Ungerer, J., & Sherman T. (1986). Defining the social deficits of autism: The contribution of non-verbal communication measures. *Journal of Child Psychology and Psychiatry, 27*(5), 657–669.

Nelson, C. A., & de Haan, M. (1996). Neural correlates of infants' visual responsiveness to facial expressions of emotion. *Developmental Psychobiology, 29,* 577–595.

Ohnishi, T., Matsuda, H., Hashimoto, T., Kunihiro, T., Nishikawa, M., Uema, T., et al. (2000). Abnormal regional cerebral blood flow in childhood autism. *Brain, 123,* 1838–1844.

Pandya, D. N., & Yererian, E. H. (1996). *Morphological correlations of human and monkey frontal lobe.* In A. R. Damasio, H. Damasio, & Y. Christen (Eds.), *Neurobiology of decision making* (pp. 13–46). New York: Springer.

Pelphrey, K. A., Mitchell, T. V., McKeown, M. J., Goldstein, J., Allison, T., & McCarthy, G. (2003). Brain activity evoked by the perception of human walking: Controlling for meaningful coherent motion. *Journal of Neuroscience, 23,* 6819–6825.

Pelphrey, K. A., Morris, J. P., & McCarthy, G. (2004). Grasping the intentions of others: The perceived intentionality of an action influences activity in the superior temporal sulcus during social perception. *Journal of Cognitive Neuroscience, 16,* 1706–1716.

Pelphrey, K. A., Morris, J. P, & McCarthy, G. (2005). Neural basis of eye gaze processing deficits in autism. *Brain, 128*(5), 1038–1048.

Pelphrey, K. A., Morris, J. P., Michelich, C. R., Allison, T., & McCarthy, G. (2005). Functional anatomy of biological motion perception in posterior temporal cortex: An fMRI study of eye, mouth and hand movements. *Cerebral Cortex, 15,* 1866–1876.

Pelphrey, K. A., Singerman, J. D., Allison, T., & McCarthy, G. (2003). Brain activation evoked by perception of gaze shifts: The influence of context. *Neuropsychologia, 41,* 156–170.

Pelphrey, K. A., Viola, R. J., & McCarthy, G. (2004). When strangers pass: Processing of mutual and averted social gaze in the superior temporal sulcus. *Psychological Science, 15,* 598–603.

Peltola, M. J., Leppänen, J. M., Mäki, S., & Hietanen, J. K. (2009). Emergence of enhanced attention to fearful faces between 5 and 7 months of age. *Scan, 4,* 134–142.

Perrett, D. I., Rolls, E. T., & Caan, W. (1979). Temporal lobe cells of the monkey with visual responses selective for faces. *Neuroscience Letters,* S358.

Perrett, D. I., Rolls, E. T., & Caan, W. (1982). Visual neurons responsive to faces in the monkey temporal cortex. *Experimental Brain Research, 47,* 329–342.

Perrett, D. I., Smith, P. A. J., Potter, D. D., Mistlin, A. J., Head, A. S., Milnder, A. D., et al. (1984). Neurones responsive to faces in the temporal cortex: Studies of functional organization, sensitivity to identity, and relation to perception. *Human Neurobiology, 3*(4), 197–208.

Perrett, D. I., Smith, P. A. J., Potter, D. D., Mistlin, A. J., Head, A. S., Milner, A. D., et al. (1985). Visual cells in the temporal cortex sensitive to face view and gaze direction. *Proceedings of the Royal Society of London Series, 223,* 293–317.

Phillips, A. T., Wellman, H. M., & Spelke, E. S. (2002). Infants' ability to connect gaze and emotional expression to intentional action. *Cognition, 85,* 53–78.

Puce, A., Allison, T., Asgari, M., Gore, J. C., & McCarthy, G. (1996), Differential sensitivity of human visual cortex to faces, letter strings, and textures: A functional MRI study. *Journal of Neuroscience, 16,* 5205–5215.

Rolls, E. T. (1981). Responses of amygdaloid neurons in the primate. In Y. Ben-Ari (Ed.), *The amygdaloid complex* (pp. 383–393). Amsterdam: Elsevier.

Rolls, E. T. (1995). Central taste anatomy and neurophysiology. In R. L. Doty (Ed.), *Handbook of olfaction and gestation* (pp. 549–573). New York: Dekker.

Rolls, E. T. (2000). The orbitofrontal cortex and reward. *Cerebral Cortex, 10,* 284–294.

Rolls, E. T. (2009). Functional neuroimaging of umami taste: What makes umami pleasant? *American Journal of Clinical Nutrition, 90,* 804–813.

Saxe, R., Xiao, D. K., Kovacs, G., Perrett, D. I., & Kanwisher, N. (2004). A region of right posterior superior temporal sulcus responds to observed intentional actions. *Neuropsychologia, 42,* 1435–1446.

Schumann, C. M., Hamstra, J., Goodlin-Jones, B. L., Lotspeich, L. J., Kwon, H., Buonocore, M. H., et al. (2004). The amygdala is enlarged in children but not adolescents with autism; the hippocampus is enlarged at all ages. *Journal of Neuroscience, 24,* 6392–6401.

Senju, A., Johnson, M. H., & Csibra, G. (2006). The development and neural basis of referential gaze perception. *Social Neuroscience, 1*(3–4), 220–234.

Simion, F., Regolin, L., & Bulf, H. (2008). A predisposition for biological motion in the newborn baby. *Proceedings of the National Academy of Sciences, 105,* 809–813.

Sorce, J. F., Emde, R. N., Campos, J., & Klinnert, M. D. (1985). Maternal emotional signaling: Its effects on the visual cliff behavior of 1-year-olds. *Developmental Psychology, 21,* 195–200.

Vander Wyk, B. C., Hudac, C. M., Carter, E. J., Sobel, D. M., & Pelphrey, K. A. (2009). Action understanding in the superior temporal sulcus region. *Psychological Science, 20,* 771–777.

Vuilleumier, P., & Pourtois, G. (2007). Distributed and interactive brain mechanisms during emotion face perception: Evidence from functional neuroimaging. *Neuropsychologia, 45,* 174–194.

Wing, L. (1981). Asperger's syndrome: A clinical account. *Psychological Medicine.* *11*(1), 115–129.

Zeki, S., Watson, J. D., Lueck, C. J., Friston, K. J., Kennard, C., & Frackowiak, R. S. (1991). A direct demonstration of functional specialization in human visual cortex. *Journal of Neuroscience, 11,* 641–649.

Zilbovicius, M., Boddaert, N., Belin, P., Poline, J. B., Remy, P., & Mangin, J. F. (2000). Temporal lobe dysfunction in childhood autism: A PET study. *American Journal of Psychiatry, 157*(12), 1988–1993.

CHAPTER 14

Genetics of Asperger Syndrome

Susan E. Folstein

When a condition is defined only by a behavioral phenotype, it is difficult to study its underlying genetics. This is a problem for all of psychiatry, but despite this difficulty we have made some headway for several conditions, including autism. Sometimes it has been helpful to separate the phenotype into subgroups based on particular clinical features. This is one of the motivations for separating from the spectrum of autism severity, cases such as those described by Hans Asperger: the possibility that it may be an etiologically separate entity or at least have some genetic or pathophysiological differences from more severe autism. This effort has encountered several difficulties. First, there has been no agreement on how to define what has come to be called (Wing, 1981) *Asperger syndrome* (AS). Wing's criteria are similar to those of Asperger, as are those of Gillberg (Gillberg & Gillberg, 1989). As described by Wing, they are identical to the features of autism as described by Kanner, except for the requirement of volubility of talk about circumscribed interests and normal measured IQ. Cases meeting criteria for AS often meet the fourth edition of the *Diagnostic and Statistical Manual of Mental Disorders* (DSM-IV; American Psychiatric Association, 1994) criteria for autism. Because the diagnosis of autism takes precedence, the cases that meet only criteria for AS are quite mild. Different diagnostic criteria result in estimates of prevalence that are very different. Studies using DSM-IV criteria and adequate ascertainment sources usually find about 1 case per thousand. Studies using Gillberg's criteria obtain much higher rates, up to 3.5 per thousand (Fombonne, 2009).

441

Another difficulty is that the clinical features of AS, at least as written in DSM-IV, overlap substantially with several other diagnostic entities: autism with normal IQ, schizoid personality disorder, schizotypal personality disorder, and some aspects of schizophrenia. Schizotypal disorder is virtually defined by its occurrence in families found through schizophrenic index cases (Kendler, McGuire, Gruenberg, et al., 1995). There are also important commonalities with mood and anxiety disorders, including obsessive–compulsive disorder (OCD). AS is not confused with these conditions, but rather these conditions are very often comorbid with AS. The phenotypic and genetic relationship to schizophrenia, on the one hand, and mood and anxiety disorders, on the other, is now being explored.

Despite the possible etiological and phenotypic relationships to schizophrenia and mood and anxiety disorders, there are many reasons to think that AS is part of the spectrum of severity of autistic disorder. It is near the mild end of the autism spectrum, a spectrum that ranges from nonverbal cases with severe mental retardation at one end to the individual traits that make up the broader autism phenotype at the other. The clinical features of AS, as described in most proposed criteria, are nearly identical to those for autism, but milder. Furthermore, most studies comparing AS with normal-IQ autism have found only minor, if any, differences in outcome, cognitive features, or neuroimaging. This body of literature was a substantial part of the motivation to move away from diagnostic subcategories in DSM-5 (American Psychiatric Association, 2013).

In this chapter, we review several aspects of genetic interest: the family history; the relationships of AS to schizophrenia and to mood and anxiety disorders; molecular biology studies that have included cases with AS; and finally, some possible ways of formulating the relationship between AS, autism, and these other conditions.

FAMILY HISTORY STUDIES OF ASPERGER SYNDROME

Familial Aggregation of Asperger Syndrome in Families with Autism

Perhaps the first relevant family history study is that of (DeLong & Dwyer, 1988). They systematically studied the first- and second-degree relatives of 51 cases of autism and pervasive developmental disorder (PDD). Those cases with IQs above 70 were more likely to have relatives with AS (13 of 19 families) than probands with lower IQs (2 of 25 families).

In a family history study of probands with autism diagnosed by Kanner (Piven, Gayle, Chase, Fink, Landa, et al., 1990), the parents of adult probands with autism were interviewed about their nonautistic children. Parents described behaviors in three of their nonautistic children (4.4%) that seem likely to represent AS, although we did not label it as such in the publication. These three individuals were extremely eccentric in their habits, socially isolated, and had restricted and unusual interests. All had normal intelligence, normal early language development, and were never thought, as children, to have autism.

In the Baltimore Family Study of autism (unpublished data, S. Folstein), all adolescent and adult siblings of 90 probands with autism were directly interviewed and tested on measures of social language, personality, and cognition. Two of the 48 siblings (both brothers) who were old enough for all these examinations met criteria for AS (nearly 4%), as did four parents (2.2%; three fathers and one mother).

Taken together, these studies suggest that AS does aggregate in families that come to attention because of having a child with autism since the prevalence in these families is an order of magnitude higher than even the highest estimates of AS prevalence in the community (see below). Several other studies have been designed to study AS cases ascertained not through probands with autism, but directly from the clinic or community.

Aggregation of Asperger Syndrome in Families with Asperger Syndrome

The first study of this type was that of Lorna Wing in her 1981 report that drew attention to cases at the mild end of the autism spectrum of severity and pointed out their resemblance to those cases first described by Hans Asperger. She based her report on a clinical sample of 34 cases. She knew 16 fathers well enough to say that 5/16 (32%) had "to a marked degree behaviors resembling AS." Two of 24 mothers (~8%) met these qualifications. Two years later, she reported triplets who were concordant for AS (Burgoine & Wing, 1983). At least one pair of concordant monozygotic (MZ) twins has also been reported (Ishijima & Kurita, 2007).

One hundred individuals diagnosed with AS who attended a psychiatric clinic were studied (Gillberg & Cederlund, 2005) in Goteborg Sweden. First- or second-degree relatives of 66 of these were thought to have autism or AS, with varying degrees of certainty; this included 25 fathers by our count. In two families, the index case had a brother with AS.

Another study (Ghaziuddin, 2005) reported on 58 individuals with AS in a psychiatric practice and compared them with 39 cases of individuals with normal-IQ autism. Ghaziuddin used DSM-IV criteria, which resulted in subjects with AS having substantially higher IQs than those with autism, although all had IQs above 70. Since most individuals with AS also meet criteria for autism, and the autism diagnosis takes precedence in the DSM-IV schema, the resulting samples include individuals with very mild AS, which makes it difficult to match for IQ with normal-IQ individuals who meet criteria for autism.

Ghaziuddin (2005) used the Folstein/Rutter family history schedule to inquire about autism-related traits and conditions. AS families had slightly more history of AS than autism (5% vs. 3.4%), and autism families had slightly less AS than autism (2.5% vs. 10%). A substantial number of individuals also had family members with the broader autism phenotype (29% vs. 20% of AS and normal-IQ autism cases, respectively). None of the differences between AS and normal-IQ autism families was statistically significant.

Taking all the family history studies together, it seems clear that when AS cases are ascertained either through autism probands or in the community, the rates of AS and autism are higher than expected given the estimated prevalence rates of these conditions.

ASPERGER SYNDROME AND SCHIZOPHRENIA

Recently, several papers have been published that call into question the long-standing belief that autism and schizophrenia are etiologically and phenomenologically unrelated. Some of these studies have involved subjects with AS.

The first suggestion comes from Ghaziuddin's 2005 paper that compared the family histories in AS and normal-IQ autism. He found 9 cases of schizophrenia in first-degree relatives of the 58 AS families (15%) and 4 in relatives of the 39 probands with autism (10%). The findings were not significantly different for the AS versus autism families, but rates for both groups are much higher than expected from the population prevalence of schizophrenia (~1%). He used the Family History—Research diagnostic criteria (Andreasen, Endicott, Spitzer, et al., 1977) to elicit diagnoses of psychiatric disorders in family members. No one else has reported an excess of schizophrenia in autism or AS families, but no one else has inquired as carefully as Ghaziuddin, using the appropriate family history instrument. Cederlund and Gillberg (2004) reported two family members with schizophrenia in families of 100 individuals with AS, not different from population expectations. However, they abstracted clinical case notes and did not interview family members, as did Ghaziuddin.

The second piece of evidence comes from a series of studies by Judith Rapoport and her colleagues on childhood-onset schizophrenia (COS). Using the Autism Diagnostic Interview, they found that 19 (25%) of 75 individuals with COS met criteria for autism spectrum disorders (ASD) as young children, some years before the onset of symptoms that qualified them for a diagnosis of schizophrenia: autism (1 person), AS (2), and PDD (16) (Sporn, Addington, Gogtay, et al., 2004; Rapoport, Chavez, Greenstein, Addington, & Goqtay, et al., 2009). Those with and without premorbid ASD did not differ by family history or other demographic factors except that among those with premorbid ASD, more were male (79% vs. 51%; $p = .03$) and among their 12 siblings, 2 were autistic, versus none of the 29 siblings of individuals without premorbid autism ($p = .02$). No one else studying COS has reported this finding, but no one else has used the appropriate diagnostic instruments for autism.

The possible overlap between AS and schizophrenia is also suggested by a series of AS case reports. Raja and Azzoni (2007) describe six individuals with AS who developed hallucinations in adolescence. However, these were not of the schizophrenic type (voices speaking in the first person and heard outside one's head). Rather, they were more like depressive hallucinations (voices speaking in the second person or noises not clearly articulated). All six individuals exhibited overvalued ideas, but the authors did not think that any of them qualified as delusions. These individuals, when examined in early adulthood, presented as AS and not schizophrenia, but with these additional features. In my experience, and as pointed out by Wing (1981) and by Raja and Azzoni (2007), it can be difficult to differentiate between overvalued ideas, which are frequent in AS and often become more pronounced in adulthood, and delusions. The ideas of adults with AS are strongly held against evidence, but unlike delusions, are not usually idiosyncratic.

Several recent studies have compared neuropsychological test results of people with ASD or schizophrenia. The results in the two groups have been surprisingly similar for theory-of-mind tests (Murphy, 2006), neural activation using BOLD while performing social-cognitive and face-processing tasks (Pinkham, Hopfinger, Pelphrey, Piven, & Penn, 2008), and using face information for assessing social scenes (Sasson, Tsuchiya, Hurley, Couture, Penn, et al., 2007; Couture, Penn, Losh, Adolphs, Hurley, et al., 2010). Only Murphy compared AS with schizophrenia; the others compared normal IQ autism with schizophrenia.

These studies suggest that it is time to reexamine the relationship between ASD and schizophrenic spectrum disorders, as useful and important, indeed crucial, as that distinction has been for research in both disorders (Rapoport et al., 2009). There are possible links in etiology, neural mechanisms, and possibly phenomenology. Based on studies to date, it seems unlikely that any of these links is specific to AS.

ASPERGER SYNDROME AND MOOD AND ANXIETY DISORDERS

The relationship between AS and schizophrenia is different from that with mood and anxiety disorders. In the former, there may be an overlap of clinical features and possibly important overlap of etiology and mechanism. The relationship between AS and mood and anxiety disorders is much easier to discern: There is frequent comorbidity between AS and these conditions, but AS is seldom confused with them. Further, a family history of mood and anxiety disorders in family members is common.

Mood Disorders in Individuals with Autism Spectrum Disorders and Their Families

DeLong and Dwyer (1988) used Andreasen's FH-RDC to interview parents of 51 children with autism and found that among those who had a positive family history for AS, 6% also had a family history of bipolar disorder. This rate was twice as high as in the families without AS. In a follow-up to this study (DeLong & Nohria, 1994), the individuals were grouped according to those with and without evidence for a neurological disorder. When grouped in this way, most of the mood disorders occurred in the families of individuals without neurological conditions.

In the Ghaziuddin family history study (2005), both the individuals with normal-IQ autism and those with AS had similar rates of relatives with depression (60% and 52%, respectively). He did not report on anxiety disorders.

Klin and his colleagues (Klin, Pauls, Schultz, et al., 2005) studied 65 individuals with normal-IQ ASD with the main goal of comparing three different diagnostic schema for AS. One of the variables on which they compared the different schema was family history. They used the Folstein/Rutter family history interview, but not the FH-RDC (which is much more detailed for mood disorders and schizophrenia), to elicit information about all psychiatric disorders. In the sample as a whole, depression was present in about 25% of the relatives. Regardless of the diagnostic schema they imposed on their normal-IQ sample, there were few significant differences in family history between those classified with autism, AS, or PDD-NOS.

A high frequency of mood disorders has been reported not just in family members but also in individuals with autism or AS. The early case reports of mood disorders in individuals with autism are reviewed in Lainhart and Folstein (1994). Using the Schedule for Affective Disorders and Schizophrenia for School-Age Children (K-SADS) as a starting point, we (Leyfer, Folstein, Bacalman, et al., 2006) developed an informant-based psychiatric interview for autism and reported rates of mood disorder in children with autism who were between 5 and 17 years old, most less than 12. The rate of major depression in this young sample was 10%, and increased to 25% when rates of children with symptoms just below the threshold for diagnosis were included.

Munesue and his colleagues (Munesue, Ono, Mutoh, Shimoda, Nakatani, et al., 2008) studied mood disorders in 44 consecutive normal-IQ patients with ASD over age 12 seen in a clinic. Of the 16 (35% of the sample) diagnosed with a mood disorder (mostly some type of bipolar disorder), all had diagnoses of AS or PDD; none of the individuals diagnosed with autism had a mood disorder, but there were only nine such individuals. The affected individuals were more likely to have a family history of mood disorder than those unaffected with a mood disorder. Mood disorder was elicited by asking about all the DSM items in the mood disorder classification.

The aggregation of mood disorders in autism spectrum families was also reported by Mazefsky, Folstein, and Lainhart (2008). Parents of persons with autism who had a comorbid mood disorder also had a higher rate of depression than did parents of individuals with autism but without depression.

Taken together, it is clear that both probands with ASD and their family members have much higher rates of mood disorders than expected from general population prevalence rates. These disorders may be more common in families of probands with higher IQs, but the rates are probably similar in individuals with high-IQ autism or AS. Evidence is mounting that mood disorders are more frequent in family members when their child with ASD has a comorbid mood disorder, suggesting that some gene or genes for mood disorder is a susceptibility gene for ASD. The link with AS specifically is less certain. Mood disorders may, however, be more common in individuals with normal-IQ ASD and their family members.

Anxiety Disorders in Individuals with Autism Spectrum Disorder

Anxiety disorders of several types are common in both probands with autism and family members, although this area has not been studied specifically in AS. The frequency of anxiety disorders, including OCD, is very high in those with ASD, as well as in family members. Based on clinical experience, individuals with AS have a high frequency of social anxiety disorder, anticipatory anxiety, and compulsive behaviors. Probably social anxiety is more common in those with normal-IQ ASD because they have insight into their social awkwardness. Less able children with autism become upset in social situations because of the noise and confusion, but they are usually oblivious to any social requirements.

MOLECULAR STUDIES

For some time, we assumed that we would find common (i.e., not rare) mutations in common complex disorders such as autism. This was the so-called *common disease/common allele* model that uses association analysis. This approach has met with limited success. It appears that multiple rare alleles are more often found in such families. Both approaches have been used with families that contain individuals with AS.

One association study carried out with 29 families found through probands with AS in Finland has been successful (Kilpinen, Ylisaukko-Oja, Hennah, et al., 2008). No family members had autism, but there were four with schizophrenia. An association was found with a particular allele of

DISC1. An association study of 97 autism families by the same research group showed a significant association with a different allele of *DISC1.* The autism families contained 8 individuals with AS, 12 with language disorders, and 3 with schizophrenia. *DISC1* has previously been associated with schizophrenia.

The search for rare variants has involved AS cases to some extent. There appears to be an etiological link between the serotonin transporter (SERT, 5-HTT) gene (*SLC6A4*) and AS, autism, OCD, and other psychiatric conditions. *SLC6A4* has long stood apart in autism research as a candidate gene due to observed hyperserotonemia and SSRI responsiveness (Cook, Arora, Anderson, Berry-Kravis, Yan, Yeoh, et al., 1993; PMID: 7684805). Several linkage studies in autism families identified chromosome 17q11.2; *SLC6A4* is located in this region (McCauley, Li, Jiang, Olson, Crockett, et al., 2005; Stone, Merriman, Cantor, Geschwind, & Nelson, 2007; Cantor, Kono, Duvall, Alvarez-Retuerto, Alarcón, et al., 2005). Despite genetic linkage, studies to test association of common *SLC6A4* alleles with autism were inconclusive.

We therefore tested the hypothesis that rare variants at this gene might contribute to the genetic effect observed by linkage (Sutcliffe et al., 2005). This idea drew support from the known existence of numerous *SLC6A4* coding variants not associated with disease and from a report by Ozaki, Goldman, Kay, Plotnicou, Greenberg, et al., 2003), that documented a rare missense mutation (*Ile425Val*) segregating with an assortment of psychiatric phenotypes in two families. The most prominent phenotypes were AS and OCD, although various psychiatric disorders were observed in some family members. We selected cases for exon resequencing from families, most contributing to 17q11.2 linkage to enrich for genetic effects. Three novel coding mutations were identified, and a fourth previously known variant was found to be greatly enriched in this sample. The phenotype of mutation carriers was notable for having more severe restricted–repetitive and compulsive behaviors compared with the large overall sample. Subsequent functional studies of these mutations and the AS/OCD-associated *Ile425Val* variant revealed gain-of-function effects leading to elevated SERT activity and altered regulatory (Prasad, Steiner, Sutcliffe, & Blakely, 2009). The etiological link between autism, AS, and OCD was solidified by the finding that the AS/OCD mutation showed the same functional defects as the novel autism-associated mutations: elevated serotonin reuptake. Elevated reuptake at serotonergic synapses can be dampened by treatment with SSRIs, so this particular molecular mechanism is consistent with the general efficacy of SSRIs in ameliorating certain behaviors in ASD. This line of inquiry has reinforced the basis for the so-called "serotonin hypothesis" in ASD.

A recent finding in the genetics of ASD is copy number variations (CNVs). There are sequences of DNA that occur in several copies; variation in the number of copies is more common in ASD than in controls. The findings regarding CNVs further reinforce the idea that autism and AS are components of a broader, common spectrum: in families found through probands with autism, some CNVs are found in individuals with either autism or AS.

HOW SHOULD WE THINK ABOUT THE GENETIC AND GENOMIC FINDINGS IN ASPERGER SYNDROME?

Clearly, autism and AS run in families. The rates of ASD among family members of probands with ASD is much higher than expected from general population rates. This is true particularly for families in which the affected probands have been diagnosed as having either normal-IQ autism or AS. A particular mutation in at least one gene, *DISC1*, has been associated specifically with AS in the Finnish population. But except for this study, evidence from ASD molecular biology studies does not support the idea that there are gene mutations specific to AS.

It is also not clear that there is any specific relationship with AS and other psychiatric disorders that is different from the relationship between autism and disorders of mood, anxiety, OCD, and schizophrenia. It seems likely that ASD shares some susceptibility genes with these psychiatric conditions, but there is little evidence, except for the Finnish association study, that there is any specific relationship with AS, as opposed to ASD. Again, these susceptibility genes may be more frequent among families ascertained by probands with normal IQs, which of course include those with AS.

It is important to keep in mind that AS, when ascertained in the community, may include some cases with schizophrenia susceptibility genes since the phenotype is closely similar to schizotypal disorder. OCD is of particular interest because, although it not universal in autism as now diagnosed, it was universal in the cases diagnosed by Kanner. One of his two essential criteria was "an anxiously obsessive desire for the maintenance of sameness" (Kanner, 1943, p. 245).

CONCLUSIONS

It is not likely that there are genetic features specific to AS, that are different from those in normal-IQ autism. Except for a single report of an association with a particular haplotype of *DISC1* with AS in Finnish families, nearly all the genetic findings in AS research are also seen in autism, particularly in cases with classical autism and not too much cognitive impairment. Both run equally in families, and each is found in families ascertained by probands with the other diagnosis. In both there is some as-yet undetermined relationship with schizophrenia and in both there is a high rate of comorbid mood and anxiety disorders and OCD in both individuals and their family members

REFERENCES

American Psychiatric Association. (1994). *Diagnostic and statistical manual of mental disorders* (4th ed.). Washington, DC: Author.

American Psychiatric Association. (2013). *Diagnostic and statistical manual of mental disorders* (5th ed.). Arlington, VA: Author.

Andreasen, N. C., Endicott, J., Spitzer, R. L., et al. (1977). The family history method using diagnostic criteria. Reliability and validity. *Archives of General Psychiatry, 34,* 1229–1235.

Burgoine, E., & Wing, L. (1983). Identical triplets with Asperger's syndrome. *British Journal of Psychiatry, 143,* 261–265.

Cantor, R. M., Kono, N., Duvall, J. A., Alvarez-Retuerto, A., Stone, J. L., Alarcón, M., et al. (2005). Replication of autism linkage: *Fine-mapping peak at 17q21. American Journal of Genetics, 76*(6), 1050–1056.

Cederlund, M., & Gillberg, C. (2004). One hundred males with Asperger syndrome: A clinical study of background and associated factors. *Developmental Medicine and Child Neurology, 46*(10), 652–660.

Cook, E. H., Arora, R. C., Anderson, G. M., Berry-Kravis, E. M., Yan, S. Y., Yeoh, H. C., et al. (1993). Platelet serotonin studies in hyperserotonemic relatives of children with autistic disorder. *Life Sciences, 52*(25), 2005–2015.

Couture, S. M., Penn, D. L., Losh, M., Adolphs, R., Hurley, R., & Piven, J. (2010). Comparison of social cognitive functioning in schizophrenia and high functioning autism: More convergence than divergence. *Psychological Medicine, 40*(4), 569–579.

Creswick, H. A., Stacey, M. W., Kelly, R. E., Jr., et al. (2006). Family study of the inheritance of pectus excavatum. *Journal of Pediatric Surgery, 41,* 1699–1703.

DeLong, G. R., & Dwyer, J. T. (1988). Correlation of family history with specific autistic subgroups: Asperger's syndrome and bipolar affective disease. *Journal of Autism and Developmental Disorders, 18,* 593–600.

DeLong, R., & Nohria, C. (1994) Psychiatric family history and neurological disease in autistic spectrum disorders. *Developmental Medicine and Child Neurology, 36,* 441–448.

Fombonne, E. (2009). Epidemiology of pervasive developmental disorders. *Pediatric Research, 65*(6), 591–598.

Ghaziuddin, M. (2005). A family history study of Asperger syndrome. *Journal of Autism and Developmental Disorders, 35,* 177–182.

Gillberg, C., & Cederlund, M. (2005). Asperger syndrome: Familial and pre- and perinatal factors. *Journal of Autism abnd Developmental Disorders, 35,* 159–166.

Gillberg, I. C., & Gillberg, C. (1989). Asperger syndrome—some epidemiological considerations: A research note. *Journal of Child Psychology and Psychiatry, 30*(4), 631–638.

Ishijima, M., & Kurita, H. (2007) Brief report: Identical male twins concordant for Asperger's disorder. *Journal of Autism and Developmental Disorders, 37,* 386–389.

Kanner, L. (1943). Autistic disturbances of affective content. *Nervous Child, 2,* 217–250.

Kendler, K. S., McGuire, M., Gruenberg, A. M., et al. (1995). Schizotypal symptoms and signs in the Roscommon Family Study: Their factor structure and familial relationship with psychotic and affective disorders. *Archives of General Psychiatry, 52,* 296–303.

Kilpinen, H., Ylisaukko-Oja, T., Hennah, W., et al. (2008). Association of *DISC1* with autism and Asperger syndrome. *Molecular Psychiatry, 13,* 187–196.

Klin, A., Pauls, D., Schultz, R., et al. (2005). Three diagnostic approaches to Asperger syndrome: Implications for research. *Journal of Autism and Developmental Disorders, 35,* 221–234.

Lainhart, J. E., & Folstein, S. E. (1994). Affective disorders in people with autism: A review of published cases. *Journal of Autism and Developmental Disorders, 24,* 587–601.

Leyfer, O. T., Folstein, S. E., Bacalman, S., et al. (2006). Comorbid psychiatric disorders in children with autism: Interview development and rates of disorders. *Journal of Autism and Developmental Disorders, 36,* 849–861.

Mazefsky, C. A., Folstein, S. E. & Lainhart, J. E. (2008). Overrepresentation of mood and anxiety disorders in adults with autism and their first-degree relatives: What does it mean? *Autism Research, 1,* 193–197.

McCauley, J. L., Li, C., Jiang, L., Olson, L. M., Crockett, G., Gainer, K., et al. (2005). Genome-wide and ordered-subset linkage analyses provide support for autism loci on 17q and 19p with evidence of phenotypic and interlocus genetic correlates. *BMC Medical Genetics, 6,* 1.

Munesue, T., Ono, Y., Mutoh, K., Shimada, K., Nakatani, H., & Kikuchi, M. (2008). High prevalence of bipolar disorder comorbidity in adolescents and young adults with high-functioning autism spectrum disorder: A preliminary study of 44 outpatients. *Journal of Affective Disorders, 111,* 170–175.

Murphy, D. (2006). Theory of mind in Asperger's syndrome, schizophrenia, and personality disordered forensic patients. *Cognitive Neuropsychiatry, 11,* 99–111.

Ozaki, N., Goldman, D., Kaye, W. H., Plotnicov, K., Greenberg, B. D., Lappalainen, J., et al. (2003). Serotonin transporter missense mutation associated with a complex neuropsychiatric phenotype. *Molecular Psychiatry, 8*(11), 933–936.

Pinkham, A. E., Hopfinger, J. B., Pelphrey, K. A., Piven, J., & Penn, D. L. (2008). Neural bases for impaired social cognition in schizophrenia and autism spectrum disorders. *Schizophrenia Research, 99,* 164–175.

Piven, J., Gayle, J., Chase, G. A., Fink, B., Landa, R., Wzorek, M. M., et al. (1990). A family history study of neuropsychiatric disorders in the adult siblings of autistic individuals. *Journal of the American Academy of Child and Adolescent Psychiatry, 29,* 177–183.

Prasad, H. C., Steiner, J. A., Sutcliffe, J. S., & Blakely, R. D. (2009). Enhanced activity of human serotonin transporter variants associated with autism. *Philosophical Transactions of the Royal Society of London Series B, 364*(1514), 163–173.

Raja, M., & Azzoni, A. (2007). Thought disorder in Asperger syndrome and schizophrenia: Issues in the differential diagnosis. A series of case reports. *World Journal of Biological Psychiatry*, 1–9.

Rapoport, J., Chavez, A., Greenstein, D., Addington, A., & Gogtay, N. (2009). Autism spectrum disorders and childhood-onset schizophrenia: Clinical and biological contributions to a relation revisited. *Journal of the American Academy of Child and Adolescent Psychiatry*, 48, 10–18.

Sasson, N., Tsuchiya, N., Hurley, R., Couture, S. M., Penn, D. L., Adolphs, R., et al. (2007). Orienting to social stimuli differentiates social cognitive impairment in autism and schizophrenia. *Neuropsychologia*, 45, 2580–2588.

Sporn, A. L., Addington, A. M., Gogtay, N., et al. (2004). Pervasive developmental disorder and childhood-onset schizophrenia: Comorbid disorder or a phenotypic variant of a very early onset illness? *Biological Psychiatry*, 55, 989–994.

Stone, J. L., Merriman, B., Cantor, R. M., Geschwind, D. H., & Nelson, S. F. (2007). High density SNP association study of a major autism linkage region on chromosome 17. *Human Molecular Genetics*, 16(6), 704–715.

Wing, L. (1981). Asperger's syndrome: A clinical account. *Psychological Medicine*, 11, 115–129.

Author Index

Author Index

Subject Index

The letter *f* following a page number indicates figure; the letter *t* indicates table.